Pediatric Audiology
Diagnosis, Technology, and Management

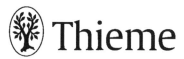

Pediatric Audiology
Diagnosis, Technology, and Management

Jane R. Madell, PhD, CCC-A/SLP, LSLS Cert. AVT
Director, Hearing and Learning Center
Co-director, Cochlear Implant Center
The Ear Institute at the New York Eye and Ear Infirmary
Professor, Clinical Otolaryngology
Albert Einstein College of Medicine
New York, New York

Carol Flexer, PhD, CCC-A, LSLS Cert. AVT
Distinguished Professor Emeritus
School of Speech-Language Pathology and Audiology
The University of Akron
Akron, Ohio

Thieme
New York • Stuttgart

Thieme Medical Publishers, Inc.
333 Seventh Ave.
New York, NY 10001

Editor: Birgitta Brandenburg
Associate Editor: Ivy Ip
Vice President, Production and Electronic Publishing: Anne T. Vinnicombe
Production Editor: Kenneth L. Chumbley, Publication Services
Vice President, International Marketing and Sales: Cornelia Schulze
Chief Financial Officer: Peter van Woerden
President: Brian D. Scanlan
Compositor: Thomson Digital
Printer: The Maple-Vail Book Manufacturing Group

Library of Congress Cataloging-in-Publication Data

Pediatric audiology: diagnosis, technology, and management / [edited by] Jane R. Madell, Carol Flexer.
    p. ; cm.
Includes bibliographical references and index.
ISBN 978-1-60406-001-0 (alk. paper)
ISBN 978-1-60406-002-7 (alk. paper)
  1. Hearing disorders in children. 2. Hearing disorders in children—Diagnosis. 3. Audiology. I. Madell, Jane Reger. II. Flexer, Carol Ann.
[DNLM: 1. Hearing Disorders. 2. Child. 3. Hearing Loss. 4. Infant. WV 271 P3715 2008]
RF291.5.C45P434 2008
618.92'09789—dc22

                                                    2007052546

Important note: Medical knowledge is ever-changing. As new research and clinical experience broaden our knowledge, changes in treatment and drug therapy may be required. The authors and editors of the material herein have consulted sources believed to be reliable in their efforts to
provide information that is complete and in accord with the standards accepted at the time of publication. However, in view of the possibility of human error by the authors, editors, or publisher of the work herein or changes in medical knowledge, neither the authors, editors, nor publisher, nor any other party who has been involved in the preparation of this work, warrants that the information contained herein is in every respect
accurate or complete, and they are not responsible for any errors or omissions or for the results obtained from use of such information. Readers are encouraged to confirm the information contained herein with other sources. For example, readers are advised to check the product information sheet included in the package of each drug they plan to administer to be certain that the information contained in this publication is accurate and that changes have not been made in the recommended dose or in the contraindications for administration. This recommendation is of
particular importance in connection with new or infrequently used drugs. Some of the product names, patents, and registered designs referred to in this book are in fact registered trademarks or proprietary names even though specific reference to this fact is not always made in the text. Therefore, the appearance of a name without designation as proprietary is not to be construed as a representation by the publisher that it is in
the public domain.

Printed in the United States of America

5 4 3 2 1

ISBN: 978-1-60406-001-0

Dedication

This book is a labor of love (in addition to a lot of hard work). It allows us to discuss, in detail, work that is near and dear to our hearts, and to which we have contributed over 75 collective years of experience as pediatric and educational audiologists.

This book would not have been written without an amazing group of chapter authors who generously contributed their time and knowledge. We are most grateful for their collegiality and expertise; it has been a privilege to work with them.

We must thank our families who have, for many years, learned to put up with us not always being around to do mom things because we were doing audiology things. (We began our careers at a time when lots of moms were still staying home and not attempting to have a career outside the home.) We thank our amazingly supportive husbands, Rob Madell and Pete Flexer, our equally amazing children, Jody, Josh, Heather, Hillari, and David, our children in-laws, James, Dawn, Joe, Josh, and Keturah, and the most special group of grandchildren, Eva, Rose, Yehuda, Rachel, Yishai, Libby, Tikva, Rebekah, and Binyamin, and those still to come (from whom we continue to learn every day.)

We could not have accomplished this work were it not for the wonderful audiologists, auditory therapists, educators, and physicians who came before us and set the stage for work with young children—the women and men who taught us to believe that anything was possible and that a hearing loss should not stop anyone from being whatever he or she wants to be.

We would know much less than we know were it not for all the very special families who have given us the privilege of allowing us to work with them day after day. Thanks to Dan Projansky who made the video possible. And finally, we want to thank our publisher, Thieme, and editors Birgitta Brandenburg and Ivy Ip, who helped us find our way.

We dedicate this book to all of them.

Jane R. Madell
Carol Flexer

Contents

DVD Contents

Introduction to the DVD—An Introduction to Testing Techniques with Jane R. Madell, PhD

Behavioral Observation Audiometry
    Introduction
    Testing

Visual Reinforcement Audiometry
    Introduction
    Testing

Conditioned Play Audiometry
    Introduction
    Testing

Speech Audiometry
    Introduction
    Testing

Cochlear Implant Surgery with Dr. George Alexiades

Special Features
    Behavioral Observation Audiometry without Audio Commentary

Foreword

With this book, two master clinicians are expressing what has become a tremendous evolution—almost a revolution—in pediatric audiology. It seems only yesterday that we were still struggling to identify children with hearing loss as early as possible, when the terms *auditory neuropathy* and *auditory dysynchony* were not part of our vocabulary, when *connexin 26* was the province only of obscure geneticists, when cochlear implants were still controversial, when no one had any idea how to habilitate a newborn baby, and when Jane Madell and I started our struggle to keep behavioral observation and visual reinforcement audiometry (VRA) in the audiology stream of consciousness.

Jane Madell and Carol Flexer are aware of the need for constant updates of the rapidly evolving technology in the field, as well as the new understandings of genetics, early education, and surgical advances. In addition to drawing on their own extensive and distinguished experiences, they have assembled contributors who are most knowledgeable in specific areas of pediatric audiology. Speaking for myself, I can't get enough information about all the advances that have appeared, seemingly overnight.

It begins with the sophisticated maturation of newborn hearing screening, with all the developments attendant on this aspect of the revolution (e.g., knowledge of diseases, genetics, medical treatment, and assessments, which mark the identification and diagnosis of a hearing disorder in the infant), and follows with all the ensuing activities that make for a successful program in identification and management of the child with hearing loss from birth. School children and teenagers are not neglected in this comprehensive report.

This vision of an ideal audiologic world is presented by two people who know whereof they speak. Jane Madell has forever fought the good fight for appropriate hearing aid and cochlear implant fittings for children, for behavioral testing of babies, and for audiologists to foster a one-on-one relationship with the children they test. She shares my insistence that all the electronic and electrophysiological applications for children's testing are only the beginning of the acquaintance one must establish with a child experiencing hearing loss. You can learn a great deal of pertinent information for habilitation by watching and playing with the child.

Carol Flexer has also fought the good fight for the child with hearing loss. She has concentrated on the auditory experience in speech and language training. Her book, *Developing Listening and Talking, Birth to Six*, expresses her message that children with hearing loss can best learn speech and language through listening with well fitted, appropriate hearing aids. Cochlear implants are also included in the emphasis on auditory development, and a chapter in this book is devoted to that experience. She has always represented what's best in audiology.

I can't think of anything they've missed in this presentation of what's new and relevant in pediatric audiology, It's going to be a great read.

Marion P. Downs, DrHS
Professor Emerita
Department of Otolaryngology
University of Colorado School of Medicine
Denver, Colorado

Preface

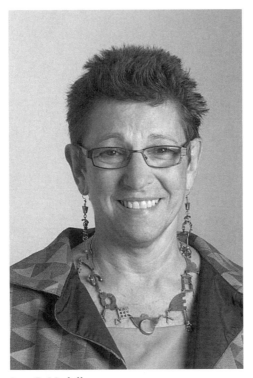

Jane R. Madell

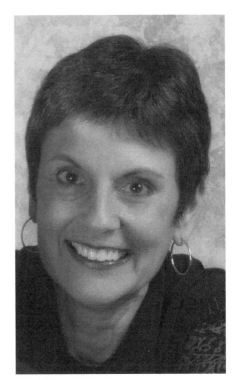

Carol Flexer

This book is intended as a text for AuD and PhD courses in pediatric and educational audiology, and also as a field guide for audiologists working in pediatric and educational audiology settings. This is a practical *how-to* book about the diagnosis and technological and educational management of infants and children with hearing disorders.

Accordingly, this text is divided into five sections:

+ Hearing Loss: Essential Information

+ Diagnosing Hearing Disorders in Infants and Children

+ Hearing Access Technology for Infants and Children

+ Educational Management of Hearing Loss

+ Disorders Requiring Special Consideration

Each chapter offers a wealth of information, and all are written by experts in specific target areas. We have also drawn on our over 75 collective years of experience as pediatric and educational audiologists to enrich this book.

We want students to keep this book as a reference when they graduate. In addition, we hope that practicing audiologists will be able to use this book as a reference when they are approaching techniques that are new to them or when they are performing behavioral diagnostic procedures that may be used only occasionally.

Even though this book cannot possibly explain every aspect of pediatric and educational audiology in detail, it can provide basic information, augmented by extensive resources, on how to move to the next level of diagnosis and management. In addition, this book includes a practical component: a DVD that demonstrates test techniques to assist both students and practicing audiologists in improving their clinical skills regarding behavioral and functional assessments of infants and children of all ages.

Other professionals working in related fields may also be interested in this book, such as speech-language pathologists, listening and spoken language specialists, including auditory-verbal therapists and teachers of children who are deaf or hard of hearing, otolaryngologists, and pediatricians.

Contributors

George Alexiades, MD, FACS
Assistant Professor
New York Medical College
Department of Otolaryngology
Division of Otology/Neurotology
The New York Eye and Ear Infirmary
New York, New York

Meredith Berger, MS
Education Specialist
The Hearing and Learning Center
The Ear Institute at the New York Eye
    and Ear Infirmary
New York, New York

Arthur Boothroyd, PhD
Distinguished Professor Emeritus
City University of New York
Scholar in Residence
San Diego State University
Distinguished Visiting Scientist
House Ear Institute
San Diego, California

Susan Cheffo, MS
Director, Educational Services
The Hearing and Learning Center
The Ear Institute at the New York Eye
    and Ear Infirmary
New York, New York

Teresa Ching, PhD
Senior Research Scientist
National Acoustic Laboratories
Chatswood, NSW Australia

Myriam De La Asuncion, AuD
Cochlear Implant Audiologist
The Hearing and Learning Center
The Ear Institute at the New York Eye
    and Ear Infirmary
New York, New York

Harvey Dillon, PhD
Director of Research
National Acoustic Laboratories
Chatswood, NSW Australia

Laura Austin Duffy, MS, CCC-A
Audiologist
Center for Childhood Communication
The Children's Hospital of Philadelphia
Philadelphia, Pennsylvania

Kris English, PhD
Associate Professor, Audiology
School of Speech–Language Pathology
The University of Akron
Akron, Ohio

M. Patrick Feeney, PhD
Chief of Audiology
Associate Professor
Otolaryngology, Head and Neck Surgery
V. M. Bloedel Hearing Research Center
University of Washington
Seattle, Washington

**Carol Flexer, PhD, CCC-A,
    LSLS Cert. AVT**
Distinguished Professor Emeritus
School of Speech-Language
    Pathology and Audiology
The University of Akron
Akron, Ohio

Kevin H. Franck, PhD, MBA, CCC-A
Director, Cochlear Implant Program
The Children's Hospital of
    Philadelphia
Assistant Professor
Department of Otolaryngology
    Head and Neck Surgery
University of Pennsylvania
    School of Medicine
Philadelphia, Pennsylvania

Maryanne Golding, PhD
Senior Research Scientist
National Acoustic Laboratories
Sydney, NSW Australia

Ronald A. Hoffman, MD, MHCM
Professor of Otolaryngology Head and
    Neck Surgery
Albert Einstein College of Medicine
Director
The Ear Institute at the New York Eye
    and Ear Infirmary
New York Medical College
New York, New York

Garima Kamo, BSc, MBA
Parent of a hearing impaired child
Cary, North Carolina

**Andrea S. Kelly, MAud,
    PhD, MNZAS**
Lecturer
Department of Audiology
School of Population Health
University of Auckland
Auckland, New Zealand

Rebecca Kooper, AuD, JD
Educational Audiology Consultant
The Hearing and Learning Center
The Ear Institute at the New York Eye
    and Ear Infirmary
New York, New York

**Jane R. Madell, PhD, CCC-A/SLP,
    LSLS Cert. AVT**
Director, Hearing and Learning Center
Co-director, Cochlear Implant Center
The Ear Institute at the New York Eye
    and Ear Infirmary
Professor, Clinical Otolaryngology
Albert Einstein College of Medicine
New York, New York

Rebecca Madore, MS, CGC
Genetic Counselor
Lahey Clinic Medical Center
Burlington, Massachusetts

Lori B. Markoff, MEd, CCC/A
Cochlear Implant Audiologist
The Hearing and Learning Center
The Ear Institute at the New York Eye
    and Ear Infirmary
New York, New York

Sarah McKay, AuD
The Center for Childhood
    Communication
The Children's Hospital of Philadelphia
Philadelphia, Pennsylvania

Simon C. Parisier, MD
Co-director, Cochlear Implant Center
The Ear Institute at the New York Eye
    and Ear Infirmary
Professor, Clinical Otolaryngology
New York Medical College
New York, New York

Beth A. Prieve, PhD
Associate Professor
Department of Communication Sciences
    and Disorders
Syracuse University
Syracuse, New York

Suzanne C. Purdy, PhD
Associate Professor
Head, Discipline of Speech Science
Department of Psychology
University of Auckland
Auckland, New Zealand

Virginia S. Ramachandran, MSW, AuD
Department of Communication
    Sciences and Disorders
Wayne State University
Division of Audiology
Department of Otolaryngology–Head
    and Neck Surgery
Henry Ford Hospital
Detroit, Michigan

Heidi L. Rehm, PhD, FACMG
Instructor of Pathology
Associate Molecular Geneticist
Laboratory for Molecular Medicine
Harvard Medical School
Partners Healthcare Center for
    Genetics and Genomics
Cambridge, Massachusetts

Ellen A. Rhoades, EdS, Cert. AVT
Auditory–Verbal Training/Consultation
    International
Plantation, Florida

Jackson Roush, PhD
Professor and Director
Division of Speech and Hearing
    Sciences
University of North Carolina School of
Medicine
Chapel Hill, North Carolina

Chris A. Sanford, PhD
Postdoctoral Fellow
Center for Hearing Research
Boys Town National Research Hospital
Omaha, Nebraska

Nicole Sislian, MA, CCC/A
Cochlear Implant Audiologist
The Hearing and Learning Center
The Ear Institute at the New York Eye
    and Ear Infirmary
New York, New York

Joseph Smaldino, PhD
Chairperson
Department of Communication
    Sciences and Disorders
Illinois State University
Normal, Illinois

Donna L. Sorkin
Vice President, Consumer Affairs
Cochlear Americas
McLean, Virginia

Brad A. Stach, PhD
Division Head
Division of Audiology
Department of Otolaryngology–Head
    and Neck Surgery
Henry Ford Hospital
Detroit, Michigan

**Arlene Stredler-Brown, MA,
    CCC-SLP, CED**
Adjunct Faculty and Senior Professional
    Research Assistant
University of Colorado
Adjunct Faculty
University of British Columbia
Project Coordinator
Marion Downs Hearing Center
University of Colorado Hospital
Boulder, Colorado

Karl R. White, PhD
Professor of Psychology
Director
National Center for Hearing
    Assessment and Management
Utah State University
Logan, Utah

Gail M. Whitelaw, PhD
Audiologist/Clinic Director
Department of Speech and
    Hearing Science
The Ohio State University
Columbus, Ohio

Elizabeth Ying, MA, CCC-SLP
Director, Hearing Habilitation
The Hearing and Learning Center
The Ear Institute at the New York Eye
    and Ear Infirmary
New York, New York

Why is Hearing Important in Children?

Carol Flexer and Jane R. Madell

Approximately 12,000 new babies with hearing loss are identified every year according to the National Institute on Deafness and Other Communication Disorders. In addition, estimates are that in the same year another 4,000 to 6,000 infants and young children between birth and 3 years of age who passed the newborn screening test acquire late onset hearing loss. Therefore, about 16,000 to18,000 new babies and toddlers are identified with hearing loss per year, making hearing loss the most common birth defect.

Numerous studies over the decades have demonstrated that when hearing loss of any degree is not adequately diagnosed and treated, it can negatively affect the speech, language, academic, emotional, and psychosocial development of young children. Therefore, the secondary effects of hearing loss, rather than the hearing loss itself, adversely affect a child's development.

Recently, there has been a surge of information and technology about testing for and managing hearing loss in infants and children. The impetus for this surge has been newborn hearing screening. As a result of identifying and treating hearing loss in neonates, we now are dealing with a vastly different population of children with hearing loss, a population that never existed before. With this new population, whose hearing loss is identified at birth, the secondary developmental and communicative deficits of hearing loss that were so common just a few years ago can be prevented. What has happened in the field of hearing loss is revolutionary, and the pediatric audiologist is in the linchpin position.

How does the pediatric audiologist of today diagnose and treat this new population of babies and children with hearing loss and their families? How does audiology, as a (health) diagnosing and treating profession, collaborate with other health-care providers, early interventionists, speech-language pathologists, teachers, and of course families, in providing quality services? The first step is to recognize that because of technology and brain neuroplasticity, everything that we used to know and believe to be true about hearing loss has changed.

This introductory section will begin at the beginning, with a discussion of the changing world for pediatric audiologists. Next, auditory neural development will be explored, along with a discussion of neuroplasticity. New meanings for the words "deaf" and "hard of hearing" will be posited. An additional topic discussed is the acoustic filter model of hearing loss.

◆ Factors Changing the Practice of Pediatric Audiology

The popular book about change, *Who Moved My Cheese?* by Spencer Johnson, MD, is particularly meaningful in the world of hearing loss. Changes brought about through technology and early hearing detection and intervention (EHDI) programs have allowed outcomes of listening and talking only dreamed of a few years ago. It is important to realize that the new outcomes available today do not invalidate the treatment decisions made by pediatric audiologists in the past. Audiologists did what was necessary with what was available at the time. For example, audiologists used to fit only one hearing aid on children who had hearing loss in both ears.

Because we now know more, we can offer better services. Audiologists do the best that can be done in today's world. Tomorrow's world will bring new possibilities, and we need to "move with the cheese." Our job as pediatric audiologists is to prepare today's babies to be the take-charge adults in the world of 2030, 2040, and 2050 . . . not in the world of 1970 or 1990 or even 2009. Because information and knowledge are the currencies of today's cultures, listening, speaking, reading, writing, and electronic technologies must be made available to our babies and children to the fullest degree possible.

◆ Relationship of Auditory Neural Development and Speech and Reading Skills

The problem with hearing loss is that it keeps sound from reaching the brain. The purpose of hearing aids and cochlear implants is to access, stimulate, and grow auditory neural connections throughout the brain as the foundation for spoken language, reading, and academics (Gordon, Papsin, and Harrison, 2004).

There is substantial evidence that "hearing" is indeed the most effective modality for the teaching of spoken language (speech), reading, and cognitive skills (Sloutsky and Napolitano, 2003; Tallal, 2004; 2005; Werker, 2006). Furthermore, with today's amplification technologies, including cochlear implants, and early identification and intervention, auditory brain access is available to babies with even the most profound deafness. This brain access allows the use of a developmental model of intervention that prevents the negative developmental outcomes of hearing loss that were so common a few years ago.

◆ Brain Development, Neuroplasticity, and Treatment of Hearing Loss in Children

Studies of brain development show that sensory stimulation of the auditory centers of the brain is critical and, indeed, influences the actual organization of auditory brain pathways (Boothroyd, 1997; Berlin and Weyand, 2003; Chermak et al, 2007). Furthermore, neural imaging has shown that the same brain areas—the primary and secondary auditory areas—are most active when a child listens and reads. That is, phonologic or phonemic awareness, which is the explicit awareness of the speech sound structure of language units, forms the basis for the development of literacy skills (Pugh, 2005; Strickland and Shanahan, 2004; Tallal, 2004).

Clearly, anything we can do to access and "program" those critical and powerful auditory centers of the brain with acoustic detail will expand children's abilities to listen and learn spoken language. As Robbins et al (2004) contend, early and ongoing auditory intervention is essential.

Important neural deficits have been identified in the higher auditory centers of the brain caused by prolonged lack of auditory stimulation; auditory stimulation directly influences speech perception and language processing in humans (Kretzmer et al; 2004; Shaywitz and Shaywitz, 2004). In order for auditory pathways to mature, acoustic stimulation must occur early and often because normal maturation of central auditory pathways is a precondition for the normal development of speech and language skills in children. Research also suggests that children receiving implants very early (around 1 year of age) may benefit more from the relatively greater plasticity of the auditory pathways, than will children who are implanted later in the developmentally sensitive period (Sharma et al, 2005). Sharma's results suggest that rapid changes in P1 latencies and changes in response morphology are not unique to electrical stimulation, but rather reflect the response of a deprived sensory system to new stimulation. Gordon et al (2003; 2004) concurred and reported that activity in the auditory pathways to the level of the midbrain can be provoked by stimulation from a cochlear implant. The hypothesis that early implantation appears to activate changes in central auditory pathways is supported by evidence provided by Gordon and colleagues.

To summarize, neuroplasticity is greatest during the first 3 $\frac{1}{2}$ years of life. The younger the infant, the greater is the neuroplasticity (Sharma et al, 2002; 2004; 2005). Rapid infant brain growth requires prompt intervention, typically including amplification and a program to promote auditory skill development. In the absence of sound, the brain reorganizes itself to receive input from other senses, primarily vision; this process is called "cross-modal reorganization" and it reduces auditory neural capacity. Early (in the first year of life) amplification or implantation stimulates a brain that is in the initial process of organizing itself, and is therefore more receptive to auditory input, resulting in greater auditory capacity. Furthermore, early implantation synchronizes activity in the cortical layers.

> **Pearl**
>
> • Identification and management of newborn hearing loss should be considered a neurodevelopmental emergency!

◆ New Meanings for the Terms "Hard of Hearing" and "Deaf"

A potential source of confusion for present-day service provision is that even though variables and outcomes have changed, the same words that have been used for centuries to describe hearing loss continue to be employed. Three of the terms used most commonly to describe hearing loss are "hearing impairment," "hard of hearing," and "deaf." These terms can have various meanings and evoke various expectations. The definitions proposed by Mark Ross, an audiologist and a person who experiences a severe to profound hearing loss, are the most useful (Ross et al, 1991). Mark Ross proposes separating audiometric degree of hearing loss from functional outcomes.

Dr. Ross uses "hearing impairment" to describe any type and degree of hearing loss. The terms "hard of hearing" and "deaf" are used functionally. These terms are not associated with time of onset of the hearing loss or with the audiometric degree of hearing loss. Using Ross's distinctions, a person is functionally hard of hearing if he or she learned language primarily auditorally and if information received from the environment is primarily auditory. This means that a person could have been born with a profound hearing loss, but if technology and auditory intervention enabled her to learn language primarily auditorally, she would be a person who is functionally hard of hearing.

A person is functionally deaf if language was learned primarily visually and information is received from the environment primarily visually. Visual input includes speech reading or lipreading, Cued Speech, and manual communication or sign language. Mark Ross further elaborates on his proposed functional definitions by stating that a child or anyone with a hearing loss who is functionally hard of hearing is much more like a typically hearing person relative to how information is acquired, than like someone who is functionally deaf. A person who is functionally hard of hearing as a result of using hearing aids or cochlear implants, accesses and develops the auditory centers of the brain in a manner similar to a person with typical hearing; she has a "hearing brain." A person who is functionally deaf does not. Educational program placement decisions must be based on the child's functional or potential listening abilities—not the degree of hearing loss. It is highly inappropriate to place a functionally hard of hearing child (even one with audiometrically profound hearing loss) in an intervention program that has a visual emphasis.

What has occurred is a paradigm shift in the way we view and manage hearing loss—from using technology to create a visual world, to using technology to create an accessible auditory world for children with hearing loss.

> **Pearl**
>
> - The cheese has moved regarding our views of deafness in the new millennium.

♦ Hearing versus Listening

There is a distinction between hearing and listening. Hearing is acoustic access to the brain; it includes improving the signal-to-noise ratio by managing the environment and using hearing technology. Listening, on the other hand, is focusing and attending to the acoustic events that are available to the child.

Sequencing is important. Hearing must be made available by audiologists before *listening* can be taught by parents, early interventions, speech-language pathologists, auditory-verbal therapists, teachers, and, of course, audiologists. That is, one can reasonably focus on developing listening skills and strategies only after acoustic events have been made available to the brain—not before.

♦ The Invisible Acoustic Filter Effect of Hearing Loss

Hearing loss of any type or degree that occurs in infancy or childhood can interfere with the development of a child's spoken language, reading and writing skills, and academic performance (Davis, 1990; Ling, 2002). That is, hearing loss can be described as an invisible acoustic filter that distorts, smears, or eliminates incoming sounds, especially sounds from a distance—even a short distance. The negative effects of a hearing loss may be apparent,

but the hearing loss itself is invisible and easily ignored or underestimated.

As human beings we are neurologically "wired" to develop spoken language (speech) and reading skills through the central auditory system. Most people think that reading is a visual skill, but recent research on brain mapping shows that primary reading centers of the brain are located in the auditory cortex—in the auditory portions of the brain (Chermak et al, 2007; Pugh 2006; Tallal, 2005). That is why many children who are born with hearing losses, and who do not have access to auditory input when they are very young (through hearing aids or cochlear implants and auditory teaching), tend to have a great deal of difficulty reading, even though their vision is fine (Robertson, 2000). Therefore, the earlier and more efficiently a pediatric audiologist can allow a child access to meaningful sound with subsequent direction of the child's attention to sound, the better opportunity that child will have to develop spoken language, literacy, and academic skills. With the technology and early auditory intervention available today, a child with a hearing loss CAN have the same opportunity as a typical hearing child to develop spoken language, reading, and academic skills.

♦ Summary

Pediatric audiologists have a key role in determining the child's future opportunities. Sound has to reach the brain before auditory-based learning can occur. All hearing losses in infants and children involve developmental and educational issues requiring audiologic intervention. Some hearing problems also involve medical issues.

The purposes of audiologic environmental and technological management strategies are to enhance the reception of clear and intact acoustic signals to access, develop, and organize the auditory centers of the brain.

> **Pitfall**
>
> - Without clear detection of the entire speech spectrum, higher levels of auditory processing are not possible, and a baby or child's outcomes will be compromised.

The pediatric audiologist needs to be ever mindful of the desired outcomes expressed by the family. The family's vision for how they want their child to communicate serves as the guide for the technological and treatment recommendations that are made. Because about 95% of children with hearing loss are born to hearing and speaking families, listening and talking likely will be desired outcomes for the vast majority of families we serve. Those outcomes require vigilant, consistent, and caring audiologic management.

In this day and age the degree of hearing loss does not determine the functional outcome for infants and children who are young enough to have brain neural plasticity; these children's auditory brain centers can be accessed, stimulated, and developed through the early use of amplification or cochlear implant technologies and appropriate specialized intervention.

Someone once said, "Neglect the future, and no one will thank you for managing the present." Our job as pediatric audiologists is to be visionary. How we audiologically diagnose and treat babies from the beginning, lays the neurologic foundation for the child's entire life.

References

Berlin, C. I., and Weyand, T. G. (2003). The brain and sensory plasticity: Language acquisition and hearing. Clifton Park, NY: Thomson Delmar Learning.

Boothroyd, A. (1997). Auditory development of the hearing child. Scandinavian Audiology Supplement, 46, 9–16.

Chermak, G. D., Bellis, J. B., and Musiek, F. E. (2007). Neurobiology, cognitive science, and intervention. In Chermak, G. D., and Musiek, F. E. (Eds.), Handbook of central auditory processing disorder: Comprehensive intervention volume II, pp. 3–28. San Diego: Plural Publishing Inc.

Davis, J. (Ed.) (1990). Our forgotten children: Hard-of-hearing pupils in the schools. Bethesda, MD: Self Help for Hard of Hearing People.

Gordon, K. A., Papsin, B. C., and Harrison, R. V. (2003). Activity-dependent developmental plasticity of the auditory brain stem in children who use cochlear implants. Ear and Hearing, 24, 485–500.

Gordon, K. A., Papsin, B. C., and Harrison, R. V. (2004). Thalamocortical activity and plasticity in children using cochlear implants. International Congress Series, 1273, 76–79.

Johnson, S. (1998). Who moved my cheese? New York: Putnam's Sons.

Kretzmer, E. A., Meltzer, N. E., Haenggeli, C. A., and Ryugo, D. K. (2004). An animal model for cochlear implants. Archives of Otolaryngology–Head & Neck Surgery, 130, 499–508.

Ling, D. (2002). Speech and the hearing impaired child. Washington, DC: Alexander Graham Bell Association of the Deaf and Hard of Hearing.

Pugh, K., Sandak, R., and Frost, S. J. (2006). Neurobiological investigations of skilled and impaired reading. In Dickinson, D., and Neuman, S. (Eds.) Handbook of early literacy research, Vol. 2. New York: Guilford.

Pugh, K. (2005). Neuroimaging studies of reading and reading disability: Establishing brain/behavior relations. Paper presented at the Literacy and Language Conference at the Speech, Language, and Learning Center, Beth Israel Medical Center, New York City, November 30, 2005.

Robertson, L. (2000). Literacy Learning for Children who are Deaf or Hard of Hearing. Washington, DC: Alexander Graham Bell Association for the Deaf and Hard of Hearing.

Robbins, A. M., Koch, D. B., Osberger, M. J., et al. (2004). Effect of age at cochlear implantation on auditory skill development in infants and toddlers. Archives of Otolaryngology Head & Neck Surgery, 130(5), 570–574.

Ross, M., Brackett, D., and Maxon, A. (1991). Assessment and management of mainstreamed hearing-impaired children. Austin, TX: Pro-Ed.

Sharma, A., Dorman, M. F., and Spahr, A. J. (2002). A sensitive period for the development of the central auditory system in children with cochlear implants: Implications for age of implantation. Ear and Hearing, 23, 532–539.

Sharma, A., Tobey, E., Dorman, et al. (2004). Central auditory maturation and babbling development in infants with cochlear implants. Archives of Otolaryngology–Head & Neck Surgery, 130, 511–516.

Sharma, A., Martin, K., Roland, P., et al. (2005). P1 latency as a biomarker for central auditory development in children with hearing impairment. Journal of the American Academy of Audiology, 16, 564–573.

Shaywitz, S. E., and Shaywitz, B. A. (2004). Disability and the brain. Educational Leadership, 61, 7–11.

Sloutsky, V. M., and Napolitano, A. C. (2003). Is a picture worth a thousand words? Preference for auditory modality in young children. Child Development, 74, 822–833.

Strickland, D. S., and Shanahan, T. (2004). Laying the groundwork for literacy. Educational Leadership, 61, 74–77.

Tallal, P. (2005). Improving language and literacy. Paper presented at the Literacy and Language Conference at the Speech, Language, and Learning Center, Beth Israel Medical Center, New York City, November 30, 2005.

Tallal, P. (2004). Improving language and literacy is a matter of time. Nature Reviews Neuroscience, 5, 721–728.

Werker, J. (2006). Infant speech perception and early language acquisition. Paper presented at the 4th Widex Congress of Paediatric Audiology, Ottawa, Canada, May 19–21, 2006.

Part I

Hearing Loss: Essential Information

Chapter 1

Hearing Disorders in Children

Brad A. Stach and Virginia S. Ramachandran

- ◆ **Conductive Hearing Disorders**

  Nature of Conductive Hearing Disorders

  Causes of Conductive Hearing Disorders

  Acquired Prenatal Conductive Disorders

  Acquired Postnatal Conductive Disorders

- ◆ **Sensory Hearing Disorders**

  Nature of Sensory Hearing Disorders

  Causes of Sensory Hearing Disorders

  Acquired Prenatal Sensory Disorders

  Acquired Perinatal and Postnatal
    Sensory Disorders

- ◆ **Neural Hearing Disorders**

  Nature of Neural Hearing Disorders

  Causes of Neural Hearing Disorder

  Auditory Neuropathy

  Other Neural Hearing Disorders

Key Points

- There are many pathological conditions that cause hearing disorders in childhood, including disease, trauma, and developmental disturbance.

- Some hearing disorders are unique to childhood; others impact children to a greater or lesser extent than they do adults.

- Conductive hearing disorder results from problems involving structures of the outer and middle ear, including congenital anomalies and otitis media and its complications.

- Sensory hearing disorder results from problems involving the cochlea, including congenital inner-ear anomalies, maternal infections such as CMV and toxoplasmosis, and acquired infections such as meningitis and mumps.

- Neural hearing disorder results from problems involving the auditory nervous system, including neoplasms and hypoxia.

- The impact of hearing disorder on speech and language development varies as a function of degree, type, configuration, and stability of hearing loss and when in the course of development hearing loss occurs.

A hearing disorder results from a disruption in function of structures that transmit an acoustic signal from the outer ear to the point of perception in the brain. Many pathologic conditions, including disease, trauma, and developmental disturbance, cause hearing disorders during childhood. In most cases, the impacts on hearing sensitivity and suprathreshold perception are predictable from the nature of the pathology.

Hearing disorders are customarily classified according to the nature of the interruption in sound transmission. Conductive hearing disorder results from a problem with transmission of mechanical energy to the cochlea, involving the structures of the outer and middle ear. Sensory hearing disorder results from a problem with the transduction of hydraulic energy to electrical energy, involving the cochlea. Neural hearing disorder results from a problem with the transmission of the electrical signal to and throughout the brain, involving the eighth cranial nerve and the central auditory nervous system pathways.

The prevalence of hearing disorders in children is relatively high compared with other childhood disorders. As many as 3 in 1000 infants are born with congenital bilateral sensorineural hearing loss. The number with significant, permanent sensorineural hearing loss in at least one ear is closer to 8 in 1000 infants. Combined with transient conductive disorder, as many as 15 in 1000 infants have some degree of hearing disorder. By the time children reach school age, from 10 to 15% fail hearing screenings, in most cases because of the residual effects of middle ear disorder.

Some hearing disorders are unique to childhood; others affect children to a greater or lesser extent than they do adults. Several factors, including type of disorder, severity, and time of onset, interact to determine the impact of childhood hearing disorder on speech and language development. Disorders that fluctuate or are transient tend to have a more subtle impact on overall hearing ability than do permanent disorders. Similarly, disorders that are unilateral are likely to have far less impact than those that are bilateral. (See Chapter 31 for a discussion of mild and unilateral hearing loss.) In general, the more severe the hearing disorder, the more likely it will be to affect normal speech and language acquisition. Interacting with type and severity of the disorder is the age of onset. Some hearing disorders are present at birth, or are congenital; others occur after birth, or are acquired. Onset of hearing disorder is also often described in relation to birth. A hearing disorder can occur before (prenatal), during (perinatal), or after (postnatal) birth.

The remainder of this chapter will focus on the characteristics of hearing disorders related to specific exogenous etiologies, which have factors that are not necessarily intrinsic to the genetic makeup of the individual. Endogenous conditions, which are inherited, are discussed in Chapter 2.

◆ Conductive Hearing Disorders

Nature of Conductive Hearing Disorders

Conductive hearing loss is caused by attenuation of sound as it travels from the outer ear to the cochlea. The roles of the outer ears and ear canals in the collection and enhancement of sound are necessarily reduced by a conductive disorder. When the middle ear mechanism is involved, its important function as an impedance matching transformer of acoustic air pressure waves to fluid motion in the cochlea is likewise disrupted. As a rule, a pathologic condition that affects the physical mass of the outer and middle ear mechanism will reduce sensitivity to higher frequency sound; one that affects the stiffness will reduce sensitivity to lower frequency sound. The net effect will be an attenuation across the frequency range of hearing.

Because conductive hearing loss acts primarily as an attenuator of sound, it has little or no impact on suprathreshold hearing. Perception of loudness, differential thresholds for pitch and loudness, temporal processing, and speech recognition ability are all normal at suprathreshold levels.

Conductive hearing disorders in children are most commonly acquired and transient. Most respond well to medical management and have negligible impact on long-term auditory function. There are two notable exceptions. First, congenital disorders, which are primarily caused by structural deformities or anomalies, can cause significant conductive hearing loss and may not be readily treatable until the child is older and skull growth is complete. Second, some children

Table 1–1   Some Causes of Conductive Hearing Disorder

Acquired Prenatal Disorders	Acquired Postnatal Disorders
Atresia	Otitis media with effusion
Middle ear anomalies	Tympanic-membrane perforation
	Cholesteatoma
	Excessive cerumen
	Otitis externa

with recurrent middle ear disorder and resultant fluctuating hearing sensitivity appear to be prone to suprathreshold hearing disorder and language/learning problems, presumably because of the inconsistency of auditory input during the critical period of language development.

Causes of Conductive Hearing Disorders

Some common causes of conductive hearing loss are listed in **Table 1–1**.

Acquired Prenatal Conductive Disorders

Outer Ear Anomalies

Atresia is the absence of an opening of the ear or external auditory meatus (for reviews, see: Declau, Cremers, and Van de Heyning, 1999; Lambert and Dodson, 1996). It is not uncommon, occurring in about 1:5,800 to 10,000 births. Bony atresia is the congenital absence of the ear canal caused by a wall of bone separating the external ear from the middle ear. Membranous atresia is the absence of a canal caused by a dense soft tissue plug obstructing the canal. Atresia is unilateral in about 70 to 85% of cases. Atresia can cause maximum conductive hearing loss (about 60 dB) depending on the density of the blockage.

Other congenital anomalies of the ear canal and outer ear can also cause conductive disorders. An abnormally small or malformed ear is known as microtia. Although microtia does not necessarily cause hearing disorder, it is often associated with abnormalities of the ear canal, including stenosis or narrowing of the ear canal. Stenosis may or may not cause a hearing disorder, but it can cause additional complications, including excessive cerumen accumulation and even cholesteatoma formation.

Middle Ear Anomalies

Abnormalities of the ear canal and pinna are often associated with middle ear anomalies (Declau, Cremers, and Van de Heyning, 1999), although they can occur in isolation. Middle ear anomalies include ossicular dysplasia, fenestral malformations, and congenital cholesteatoma. Ossicular dysplasia can result in fixation, deformity, and disarticulation of the bones, especially the incus and stapes. In cases of congenital stapes fixation the stapes footplate is fixed into the bony wall of the cochlea at the oval window. Lack of oval window development is an example of fenestral malformation. Congenital cholesteatoma is a cyst that is present in the middle ear space without any evidence of causative factors such as otitis media.

Acquired Postnatal Conductive Disorders

Otitis Media with Effusion

Otitis media is a general term to describe inflammation of the middle ear mucous membrane and tympanic membrane (for reviews, see: Bluestone, 1998; Shekelle, Takata, and Chan, 2003; Smith and Danner, 2006). Otitis media is the most common diagnosis of patients who make office visits to physicians in the United States. Estimates are that 76 to 95% of all children have one episode of otitis media by 6 years of age. The prevalence is highest during the first 2 years and declines with age. Approximately 60% of those children who have otitis media before the age of 1 year will have six or more bouts within the ensuing 2 years. Risk factors for otitis media include young age, Native American and American or Canadian Eskimo heritage, anatomic defects, exposure to smoke in the household, male gender, crowded living conditions, poor sanitation, inadequate medical care, eating in prone position, and day care. Otitis media is usually caused by Eustachian tube dysfunction secondary to upper respiratory tract infection. Swelling of the nasopharynx results in failure of the Eustachian tube to protect, clear, and equalize the pressure of the middle ear space, permitting reflux of infectious secretions from the nasopharynx into the middle ear.

Otitis media is usually defined by the presence or absence of effusion in the middle ear space, the type of effusion, and the time course of the disorder. *Otitis media with effusion* (OME) is the common term used to describe the disorder. The fluid may be referred to as serous (thin, watery, sterile), suppurative (containing pus), purulent (suppurative), mucoid (thick, viscid), and sanguineous (containing blood). Adhesive otitis media refers to severe retraction of the tympanic membrane into the middle ear space.

Acute otitis media with effusion is the term describing rapid onset of symptoms of middle ear inflammation, including redness of the tympanic membrane and otalgia. It is usually referred to as acute if it lasts fewer than 3 weeks; subacute if it lasts fewer than 3 months. Middle ear effusion is signaled by bulging and limited mobility of the tympanic membrane, otorrhea, or a fluid level behind the tympanic membrane. Other nonspecific symptoms in an infant or toddler may include fever, excessive crying, or pulling on the ears. Recurrent acute OME describes repeated episodes of acute otitis media with normal middle ear examinations between episodes. Persistent middle-ear effusion is an asymptomatic effusion that persists following treatment for acute OME. *Chronic* OME is used to describe a condition that lasts longer than 3 months. Chronic suppurative otitis media is a chronic infection of the middle ear and mastoid with a perforation of the tympanic membrane and otorrhea.

OME may resolve spontaneously or may require treatment with antibiotics or pressure-equalization tubes. Hearing loss fluctuates with the presence or absence of fluid. Untreated OME can lead to several complications, including cholesterol granuloma, adhesive otitis media, facial paralysis, labyrinthitis, acute mastoiditis, petrositis, meningitis, sigmoid sinus thrombosis, extradural abscess, brain abscess, otic hydrocephalus, and sensorineural hearing loss. Among the more common complications are tympanic membrane perforation, tympanosclerosis, and cholesteatoma (Slattery and House, 1998).

Complications of Otitis Media with Effusion

The tympanic membrane may become perforated as a result of OME because of increased pressure from fluid in the middle ear space, or from barotraumas, trauma, myringotomy, or tympanostomy tube placement (Slattery and House, 1998). Although perforations generally heal spontaneously, they may require surgical intervention to repair the damaged membrane. Drainage from perforation may cause a secondary infection of the external auditory canal or pinna. A perforation may or may not result in hearing loss, depending on its size and location.

Tympanosclerosis is a degeneration of collagenous fibrous tissues of the tympanic membrane and is a common sequela of OME, occurring in about 10% of cases (Hunter and Margolis, 1997; Slattery and House, 1998). Calcification or ossification may occur and spread to the ossicles in rare cases. Tympanosclerosis can often be observed as a horseshoe-shaped plaque on the tympanic membrane. Tympanosclerosis is not associated with significant hearing loss unless it also involves the ossicular chain.

Cholesteatomas are cysts that contain keratinizing squamous epithelium found in the middle ear, mastoid, external auditory canal, or petrous bone (for reviews, see: Bennett, Warren, Jackson, and Kaylie, 2006; Semaan and Megerian, 2006; Sie, 1996). Congenital cholesteatomas are present behind an intact tympanic membrane with no history of significant otitis media or eustachian tube dysfunction. Acquired cholesteatomas are more common and are usually a consequence of chronic otitis media. Cholesteatomas can be destructive as they grow and compete for space with the normal structures of the areas they occupy. Conductive hearing loss varies as a function of the structures involved. Average air-bone gaps are estimated to be 30 to 38 dB. Allowed to grow unchecked, cholesteatoma can erode the middle ear ossicles and cause ossicular discontinuity, creating additional conductive hearing loss. In advanced cases, sensorineural hearing loss can also occur because of cochlear erosion.

Excessive Cerumen

Excessive cerumen is an accumulation of ear wax in the ear canal (for reviews, see Roeser and Ballachandra, 1997; Roeser and Roland, 1992). Impacted cerumen completely occludes the ear canal. Excessive cerumen occurs in about 10% of children, and it may have an even greater incidence, up to 28 to 36%, in children with developmental delays. A high-frequency conductive hearing loss can occur when the ear canal is 80 to 95% occluded. A low-frequency conductive loss occurs with total occlusion of the ear canal.

Otitis Externa

Otitis externa is the broad term for inflammation or infection of the external auditory canal and auricle (for reviews, see: Bojrab, Bruderly, and Abdulrazzak, 1996; Osguthorpe and Nielsen, 2006; Rosenfeld et al, 2006). Otitis externa rarely causes hearing disorder, except in cases where it causes stenosis of the external auditory meatus. Acute diffuse otitis externa, also known as swimmer's ear, is one example of otitis externa. It is a bacterial infection that causes itching, tenderness, and pain, and may include hearing loss and aural fullness as the external auditory canal decreases in size with swelling. Several fungal, viral, and bacterial infections of the external ear have been reported; rarely, though, do they result in hearing disorder. Complications of otitis externa may include ear canal stenosis, myringitis, and tympanic membrane perforation. Ototoxicity from topical otic preparations for treatment of external otitis can also occur.

♦ Sensory Hearing Disorders

Nature of Sensory Hearing Disorders

Sensory, or sensorineural, hearing disorder is caused by a failure in the cochlear transduction of sound from the mechanical vibrations of the middle ear to neural impulses in the eighth cranial nerve. Sensory disorders can occur from any number of changes in cochlear structure and function, but the most vulnerable structures seem to be the outer hair cells of the organ of Corti, which are responsible for the exquisite sensitivity and fine-tuning of the cochlea.

Hearing sensitivity loss is the hallmark of a sensory disorder and ranges from mild to profound. Sensorineural hearing loss is usually permanent, although it can fluctuate in some cases and may be treatable in others. Depending on the cause, the loss may also be progressive.

Disorders of cochlear processes result in reduced sensitivity of the cochlear receptor cells, reduced frequency resolution, and reduced dynamic range. These complex changes in cochlear function can have a significant negative impact on suprathreshold hearing. The cause of most congenital hearing loss is genetic and is described in Chapter 2.

Causes of Sensory Hearing Disorders

Some common causes of sensory hearing disorder are listed in **Table 1–2**.

Acquired Prenatal Sensory Disorders

Inner Ear Anomalies

Inner ear malformations occur when development of the membranous and/or bony labyrinth is arrested during fetal development (Reilly, Lalwani, and Jackler, 1998). Although in many cases the arrest of development is genetic, some cases are the result of teratogenic influences during pregnancy (Irving and Ruben, 1998), including viral infections

Table 1–2   Some Causes of Sensory Hearing Disorder

Acquired Prenatal Disorders	Acquired Perinatal and Postnatal Disorders
Inner ear anomalies	PPHN/ECMO
Cytomegalovirus	Meningitis
Syphilis	Autoimmune inner-ear disorder
Rubella	Mumps
Toxoplasmosis	Measles
	Ototoxicity

such as rubella, drugs such as thalidomide, and fetal radiation exposure.

Inner ear malformations can be divided into those in which both the osseous and membranous labyrinths are abnormal and those in which only the membranous labyrinth is abnormal. The former anomalies are better understood because they can be readily identified with scanning techniques.

Included in the malformations of both membranous and osseous labyrinths are complete labyrinthine aplasia (Michel deformity), common cavity defect, cochlear aplasia and hypoplasia, and Mondini defect (Reilly, Lalwani, and Jackler, 1998). Michel deformity is a very rare malformation characterized by complete absence of membranous and osseous inner ear structures, resulting in total deafness. Common-cavity malformation comprises about one fourth of all cochlear malformations (Casselman et al, 2001). It is a membranous and osseous malformation in which the cochlea is not differentiated from the vestibule, usually resulting in substantial hearing loss. Cochlear aplasia is a rare malformation consisting of complete absence of the membranous and osseous cochlea and no auditory function, but presence of semicircular canals and vestibule. Cochlear hypoplasia is a malformation in which less than one full turn of the cochlea is developed. Cochlear hypoplasia accounts for about 15% of cochlear malformations. Mondini malformation, an incomplete partition of the cochlea, is a relatively common inner ear malformation in which the cochlea contains only about 1.5 turns, and the osseous spiral lamina is partially or completely absent. The resulting hearing loss is highly variable.

Other abnormalities of both the osseous and membranous labyrinth include anomalies of the semicircular canals, the internal auditory canals, and the cochlear and vestibular aqueducts. One example of the latter is large vestibular aqueduct syndrome, a malformation of the temporal bone that is associated with early onset hearing loss and vestibular disorders. Hearing loss is usually progressive, profound, and bilateral (Cox and MacDonald, 1996). Large vestibular aqueduct syndrome is often associated with Mondini malformation.

Included in malformations limited to the membranous labyrinth are complete membranous labyrinth dysplasia (Bing Siebenmann) and two forms of partial dysplasia, cochleosaccular dysplasia (Scheibe) and cochlear basal turn dysplasia (Alexander). The Bing Siebenmann malformation is a rare malformation that results in complete lack of development of the membranous labyrinth. Scheibe aplasia is a common inner ear abnormality in which there is failure of the organ of Corti to fully develop, collapse of the cochlear duct, adherence of Reissner's membrane to the limbus, and degeneration of the stria vascularis. Alexander aplasia is an abnormal development of the basal turn of the cochlea, with typical development in the remainder of the cochlea, resulting in low frequency residual hearing.

Cytomegalovirus

Cytomegalovirus (CMV) is the largest known member of human herpesvirus family and is the most common fetal viral illness (for review, see Fowler and Boppana, 2006; Gaytant et al, 2002; Pass, 2006; Pass et al, 2006). Congenital infection is the result of transplacental transmission of CMV and is known as cytomegalic inclusion disease. Sensorineural hearing loss is the most common clinical finding of congenital CMV. Other findings include microcephaly, petechiae (small purple spots on a body surface), intrauterine growth retardation, enlargement of the liver and spleen, and inflammation of the choroid and retina (chorioretinitis). Hearing loss is of variable severity and can be bilateral or unilateral. The most commonly found configuration is flat (Dahle et al, 2000). Threshold fluctuations are common (more than 20% of cases) and hearing loss is often progressive (more than 15%). The presence of petechiae and intrauterine growth retardation in symptomatic neonates are factors that independently predict presence of hearing loss (Rivera et al, 2002). Approximately 10 to 15% of congenitally infected infants are symptomatic at birth. Children with symptomatic congenital CMV are at greater risk for hearing impairment (22 to 65%) than those with asymptomatic infection (6 to 23%), and hearing loss tends to appear earlier and with greater severity (Fowler and Boppana, 2006).

Congenital Syphilis

Congenital syphilis is a bacterial infection that is transmitted from mother to fetus in utero, or through contact with a genital lesion during delivery (for review, see: Ingall, Sanchez, and Baker, 2006; Irving and Ruben, 1998; Pletcher and Cheung, 2003). The disease occurs in 11.2 cases per 100,000 live births (Centers for Disease Control and Prevention, 2004). Congenital syphilis is categorized by its time of occurrence into early and late stages. In early congenital syphilis, occurring within the first 2 years of life, severity can range from severe multiorgan involvement to minor symptoms. Although rarely observed in the United States, late congenital syphilis includes symptoms known as Hutchinson's triad, which are small notched teeth, hearing loss, and interstitial keratitis. Typical hearing loss is a rapid symmetric progression from high-frequency sensory loss to complete bilateral deafness. Hearing loss can also involve neural or conductive components. Vestibular function may also be severely affected. Hennebert's sign, in which nystagmus is observed as a result of pressure applied to the external auditory canal, is often found in otosyphilis.

Maternal Rubella

Maternal rubella occurs when an infected mother transmits the rubella virus to the fetus (for review, see Banatvala and Brown, 2004; Cooper and Alford, 2006; Irving and Ruben, 1998). Expression of symptoms of maternal rubella infection, called congenital rubella syndrome or Gregg syndrome, includes a wide variety of defects, usually affecting hearing, vision, and heart function, and often involving mental retardation and microcephaly. Subclinical infections are more common than those that are symptomatic at birth. However, 70% of infants who are asymptomatic at birth will develop symptoms within the first 5 years of life. Hearing loss is the most common manifestation of congenital rubella, occurring in up to 80% of infected children. Hearing loss ranges from unilateral mild loss to bilateral profound deafness; severe bilateral losses are more common. Configuration of the hearing loss is usually flat, and hearing sensitivity may be asymmetric. Children with normal pure tone thresholds may demonstrate abnormal auditory brainstem responses (Niedzielska, Katska, and Szymula, 2000). Once transmission has occurred, fetal infection is chronic. Infection tends to persist throughout fetal life and after birth and continues to cause pathology in the child.

Toxoplasmosis

Toxoplasmosis is an infection caused by the parasite *Toxoplasma gondii* (for review, see Jones, Lopez, Wilson, Schulkin, and Gibbs, 2001; Rorman, Zamir, Rilkis, and Ben-David, 2006). The parasite can be transmitted to humans by ingestion of raw or inadequately cooked infected meat or foods that have come in contact with infected meat, ingestion of parasites that cats have passed in their feces, or transplacental transmission of the infection from a woman to her unborn fetus. Despite increasing probability of infection with pregnancy progression, consequences are more severe when fetal infection occurs in early stages of pregnancy. Although most newborns (70 to 90%) infected with congenital toxoplasmosis are asymptomatic at birth, up to 80% of these children develop sequelae later in life. Those who are symptomatic often have a classic triad of chorioretinitis, intracranial calcifications, and hydrocephalus. The disease course may also include cognitive abnormalities of variable severity, seizures, or learning disabilities with onset after several months or years. Auditory disorder can occur from mastoid and cochlear inflammation and involvement of the auditory brainstem. Resulting disorder is a sensory or neural hearing loss that may range from mild unilateral loss (Wilson et al, 1980) to bilateral deafness (Sever et al, 1988).

Acquired Perinatal and Postnatal Sensory Disorders

Persistent Pulmonary Hypertension of the Newborn Extracorporeal Membrane Oxygenation

Persistent pulmonary hypertension of the newborn (PPHN), also known as persistent fetal circulation, is a condition wherein the infant's blood flow bypasses the lungs, thereby eliminating oxygen supply to the organs of the body (for review, see: Perreault, 2006; Verklan, 2006). PPHN is associated with perinatal respiratory problems such as meconium aspiration or pneumonia. Sensorineural hearing loss is a common complication of PPHN and has been found in from 32% (Kawashiro et al, 1996) to 37% of surviving children. Hearing loss ranges from high-frequency unilateral loss to severe-to-profound bilateral loss and is progressive in many cases.

PPHN is treated by administration of oxygen or oxygen and nitric oxide via a mechanical ventilator. Extracorporeal membrane oxygenation (ECMO) is a treatment for PPHN that involves diverting blood from the heart and lungs to an external bypass where oxygen and carbon dioxide are exchanged before reentering the body. When ECMO is applied as part of respiratory management, it has been associated with hearing loss in up to 75% of cases (Kawashiro, Tsuchihashi, Koga, Kawano, and Itoh, 1996; Lasky, Wiorek, and Becker, 1998; Mann and Adams, 1998). Hearing loss is often progressive.

Meningitis

Meningitis is an inflammation of the membranes that surround the brain and spinal cord. There are three types of meningitis: bacterial, aseptic, and viral. The greatest frequency of hearing loss occurs in cases of bacterial meningitis (Bao and Wong, 1998); estimates range from 5 to 35% of cases. Other common signs and symptoms of bacterial meningitis include fever, seizures, neck stiffness, and altered mental status. (For reviews, see Saez-Llorens and McCracken, 2003). Hearing disorder ranges from mild to profound sensitivity loss or total deafness, may be unilateral or bilateral, and may be progressive. Most involvement is thought to be cochlear, but central auditory involvement may occur in some individuals (Bedford et al, 2001; Cherukupally and Eavey, 2004; Hodgson et al, 2001; Hugosson et al, 1997; Koomen et al, 2003; Kutz, et al, 2006). Hearing loss is usually permanent, although there have been reports of some recovery of hearing over time in some individuals (Bao and Wong, 1998). Cochlear osteoneogenesis, or bony growth in the cochlea may occur following meningitis, complicating possible cochlear implantation (Dodds, Tyszkiewicz, and Ramsden, 1997; Fishman and Holliday, 2000). There have been reports of meningitis following cochlear implantation, especially with use of a positioner during implantation (Callanan and Poje, 2004). Elimination of use of positioners as well as requiring meningitis vaccination prior to cochlear implantation, has reduced meningitis occurrence.

Autoimmune Inner Ear Disease

Autoimmune inner ear disease (AIED) is a syndrome of potentially reversible, bilateral, rapidly progressive, and often fluctuating sensory hearing loss that may be associated with vestibular symptoms mimicking Meniere's disease (for review, see Bovo, Aimoni, and Martini, 2006; Harris, 1998; Matteson et al, 2003; Ryan, Harris, and Keithley, 2002). Symptoms are thought to be consequences of immune-mediated inflammation in the inner ear. The disorder may be specific to the ear or may occur as a manifestation of a systemic immune-mediated inflammatory disorder such as rheumatoid arthritis, systemic lupus erythematous, inflammatory bowel disease, polyarteritis nodosa, or Cogan's syndrome. Hearing sensitivity is generally responsive to immunosuppressive drugs such as steroids. AIED is associated with sensory hearing loss that is generally bilateral, asymmetric, and rapidly progressive.

Viral Infections

Mumps is a viral infection that attacks a variety of organs, especially the salivary glands (for a review of mumps and hearing loss, see McKenna, 1997). Although the incidence in the United States of hearing loss associated with mumps is low because of vaccination, it continues to occur in other areas of the world (Kawashima et al, 2005), and outbreaks have occurred in the United States as recently as 2006 (Centers for Disease Control and Prevention, 2006). Infection following vaccination for mumps has also been known to occur. Mumps is the most common cause associated with unilateral acquired sensorineural hearing loss in children. The typical pattern of sensory hearing loss is unilateral and profound, with sudden onset. Endolymphatic hydrops is also a common manifestation of mumps virus.

Measles is a highly contagious viral illness that characteristically causes symptoms of rash, cough, fever, conjunctivitis, photophobia, and Koplik spots (white spots on the membranous surfaces of the mouth) (McKenna, 1997; Rima and Duprex, 2006). Hearing loss is a common complication of the measles virus. Before vaccination in the United States became widespread, measles accounted for 5 to 10% of all cases of profound, bilateral, sensorineural hearing loss. Measles is still a significant cause of hearing loss and deafness in other parts of the world (Lasisi, Ayodele, and Ijaduola, 2006). Sensory hearing loss from measles virus is typically severe, permanent, and bilateral, although milder hearing loss can occur. Conductive hearing loss from otitis media is also a common complication of measles, which may be due to immunosuppression following viral infection.

Ototoxicity

Ototoxicity is hearing loss from the toxic effects of drugs on the inner ear (Irving and Ruben, 1998; Roland and Cohen, 1998; Roland, 2004; Rybak and Whitworth, 2005). Aminoglycoside antibiotics (streptomycin, gentamycin, dihydrostreptomycin, neomycin, kanamycin, erythromycin, and vancomycin), loop diuretics (furosemide), antineoplastic agents (cisplatin), salicylates, and antimalarial drugs (quinine) can all damage the cochlea. Effects relate to the level of the drug in the system, synergistic effects of these drugs in combination, potentiation of effect caused by coexisting renal disease, and hereditary susceptibility in the case of aminoglycosides. Children and neonates are considered to be at lower risk for ototoxicity than are adults in most cases. One exception is in the case of cisplatin-induced hearing loss, which has a higher incidence and increased severity in children. Hearing loss from ototoxicity is generally symmetric sensory loss that progresses from higher to lower frequencies with increased drug exposure. Some hearing loss also involves neural components with certain drug classes.

Table 1–3   Some Causes of Neural Hearing Disorder

Causes of Neural Disorders
Neoplasms
Hydrocephaly
Hypoxia
Hyperbilirubinemia

◆ Neural Hearing Disorders

Nature of Neural Hearing Disorders

Neural hearing disorders tend to be divided into two groups: retrocochlear disorders and auditory processing disorders. When a disorder is caused by an active, measurable disease process, such as a neoplasm, or from damage caused by trauma or stroke, it is often referred to as a retrocochlear disorder. That is, retrocochlear disorders result from structural lesions of the nervous system. Neural hearing disorders in children from retrocochlear pathology are relatively rare. When they do occur, the hearing disorder is characterized by patterns of abnormality consistent with those found in adults with similar lesions (Bergman et al, 1984; Goodglass, 1967; Jerger, 1987). Children with intra- and extra-axial neoplasms have abnormal, degraded monotic speech perception, and those with temporal lobe lesions have abnormal dichotic speech perception. Although most children and adults tend to exhibit similar patterns of abnormality, some children with central nervous system lesions may have auditory deficits that are more generalized and less severe than in adults with similar lesions (Woods, 1984). Regardless, the morbidity and mortality of tumors in young children is significantly greater than in adults.

When an impairment is due to developmental disorder or delay, it is often referred to as an auditory processing disorder (APD). That is, APDs result from functional lesions of the nervous system. The term *APD* is also used to describe the functional consequence of a retrocochlear disorder.

The most common symptom of neural hearing disorder is difficulty extracting a signal of interest from a background of noise. Although the basis for the disorder is not always clear, it most often results in an inability to structure auditory space appropriately. This spatial hearing deficit usually translates into difficulty hearing in noise, which becomes particularly obvious in a classroom setting. Another common symptom is difficulty localizing a sound source, especially in the presence of background noise. Perhaps as a consequence of these symptoms, children and their parents and teachers are also likely to describe behaviors such as inattentiveness and distractibility. Auditory processing disorders are discussed in detail in Chapter 16.

Causes of Neural Hearing Disorder

Some common causes of neural hearing disorder are listed in **Table 1–3**.

Auditory Neuropathy

Auditory neuropathy is a term that is used to describe disorders that are operationally defined based on a constellation of clinical findings. That constellation varies necessarily as a function of age. In older children, auditory neuropathy is defined by an absent auditory brainstem response (ABR), poor speech perception, varying levels of hearing sensitivity loss, absence of acoustic reflexes, and a preservation of some cochlear function as evidenced by the preservation of otoacoustic emissions (OAEs) and/or cochlear microphonics. In infants, auditory neuropathy is defined by absent ABR and preserved OAEs and/or cochlear microphonics.

It is becoming apparent that the term *auditory neuropathy*, as it is defined clinically, may represent at least two fairly different disorders, one sensory and the other neural (Rapin and Gravel, 2006). The auditory neuropathy of sensory origin—AN(S)—is probably a sensory hearing disorder that represents a transduction problem, with the failure of the cochlea to transmit signals to the auditory nerve. The most likely origin of AN(S) is the inner hair cells, a concept that has been reported both in patient populations (Konrádsson, 1996; Loundon et al, 2005) and in animal models (Harrison, 1998). Preservation of the otoacoustic emissions and cochlear microphonic represents normal function of outer hair cells without any inner hair cells to sensitize. In cases of AN(S), the absence of an ABR is a reflection of the sensitivity loss of the system and accurately predicts substantial hearing loss. Hearing loss from AN(S) acts like any other sensitivity loss in terms of its influence on speech and language acquisition and its amenability to hearing aids and cochlear implants.

Auditory neuropathy of neural origin—AN(N)—was first described as a specific disorder of the auditory nerve that results in a loss of synchrony of neural firing (Starr et al, 1996). Because of the nature of the disorder, it is also referred to as auditory dys-synchrony (Berlin et al, 2001). The cause of auditory neuropathy is often unknown, although it may be observed in cases of syndromic peripheral pathologies (e.g., Freidreich's ataxia, Charcot-Marie-Tooth syndrome). The age of onset is usually before 10 years. Hearing sensitivity loss ranges from normal to profound and is most often flat or reverse-sloped in configuration. Hearing loss often fluctuates and is progressive in some children. Speech perception is often substantially poorer than what would be expected from the audiogram (Sininger and Oba, 2001). AN(N) may not be as amenable to conventional amplification and implant treatment as that of sensory origin.

Other Neural Hearing Disorders

Neoplasm

Unlike in adults, tumors of the posterior fossa in children are less likely to be acoustic schwannoma and more likely to be intrinsic tumors such as gliomas and medulloblastomas (for review, see Angeli and Brackmann, 1998). These tumors of the cerebellopontine angle are benign and affect the auditory system when they impinge on the eighth cranial nerve. The most common form of acoustic tumor in children is that found in association with neurofibromatosis type 2 (NF2). NF2 is characterized by bilateral cochleovestibular schwannomas. The schwannomas are faster growing and more virulent than the unilateral type. This is an autosomal dominant disease and is associated with other intracranial tumors. Hearing loss in NF2 is not particularly different from a unilateral type of schwannoma, except that it is bilateral and often progresses more rapidly.

Hydrocephaly

The cause of neural hearing disorders in children has also been attributed to more diffuse sources, including hydrocephaly, hypoxia, and hyperbilirubinemia. In hydrocephaly, the most common finding is one of neuromaturational delay of the auditory system as measured on the auditory brainstem response. This is usually due to enlarged ventricles and is not associated with permanent changes in auditory function.

Hypoxia

Hypoxia is a deficiency in the amount of oxygen in the body. Hearing disorder is often associated with hypoxia, although the effects of respiratory distress in neonates are difficult to separate from other possible factors such as kernicterus, treatment with ototoxic medications, and low birth weight (Roizen, 2003; Yoshikawa, Ikeda, Kudo, and Kobayashi, 2004). Disorders of auditory neural function are often diffuse, although progressive sensorineural hearing loss can occur as a result.

Hyperbilirubinemia

Hyperbilirubinemia is an excess of bilirubin in the blood that can be caused by many factors (for review, see: Shapiro, 2003). Hyperbilirubinemia is associated with auditory neuropathy and other neural hearing disorders. The clinical spectrum of bilirubin-induced auditory toxicity ranges from transient auditory dysfunction to permanent sensory hearing loss. Audiometric findings include predominantly high frequency bilateral and symmetric hearing loss with recruitment and abnormal loudness growth. Auditory nerve and generalized auditory brainstem dysfunction may occur (Amin, 2004; Sharma et al, 2006). Other more diffuse APDs have also been associated with hyperbilirubinemia.

References

Angeli, S. I., and Brackmann, D. E. (1998). Posterior fosa tumors in children. In A. K. Lalwani and K. M. Grundfast (Eds.), Pediatric otology and neurotology (pp. 489–504). Philadelphia: Lippincott-Raven Publishers.

Amin, S. B. (2004). Clinical assessment of bilirubin-induced neurotoxicity in premature infants. Seminars in Perinatology, 28, 340–347.

Banatvala, J. E., and Brown, D. W. G. (2004). Rubella. Lancet, 363, 1127–1137.

Bao, X., and Wong, V. (1998). Brainstem auditory-evoked potential evaluation in children with meningitis. Pediatric Neurology, 19, 109–112.

Bedford, H., de Louvois, J., Halket, S., Peckham, C., Hurley, R., and Harvey, D. (2001). Meningitis in infancy in England and Wales: follow up at age 5 years. British Medical Journal, 323, 533–536.

Bennett, M., Warren, F., Jackson, G. C., and Kaylie, D. (2006). Congenital cholesteatoma: theories, facts, and 53 patients. Otolaryngologic Clinics of North America, 39, 1081–1094.

Bergman, M., Costeff, H., Koren, V., Koifman, N., and Reshef, A. (1984). Auditory perception in early lateralized brain damage. Cortex, 20, 233–242.

Berlin, C., Hood, L., and Rose, K. (2001). On renaming auditory neuropathy as auditory dys-synchrony. Audiology Today, 13, 15–17.

Bluestone, C. D. (1998). Otitis media: a spectrum of diseases. In A. K. Lalwani and K. M. Grundfast (Eds.), Pediatric otology and neurotology (pp. 233–240). Philadelphia: Lippincott-Raven Publishers.

Bojrab, D. I., Bruderly, T., and Abdulrazzak, Y. (1996). Otitis externa. Otolaryngologic Clinics of North America, 29, 761–782.

Bovo, R., Aimoni, C., and Martini, A. (2006). Immune-mediated inner ear disease. Acta Oto-Laryngologica, 126, 1012–1021.

Callanan, V., and Poje, C. (2004). Cochlear implantation and meningitis. International Journal of Pediatric Otorhinolaryngology, 68, 545–550.

Casselman, J. W., Offeciers, E. F., De Foer, B., Govaerts, P., Kuhweide, R., and Somers, T. (2001). CT and MR imaging of congenital abnormalities of the inner ear and internal auditory canal. European Journal of Radiology, 40, 94–104.

Centers for Disease Control and Prevention. (2004). Congenital syphilis—United States, 2002. Morbidity & Mortality Weekly Report, 53, 716–719.

Centers for Disease Control and Prevention. (2006). Brief report: update: mumps activity–United States, January 1–October 7, 2006. Morbidity & Mortality Weekly Report, 55, 1152–1153.

Chavez-Bueno, S., and McCracken, G. H. (2005). Bacterial meningitis in children. Pediatric Clinics of North America, 52, 795–810.

Cherukupally, S. R., and Eavey, R. (2004). Vaccine-preventable pediatric postmeningitic sensorineural hearing loss in southern India. Otolaryngology-Head and Neck Surgery, 130, 339–343.

Cooper, L. Z., and Alford, C. A. (2006). Rubella. In J. S. Remington, J. O. Klein, C. B. Wilson, and C. J. Baker (Eds.), Infectious diseases of the fetus and newborn infant (pp. 893–926). Philadelphia: Elsevier Saunders.

Cox, L. C., and MacDonald, C. B. (1996). Large vestibular aqueduct syndrome: a tutorial and three case studies. Journal of the American Academy of Audiology, 7, 71–76.

Dahle, A. J., Fowler, K., Wright, J. D., Boppana, S., Britt, W. J., and Pass, R. F. (2000). Longitudinal investigation of hearing disorders in children with congenital cytomegalovirus. Journal of the American Academy of Audiology, 11, 283–290.

Declau, F., Cremers, C., and Van de Heyning, P. (1999). Diagnosis and management strategies in congenital atresia of the external auditory canal. British Journal of Audiology, 33, 313–327.

Dodds, A., Tyszkiewicz, E., and Ramsden, R. (1997). Cochlear implantation after bacterial meningitis: the dangers of delay. Archives of Disease in Childhood, 76, 139–140.

Fishman, A. J., and Holliday, R. A. (2000). Principles of cochlear implant imaging. In S. B. Waltzman and N. L. Cohen (Eds.), Cochlear implants (pp. 79–107). New York: Thieme Medical Publishers, Inc.

Fowler, K. B., and Boppana, S. B. (2006). Congenital cytomegalovirus (CMV) infection and hearing deficit. Journal of Clinical Virology, 35, 226–231.

Gaytant, M. A., Steegers, E. A. P., Semmekrot, B. A., Merkus, H., and Galama, J. M. D. (2002). Congenital cytomegalovirus infection: review of the epidemiology & outcome. Obstetrical and Gynecological Survey, 57, 245–256.

Goodglass, H. (1967). Binaural digit presentation and early lateral brain damage. Cortex, 3, 295–306.

Harris, J. P. (1998). Autoimmune inner ear diseases. In A. K. Lalwani and K. M. Grundfast (Eds.), Pediatric otology and neurotology (pp. 405–419). Philadelphia: Lippincott-Raven Publishers.

Harrison, R. V. (1998). An animal model of auditory neuropathy. Ear and Hearing, 19, 355–361.

Hodgson, A., Smith, T., Gagneux, S., Akumah, I., Adjuik, M., Pluschke, G., et al. (2001). Infectious diseases: survival and sequelae of meningococcal meningitis in Ghana. International Journal of Epidemiology, 30, 1440–1446.

Hugosson, S., Carlsson, E., Borg, E., Brorson, L. O., Langeroth, G., and Olcen, P. (1997). Audiovestibular and neuropsychological outcome of adults who had recovered from childhood bacterial meningitis. International Journal of Pediatric Otorhinolaryngology, 42, 149–167.

Hunter, L. L., and Margolis, R. H. (1997). Effects of tympanic membrane abnormalities on auditory function. Journal of the American Academy of Audiology, 8, 431–446.

Ingall, D., Sanchez, P. J., and Baker, C. J. (2006). Syphilis. In J. S. Remington, J. O. Klein, C. B. Wilson and C. J. Baker (Eds.), Infectious diseases of the fetus and newborn Infant (pp. 545–580.). Philadelphia: Elsevier Saunders.

Irving, R. M., and Ruben, R. J. (1998). The acquired hearing losses of childhood. In A. K. Lalwani and K. M. Grundfast (Eds.), Pediatric otology and neurotology (pp. 375–385). Philadelphia: Lippincott-Raven Publishers.

Jerger, S. (1987). Validation of the pediatric speech intelligibility test in children with central nervous system lesions. Audiology, 26, 298–311.

Jones, J. L., Lopez, A., Wilson, M., Schulkin, J., and Gibbs, R. (2001). Congenital toxoplasmosis: a review. Obstetrical & Gynecological Survey, 56, 296–305.

Kawashima, Y., Ihara, K., Nakamura, M., Nakashima, T., Fukuda, S., and Kitamura, K. (2005). Epidemiological study of mumps deafness in Japan. Auris Nasus Larynx, 32, 125–128.

Kawashiro, N., Tsuchihashi, N., Koga, K., Kawano, T., and Itoh, Y. (1996). Delayed post-neonatal intensive care unit hearing disturbance. International Journal of Pediatric Otorhinolaryngology, 34, 35–43.

Konrádsson, K. S. (1996). Bilaterally preserved otoacoustic emissions in four children with profound idiopathic unilateral sensorineural hearing loss. Audiology, 35, 217–227.

Koomen, I., Grobbee, D. E., Roord, J. J., Donders, R., Jennekens-Schinkel, A., and van Furth, A. M. (2003). Hearing loss at school age in survivors of bacterial meningitis: assessment, incidence, and prediction. Pediatrics, 112, 1049–1053.

Kutz, J. W., Simon, L. M., Chennupati, S. K., Giannoni, C. M., and Manolidis, S. (2006). Clinical predictors for hearing loss in children with bacterial meningitis. Archives of Otolaryngology-Head and Neck Surgery, 132, 941–945.

Lambert, P. R., and Dodson, E. E. (1996). Congenital malformations of the external auditory canal. Otolaryngologic Clinics of North America, 29, 741–760.

Lasisi, O. A., Ayodele, J. K., and Ijaduola, G. T. A. (2006). Challenges in management of childhood sensorineural hearing loss in sub-Saharan Africa, Nigeria. International Journal of Pediatric Otorhinolaryngology, 70, 625–629.

Lasky, R. E., Wiorek, L., and Becker, T. R. (1998). Hearing loss in survivors of neonatal extracorporeal membrane oxygenation (ECMO) therapy and high-frequency oscillatory (HFO) therapy. Journal of the American Academy of Audiology, 9, 47–58.

Loundon, N., Marcolla, A., Roux, I., Rouillon, I., Denoyelle, F., et al. (2005). Auditory neuropathy or endochlear hearing loss? Otology & Neurotology, 26, 748–754.

Mann, T., and Adams, K. (1998). Sensorineural hearing loss in ECMO survivors. Journal of the American Academy of Audiology, 9, 367–370.

Matteson, E. L., Fabry, D. A., Strome, S. E., Driscoll, C. L., Beatty, C. W., and McDonald, T. J. (2003). Autoimmune inner ear disease: diagnostic and therapeutic approaches in a multidisciplinary setting. Journal of the American Academy of Audiology, 14, 225–230.

McKenna, M. J. (1997). Measles, mumps, and sensorineural hearing loss. Annals of the New York Academy of Sciences, 830, 291–298.

Niedzielska, G., Katska, E., and Szymula, D. (2000). Hearing defects in children born of mothers suffering from rubella in the first trimester of pregnancy. International Journal of Pediatric Otorhinolaryngology, 54, 1–5.

Osguthorpe, J. D., and Nielsen, D. R. (2006). Otitis externa: review and clinical update. American Family Physician, 74, 1510–1516.

Pass, R. F. (2006). Congenital cytomegalovirus infection and hearing loss. Herpes, 12, 50–55.

Pass, R. F., Fowler, K. B., Boppana, S. B., Britt, W. J., and Stagno, S. (2006). Congenital cytomegalovirus infection following first trimester maternal infection: symptoms at birth and outcome. Journal of Clinical Virology, 35, 216–220.

Perreault, T. (2006). Persistent pulmonary hypertension of the newborn. Pediatric Respiratory Reviews, 7S, S175–S176.

Pletcher, S. D., and Cheung, S. W. (2003). Syphilis and otolaryngology. Otolaryngologic Clinics of North America, 36, 595–605.

Rapin, I., and Gravel, J. S. (2006). Auditory neuropathy: a biologically inappropriate label unless acoustic nerve involvement is documented. Journal of the American Academy of Audiology, 17, 147–150.

Reilly, P. G., Lalwani, A. K., and Jackler, R. K. (1998). Congenital anomalies of the inner ear. In A. K. Lalwani and K. M. Grundfast (Eds.), Pediatric otology and neurotology (pp. 201–210). Philadelphia: Lippincott-Raven Publishers.

Rima, B. K., and Duprex, W. P. (2006). Morbilliviruses and human disease. Journal of Pathology, 208, 199–214.

Rivera, L. B., Boppana, S. B., Fowler, K. B., Britt, W. J., Stagno, S., and Pass, R. F. (2002). Predictors of hearing loss in children with symptomatic congenital cytomegalovirus infection. Pediatrics, 110, 762–767.

Roeser, R. J., and Ballachandra, B. B. (1997). Physiology, pathophysiology, and anthropology/epidemiology of human earcanal secretions. Journal of the American Academy of Audiology, 8, 391–400.

Roeser, R. J., and Roland, P.S. (1992). What audiologists must know about cerumen and cerumen management. American Journal of Audiology, 1, 27–35.

Roizen, N. J. (2003). Nongenetic causes of hearing loss. Mental Retardation & Developmental Disabilities Research Reviews, 9, 120–127.

Rol, J. T., Jr., and Cohen, N. L. (1998). Vestibular and auditory ototoxicity. In C. W. Cummings (Ed.), Otolaryngology—head and neck surgery (3rd ed., pp. 3186–3197). St. Louis: Mosby Year Book.

Roland, P. S. (2004). New developments in our understanding of ototoxicity. Ear, Nose & Throat Journal, 83, 15–17.

Rorman, E., Zamir, C. S., Rilkis, I., and Ben-David, H. (2006). Congenital toxoplasmosis: prenatal aspects of *Toxoplasma gondii* infection. Reproductive Toxicology, 21, 458–472.

Rosenfeld, R. M., Brown, L., Cannon, C. R., Dolor, R., Ganiats, T. G., Hannley, M., et al. (2006). Clinical practice guideline: acute otitis externa. Otolaryngology-Head and Neck Surgery, 134, S4–S23.

Ryan, A. F., Harris, J. P., and Keithley, E. M. (2002). Immune-mediated hearing loss: basic mechanisms and options for therapy. Acta Otolaryngologica Supplement 548, 38–43.

Rybak, L. P., and Whitworth, C. A. (2005). Ototoxicity: therapeutic opportunities. Drug Discovery Today, 10, 1313–1321.

Saez-Llorens, X., and McCracken, G. H. (2003). Bacterial meningitis in children. (Seminar). Lancet, 361, 2139–2148.

Semaan, M. T., and Megerian, C. A. (2006). The pathophysiology of cholesteatoma. Otolaryngologic Clinics of North America, 39, 1143–1159.

Sever, J. L., Ellenberg, J. H., Ley, A. C., Madden, D. L., Fuccillo, D. A., Tzan, N. R., et al. (1988). Toxoplasmosis: maternal and pediatric findings in 23,000 pregnancies. Pediatrics, 82, 181–192.

Shapiro, S. M. (2003). Bilirubin toxicity in the developing nervous system. Pediatric Neurology, 29, 410–421.

Sharma, P., Chhangani, N. P., Meena, K. R., Jora, R., Sharma, N., and Gupta, B. D. (2006). Brainstem evoked response audiometry (BAER) in neonates with hyperbilirubinemia. Indian Journal of Pediatrics, 73, 413–416.

Shekelle, P., Takata, G., and Chan, L. S. (2003). Diagnosis, natural history and late effects of otitis media with effusion. Summary, Evidence report/technology assessment No. 55 (No. 02-E025). Rockville, MD: Agency for Healthcare Research & Quality.

Sie, K. C. Y. (1996). Cholesteatoma in children. Pediatric Clinics of North America, 43, 1245–1252.

Sininger, Y., and Oba, S. (2001). Patients with auditory neuropathy: who are they and what can they hear? In Y. Sininger and A. Starr (Eds.), Auditory neuropathy (pp. 15–36). San Diego: Singular Thomson Learning.

Slattery, W. H. I., and House, J. W. (1998). Complications of otitis media. In A. K. Lalwani and K. M. Grundfast (Eds.), Pediatric otology and neurotology (pp. 251–263). Philadelphia: Lippincott-Raven Publishers.

Smith, J. A., and Danner, C. J. (2006). Complications of chronic otitis media and cholesteatoma. Otolaryngologic Clinics of North America, 39, 1237–1255.

Starr, A., Picton, T. W., Sininger, Y., Hood, L. J., and Berlin, C. I. (1996). Auditory neuropathy. Brain, 119, 741–753.

Verklan, M. T. (2006). Persistent pulmonary hypertension of the newborn: not a honeymoon anymore. Journal of Perinatal & Neonatal Nursing, 20, 108–112.

Wilson, C. B., Remington, J. S., Stagno, S., and Reynolds, D. W. (1980). Development of adverse sequelae in children born with subclinical congenital *Toxoplasma* infection. Pediatrics, 66, 767–774.

Woods, B.T. (1984). Dichotic listening ear preference after childhood cerebral lesions. Neuropsychologia, 22, 303–310.

Yoshikawa, S., Ikeda, K., Kudo, T., and Kobayashi, T. (2004). The effects of hypoxia, premature birth, infection, ototoxic drugs, circulatory system and congenital disease on neonatal hearing loss. Auris Nasus Larynx, 31, 361–368.

Chapter 2

Genetics of Hearing Loss

Heidi L. Rehm and Rebecca Madore

♦ **Basic Genetics and Inheritance Patterns**

♦ **Causes of Permanent Hearing Loss**

♦ **Nonsyndromic Genetic Hearing Loss**

Connexin Hearing Loss
DFNB4 Hearing Loss
Mitochondrial Hearing Loss
Auditory Dys-synchrony/Neuropathy

♦ **Syndromic Forms of Genetic Hearing Loss**

Alport Syndrome
Branchio-Oto-Renal Syndrome
CHARGE Syndrome
Jervell and Lange-Nielsen Syndrome
Neurofibromatosis Type 2
Pendred Syndrome
Usher Syndrome
Waardenburg Syndrome

♦ **Genetic Testing for Hearing Loss**

♦ **Genetic Counseling for Hearing Loss**

♦ **Gene Therapy for Hearing Loss**

♦ **Summary**

Key Points

- More than half of childhood hearing loss is genetic.

- Any child with sensorineural hearing loss (SNHL) should have a genetic evaluation.

- Approximately 70% of genetic SNHL is nonsyndromic.

- In most cases of genetic hearing loss, there is no family history.

- The most common cause of congenital nonsyndromic SNHL is mutations in the *GJB2* (connexin 26) gene.

- Symptoms such as vision loss, thyroid problems, fainting episodes, and hematuria may be indications that hearing loss is part of a genetic syndrome.

- Clinical genetic testing is available for several genes associated with syndromic and nonsyndromic hearing loss.

- Genetic counseling is highly recommended for individuals and families before and after pursuing genetic testing for hearing loss.

The prevalence of congenital (present at birth) hearing loss is estimated at 3 in 1000 births, making it the most frequently occurring birth defect (NCHAM, 2006). Over the last 10 years, our understanding of the genetics of hearing and deafness has grown exponentially. Among the most significant advances is the discovery that approximately half of nonsyndromic recessive hearing loss is caused by mutations in the *GJB2* gene, which encodes the connexin 26 protein (Cx26). Genetic testing for *GJB2* mutations has been available for several years and substantially increases the likelihood of obtaining an etiology for congenital hearing loss. The ability to diagnose the cause of hearing loss has an impact on the medical decisions made by patients, their families, and their physicians. Knowledge gained from a genetic evaluation and appropriate genetic testing can simplify the diagnosis, prognosis, and treatment decisions offered by the physician. Furthermore, this information helps individuals understand the cause and heritability of their hearing loss.

◆ Basic Genetics and Inheritance Patterns

Genetic information is packaged inside virtually every cell of the body into structures called chromosomes. There are 23 pairs of chromosomes in each cell. One chromosome from each pair is from the mother and the other is from the father. Genes are segments of the chromosome that provide the body with instructions for growth and development. Just as there are two copies of each chromosome, there are also two copies of every gene. A genetic condition is the result of a change (mutation) in a gene that alters the body's instructions. Some genetic diseases arise when only one copy of a gene is altered. This is referred to as a dominant genetic condition, as the altered gene "dominates" over the normal copy. Other genetic conditions, referred to as recessive, arise only when both copies (one from each parent) of a gene have undergone a mutation. If something is said to be "inherited," it means it is passed on from one or both parents to the child, though parents or other family members may not be clinically affected. **Figs. 2–1** to **2–4** discuss these forms of inheritance.

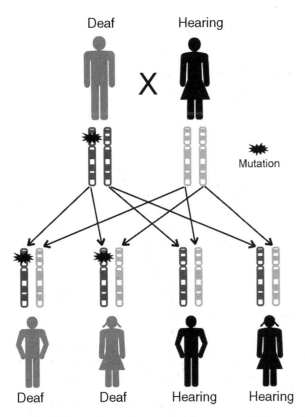

Figure 2–1 Dominant inheritance. When a mutation is passed in a dominant way, it means that only one mutation is needed to cause hearing loss. Hearing loss also appears in each generation (e.g., grandparent, parent, child). Therefore, if a person has one dominant mutation, he will have hearing loss. That also means that *every* child of that person will have a 50% (or 1 in 2) chance of having the mutation and hearing loss.

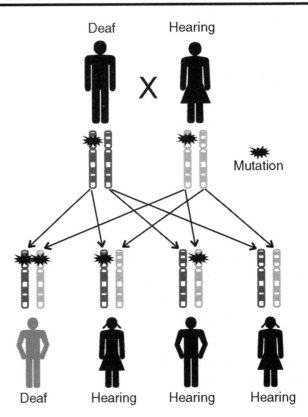

Figure 2–2 Recessive inheritance. Mutations in both copies of a gene (one from each parent) are required to cause recessive hearing loss. Individuals with just one recessive mutation are called carriers and do not have hearing loss. If each parent has one recessive mutation, each child has a 25% (or 1 in 4) chance of having hearing loss and a 50% chance of being an unaffected carrier. Hearing loss that is inherited in a recessive pattern often appears without any family history.

◆ Causes of Permanent Hearing Loss

There are many causes of permanent hearing loss, which can be broadly grouped into genetic and nongenetic etiologies. Historical estimates indicate that approximately half of children identified with a permanent hearing loss have a genetic cause and the other half have an environmental or unknown cause (Toriello et al, 2004). Genetic causes of hearing loss may be classified as syndromic or nonsyndromic. Approximately one third of genetic hearing loss is syndromic, indicating that it is associated with additional medical problems. In contrast, the majority of children with genetic hearing loss have no associated medical problems. In these cases, the loss is classified as nonsyndromic.

Genetic hearing loss can also be subdivided by mode of inheritance; about 77% of cases of hereditary hearing loss are recessive, 22% are dominant, and 1% are X-linked (Morton, 1991). In addition, a small fraction (less than 1%) represents those families with mitochondrial inheritance in which the trait is passed through the maternal lineage. These patterns of inheritance are discussed in **Fig. 2–1**, **Fig. 2–2**, **Fig. 2–3**, **and Fig. 2–4** and the breakdown of different forms of hearing loss is illustrated in **Fig. 2–5**. In all cases of genetic, or

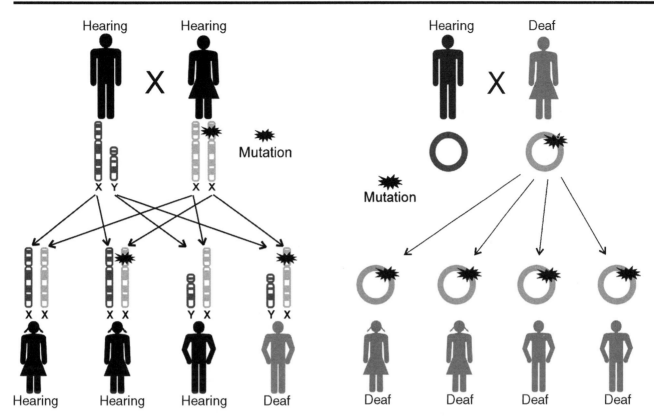

Figure 2–3 X-linked inheritance. The X and Y chromosomes are called sex chromosomes because they determine gender. Women have two X chromosomes; men have one X and one Y chromosome. If a mutation is said to be X-linked, it means it occurs only on the X chromosome. Since women have two X chromosomes, if one X chromosome has a recessive mutation, the second chromosome can provide a functioning copy of the gene, and hearing loss will often not develop. In men, the Y chromosome cannot provide a normal copy of the gene so hearing loss will occur. Therefore, hearing loss resulting from X-linked mutations is usually seen only in males. If the mother has a mutation on one copy of her X chromosomes, each female child has a 50% chance of being a carrier (but will not have hearing loss) and each male child will have a 50% chance of having hearing loss.

Figure 2–4 Mitochondrial inheritance. Mitochondrial genes are found inside the mitochondria, which are found within each of our cells. Unlike most of our genes, which are passed on by each parent, mitochondria are passed on by the mother only. This means that if the mother has hearing loss mutation in one of her mitochondrial genes, she will pass it on to all of her children and they may have hearing loss. If the father has a hearing loss mutation in one of his mitochondrial genes, he will not pass it on to any of his children and thus they will not have hearing loss.

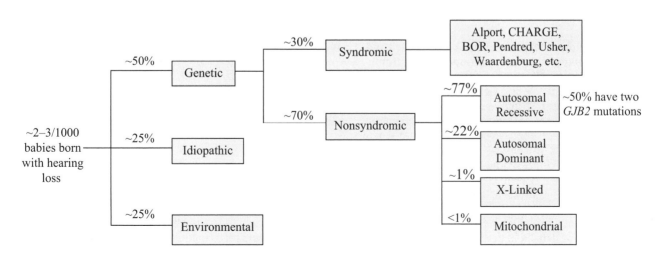

Figure 2–5 Breakdown of etiologies of hearing loss.

"inherited," hearing loss, the gene mutation is present at birth. However, in many cases, particularly for gene mutations with dominant inheritance, the hearing loss may not begin until late childhood or adulthood.

Because a large proportion (77%) of nonsyndromic genetic hearing loss is recessive, where each parent is a carrier of a mutation but has normal hearing, there are many instances when a couple with no family history of hearing loss will give birth to a child with hearing loss. The underlying cause of hearing loss in these cases can be especially difficult to determine because the loss may be either genetic or acquired. It is therefore important to be aware of nongenetic causes of hearing impairment that are discussed in Chapters 1 and 2. Recognition of nongenetic causes is critical, for in some cases there are interventions that can either resolve the hearing loss or stop its progression.

Pitfall

- Unfortunately, diagnosis of the etiology of hearing loss remains difficult even if environmental causes have been ruled out, as the current paucity of molecular diagnostic tests makes it difficult to positively conclude that a patient's hearing loss has genetic origins. In addition, even when an environmental risk factor is present, a definitive association with hearing loss can be difficult.

As such, a genetics evaluation is a very important part of the child's workup and is recommended for all children with SNHL (Panel, 2002). Approaches used by clinical geneticists and genetic counselors to aid in a genetics evaluation include review of the family history as well as pregnancy and neonatal histories. A complete review of the child's medical and developmental histories and a complete physical and dysmorphology examination is necessary to identify specific risk factors as well as clinical findings that may indicate a syndromic form of hearing loss.

Currently, more than 270 genes have been identified and found to be associated with syndromic and nonsyndromic forms of hearing loss (OMIM, 2004), and more are expected to be discovered as time goes on. Despite this growing understanding of genetic hearing loss, very few molecular tests have been available to aid in the diagnosis of genetic forms of hearing loss. This tends to be less important when dealing with syndromic hearing loss, which may be accompanied by an array of defining symptoms. However, for nonsyndromic hearing loss, as well as in instances when the signs and symptoms of a particular syndrome do not begin until after birth such as retinitis pigmentosa in Usher syndrome and thyroid abnormalities in Pendred syndrome, the use of genetic testing can aid in determining the causative gene and mode of inheritance and predict the development of any associated clinical findings.

◆ Nonsyndromic Genetic Hearing Loss

Most genetic hearing loss is nonsyndromic. In these cases, the only clinical finding is hearing loss, except that some patients may have accompanying vestibular symptoms. Although hearing loss and vestibular dysfunction do not always occur together, the existence of many disorders involving both the auditory and vestibular systems reflects their close anatomic proximity, structural similarity, and common developmental origin. Unfortunately, the diagnosis of vestibular problems is often challenging, especially at young ages.

Pearl

- An early clue to vestibular problems can be a delay in walking (Angeli, 2003).

One of the difficulties in studying nonsyndromic hearing loss, and discovering the underlying genetic causes, is the immense genetic heterogeneity in nonsyndromic forms of hearing loss. Although subtle pathologic differences may allow clinical differentiation between certain subtypes of nonsyndromic hearing loss, there is still a plethora of genes whose dysfunction can result in highly similar clinical presentations. In fact, mapping efforts have located more than 120 independent loci (gene locations) for nonsyndromic hearing loss (Van Camp and Smith, 2004). Each locus is labeled "DFN" followed by "A" for dominant inheritance, "B" for recessive, or no additional letter for X-linked. A unique number is then added to the locus designation to indicate the sequential order in which the genes were mapped.

Pearl

- In general, autosomal recessive forms of hearing loss are usually prelingual, and autosomal dominant ones often result in progressive, postlingual hearing loss. This likely reflects the fact that most recessive disorders represent a complete loss of a gene's function, whereas dominant disorders may mechanistically represent an interaction between the activity of the normal gene product and the activity of the mutant product.

The responsible gene has been identified in 40 of these nonsyndromic loci, covering 22 forms of autosomal dominant hearing loss, 23 forms of autosomal recessive hearing loss, 1 form of X-linked recessive hearing loss, and 2 forms of mitochondrially inherited hearing loss. The discrepancy in these numbers reflects the fact that different mutations in some of these genes (e.g., *GJB2* (connexin 26), *GJB6*, *MYO7A*, *MYO6*, *TMC1*, *TECTA*) can cause both recessive and dominant forms of hearing loss. For a full summary of hearing loss loci, refer to the frequently updated Hereditary Hearing Loss home page, which contains tables summarizing the details of these nonsyndromic loci, as well as a wealth of other information for the research community and others interested in hereditary hearing loss (Van Camp and Smith, 2004).

Connexin Hearing Loss

DFNB1 was the first recessive hearing loss locus identified in 1994, and the responsible gene, *GJB2*, encodes the gap junction β 2 protein, known as connexin 26. Mutations in the *GJB2* gene are the most common cause of SNHL, responsible for 12 to 24% of permanent childhood SNHL (Putcha et al, 2007). This gene represents a common cause of hearing loss across the world, though different regions have distinct common mutations. For instance, two frameshift mutations, 35delG and 167delT, are more commonly identified in Caucasians (carrier rate 2.5% in the United States) and Ashkenazi Jews (4%), respectively. A third frameshift mutation, 235delC, is prevalent in Asians with a carrier frequency of 1%. A database of most published mutations can be found online at the Connexins and Deafness Web site (Smith, 2005; Calvo et al, 2007).

Hearing loss caused by *GJB2* mutations is typically congenital, though roughly 4% are now thought to be delayed in onset (Norris et al, 2006). The severity of hearing loss ranges from mild to profound; certain mutations, such as M34T and V37I, are associated with a milder hearing loss (ranging from normal to moderate) (Snoeckx et al, 2005). In addition, a recent study by Kenna and colleagues found progression of hearing loss in about 19% of patients with two *GJB2* mutations (Rehm and Kenna, unpublished data).

On some occasions mutations in the connexin 26 gene can be inherited in an autosomal dominant rather than a recessive pattern. Dominant sensorineural hearing loss caused by *GJB2* mutations is generally early onset, moderate to severe, and frequently demonstrates a progressive course. Some of these dominant mutations can also cause syndromic rather than nonsyndromic hearing loss in which patients have variable types of skin findings such as Vohwinkel or KID syndrome.

In addition to *GJB2*, other gap junction genes also play a role in the development of hearing loss such as *GJB6*, encoding the connexin 30 protein. Located directly adjacent to the *GJB2* gene, the *GJB6* gene is located in a region that is known to be deleted in some patients with a single *GJB2* mutation. In the United States, only 1% of individuals with hearing loss have this mutation, and it almost always is present in combination with a single connexin 26 mutation (Putcha et al, 2007). Higher frequencies have been reported in individuals of Spanish, French, and Ashkenazi Jewish descent and a few cases of SNHL have been associated with two copies of the *GJB6* deletion in the absence of a *GJB2* gene mutation (Schrijver and Gardner, 2006).

DFNB4 Hearing Loss

Mutations in the *SLC26A4* gene (also called PDS) are associated with both a syndromic form of hearing loss called Pendred syndrome (see later section) as well as a nonsyndromic form called DFNB4. DFNB4 patients have autosomal recessive, nonsyndromic SNHL with enlarged vestibular aqueducts (EVA) and/or Mondini malformations, but do not manifest the thyroid abnormalities seen in Pendred syndrome. Hearing loss tends to be congenital, bilateral, severe to profound SNHL, though mild to moderate loss can also been seen; progression and fluctuation are not uncommon (Smith, 2006c). On rare occasions hearing loss onset can occur in childhood. For cases of hearing loss with EVA, about 50% of cases from multiplex families (more than one family member affected) and 20% of singleton cases have mutations in the *SLC26A4* (or *PDS*) gene (Smith, 2006c).

Mitochondrial Hearing Loss

There are many mitochondrial syndromes in which hearing loss is a component (often associated with neuromuscular disease); however, two forms of mitochondrial hearing loss are usually nonsyndromic. These are caused by mutations in the *MTRNR1* (encoding 12S rRNA) and *MTTS1* (encoding tRNAser[(UCN)]) mitochondrial genes. Due to their location on the mitochondrial chromosome, families with mutations in these genes show maternal inheritance of hearing loss (see **Fig. 2–4** for an explanation of maternal inheritance). However, this pattern of inheritance may not be clear in some families. For instance, some individuals with certain mutations in the *MTRNR1* gene, such as the 1555A>G and 1494C>T mutations, may develop hearing loss only when exposed to aminoglycoside antibiotics (e.g., gentamicin, neomycin, amikacin, tobramycin). The 1555A>G mutation is present in variable percentages of the hearing impaired population based on geographic and/or ethnic origin: 0.6% Caucasian (Li et al, 2004), 0.7% German (Kupka et al, 2002), 3.5% Asian (Usami et al, 2000), 20% Spanish (del Castillo, 2003a).

People can lose their hearing because of treatment with high doses of aminoglycoside antibiotics even if they do not have any of these mutations. Also, a person with one of these mutations can develop hearing loss even with no exposure to aminoglycoside antibiotics. Hearing loss from mitochondrial mutations is highly variable and can begin any time from birth to the late adulthood, can be flat, sloping, or high frequency, or can progress, remain stable, or fluctuate (Li et al, 2004; Pandya, 2004). Identifying an *MTRNR1* mutation as the etiology of hearing loss in one individual allows maternally related relatives to prevent exposures that could result in their hearing loss.

Auditory Dys-synchrony/Neuropathy

Auditory dys-synchrony (AD/AN), also called auditory neuropathy, is a complex type of hearing loss with multiple etiologies, including environmental (e.g., hyperbilirubinemia, prematurity, and hypoxia) and genetic. More information about AD/AN can be found in Chapter 32. Some syndromes such as Charcot-Marie-Tooth and Friedreich's ataxia (OMIM, 2004) are associated with AD/AN. In addition, two genes, the *OTOF* gene, encoding otoferlin (Yasunaga et al, 1999), and the *PJVK* gene, encoding pejvakin, are known to be associated with nonsyndromic forms of genetic AD/AN

(Delmaghani et al, 2006). Individuals with mutations in *OTOF* can present with AD/AN or a pure SNHL. The hearing loss is typically prelingual and moderate to profound; a variety of audiometric shapes are observed, including flat, rising, sloping, and bowl-shaped (Varga et al, 2006). Recently, several families have been identified with a unique form of hearing loss that manifests only in the presence of a fever (Varga et al, 2006; Kelly and Rehm, unpublished data). The genetic basis for this appears to be temperature-sensitive mutations in the *OTOF* gene. Another mutation in *OTOF*, Q829X, is common in the Spanish population and is believed to be responsible for 3% of recessive cases of deafness in this region (Migliosi et al, 2002). In addition, like most patients with AD/AN, patients with *OTOF* mutations appear to do well with cochlear implants (Rodriguez-Ballesteros et al, 2003).

◆ Syndromic Forms of Genetic Hearing Loss

Approximately 30% of patients with childhood hearing loss also have additional clinical and physical findings that define a particular syndrome. More than 400 such syndromic forms of hearing loss have been characterized; the most complete collection of these disorders is found in Toriello and colleagues' *Hereditary Hearing Loss and Its Syndromes* (2004). Some of these syndromes are reviewed below and listed in **Table 2–1** with their accompanying phenotype, responsible gene, and availability of clinical testing. An excellent source of up-to-date, freely available information on these and other genetic disorders can be found through the GeneTests Web site, where experts in the field contribute comprehensive reviews, called "GeneReviews" of many genetic disorders (GeneTests, 2007). This Web site can also be queried to determine the availability of gene testing for any genetic disorder.

Alport Syndrome

Alport syndrome (AS) is characterized by renal, cochlear, and ocular involvement and can be inherited in an X-linked (80% XLAS), autosomal recessive (15% ARAS), or autosomal dominant (5% ADAS) manner (Kashtan, 2007). Its prevalence is estimated to be 1 in 50,000 live births (Levy and Feingold, 2000). The characteristic symptom of the disease is microscopic hematuria (blood in the urine), which can progress to end-stage renal disease. The associated hearing loss is never congenital and initially affects the high frequencies with progression to all frequencies over time. Onset occurs by late

Table 2–1   Selected Hearing Loss Syndromes

Syndrome	Features (besides hearing loss)	Inheritance Pattern(s)	Gene(s)	Available Gene Tests*
Alport syndrome	Nephritis, ocular abnormalities	80% XL 15% AR 5% AD	XLAS: *COL4A5* ARAS: *COL4A3* ADAS: *COL4A4*	Europe only
Branchio-oto-renal syndrome	Branchial remnants, renal anomalies	AD	*EYA1*	Yes
CHARGE syndrome	Ocular, ear, and heart defects, delayed growth and development, genital abnormalities	Sporadic or AD	*CHD7*	Yes
Jervell and Lange-Nielsen syndrome	Cardiac conduction defects	AR	JLN1: *KCNQ1* JLN2: *KCNE1*	Yes
Neurofibromatosis type 2	Acoustic neuromas	AD or sporadic	*NF2*	Yes
Pendred syndrome	Thyroid goiter	AR	*SLC26A4* (PDS)	Yes
Usher syndrome	Retinitis pigmentosa, vestibular problems	AR	USH1B: *MYO7A* USH1C: *USH1C* USH1D: *CDH23* USH1E: Unknown USH1F: *PCDH15* USH1G: *USH1G* USH2A: *USH2A* USH2C: *GPR98* USH3: *CLRN1*	Yes
Waardenburg syndrome	Pigmentary abnormalities of the skin, hair, and eyes	AD or sporadic	WS1: *PAX3* WS2: *MITF*, *SNAI2* WS3: *PAX3* WS4: *END3*, *EDNRB*, *SHOX10*	Yes

Abbreviations: AD, autosomal dominant; AR, autosomal recessive; XL, X-linked.

Note: For up-to-date information about test availability go to www.genetests.org.

childhood or early adolescence in individuals with ARAS or males with XLAS, whereas onset is later in individuals with ADAS. Females with XLAS tend to have milder hearing loss and other symptoms, if they have any at all. Although only present in 15 to 20% of patients, the identification of anterior lenticonus, a defect of the lens of the eye, is virtually pathognomonic for Alport syndrome (Kashtan, 2007).

Branchio-Oto-Renal Syndrome

Branchio-oto-renal syndrome (BOR) is a genetic disorder that includes branchial and kidney malformations and hearing loss. The condition is inherited in an autosomal dominant pattern with a prevalence estimated to be 1 in 40,000 to 700,000 individuals (Fraser, 1976; Fraser, Sproule, and Halal, 1980). Expression of the disease is highly variable, even among members of the same family. Malformations of the branchial arches can include cupping of the outer ear, ear pits in front of, or on, the outer ear, tags of skin in front of the ear, and cysts or fistulas on the neck. Renal abnormalities can range from mild renal hypoplasia to bilateral renal agenesis; however, many individuals with BOR have either no renal disease or do not experience symptoms of their renal anomalies. On rare occasions, individuals with BOR may also have blocked tear ducts that interfere with tear flow and require surgical repair. Most individuals with BOR (more than 90%) have some degree of hearing loss, and some also have radiologic abnormalities such as enlarged vestibular aqueducts (Kemperman et al, 2004). The type of loss can be mixed (52%), conductive (33%), or sensorineural (29%); severity ranges from mild to profound and the loss can either be nonprogressive (about 70%) or progressive (about 30%) (Smith, 2006). Approximately 40% of individuals have a mutation in *EYA1* (Chang et al, 2004), fewer than 1% have a mutation in *SIX1* (Ruf et al, 2004), and others likely have mutations in additional genes yet to be discovered.

CHARGE Syndrome

CHARGE is a mnemonic that stands for the major features of the disease: **c**oloboma, **h**eart defects, choanal **a**tresia, **r**etarded growth and development, **g**enital abnormalities, and **e**ar anomalies (Lalani, 2006a). Hearing loss is one of the most common features of CHARGE syndrome and can be sensorineural or conductive because of the presence of Mondini and/or ossicular malformations, respectively. The sensorineural component of the hearing loss can vary from mild to profound and the conductive component may fluctuate with middle ear disease, which is common in these patients. The prevalence of CHARGE syndrome is about 1 in 8500 (Issekutz et al, 2005). The majority of individuals with CHARGE syndrome have a mutation in the *CDH7* gene; most cases arise from new mutations, though autosomal dominant inheritance can be observed (Lalani, 2006b).

Jervell and Lange-Nielsen Syndrome

Individuals with Jervell and Lange-Nielsen syndrome (JLNS) have congenital deafness and cardiac conduction defects referred to as prolonged QTc intervals (long QT). Long QT is associated with arrhythmias that can result in fainting or sudden death; however, several methods of cardiac management are available. Although the overall prevalence is rare, as many as 1 in 250 deaf children may have JLNS (Schwartz, Periti, and Malliani, 1975). JLNS is inherited in an autosomal recessive pattern and is caused by mutations in *KCNQ1* (JLNS1; 90% of cases) or *KCNE1* (JLNS2; fewer than 10% of cases) (Daley et al, 2004). Parents and siblings of a child with JLNS may have an autosomal dominant form of long QT, without hearing loss, called Romano-Ward syndrome.

Neurofibromatosis Type 2

Neurofibromatosis type 2 (NF2) is a rare disease characterized by bilateral acoustic neuromas (benign tumors of the auditory and vestibular nerves), which lead to tinnitus, hearing loss, and balance dysfunction. The average age of onset is typically 18 to 24 years and the disease is usually unilateral (Evans, 2006). Other tumors of the central nervous system can also develop. NF2 is inherited in an autosomal dominant pattern, and with exhaustive testing, a mutation can be identified in the *NF2* gene in most patients. However, many patients have a new mutation and therefore have no family history for the disorder.

Pendred Syndrome

Pendred syndrome is an autosomal recessive disease that consists of hearing loss associated with temporal bone anomalies and later development of thyroid goiter (which can be hypothyroid or euthyroid). Soon after the discovery that Pendred syndrome is caused by mutations in the *SLC26A4* (PDS) gene, Usami et al (1999) recognized that many with *SLC26A4* gene mutations are nonsyndromic and do not have thyroid abnormalities (referred to as DFNB4). The temporal bone abnormalities consist of dilation of the vestibular aqueduct (commonly referred to as enlarged vestibular aqueduct or EVA) with or without cochlear hypoplasia, such as a common cavity or Mondini's malformation) (Goldfeld et al, 2005). The hearing loss in Pendred syndrome and DFNB4 tends to be congenital, bilateral, severe to profound SNHL, though mild to moderate severity and unilateral loss can also been seen, and progression and fluctuation are not uncommon (Smith, 2006c). On rare occasions hearing loss onset can occur in childhood. The exact prevalence of Pendred syndrome and DFNB4 hearing loss is not known, but it appears to be a relatively common cause, particularly in patients with temporal bone abnormalities.

Usher Syndrome

Usher syndrome is characterized by sensorineural hearing loss and retinitis pigmentosa (RP), with or without vestibular abnormalities. A recent study suggested that as many as 20% of children with cochlear implants have Usher syndrome (Smith, 2006a). The disease is divided into three types based on the onset and severity of hearing loss and RP as well as the presence (USH1) or absence (USH2) of vestibular problems (dizziness, loss of balance and coordination, delayed walking) (Keats and Lentz, 2006a; 2006b). RP is a progressive degeneration of the rod and cone functions of the retina. It first causes night blindness and tunnel vision and later results in loss of day vision, although most individuals do not usually become completely blind (Kimberling and Moller, 1995). All three types of Usher syndrome are inherited in an autosomal recessive pattern.

Waardenburg Syndrome

Waardenburg syndrome (WS) is characterized by hearing loss and changes in pigmentation of the hair, skin, and eyes. Eye color can either be pale blue, a combination of two colors in one eye, or a different color in each eye (referred to as heterochromia irides). The eyes appear widely spaced because of the lateral displacement of the inner canthi (dystopia canthorum) in some types of WS. Distinctive hair coloring such as a patch of white hair or premature graying is another common sign of the condition. There are four types of Waardenburg syndrome, which are distinguished by their physical characteristics: WS1, WS2, WS3 (Klein-Waardenburg syndrome), and WS4 (Waardenburg-Shah).Types I and II are the most common, and individuals with WS1 can have all of the above described characteristics. Close to 60% of WS1 patients have hearing loss, which is usually congenital bilateral profound SNHL, though other types, including unilateral cases, are seen (Milunsky, 2006). Mutations in the PAX3 gene are responsible for WS1, and WS3 (WS3 also includes upper limb abnormalities). Individuals with WS2 have hearing loss and pigmentation abnormalities but do not have dystopia canthorum. Individuals with WS4 have the pigmentary abnormalities, dystopia canthorum, and Hirschsprung disease (inadequate muscular movement of the bowel leading to severe constipation and intestinal blockage). The features of Waardenburg syndrome vary among affected individuals, even among members in the same family. The prevalence of Waardenburg syndrome is estimated to be 1 in 20,000 to 40,000 individuals; about 3% of people who are deaf have this condition (Milunsky, 2006). The disorder is usually inherited in an autosomal dominant pattern, although autosomal recessive inheritance has been described for WS2, WS3, and WS4.

◆ Genetic Testing for Hearing Loss

The presence of only a small subset of clinically available genetic tests for hearing loss makes identification of a genetic etiology challenging; however, some genetic tests can be very informative.

> **Special Consideration**
>
> • In almost all cases of childhood SNHL, it is suggested that GJB2 gene (connexin 26 gene) testing be ordered because it is substantially more common than any other cause of SNHL and the audiologic characteristics can be quite variable, ranging from mild to profound hearing loss.

It is even worthwhile to order this test if the patient passed a newborn screen, yet developed hearing loss in early childhood, because an estimated 4% percent of cases present after birth (Green et al, 2000; Norris et al, 2006)

If a child has a history of exposure to aminoglycoside antibiotics, a family history of hearing loss consistent with maternal inheritance, or is of Spanish or Chinese ethnicity, testing for mitochondrial mutations in the MTRNR1 (12S rRNA) and MTTS1 (tRNAser(UCN)) genes would be appropriate. Testing for mutations in the SLC26A4 (PDS) gene is indicated if the child has abnormalities of the temporal bone, such as EVA or a Mondini malformation. In a child with a diagnosis of auditory neuropathy/dys-synchrony, testing for OTOF and PJVK gene mutations may be appropriate, particularly if there are other affected siblings. Patients with mutations in OTOF appear to do well with cochlear implants but not with hearing aids, so diagnosis of this etiology can be useful in management of the hearing loss (Varga et al, 2003).

Some individuals with hearing loss also experience vestibular problems. At early stages this may manifest as delayed walking. At older ages, patients may complain of dizziness, vertigo, or other troubles with balance. Nonetheless, if there is evidence of vestibular problems, certain tests such as COCH, when the hearing loss begins later in life (15 to 65 years), or, MYO7A, when the hearing loss is congenital, may be indicated. The importance of screening for MYO7A mutations in a child with severe to profound hearing loss and delayed walking is that children who test positive will likely go on to develop Usher syndrome, which is associated with progressive blindness (see section on Usher syndrome).

> **Pearl**
>
> • An early diagnosis of Usher syndrome would prompt initiation of dietary supplementation, which may slow the progression of vision loss (Berson et al, 1993) as well as aid in managing the hearing loss (i.e., cochlear implants would be preferred over sign language).

Although rare, one additional form of childhood hearing loss, for which gene testing is available, is DFN3, caused by mutations in the POU3F4 gene. Unlike most forms of nonsyndromic hearing loss that are strictly sensorineural, these patients can have conductive, sensorineural, or mixed hearing loss. In addition, the patients often have radiologic abnormalities of the temporal bone and can manifest a perilymphatic gusher during stapedectomy (Chee, Suhailee, and Goh 2006).

A summary of all currently available gene tests for nonsyndromic hearing loss is listed in **Table 2–2** along with the most typical type of hearing loss observed. For ongoing updates of available tests, refer to the GeneTests Web site (GeneTests, 2007).

Table 2–2 Clinically Available Gene Tests Indicated for Types of Nonsyndromic Hearing Loss

Hearing Loss Type	Available Gene Tests
Congenital/prelingual SNHL	*GJB2, GJB6, MTRNR1, MTTS1*
Congenital/prelingual SNHL with EVA	*SLC26A4 (PDS)*
Congenital auditory neuropathy/dys-synchrony	*OTOF, PJVK*
Congenital/prelingual SNHL with vestibular symptoms (*i.e.*, delayed walking may be first sign)	*MYO7A*
SNHL with aminoglycoside exposure	*MTRNR1*
SNHL with maternal (mitochondrial) inheritance	*MTRNR1, MTTS1*
SNHL +/ − conductive HL (perilymphatic gusher on stapedectomy)	*POU3F4*
Dominantly inherited congenital/prelingual SNHL	*GJB2*
Dominantly inherited postlingual, progressive, sloping SNHL	*GJB2, MYO7A*
Dominantly inherited postlingual, low frequency SNHL	*WFS1, MYO7A*
Dominantly inherited postlingual, progressive, vestibular symptoms	*COCH*

Abbreviations: SNHL, sensory neural hearing loss; EVA, enlarged vestibular aqueducts; HL, hearing loss.

♦ Genetic Counseling for Hearing Loss

As with any condition that may be genetic, it is recommended that families see a genetic counselor. Genetic counseling is the process of providing individuals and families with information on the nature, inheritance, and implications of genetic conditions to help them make informed medical and personal decisions. The process also includes supportive counseling, advocating for the clients and their families, and referring them to community or state support services when needed. Individuals may choose to pursue genetic counseling for various reasons and at different times. Some individuals may chose to seek genetic counseling when the child is first diagnosed and they are trying to understand the cause and make critical decisions about managing the hearing loss. Others may seek genetic counseling when considering family planning or to obtain updated information about genetic testing or research opportunities. Genetic counselors can provide information about recurrence risks, preimplantation genetic diagnosis, or prenatal diagnostic testing.

If genetic testing is pursued, a genetic counselor can discuss the benefits and limitations of genetic testing, including the possible test results, as well as help the family interpret the results of testing when they are received. A potential benefit of genetic testing is that identifying mutations may help to rule out, or predict the development of, additional clinical features, depending on whether a nonsyndromic or syndromic etiology is identified. Identifying the genetic etiology may also help determine whether the hearing loss will progress and may help determine how best to manage the hearing loss. In addition, identification of a genetic cause allows families to know the recurrence risk (chance of having future children with hearing loss). For example, if a hearing couple has a child with hearing loss, the recurrence risk of having a second child with hearing loss is about 17.5%, which takes into account the possibility that it may be either genetic or environmental in origin (Green et al, 1999). This risk drops slightly to about 14% if connexin 26 testing is negative (Smith, 2002). In contrast, if genetic testing is positive, more informative risk assessments can be provided.

Pitfall

- Potential limitations of genetic testing are that the test (in the case of a negative result) does not rule out a genetic cause for hearing loss.

As described above, many genes are associated with hearing loss, and currently there is testing for only a handful of them. Genetic testing may also give unclear results. For instance, if a child with nonsyndromic sensorineural hearing loss is found to have one connexin 26 mutation, as is the case 10 to 50% of the time (del Castillo, 2003b), connexin 26 may be in fact responsible for causing the hearing loss, but the second mutation was not detected. However, the child may simply be a carrier for the connexin 26 mutation, and another unidentified cause, genetic or environmental, may be responsible for the hearing loss. In these cases it is not possible to differentiate these possible explanations in any given child. Also, genetic testing cannot always predict the characteristics of the hearing loss such as age of onset, progression, or how severe the loss or associated signs and symptoms will be.

◆ Gene Therapy for Hearing Loss

Much hope has been placed on the concept of gene therapy for genetic disorders. Unfortunately, gene therapy has not been realized to its full potential because of some very significant practical challenges. These include challenges in the successful development of methods to put the correct gene into the cells that need it as well as in figuring out ways to maintain the cells with the new genetic material (our body often sees the changed cells as foreign bodies and destroys them). Despite these challenges, there are success stories, some involving immune related diseases where gene therapy can be performed on blood cells that are taken out of the person and put back after genetic alteration.

Although gene therapy has not advanced as quickly as hoped, advances have been made with some of these accomplishments specific to hearing loss. For example, methods have been developed to stably incorporate genetic material into the hair cells of mammals, including mice and guinea pigs. In one study, the addition of the *Atoh1* gene caused the ear to regenerate new hair cells in a guinea pig whose hearing had been destroyed by ototoxic damage. Early studies are now under way to use similar approaches to restore function to mammals with genetically based hearing loss. Such approaches have been used to successfully restore vision to dogs with an early form of genetic blindness (Acland et al, 2005). This holds promise for the ability to prevent blindness in patients diagnosed early with Usher syndrome. Early work on Usher syndrome gene therapy has already begun and the correction of retinal abnormalities in mice with Usher syndrome has been demonstrated (Hashimoto et al, 2007). Furthermore, recent studies suggest that a future approach to correction of connexin 26–based hearing loss could be to upregulate the neighboring connexin 30 gene in patients (Ahmad et al, 2007). Despite these encouraging advances, it will probably be 10 or more years before such approaches may begin to be used in humans.

◆ Summary

Substantial advancements have been made in understanding, diagnosing, and treating hearing loss. In particular, much has been learned from the discovery of a portion of the genes responsible for hearing loss. This understanding will increase as additional genes are identified and their functions elucidated. Although the cost of genetic testing is still quite high, technologies are improving. This brings costs down and allows better integration of genetic screening into the evaluation of a child with hearing loss. Such integration will lead to improved diagnoses and more tailored strategies for managing, and eventually curing, hearing loss.

Discussion Questions

1. If your patient is the only individual in his family with hearing loss, can it be genetic?

2. If a couple has a child with congenital SNHL from two mutations in the connexin 26 gene, what is their chance of having a second child with SNHL?

3. If a child tests negative for connexin 26 gene mutations, could his hearing loss still be genetic? What is the chance that the parents will have a second child with hearing loss?

4. You have been seeing Michael since he failed his newborn hearing screen and was found to have a bilateral, profound SNHL. He is now 10 years old and at his last appointment his mother mentioned he was having trouble seeing at night and has always been clumsy. Is there anything to be concerned about? Could these problems be related to his hearing loss? If so, what should you do?

5. A deaf couple shares with you that they are currently pregnant and state that they are interested in knowing the genetic status for deafness in the fetus because they feel they cannot continue a pregnancy that will result in the birth of a hearing child. How would you respond?

References

Acland, G. M., Aguirre, G. D., Bennett, J., et al. (2005). Long-term restoration of rod and cone vision by single dose rAAV-mediated gene transfer to the retina in a canine model of childhood blindness. Molecular Therapy, 12, 1072–1082.

Ahmad, S., Tang, W., Chang, Q., et al. (2007). Restoration of connexin26 protein level in the cochlea completely rescues hearing in a mouse model of human connexin30-linked deafness. Proceedings of the National Academy of Science U S A, 104, 1337–1341.

Angeli, S. (2003). Value of vestibular testing in young children with sensorineural hearing loss. Archives of Otolaryngology Head and Neck Surgery, 129, 478–482.

Berson, E. L., Rosner B., Sandberg, et al. (1993). A randomized trial of vitamin A and vitamin E supplementation for retinitis pigmentosa. Archives of Ophthalmology 111, 761–772.

Calvo, J. R. R., Gasparini, P., and Estivill, X. (2007). Connexins and Deafness Homepage, Deafness Research Group (CRG). http://davinici.crg.es/deafness

Chang, E. H., Menezes, M., Meyer, N. C., et al. (2004). Branchio-oto-renal syndrome: the mutation spectrum in EYA1 and its phenotypic consequences. Human Mutation, 23, 582–589.

Chee, N. W., Suhailee, S., and Goh, J. (2006). Clinics in diagnostic imaging (111): X-linked congenital mixed deafness syndrome. Singapore Medical Journal, 47, 822–824; quiz 825.

Daley, S. M., Tranebjærg, L., Samson, R. A., and Green, G. E. (2004). Jervell and Lange-Nielsen Syndrome. In GeneReviews at GeneTests: Medical Genetics Information Resource (database online), University of Washington, Seattle. Available at http://www.genetests.org. Accessed April 2007.

del Castillo, F. J., Rodriguez-Ballesteros, M., Martin, Y., et al. (2003a). Heteroplasmy for the 1555A>G mutation in the mitochondrial 12S rRNA gene in six Spanish families with non-syndromic hearing loss. Journal of Medical Genetics, 40, 632–636.

del Castillo, I., Moreno-Pelayo, M.A., del Castillo, et al. (2003b). Prevalence and evolutionary origins of the del(GJB6-D13S1830) mutation in the DFNB1 locus in hearing-impaired subjects: a multicenter study. American Journal of Human Genetics, 73, 1452–1458.

Delmaghani, S., del Castillo, F. J., Michel, V., et al. (2006). Mutations in the gene encoding pejvakin, a newly identified protein of the afferent auditory pathway, cause DFNB59 auditory neuropathy. Nature Genetics, 38, 770–778.

Evans, D. G. (2006). Neurofibromatosis 2. In GeneReviews at GeneTests: Medical Genetics Information Resource (database online), University of Washington, Seattle. Available at http://www.genetests.org. Accessed April 2007.

Fraser, F. C., Sproule, J. R., and Halal, F. (1980). Frequency of the branchio-oto-renal (BOR) syndrome in children with profound hearing loss. American Journal of Medical Genetics, 7, 341–349.

Fraser, G. (1976). The causes of profound deafness in childhood. Baltimore: Johns Hopkins University Press.

GeneTests. (2007). GeneTests: Medical Genetics Information Resource (database online). University of Washington, Seattle. Available at http://www.genetests.org. Accessed April 2007.

Goldfeld, M., Glaser, B., Nassir, E., Gomori, J. M., Hazani, E., and Bishara, N. (2005). CT of the ear in Pendred syndrome. Radiology, 235, 537–540.

Green, G. E., Scott, D. A., McDonald, J. M., Woodworth, G. G., Sheffield, V. C., and Smith, R. J. (1999). Carrier rates in the midwestern United States for GJB2 mutations causing inherited deafness. JAMA, 281, 2211–2216.

Green, G. E., Smith, R. J., Bent, J. P., and Cohn, E. S. (2000). Genetic testing to identify deaf newborns. JAMA, 284, 1245.

Hashimoto, T., Gibbs, D., Lillo, C., et al. (2007). Lentiviral gene replacement therapy of retinas in a mouse model for Usher syndrome type 1B. Gene Therapy 14, 584–594.

Issekutz, K. A., Graham, J. M. Jr., Prasad, C., Smith, I. M., and Blake, K. D. (2005). An epidemiological analysis of CHARGE syndrome: preliminary results from a Canadian study. American Journal of Medical Genetics A., 133, 309–317.

Kashtan, C. E. (2007). Collagen IV-Related Nephropathies (Alport syndrome and thin basement membrane nephropathy). In GeneReviews at GeneTests: Medical Genetics Information Resource (database online), University of Washington, Seattle. Available at http://www.genetests.org. Accessed April 2007.

Keats, B. J., and Lentz, J. (2006a). Usher Syndrome Type I. In GeneReviews at GeneTests: Medical Genetics Information Resource (database online), University of Washington, Seattle.

Keats, B. J., and Lentz, J. (2006b). Usher Syndrome Type II. In GeneReviews at GeneTests: Medical Genetics Information Resource (database online), University of Washington, Seattle. Available at http://www.genetests.org. Accessed April 2007.

Kemperman, M. H., Koch, S. M., Kumar, S., Huygen, P. L., Joosten, F. B., and Cremers, C. W. (2004). Evidence of progression and fluctuation of hearing impairment in branchio-oto-renal syndrome. International Journal of Audiology, 43, 523–532.

Kimberling, W. J., and Moller, C. (1995). Clinical and molecular genetics of Usher syndrome. Journal of the American Academy of Audiology, 6, 63–72.

Kupka, S., Braun, S., Aberle, S., et al. (2002). Frequencies of GJB2 mutations in German control individuals and patients showing sporadic non-syndromic hearing impairment. Human Mutation, 20, 77–78.

Lalani, S. R., Hefner, M., Belmont, J. W., and Davenport, S. L. (2006a). CHARGE Syndrome. In GeneReviews at GeneTests: Medical Genetics Information Resource (database online), University of Washington, Seattle. Available at http://www.genetests.org. Accessed April 2007.

Lalani, S.R., Safiullah, A. M., Fernbach, S. D., et al. (2006b). Spectrum of CHD7 mutations in 110 individuals with CHARGE syndrome and genotype-phenotype correlation. American Journal of Human Genetics, 78, 303–314.

Levy, M., and Feingold, J. (2000). Estimating prevalence in single-gene kidney diseases progressing to renal failure. Kidney International, 58, 925–943.

Li, R., Greinwald, J. H, Jr., Yang, L., Choo, D. I., Wenstrup, R. J., and Guan, M. X. (2004). Molecular analysis of the mitochondrial 12S rRNA and tR-NASer(UCN) genes in paediatric subjects with non-syndromic hearing loss. Journal of Medical Genetics, 41, 615–620.

Migliosi, V., Modamio-Hoybjor, S., Moreno-Pelayo, et al. (2002). Q829X, a novel mutation in the gene encoding otoferlin (OTOF), is frequently found in Spanish patients with prelingual non-syndromic hearing loss. Journal of Medical Genetics, 39, 502–506.

Milunsky, J. M. (2006). Waardenburg Syndrome Type I. In GeneReviews at GeneTests: Medical Genetics Information Resource (database online), University of Washington, Seattle. Available at http://www.genetests.org. Accessed April 2007.

Morton, N. E. (1991). Genetic epidemiology of hearing impairment. Annals of New York Academy of Science, 630, 16–31.

NCHAM (2006). National Center for Hearing Assessment and Management.

Norris, V. W., Arnos, K., Hanks, W., Xia, X., Nance, W., and Pandya, A. (2006). Does universal newborn hearing screening identify all children with GJB2 (Connexin 26) deafness? Penetrance of GJB2 deafness. Ear and Hearing, 27, 732–741.

OMIM (2004). Online Mendelian Inheritance in Man. McKusick-Nathans Institute for Genetic Medicine, Johns Hopkins University (Baltimore, MD) and National Center for Biotechnology Information, National Library of Medicine (Bethesda, MD).

Pandya, A. (2004). Nonsyndromic Hearing Loss, Mitochondrial. In GeneReviews at GeneTests: Medical Genetics Information Resource (database online), University of Washington, Seattle. Available at http://www.genetests.org. Accessed April 2007.

Panel (Genetic Evaluation of Congenital Hearing Loss Expert Panel) (2002). Genetics evaluation guidelines for the etiologic diagnosis of congenital hearing loss. Genetics in Medicine, 4, 162–171.

Putcha, G. V., Bejjani, B. A., Bleoo, S., et al. (2007). A multicenter study of the frequency and distribution of GJB2 and GJB6 mutations in a large North American cohort. Genetics in Medicine, 7, 413–426.

Rodriguez-Ballesteros, M., del Castillo, F. J., Martin, Y., et al. (2003). Auditory neuropathy in patients carrying mutations in the otoferlin gene (OTOF). Human Mutation 22, 451–456.

Ruf, R. G., Xu, P. X., Silvius, D., Otto, E. A., Beekmann, F., Muerb, U. T., et al. (2004). SIX1 mutations cause branchio-oto-renal syndrome by disruption of EYA1-SIX1-DNA complexes. Proceedings of the National Academy of Science U S A, 101, 8090–8095.

Schrijver, I., and Gardner, P. (2006). Hereditary sensorineural hearing loss: advances in molecular genetics and mutation analysis. Expert Review Molecular Diagnosis, 6, 375–386.

Schwartz, P. J., Periti, M., and Malliani, A. (1975). The long Q-T syndrome. American Heart Journal, 89, 378–390.

Smith, R. (2006a). Congenital Deafness-GJB2 and Usher Syndrome Type1. First International Symposium on Usher Syndrome and Related Disorders October 3-6, 2006. Omaha, Nebraska.

Smith, R. J. (2006b). Branchiootorenal Syndrome. In GeneReviews at GeneTests: Medical Genetics Information Resource (database online), University of Washington, Seattle.

Smith, R. J., and Robin, N. H. (2002). Genetic testing for deafness—GJB2 and SLC26A4 as causes of deafness. Journal of Communication Disorders, 35, 367–377.

Smith, R. J., and Van Camp, G. (2005). Nonsyndromic Hearing Loss and Deafness, DFNB1. In GeneReviews at GeneTests: Medical Genetics Information Resource (database online), University of Washington, Seattle. Available at http://www.genetests.org. Accessed April 2007.

Smith, R. J., and Van Camp, G. (2006c). Pendred Syndrome/DFNB4. In GeneReviews at GeneTests: Medical Genetics Information Resource (database online), University of Washington, Seattle. Available at http://www.genetests.org. Accessed April 2007.

Snoeckx, R. L., Huygen, P. L., Feldmann, D., et al. (2005). GJB2 mutations and degree of hearing loss: a multicenter study. American Journal of Human Genetics, 77, 945–957.

Toriello, H. V., Reardon, W., and Gorlin, R. J. (2004). Hereditary hearing loss and its syndromes. Oxford: Oxford University Press.

Usami, S., Abe, S., Akita, J., et al. (2000). Prevalence of mitochondrial gene mutations among hearing impaired patients. Journal of Medical Genetics, 37, 38–40.

Usami, S., Abe, S., Weston, M. D., Shinkawa, H., Van Camp, G., and Kimberling, W. J. (1999). Non-syndromic hearing loss associated with enlarged vestibular aqueduct is caused by PDS mutations. Human Genetics 104, 188–992.

Van Camp, G., and Smith, R. J. H. (2004). Hereditary Hearing Loss Homepage.

Varga, R., Avenarius, M. R., Kelley, P. M., et al. (2006). OTOF mutations revealed by genetic analysis of hearing loss families including a potential temperature sensitive auditory neuropathy allele. Journal of Medical Genetics, 43, 576–581.

Varga, R., Kelley, P. M., Keats, B. J., et al. (2003). Non-syndromic recessive auditory neuropathy is the result of mutations in the otoferlin (OTOF) gene. Journal of Medical Genetics, 40, 45–50.

Yasunaga, S., Grati, M., Cohen-Salmon, M., et al. (1999). A mutation in OTOF, encoding otoferlin, a FER-1-like protein, causes DFNB9, a nonsyndromic form of deafness. Nature Genetics, 21, 363–369.

Chapter 3

Medical Evaluation and Management of Hearing Loss in Children

George Alexiades and Ronald A. Hoffman

♦ **Medical Evaluation of Child Newly Identified with Sensorineural Hearing Loss**

History

Physical Examination

Laboratory Testing

♦ **Disease Entities Causing Sensorineural Hearing Loss**

Vestibulocochlear Abnormalities

Perilymphatic Fistula

Large Vestibular Aqueduct Syndrome

Ototoxic Medications

Infections

Neoplasms

♦ **Disease Entities Causing Conductive Hearing Loss**

Otitis Media with Effusion

Complications of Chronic Otitis Media

Aural Atresia

Key Points

- Proper diagnosis of hearing loss in children is predicated on a thorough history, good physical examination, and proper imaging studies.

- Most congenital hearing loss is hereditary.

- Constant vigilance by parents, pediatricians, and teachers is necessary because much hearing loss develops later in childhood.

Sensorineural hearing loss (SNHL) is the most common birth disorder in the United States (2004 National Consensus Conference on Effective Educational and Health Care Interventions for Infants and Young Children with Hearing Loss). Severe to profound SNHL occurs in 1 to 2 children per 1000 live births and another 2 to 3 per 1000 babies are born with partial hearing loss. The cumulative incidence of otitis media with effusion, associated with conductive hearing loss (CHL), is 80% by the age of 4 years (Louis et al. 2005). The proper identification and medical management of these children with hearing loss are a priority if speech and language deficits are to be minimized and progressive otologic disease avoided.

The most important aspect of managing a child with hearing loss is early identification. Universal newborn hearing screening, implemented in most states, allows for the early identification of most children with hearing loss. However, constant vigilance by parents, pediatricians, and teachers is necessary because much hearing loss develops later in childhood.

Congenital sensorineural hearing loss (CSHL) is defined as hearing loss that is present at birth. CHL is not synonymous with hereditary hearing loss, though they are mistakenly used interchangeably. Much hereditary hearing loss manifests itself later in childhood, and much CSHL is due to nongenetic causes. Approximately 60% of CSHL is believed to be hereditary (Morton, 1991). If a child passes newborn hearing screening, but there is a family history of hearing loss, that child must be tested serially over time.

Neonatal hearing loss may be syndromic or nonsyndromic. Syndromic hearing losses occur in association with other clinical features, though they are not exclusively hereditary (e.g., fetal alcohol syndrome). Approximately 70% of hereditary hearing loss is nonsyndromic (Lalwani, 1999), where hearing loss is the only clinical manifestation. Of these, the inheritance pattern is autosomal recessive in 75% of the cases, autosomal dominant in 10 to 20%, X-linked in 2 to 3%, and mitochondrial in 1% (Doyle, 2003). The most common cause of hereditary hearing loss is connexin 26 mutation, which accounts for up to 80% of autosomal recessive nonsyndromic hearing loss (Denoyelle, 1997). Hearing loss with connexin 26 mutation can be of any degree, and these children are usually otherwise healthy and normal.

> **Pearl**
>
> - Most hereditary hearing loss is nonsyndromic and autosomal recessive, and connexin 26 mutation is the most common disorder.

◆ Medical Evaluation of Child Newly Identified with Sensorineural Hearing Loss

History

When a neonate with a newly identified SNHL is seen, the physician begins with a detailed history. That history includes:

- *Birth history* Were there any perinatal factors such as prematurity, fetal distress, pregnancy-related illnesses, drug treatments during pregnancy, low birth weight, the need for neonatal intensive care unit (NICU), intravenous ototoxic antibiotics, or kernicterus (a high bilirubin) that might predispose the baby to hearing loss?

- *Family history* Is there a family history of hearing loss that would suggest a genetic cause?

- *Medical history* Is there any known history of cytomegalovirus, herpes, or syphilis? Has the child had perinatal meningitis?

> **Pearl**
>
> - The history is the most important piece in identifying the etiology of hearing loss.

Physical Examination

A physical examination is performed to be sure there are no physical stigmata associated with syndromic hearing loss. For example, widespread eyes, heterochromia iridis (multicolored eyes), and a white forelock of hair are typical of Waardenburg's syndrome. A hypoplastic malar eminence is a facial deformity

that may suggest Treacher-Collins syndrome. The outer and middle ears are carefully examined with an otoscope or operating microscope to ensure there is no atresia of the external ear or middle ear pathology, such as an effusion (fluid). A middle ear effusion is a major cause of false-positive neonatal hearing screening: the child fails the screen, but in fact there is no SNHL.

Laboratory Testing

The use of laboratory testing to diagnose SNHL at birth is controversial because the yield of useful information is low. Genetic testing may provide a diagnosis for hearing loss and may help to predict the likelihood of parents having another child with hearing loss, but does not influence how the child is managed clinically.

Children who are identified as having a severe to profound SNHL should all undergo ophthalmologic examination to rule out Usher's syndrome, which is characterized by SNHL and progressive vision loss. Today, earlier identification of these children is possible with an electroretinogram, which can identify these patients before there are any visible retinal changes (Young, Mets, and Hain, 1996).

An electrocardiogram is necessary to diagnose Jervell Lange-Neilson syndrome, which can lead to a potentially fatal cardiac arrhythmia if left untreated. Serologic studies (blood tests) have proven disappointing and, other than for genetic testing, are not recommended.

Imaging studies of the inner ear (CT scan, MRI scan) may provide useful information, particularly regarding the anatomy of the inner ear. However, these are of no pragmatic value during the first 2 years of life when the only issue is amplification. As the child matures, the identification of large vestibular aqueduct syndrome (LVAS) may influence behavioral modification, since minor head trauma is associated with further loss. When cochlear implantation becomes an alternative, preoperative imaging is essential (see Chapter 19).

If a child has had stable SNHL that then progresses over time, receives no benefit from amplification, or if there is a fluctuating SNHL, the evaluation algorithm changes and becomes more proactive. Such children should be imaged to identify a cochlear abnormality that may be associated with a perilymphatic fistula, which is a microscopic leak of fluid from the inner ear. Middle ear exploration and repair of the fistula may be warranted in such cases. Blood tests should also be performed to rule out autoimmune disorders, syphilis, or Lymes disease. If hearing loss is unilateral, a cerebellopontine angle tumor must be ruled out.

In all cases where a child is identified with an SNHL, whether stable or progressive, that child should be followed with at least yearly audiograms and examinations. At the initial stages of identification of hearing loss, more frequent audiograms (including auditory brainstem response and otoacoustic elements) are required to document the stability of hearing loss.

> **Controversial Point**
>
> - Laboratory testing in the workup of SNHL in children is not productive.

◆ Disease Entities Causing Sensorineural Hearing Loss

Vestibulocochlear Abnormalities

Vestibulocochlear dysplasias cover a wide variety of abnormalities in the inner ear. These may range from isolated semicircular canal abnormalities with little to no impact on hearing, to a common cavity deformity, where there is one spherical cavity for both the auditory and vestibular systems and a resultant severe to profound SNHL. It is important to identify these abnormalities, as they may have a significant impact on cochlear implantation and postoperative performance. In addition, cochlear dysplasias are associated with a real incidence of perilymphatic fistula, usually through a hole in the footplate of the stapes.

Perilymphatic Fistula

A perilymphatic fistula (PLF) is an abnormal communication between the perilymphatic space and the middle ear cavity. A PLF may occur through the round window, oval window, or both. PLF usually occurs as a result of head trauma or barotrauma. Patients suffer a sudden, progressive, or fluctuating SNHL with or without vestibular symptoms. The key to the diagnosis in an older child or adult is the history. For example, the patient who experiences severe pain on airplane descent with sudden hearing loss and vertigo has a PLF until proven otherwise.

Children, on the other hand, are not likely to be able to provide a history of head trauma, which they experience regularly. Moreover, in the presence of a cochlear malformation, children may suffer from spontaneous PLF, unassociated with head or barotrauma. The key to the diagnosis in a child is the detection of a cochlear malformation. The diagnosis of a spontaneous PLF in a child without a cochlear malformation is highly controversial. The treatment algorithm for a child with a progressive or fluctuating SNHL with a suspected PLF is outlined in **Fig. 3–1**.

Large Vestibular Aqueduct Syndrome

Large vestibular aqueduct syndrome (LVAS) is a specific type of inner ear abnormality. In this syndrome, the vestibular aqueduct, the bony channel that houses the endolymphatic duct, is abnormally enlarged. It is the most common inner ear abnormality found on computed tomography (CT) scans; its incidence is 4 to 10% in children with SNHL (Madden et al, 2003). Genetic testing should be performed to diagnose

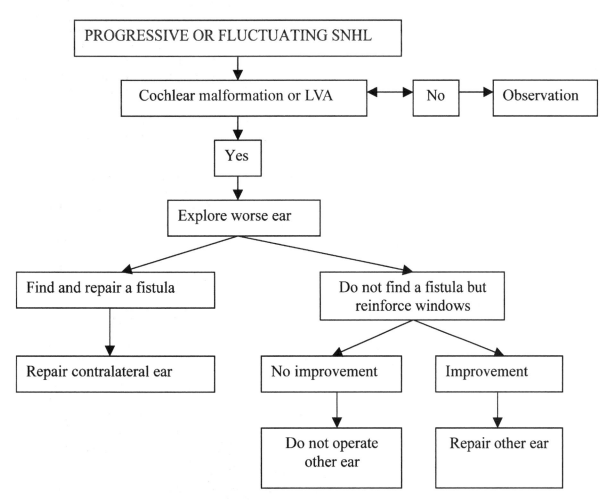

Figure 3–1 Algorithm for medical management of a child with a progressive or fluctuating sensorineural hearing loss. SNHL, sensorineural hearing loss; LVA, large vestibular aqueduct.

Pendred syndrome, which is categorized by abnormal iodine incorporation and resultant enlargement of the thyroid gland, and is associated with LVAS in up to 50% of cases (Berrettini et al, 2005). Conversely, almost all patients with Pendred syndrome have an inner ear abnormality, usually LVAS. LVAS is associated with a progressive, fluctuating, or sudden SNHL. Stepwise SNHL is often precipitated by minor head trauma. Therefore, it is recommended that these children abstain from participating in contact sports, as this may result in an acute drop in hearing.

Ototoxic Medications

Many medications have been identified as ototoxic in nature, yet are still used because they effectively treat specific medical conditions. The most common class of ototoxic medications used is the aminoglycoside antibiotics, most commonly gentamicin. These drugs are used quite frequently in neonates with suspected sepsis or meningitis. Moreover, they are used commonly in developing nations because they are potent and inexpensive. Although newer, nonototoxic antibiotics have been developed that cover similar organisms, aminoglycosides are often necessary to treat resistant organisms or serious infections.

Many chemotherapeutic agents are also ototoxic. The most common is cisplatin, used for a variety of pediatric malignancies. Ototoxic hearing loss begins with a high frequency deficit. It is important to obtain a baseline audiogram before treatment, and to follow up with audiograms throughout the treatment. Evolving hearing loss may necessitate a change to another, less ototoxic agent.

Infections

Meningitis is an inflammation of the lining of the brain, which is often caused by bacteria. Today, *Streptococcus pneumoniae* and *Neisseria meningitides* are the most common organisms causing meningitis. With the advent of the *Haemophilus influenza* vaccine, meningitis from this bacterium has been virtually eliminated. The cochlear aqueduct is a connection between the basal turn of the cochlea and the cerebrospinal fluid space surrounding the brain. On occasion, particularly in young children, the cochlear aqueduct is large and open. The bacteria that cause meningitis can gain access to the inner ear from the infected cerebrospinal fluid via the cochlear aqueduct, resulting in severe to profound hearing loss. Moreover, these bacteria are highly irritative and can cause new bone to form in the cochlea, so-called labyrinthitis ossificans (Hartnick et al, 2001). This dynamic process begins immediately after the infection, and can result in significant blockage of the cochlea in as little as 6 weeks (Tinling, 2004). It is imperative that these patients be "fast tracked" through the cochlear implant evaluation process and, if indicated, an implant be inserted as quickly as possible. Should too much time pass, significant ossification of the cochlea can result in an incomplete electrode insertion or, in some cases, preclude implantation altogether.

Neoplasms

Neoplasms in the cerebellopontine angle or internal auditory canal are rare in children and comprise only 1% of all intracranial lesions. The most common neoplasms in this area are neurofibromatosis type 2, arachnoid cysts, epidermoid cysts, and meningiomas (Ruggieri et al, 2005). Rarely, an isolated acoustic neuroma will be encountered in a child. Children with such intracranial neoplasms usually present with unilateral SNHL or imbalance, and in the case of neurofibromatosis type 2, frequently have ocular or motor dysfunction caused by the multicentricity of the disease. Rarely, malignant neoplasms of the cerebellopontine angle cause unilateral SNHL such as medulloblastomas and glioblastomas. When a child presents with a new or progressive unilateral SNHL, magnetic resonance imaging with gadolinium contrast enhancement is indicated for diagnosis.

◆ Disease Entities Causing Conductive Hearing Loss

Otitis Media with Effusion

Acute suppurative otitis media is the most common infection worldwide and the most common indication for antibiotics in children. Otitis media with effusion (OME) is fluid in the middle ear space, without the signs and symptoms of infection (pain, fever, and redness of the tympanic membrane). OME can cause hearing loss of up to 30 dB. There is a general consensus that OME is overtreated. Decongestants may be indicated if a child suffers with allergies or a sinus condition. Antibiotics are not generally useful. Although oral steroids may resolve OME, the recurrence rate is high and their use in children controversial. Current guidelines recommend waiting a minimum of 3 months for OME to clear spontaneously before considering insertion myringotomy tubes.

Multiple studies have been done on the long-term effect on language development of placing ventilation tubes in children with less than 3 months of OME, as opposed to later insertion. The data clearly show that early insertion of ventilation tubes does not favorably affect speech and language skills long term (Paradise et al, 2005; Louis et al, 2005). However, no studies have been undertaken in children with underlying SNHL, learning disabilities, or speech and language delay. It is the authors' opinion that in these children more aggressive medical management is appropriate.

Complications of Chronic Otitis Media

Chronic otitis media with effusion and/or recurrent suppurative otitis media improperly treated over time can lead to serious pathologic sequelae, including tympanic membrane perforations, adhesive otitis media, cholesteatoma, ossicular destruction, and, in each case, significant CHL. Tympanic membrane perforations most often occur in children secondary to prolonged placement of ventilating tubes. Occasionally, perforations result from repeated ruptures of the tympanic membrane caused by acute suppurative otitis media. Surgical repair of tympanic membrane perforation should be delayed, if possible, until normal eustachian tube (ET) function has been established. There is no test for adequacy of ET function. If there is a perforation in one ear the opposite ear can be used as a measure. If the opposite remains free of fluid or infection through a winter, it can be assumed the child has adequate ET function. If perforations are bilateral, one ear should be repaired and observed over a similar period of time. Occasionally, surgery will be mandated by chronic infection. Hearing loss alone is rarely an indication for surgery, because these ears can usually be fit with hearing aids.

Chronic suppurative otitis media is a chronic infection of the middle ear and mastoid bone and is rare in young children; it usually results in a chronic tympanic membrane perforation and intermittent ear drainage. Ossicular erosion can occur and may result in a maximum CHL. Chronic suppurative otitis media is usually treated surgically.

Cholesteatoma is a cyst formed from normal skin trapped in the middle ear space. Usually, there is no skin in the middle ear, only in the external auditory canal and on the lateral surface of the tympanic membrane. There are three types of cholesteatoma: congenital, primary acquired, and secondary acquired. Congenital cholesteatoma occurs when a nest of skin becomes trapped in the middle ear space, behind an intact tympanic membrane, during fetal development. The congenital cholesteatoma is usually asymptomatic and is discovered coincidentally on routine physical examination. It presents as a white "pearl" anterior to the short process of the malleus. To make this diagnosis, there has to have been no history of tympanic membrane perforation or placement of a myringotomy tube.

Primary acquired cholesteatoma is the most common type of cholesteatoma and results when skin shed from the lateral surface of the tympanic membrane collects in a retraction pocket. Retraction pockets usually arise from the weakest part of the tympanic membrane, called the pars flaccida, located above the short process of the malleus. Secondary acquired cholesteatoma occurs when the skin from the lateral surface of the tympanic membrane migrates through a tympanic membrane perforation and grows within the middle ear space. Regardless of the type, cholesteatoma gradually enlarge and can be destructive of surrounding structures. CHL caused by ossicular destruction is common. In advanced cases, cholesteatoma can press on the facial nerve, injuring it and causing a facial paralysis. Cholesteatoma becomes particularly aggressive when it gets infected and can lead to meningitis or a brain abscess. The treatment of cholesteatoma is surgical. The abnormal skin must be completely removed from the middle ear and mastoid. The tympanic membrane can be repaired and damaged ossicles replaced. There is usually some residual CHL.

Pitfall

- Congenital cholesteatoma can be easily missed on a physical medical exam.

Adhesive otitis media occurs when the tympanic membrane collapses completely and becomes fixed to the ossicles and other middle ear structures. If left untreated, it leads to retraction cholesteatoma. The ossicles can be destroyed by cholesteatoma, as mentioned above, or can be fixed by an abnormal scarring and calcification called tympanosclerosis. The resultant CHL can range from mild to moderate. Fixation of the stapes in children can occur because of tympanosclerosis, otosclerosis, or congenital fixation (Welling et al, 2003). Hearing loss from any of the aforementioned etiologies can be corrected with either surgery or a hearing aid. Appropriate management of hearing loss is dependent upon the age of the child, the status of the ET, and the etiology of hearing loss.

Aural Atresia

Aural atresia is a malformation of the external auditory canal and the middle ear. The clinical presentation is very variable and the extent of abnormality is defined with computed tomography. In the mildest form, the external auditory canal will be very narrow and threadlike. In more advanced cases there may be no external auditory canal and the ossicles may be severely deformed or completely absent. There may be no oval window at all and the facial nerve might take an extremely anomalous course. Aural atresia can be unilateral or bilateral, and can be an isolated finding or in association with a syndrome. Aural atresia results in a maximal CHL in the affected ear. Occasionally, a SNHL may coexist. Aural atresia is often found in conjunction with microtia, a malformation of the external ear that can range from a small pinna to total absence of the pinna.

There is controversy in the management of aural atresia, as there are considerable complications with its surgical repair. The course of the facial nerve is very variable in these children and is at risk during the atresia repair, especially in inexperienced hands (Jahrsdoerfer and Lambert, 1998). Restenosis of the external auditory canal after surgery has been reported in up to 32% of cases (Shih, and Crabtree, 1993). Closure of air-bone gaps to within 30 dB occurs in only 60 to 70% of cases, regardless of the type of ossicular reconstruction (Teufert and De la Cruz, 2004). Many advocate the use of a bone anchored hearing aid (BAHA), as hearing improvement is more consistent and there are fewer complications.

Controversial Point

- The surgical repair of aural atresia, especially in unilateral cases, is controversial.

Discussion Questions

1. What are the most common causes of congenital and acquired hearing loss?

2. What are the most common causes of CHL in children?

3. How should CHL be managed?

References

Berrettini, S., Forli, F., Bogazzi F. et al. (2005). Large vestibular aqueduct syndrome: audiological, radiological, clinical, and genetic features. American Journal of Otolaryngology, 26, 363–371.

Hartnick, C. J., Kim, H. H., Chute, P. M., and Parisier, S. C. (2001). Preventing labyrinthitis ossificans: the role of steroids. Otolaryngology-Head and Neck Surgery, 127, 180–183.

Jahrsdoerfer, R. A., and Lambert, P. R. (1998). Facial nerve injury in congenital aural atresia surgery. American Journal of Otolaryngology, 19, 283–287.

Louis, J., Burton, M. J., Felding, J. U., Ovesen, T., Rovers, M. M., and Williamson, I. (2005). Grommets (ventilation tubes) for hearing loss associated with otitis media with effusion in children. Cochrane Database System Review, 25, CD001801.

Madden, C., Halsted, M., Benton, C., Greinwald, J., and Choo, D. (2003). Enlarged vestibular aqueduct syndrome in the pediatric population. Otology and Neurotology, 24, 625–632.

Paradise, J. L., Campbell, T. F., Dollaghan, et al. (2005). Developmental outcomes after early or delayed insertion of tympanostomy tubes. New England Journal of Medicine, 11, 576–586.

Ruggieri, M., Iannetti, P., Polizzi, A., La Mantia, I., Spalice, A., Giliberto, O., et al. (2005). Earliest clinical manifestations and natural history of neurofibromatosis type 2 (NF2) in childhood: a study of 24 patients. Neuropediatrics, 36, 21–34.

Shih, L., and Crabtree, J. A. (1993). Long-term surgical results for congenital aural atresia. Laryngoscope, 103, 1097–1102. Review.

Teufert, K. B., and De la Cruz, A. (2004). Advances in congenital aural atresia surgery: effects on outcome. Otolaryngology Head and Neck Surgery, 131, 263–270.

Tinling, S. P., Colton, J., and Brodie, H. A. (2004). Location and timing of initial osteoid deposition in postmeningitic labyrinthitis ossificans determined by multiple fluorescent labels. Laryngoscope, 114, 675–680.

Welling, D. B., Merrell, J. A., Merz, M., and Dodson, E. E. (2003). Predictive factors in pediatric stapedectomy. Laryngoscope, 113, 1515–1519.

Young, N. M., Mets, M. B., and Hain, T. C. (1996). Early diagnosis of Usher syndrome in infants and children. American Journal of Otology, 17, 30–34.

Chapter 4

Newborn Hearing Screening

Karl R. White

♦ **Factors Contributing to the Expansion of Newborn Hearing Screening Programs**

Policy Initiatives

Federal Funding for Early Hearing Detection and Intervention Initiatives

Successful Implementation of Screening Programs

Technological Advances

Endorsements by Professional and Advocacy Groups

Legislation Related to Newborn Hearing Screening

♦ **Establishing and Operating Successful Newborn Hearing Screening Programs**

Creating Stakeholder Support

Selecting Equipment and Protocols for the Hospital

Dealing with Procedural Issues

Communicating with Stakeholders

Training Newborn Hearing Screeners

Operating an Efficient Program

Managing Data and Patient Information

Program Coordination

Key Points

- The percentage of newborns screened for hearing loss before hospital discharge has increased from fewer than 5% in 1993 to more than 95% in 2006.

- Forty-one states have passed legislation requiring newborn hearing screening, and many governmental and professional organizations endorse hearing screening for all newborns.

- Newborn hearing screening is only the first step (and probably the easiest) in the process of identifying and providing appropriate services to infants and young children with hearing loss (other important steps include diagnostic evaluation, early intervention, family support, tracking and data management, and coordination with the child's primary health care provider).

- Equipment, protocols, and procedures used in successful newborn hearing screening programs vary widely depending on the circumstances of the hospital and preferences of those running the program—there is no one best approach.

- The most successful programs are excellent at involving and communicating with a range of stakeholders (e.g., hospital staff and administrators, primary health care providers, parents, and hearing health professionals).

During the past 15 years (**see Fig. 4–1**) the percentage of newborns being screened for hearing loss has increased from 3 to 95% (NCHAM 2007a). What has contributed to such a dramatic increase and what can we learn from these initiatives that will enable us to continue to refine and improve our programs for identifying and serving infants and young children with permanent hearing loss?

♦ Factors Contributing to the Expansion of Newborn Hearing Screening Programs

First, it is important to understand that a variety of factors interacted in a synergistic manner to achieve the growth shown in **Fig. 4–1**: (1) policy initiatives by government, professional associations, and advocacy groups; (2) financial assistance from the federal government; (3) improvements in technology; (4) legislative initiatives; and (5) the demonstrated success of early implementations.

Policy Initiatives

The federal government has been advocating for earlier identification of permanent hearing loss for many years. For example, the Babbidge Report (1965) issued by the U.S.

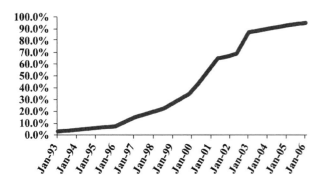

Figure 4–1   Percentage of newborns screened in United States for hearing loss from 1993 through 2006.

Department of Health, Education and Welfare recommended the development and nationwide implementation of "universally applied procedures for early identification and evaluation of hearing impairment" (p. C-10). A short time later, based on the pioneering work of Marion Downs (Downs and Sterritt, 1964, 1967), the Joint Committee on Infant Hearing (JCIH) was established in 1969 by a group of professional associations (e.g., American Speech Language and Hearing Association, American Academy of Pediatrics, among others). Even though the JCIH had little or no budget and no formal authority, the committee has become a powerful force in advocating for earlier identification and better treatment of congenital hearing loss (Olusanya et al, 2006; JCIH, 2007).

As new hearing screening technologies became available in the late 1980s, the federal government began devoting more resources to reducing the age at which hearing loss was identified. These efforts were supported in part by a recommendation from the congressionally mandated Commission on Education of the Deaf that "the Department of Education, in collaboration with the Department of Health and Human Services, should . . . assist states in implementing improved screening procedures for each live birth···" (Toward Equality, 1988).

A few years later, Healthy People 2000 (US Department of HHS, 1990) included an objective to "reduce the average age at which children with significant hearing impairment are identified to no more than 12 months." This report went on to state:

> It is difficult, if not impossible, for many [children with congenital hearing loss] to acquire the fundamental language, social, and cognitive skills that provide the foundation for later schooling and success in society. When early identification and intervention occur, hearing impaired children make dramatic progress, are more successful in school, and become more productive members of society. The earlier intervention and habilitation begin, the more dramatic the benefits. (p. 460)

Although the concept underlying the objective was similar to what people had been advocating for several decades, the inclusion of a goal related to early identification of hearing loss in Healthy People 2000 broke new ground because it required that progress toward each objective be tracked and reported at regular intervals.

In March 1993, the National Institutes of Health (NIH) convened a Consensus Development Panel to review the extant evidence on early identification of hearing loss and make recommendations to improve practice. The panel concluded that, "All hearing impaired infants should be identified and treatment initiated by 6 months of age . . . [T]he consensus panel recommends screening of all newborns . . . for hearing impairment prior to discharge." (NIH, 1993).

Some people expected immediate implementation of universal newborn hearing screening programs as a result of the NIH recommendation. Such was not to be the case, however, as critics of the panel pointed out that the research evidence and experience for such broad-scale implementation were lacking. For example, Bess and Paradise (1994) concluded that "the Consensus Panel's recommendation of universal infant screening falls short of being justified on grounds of practicability, effectiveness, cost, and harm-benefit ratio." Two years later the prestigious United States Preventive Services Task Force (1996) noted that "congenital hearing loss is a serious health problem associated with developmental delay in speech and language function," but concluded that "there is little evidence to support the use of routine, universal screening for all neonates." Similarly, in a 1999 article in *Pediatrics*, Paradise concluded that,

> universal newborn hearing screening in our present state of knowledge is not necessarily the only, or the best, or the most cost-effective way to achieve [early identification of hearing loss], and more importantly, . . . the benefits of universal newborn hearing screening may be outweighed by its risks.

Federal Funding for Early Hearing Detection and Intervention Initiatives

The policy initiatives of the late 1980s and early 1990s led to significantly more federal funding for research, demonstration, and technical assistance projects focused on reducing the age at which congenital hearing loss was identified. One of the best known was the Rhode Island Hearing Assessment Project (White and Behrens, 1993), but there were many others (e.g., Barsky-Firkser and Sun, 1997; Finitzo, Albright, and O'Neil, 1998; Mason and Herrmann, 1998; Mehl and Thomson, 1998; Vohr, et al, 1998).

Successful Implementation of Screening Programs

By the mid-1990s the percentage of newborns being screened for hearing loss had increased dramatically (from fewer than 3% in 1993 to 15% in 1996 to 22% in 1998; see **Fig. 4–1**). By 1998 dozens of large-scale universal newborn hearing screening programs had become operational in various states (White, 1997). These projects provided the data and the experience to sustain the momentum that had started during the early 1990s.

Technological Advances

The growth of newborn hearing screening programs was directly linked to the technological breakthroughs in hearing screening equipment that occurred during the late 1980s and early 1990s. Without the improvements in automated auditory brainstem response (AABR; Herrmann, et al, 1995) and otoacoustic emissions (OAE)) (Kemp, 1978; Lonsbury-Martin and Martin, 1990; Kemp and Ryan, 1993), all of the policy initiatives, federally funded projects, and clinical screening programs that combined to demonstrate the practicality of newborn hearing screening programs would never have happened.

Endorsements by Professional and Advocacy Groups

The demonstrated feasibility of hospital-based screening, coupled with the results of research, led to more endorsements for universal newborn hearing screening by other government, professional, and advocacy organizations. For example, in 1999 the American Academy of Pediatrics "[endorsed] the goal of universal detection of hearing loss in infants before 3 months of age . . . [which] requires universal screening of all infants." Other organizations, including the American Speech-Language-Hearing Association, the American Academy of Audiology, March of Dimes, and the American College of Medical Genetics, soon followed suit (NCHAM 2007b). Also in 1998, the federal Maternal and Child Health Bureau (MCHB, 2002) began requiring states to report "percent of newborns screened for hearing impairment before hospital discharge" as one

of a handful of core performance measures that states reported annually to receive federal MCHB block grant funding. By the end of 2001, every state had established an early hearing detection and intervention (EHDI) program, which was responsible for setting up newborn hearing screening programs and linking babies referred from those programs to diagnostic, early intervention, family support, and other health care services.

Legislation Related to Newborn Hearing Screening

The factors described above created an atmosphere in which newborn hearing screening programs could be implemented, but legislative action in many states expanded the reach of these programs and increased the probability that they would be continued. The first legislation related to newborn hearing screening was passed in Hawaii in 1990. Spurred on by the demonstrated success of newborn hearing screening programs, 41 states now have statutes requiring newborn hearing screening. The increase in legislative activity was probably influenced by the publication of the Position Statement by the American Academy of Pediatrics in February 1999 and the publication in prestigious journals in 1998 of major articles about the feasibility and benefits of implementing large-scale universal newborn hearing screening programs (e.g., Finitzo, Albright, and O'Neil, 1998; Moeller, 2000; Mehl and Thomson, 1998; Yoshinaga-Itano, et al, 1998). Key provisions of each statute are summarized in **Table 4–1**; the exact wording is available at www.infanthearing.org/legislative/index.html.

Table 4–1 Newborn Hearing Screening Legislation in the United States

State	Year Passed	Requires Screening of:	Advisory Committee	Covered by Health Insurance	Report Results to State	Provide Educational Materials	Informed Consent by Parents
AK	2006	All babies		Yes	Yes	Yes	
AR	1999	Hospitals >50 births	Yes	Yes	Yes	Yes	
AZ	2007	All babies	Yes		Yes	Yes	
CA	2006	All babies		Medicaid		Yes	Yes
CO	1997	85% of newborns	Yes			Yes	
CT	1997	All babies		Yes		Yes	
DE	2005	All babies		Yes	Yes	Yes	
FL	2000	All babies		Yes		Yes	
GA	1999	95% of newborns	Yes			Yes	
HI	1990	All babies			Yes		
IA	2003	All babies			Yes		
IL	1999	All babies	Yes			Yes	
IN	1999	All babies	Yes	Yes	Yes	Yes	
KS	1999	All babies					Yes
KY	2000	Hospitals >40 births	Yes		Yes		
LA	1999	All babies	Yes				
ME	1999	>85%	Yes	Yes	Yes	Yes	
MD	1999	All babies	Yes	Yes	Yes	Yes	
MA	1997	All babies	Yes	Yes	Yes		
MN	2007	All babies	Yes		Yes		Yes
MS	1997	All babies	Yes		Yes	Yes	
MO	1999	All babies	Yes	Yes	Yes	Yes	
MT	2001	All babies	Yes		Yes		
NE	2000	>95%		Yes	Yes	Yes	

(Continued)

Table 4–1   *(Continued)*

NV	2000	Hospitals >500 births			Yes	Yes	
NJ	2000	All babies	Yes	Yes	Yes	Yes	Yes
NM	2001	All babies					
NY	1999	Hospitals >400 births			Yes		
NC	1999	All babies			Yes	Yes	
OH	2002	All babies	Yes	Yes	Yes	Yes	
OK	2000	All babies					
OR	1999	Hospitals >200 births	Yes		Yes	Yes	
PA	2001	85% of newborns	Yes		Yes	Yes	
RI	1992	All babies		Yes			
SC	2000	Hospitals >100 births	Yes	Yes	Yes	Yes	
TX	1999	Hospitals >100 births		Yes	Yes	Yes	Yes
UT	1998	All babies	Yes		Yes	Yes	
VA	1998	All babies	Yes	Yes	Yes	Yes	
WV	1998	All babies	Yes	Yes	Yes		
WI	1999	88% of newborns			Yes		
WY	1999	All babies				Yes	Yes

◆ Establishing and Operating Successful Newborn Hearing Screening Programs

As a result of work done by JCIH (JCIH, 2000), MCHB, and the Centers for Disease Control and Prevention (CDC, 2004), most people stopped using the phrase, "universal newborn hearing screening" and began referring to "early hearing detection and intervention" (EHDI) programs. The change in how these programs are described is important, because it underscores that to successfully identify and serve infants and young children with congenital hearing loss, successful screening programs must be coupled with timely audiologic diagnosis; appropriate medical, audiologic, and educational intervention; coordination with the child's primary health-care provider (often referred to as the child's medical home); and EHDI tracking and data management systems. (Other chapters in this book describe these important aspects of the EHDI system in more detail.)

During the 15 years after the recommendation by NIH that all newborns should be screened before being discharged from the hospital, the techniques, procedures, equipment, and support systems for newborn hearing screening have continued to evolve, and the goal of screening all newborns for hearing loss, which many thought was completely unrealistic in 1993, has been largely attained. The remainder of this chapter summarizes some of the

most important considerations and lessons learned about operating a successful newborn hearing screening program.

Creating Stakeholder Support

A successful newborn hearing screening program requires support from dozens of stakeholders, including hospital administrators, primary health care providers, nurses, and parents. All of these people should know that the endorsement of universal newborn hearing screening by so many authoritative groups accompanied by so many successful programs throughout the country and the ready availability of relatively inexpensive equipment and procedures, means that newborn hearing screening has become the de facto "standard of care." Hospitals run a significant liability risk if they do not screen all newborns for hearing loss (see White, 2003).

Primary Health-Care Providers

Most hospitals have a pediatric committee, a medical policy committee, or other such groups that make decisions about what constitutes standard of care in that hospital. Physicians in that group need to understand the benefits associated with newborn hearing screening and how it is done. Physicians, nurse practitioners, and physician assistants in the community who care for babies also need to understand why newborn hearing screening is important and how the process is supposed to work. Ideally, every newborn should have a health-care provider who knows that baby and its circumstances and is responsible for ensuring that it receives consistent and appropriate health care. Often referred to as the baby's "medical home," the baby's primary health-care provider is the key to an effective early hearing detection and intervention program (AAP 2002). Because the baby's primary care physician is responsible for the total health care of the baby, he or she needs to be assured that newborn hearing screening will not interfere with or complicate other health-care activities.

Nurses

If the nurses working in the newborn nursery are not convinced that newborn hearing screening should be happening, it will be almost impossible to have a successful program. If the nurses want newborn hearing screening, they can often convince the physicians and administrators to give it a try. In fact, some of the earliest successful hospital-based newborn hearing screening programs were started and largely operated by nursing staff.

Selecting Equipment and Protocols for the Hospital

One of the first decisions in setting up a newborn hearing screening program is deciding what equipment to use and what type of basic screening protocol to follow. The good news is that there are a lot of options, and almost all have been successfully implemented at one hospital or another. The bad news is that because there are so many options, some people unnecessarily delay the implementation of the screening program to sort through them all.

The best approach is to talk to people who have tried some of the most frequently used options; devote some brief, but intensive, study time to what type of equipment and protocol is best for your hospital; and then make your choice and move ahead. Waiting to identify the "perfect" solution for every aspect of the program will unnecessarily delay getting started. Adjustments to initial decisions can always be made later.

Which Equipment Is Best?

In the past 10 years, a variety of types of equipment have been developed that can be used successfully in universal newborn hearing screening programs. Transient evoked otoacoustic emissions, distortion product otoacoustic emissions, and automated (auditory brainstem response, ABR) equipment have all demonstrated their practicality and effectiveness in hospital-based newborn hearing screening programs. Each type of equipment has its proponents, and debates about which technique is best are sometimes quite energetic. It is clear, however, that the particular brand and type of equipment selected is not the most important issue in whether the program will be successful. Equipment continues to be modified and improved, and it is almost certain that better, faster, and easier-to-use equipment will become readily available. That is no reason, however, to delay implementing a program. Currently available equipment is more than adequate for operating a successful newborn hearing screening program. A brief summary of the issues to be considered in selecting equipment, as well as a listing of names and contact information for different manufacturers, are available at www.infanthearing.org.

How Many Tests Should Be Included in the Screening Protocol?

The purpose of any screening program is to select a subgroup from the general population, which is at higher risk of having a particular condition, so that a more in-depth diagnostic assessment can be done with members of that group. Therefore, some false positives (i.e., infants with normal hearing who do not pass the screening test) and occasional false negatives (infants who pass the screening test but do have a hearing loss) are expected. If only one screening test is done for each baby before hospital discharge, as many as 10 to 15% of the babies may not pass. Therefore, many hospitals require two or more screening tests if babies do not pass at first. Sometimes this is done with the same type of equipment; sometimes with different types of equipment. Furthermore, some hospitals do a two-stage screening with different types of equipment before the baby is discharged from the hospital; others do a single stage before the baby is discharged and then follow with an outpatient screen several days later. Deciding which protocol is best for a given situation is usually based on factors such as the following:

◆ How long babies typically stay in the hospital before discharge

◆ How difficult it is in this area to get parents to come back for re-screens

◆ The availability of different types of equipment

◆ Who is doing the screening

> **Pearl**
>
> • More important than the type of equipment used or the protocol being followed is having someone in charge of the program who is passionate about the importance of newborn hearing screening and completely committed to the success of the program.

The fact that successful programs currently use such a variety of protocols suggests that no one protocol is really best for all situations. Regardless of the protocol selected, it is best to have a written document to guide the activities of all people associated with the program. Examples of several such written protocols can be found at www.infanthearing.org.

Dealing with Procedural Issues

Regardless of the technology and protocol used, several procedural issues are important for an efficient, successful program. It is often useful, and in fact, many hospitals require a written summary describing how the program typically addresses issues such as the following.

Who Is in Charge?

If everyone is responsible for a task, it often remains unfinished. Thousands of hospitals have demonstrated that newborn hearing screening can easily be incorporated into the routine of a hospital. Just like any other procedure, however, it takes attention to detail and someone who is ultimately

Table 4–2 Who Does Newborn Hearing Screening as Reported by Early Hearing Detection and Intervention Program Coordinators?

Audiologists	67%
Physicians	5%
Nursing staff	95%
Trained volunteers	36%
Trained technicians	85%

Note: Percentages sum to more than 100% because many coordinators reported that more than one group of people screened in the same hospital.

responsible to make sure that all of the specifics are done. The person responsible for day-to-day operation of the program does not need specific professional certification, but he or she needs to have good connections with the nursery, understand how screening happens, and most of all be committed to the success of the program. Instead of looking for reasons why newborn hearing screening will not work, that person needs to be committed to its success. Depending on how the program is organized, most hospitals find that this person will require 2 to 6 hours per week per 1000 births to coordinate and manage the overall program.

Who Will Do the Screening?

Reports from hundreds of operational programs provide clear evidence that newborn hearing screening can be performed by a wide variety of people, including nurses, audiologists, technicians, health-care assistants, volunteers, and students **(see Table 4–2).** Some states have laws regarding who can screen for hearing and how they must be supervised; others do not. Regardless of who does the screening, they must be properly trained and supervised and data should be kept on each screener's performance to enable timely and appropriate training and assistance when needed.

When Should Screening Be Done?

All other things being equal, newborn hearing screening is faster and easier if babies are quiet and the environment is not too chaotic. Because of this, most screening is done in the early morning or during the night when fewer people (doctors, visiting relatives, nurses, parents, etc.) want access to the baby. However, depending on who is screening, their other responsibilities, and how the hospital's nursery is organized, screening can be done successfully at other times. Whatever decision is made, dozens of other hospitals are doing it at approximately the same time. The conclusion? There really is no wrong time to do newborn hearing screening.

How Do You Ensure Every Baby Is Screened?

There are many procedures to ensure that no babies are missed. Setting up a system to log the birth and screening of every baby, making sure screeners are available to screen

every baby before discharge, and incorporating the hearing screening into the discharge plan should all be considered. Because some hospitals discharge babies after very short stays, seven-day-a-week coverage is usually needed. Many screening program coordinators have found that it is more efficient to incorporate screening duties into the job responsibilities of existing personnel than it is to hire dedicated screening staff.

Should Screening Be Done with Parents Present?

If parents are present for the screening, they will have questions and want to discuss the process. This is wonderful from an educational perspective, but it requires more time and, consequently, increases the cost of the screening program. If you can afford it and want to provide the extra education, it's a great thing to do, but be mindful of the extra time required. Even if parents are not routinely present for screening, if they ask to watch, they should certainly be accommodated. It is important to make sure parents are involved and supported at every opportunity.

Should Parents Be Required to Give Written Permission for Screening?

There are really two different, but related, questions here. First, should there be procedures to ensure that parents understand what happens during newborn hearing screening so they can make an informed decision about whether they want their baby to be screened? Second, should parents be required to sign a written permission before their baby is screened? The answer to the first question is definitely yes; the answer to the second is probably no. With regard to the first question, every effort should be made to educate parents about newborn hearing screening before it happens (what it is, why it is important, how it is done, etc.). This can be done with information in the preadmission materials, prenatal classes, media materials, or placed in the baby's crib. If, based on this information, parents do not want to have their baby screened, they have the right to refuse (it is a good idea to require that they give you a written documentation of that refusal, which is kept on file).

With regard to the second question, it is important to remember that newborn hearing screening is not an experimental research procedure. If it were, written parental permission would be required for every baby screened. Although it requires extra time (in some cases, more than the total time required to do screening), a few hospitals still obtain written permission from parents before screening the baby. This does provide an opportunity to explain to parents exactly what the screening is and why it is important, but this could be done faster in other ways. Also, some states have laws or regulations regarding such issues.

Communicating with Stakeholders

Many people have a stake in the results of a newborn hearing screening program. It is essential for the success of the program to make sure these people receive timely information. In many cases, it is also important to document that communication has occurred and to have a system to quickly and accurately retrieve information that has been communicated.

Communicating with Parents

Parents are among the most important stakeholders, because they are the ones who have long-term responsibility for ensuring that the baby receives appropriate care. They are also the ones who have the strongest feelings (but usually limited experience) about what it means to have a child with a hearing loss. It is essential that each parent be told the results of their baby's hearing screening test and this should involve more than just saying that the baby passed or failed. Instead, parents need to know what the result means and what the next steps should be. Even when the baby passes a screening test, it is a great opportunity to help parents understand the importance of monitoring language development and of being aware of the indicators of hearing loss that might occur later. Most successful newborn hearing screening programs use a variety of materials to educate, inform, and follow up with parents. For example, a 6-minute movie that explains how newborn hearing screening is done, why it is important, what the results mean, and what should happen next is available as a free download in both English and Spanish from NCHAM at www.infanthearing.org. Such a video can be used during birthing classes so that mothers know what to expect when the screening is done. Other examples of parent information include information pamphlets about the screening program, parent education materials, letters sent to parents about the results of the test, and cards used to make return appointments for rescreens or diagnostic evaluations (examples of such materials currently being used in other programs are available at www.infanthearing.org).

It is best if parents can be told about the results of the newborn hearing screening test before the baby is discharged. Then, any needed additional screening or testing can be scheduled before they leave the hospital, and parents can have their questions answered and any misunderstandings clarified. Some health-care providers want to be involved in communicating results of screening tests to parents, others do not. Therefore, make sure you have discussed your procedures for informing parents with health-care providers in your community.

Some people have worried about creating unnecessary anxiety in parents or disrupting family functioning, because most babies who fail the initial newborn hearing screening test will have normal hearing. There is no evidence that this is really a problem (Tueller, 2006). To avoid creating unnecessary anxiety, make sure parents understand that the screening test is not a diagnostic evaluation and that a referral for further testing does not mean that the baby has a hearing loss.

The activities associated with a newborn hearing screening program also provide an ideal opportunity to help parents understand the importance of language development. Just because a child has passed a newborn hearing screening test does not mean that there will not be future problems with hearing or language development. Materials distributed in conjunction with the newborn hearing screening should emphasize the need to monitor their child's language development and what parents should do if the child does not achieve developmental milestones in a timely manner. It should also be made clear that the newborn hearing screening test provides information about the status of the infant's hearing at the time of discharge. Common childhood diseases can later cause fluctuating or permanent hearing loss that will interfere with language development. Educational materials should emphasize the importance of parents requesting another hearing evaluation if they have any concerns about their child's language development.

Pitfall

- Some parents mistakenly assume that babies who pass the newborn hearing screening test will always have normal hearing. Babies can have normal hearing at birth and acquire permanent hearing loss later in life.

Communicating with Health-Care Providers

From the very beginning, the child's primary health-care provider needs to understand how newborn hearing screening contributes to better health care. Distributing written materials to all primary health-care providers in the community who see children is a good beginning. It may be useful to do some screening of babies when health-care providers typically make their rounds (as long as you don't interfere or take their babies while they are trying to examine them). Just being there and doing your work will prompt a lot of questions and understanding of what is involved in newborn hearing screening. As babies with hearing loss are identified, be sure to communicate the results to that baby's physician. Periodically, reports to the hospital's pediatric committee, or a newsletter to inform the hospital's medical staff about the success of the program can be sent. Including anonymous case histories or personal experiences of families whose babies have been helped by the program are particularly useful in such reports and newsletters.

It is also important to have a system to notify each health-care provider about the screening results for his or her patients. Although this is particularly important for babies who do not pass the initial screening, it is best to provide information about all of his patients, along with a clear recommendation of what should happen next. Few things will undermine the success of a newborn hearing screening program as much as the baby's health-care provider telling the parent during a well-baby check that it is really not that important to follow up with the outpatient screen or diagnostic evaluation procedures. Thus, it is critical for health-care providers to encourage parents to complete recommended testing as quickly as possible. Additionally, if parents have concerns about their baby's hearing or language development, they should be encouraged to see an audiologist who has experience working with infants and young children.

When a baby fails the newborn hearing screening, medical evaluation is an essential part of the diagnostic process, and health-care providers need to understand that they are a critical part of that multidisciplinary team. It is also important that everyone involved in the baby's medical management understand how detrimental it is when the diagnostic process requires several months, instead of being completed within a few weeks. For babies without other medical complications, the goal should be to have a definitive diagnosis, fit the hearing aids (if parents choose to do so), and begin early intervention within a few weeks of birth. For that to happen, however, all members of the team have to recognize the importance of early diagnosis and intervention and then work together to make it happen as quickly as possible.

Communicating with Hospital Administrators and Staff

Hospital administrators, risk managers, nursery supervisors, and community education staff, among others, also need to be kept informed about the newborn hearing screening program. If various people in the hospital are receiving the information they need on a timely basis, the continuation of the newborn hearing screening program is almost guaranteed because the benefits will be well documented and many different groups can work to support and improve the program. It is also important to make sure that hearing screening results are a part of the child's permanent medical record.

Having an effective data management system in place is important to be able to produce reports on a predetermined schedule or on request showing such things as the percentage of babies screened, the percentage who passed prior discharge, the percentage who are referred from the initial screening who eventually receive diagnostic evaluations, and the number of babies identified with permanent hearing loss. It is also useful to produce a monthly report summarizing the successes of the program, the challenges that still need to be addressed, and the strategies for resolving those challenges. It is particularly valuable to highlight the human side of any success stories so administrators see that people's lives are better off as a result of this program. Many administrators will also want to know more about program costs. A simple, but complete, cost analysis of the program after the first year, and then at periodic intervals thereafter, is very useful.

Pearl

- Accurate reporting about key variables related to the newborn hearing screening program is valuable in identifying weaknesses and improving the program as well as building support among various stakeholders.

Training Newborn Hearing Screeners

Regardless of which screening equipment or protocol is used, screeners will become proficient much faster if there is hands-on, competency-based training at the beginning.

Sales representatives can demonstrate how to operate the equipment, but the best training is done by people who are experienced screeners. Ideally, such training should include ample time for the people being trained to do supervised screening. Once a person acquires skill with the screening equipment, it is easily remembered.

The number of screeners needed to operate a universal newborn hearing screening program depends on the annual number of births and how the program is organized. Because some babies are discharged just a few hours after being born, 7-day-a-week coverage will be needed. However, the total amount of screening time is relatively small. Many hospitals make the mistake of training too many people (e.g., all of the nursing staff). Not only does this require extra time for training and supervision, but it often results in a less efficient program because responsibility for screening babies is diffused and the quality of screening suffers.

Although it is often said that practice makes perfect, it is more accurate to say that practice makes permanent. Consequently, it is important to provide timely feedback to people who are just learning to screen so errors can be corrected before they become ingrained. Subsequently, there should be regular one-on-one observation and feedback. A regular report which shows screener's performance with regard to variables such as the number of babies screened, babies passed, invalid tests, and screens completed per hour of work, can be useful in identifying screeners who are having difficulty and need assistance. Such supervision should be organized so that it is viewed as assistance instead of punishment.

Operating an Efficient Program

Regardless of the type of technology or protocol used, the goal of newborn hearing screening is to create the smallest reasonable subset of the general population that still contains all of the infants with hearing loss. In other words, without missing any babies, it is generally best to minimize the number of infants who fail the screening test and are referred for a diagnostic evaluation. The following strategies should be considered.

Do Screening when Babies Are Quiet

Even though it is possible to screen babies who are awake and restless, screening is easier and quicker when the baby is quiet (or even asleep), happy, well fed, and comfortable. Therefore, if possible, most screening should be done when babies are most likely to be in this optimal state. When and where screening is done will depend on other activities, routines, and available space at the hospital.

Test a Second Time before Discharge for Babies Who Do Not Pass at First

Typically, the first attempt to screen the baby is made shortly after birth. It is best not to spend too much time with the baby during this initial attempt. If the baby passes (as the majority will do), screening is finished. If not, wait several hours and try again. Regardless of the equipment or protocol being used, these second efforts before discharge can substantially reduce the number of babies who need to come in for outpatient screens or diagnostic procedures. Instead of spending 30 minutes with the baby during an initial attempt, it is much more efficient to make a quick first attempt, followed by a second or even third attempt a few hours later. It is not appropriate (and not an efficient use of time) to screen a particular baby more than three times in each ear before discharge.

Minimize Noise and Confusion in the Screening Area

None of the screening equipment requires extraordinary measures to make the screening area quiet. For example, newborn hearing screening is routinely being done in crowded and noisy neonatal intensive care units. However, other things being equal, screening will be faster and more effective if the screening area is relatively quiet. In other words, where possible, do the screening when physicians are not making their rounds, do not screen directly under a ventilator fan, and screen in an area that is not adjacent to a bathroom where running water creates unnecessary noise. Where sensible and inexpensive modifications can be done to reduce noise (e.g., carpeting on the floor, curtains on windows), they can make screening more efficient.

Have Backup Equipment and Supplies Readily Available

Because some babies are discharged after just a few hours in the nursery, arrangements should be made to have backup equipment in case there is a breakdown. Most newborn hearing screening equipment is extremely reliable. However, if the equipment unexpectedly stops operating and it takes 3 days to get a replacement, 10% of the babies born at the hospital that month will be missed.

Pitfall

- It is possible to become so fixated on achieving very low "fail" rates that the quality of the program suffers. Remember, the object of a newborn hearing screening program is to find babies with permanent hearing loss, not to have every baby pass the screening test.

Although such babies can come back for screening, it is extra work for everyone and unlikely to be completely successful. Thus, it is best to have made arrangements to obtain replacement or loan equipment within a very short time from the salesperson, a neighboring hospital, or a nearby university. It is also important to have sufficient supplies.

Managing Data and Patient Information

To identify babies with hearing loss and enroll them in appropriate intervention programs as early as possible requires coordination with the baby's medical home, one or more audiologists, and various state and local agencies who are responsible for providing services to infants and young children with hearing loss. The screening that happens before hospital discharge is only the first step. Most screening program managers report that keeping track of what happens in the screening program and managing babies through the referral and diagnostic process is the most challenging part of an EHDI program. Data and patient information management includes keeping track of which babies have been screened, what screening or diagnostic procedures should happen next, and which babies have missed appointments and need to be located. It also involves generating reports for program management, accountability, and program continuation, and generating letters to parents and physicians concerning the outcome of various screening and evaluation procedures. If such data and patient information management is not handled appropriately, it can be much more time consuming than the actual screening.

Arranging for a data and patient information management system is the kind of task on which it is easy to procrastinate. The amount of information that needs to be managed continues to multiply as more and more babies are born. If a system is not in place when the screening programs starts, you will soon find that you are overwhelmed, and the whole system begins to collapse in piles of paper and yellow sticky notes.

Summarizing data from individuals into understandable reports, generating letters to parents and pediatricians at different times based on the most recent outcomes, and sending reminders about upcoming and overdue screening and diagnostic activities are all easily done with a computer-based program. Information about several complete data and patient information packages that can be used by hospitals is available at www.infanthearing.org.

Program Coordination

The person in charge of the early identification of hearing loss program needs a continual flow of information, including:

- The number of babies born at the hospital
- The percentage of babies successfully screened
- The percentage of babies who fail the screening test
- The percentage of babies rescreened and/or diagnosed
- The number of babies identified with hearing loss
- How well each of the screeners is functioning

Regular and timely summaries of such information are critical if the program is to be successful. There should be regular coordination meetings (at least monthly) to review such information. This meeting should be attended by the program coordinator, a representative of the screening staff, the nursery coordinator, an audiologist who is involved with the program, and a health-care provider who cares for newborns at that hospital. The purpose of the meeting is to review the functioning of the program during the previous time period to make sure that its goals are being accomplished. Results from a computer-based data and patient information management program will provide all of the necessary data, but the meeting must still be convened, minutes taken, and follow-up done.

Over the long term, an efficient hearing identification program will identify about 3 babies per 1000 with permanent hearing loss. However, because hearing loss is a low-incidence condition, it may take 10,000 or more babies to achieve that average. In other words, it is not unusual for a hospital to screen 1000 babies and not find a single infant with permanent hearing loss. That same hospital, however, may find 5 or 6 infants in the next 1000.

Pearl

- Don't be discouraged if it takes a while to identify the first baby with a hearing loss.

Discussion Questions

1. What factors have contributed to the dramatic increase in percentage of newborns screened for hearing loss during the past 15 years?

2. What other components of an EHDI system are important to have in place to make newborn hearing screening effective?

3. Why is it important for stakeholders to know that newborn hearing screening is now considered to be a medical "standard of care"?

4. In what ways does an effective data management and tracking system contribute to a successful newborn hearing screening program?

5. Assume you are consulting with a hospital that has an unusually high percentage of newborns who fail the newborn hearing screening test. What factors would you suggest that they consider to achieve a more reasonable percentage of newborns who fail the test?

6. Why is it important to have screeners available to do newborn hearing screening seven days per week?

7. What information do parents need to know about their baby's newborn hearing screening test and when do they need to know it?

References

American Academy of Pediatrics (AAP). (1999). Newborn and infant hearing loss: detection and intervention. Pediatrics 103, 527–530.

American Academy of Pediatrics. (2002). The Medical Home Policy Statement. Pediatrics 110(1). www.aap.org/policy/s060016.html. Last accessed December 18, 2002.

Babbidge, H. (1965). Education of the deaf in the United States: report of the Advisory Committee on Education of the Deaf. Washington, DC: U.S. Government Printing Office.

Barsky-Firkser, L., and Sun, S. (1997). Universal newborn hearing screenings: a three-year experience. Pediatrics 99, E4.

Bess, F. H., and Paradise J. L. (1994). Universal screening for infant hearing impairment: not simple, not risk-free, not necessarily beneficial, and not presently justified. Pediatrics 93, 330–334.

Centers for Disease Control and Prevention (CDC). (2004). National EHDI Goals. www.cdc.gov/ncbddd/ehdi/nationalgoals.htm.

Downs, M. P., and Sterritt, G. M. (1964). Identification audiometry for infants: a preliminary report. Journal of Auditory Research, 4, 69–80.

Downs, M. P., and Sterritt, G. M. (1967). A guide to newborn and infant hearing screening programs. Archives of Otolaryngology, 85, 37–44.

Finitzo, T., Albright, K., and O'Neal, J. (1998). The newborn with hearing loss: detection in the nursery. Pediatrics, 102, 1452–1460.

Herrmann, B. S., Thornton, A. R., and Joseph, J. M. (1995). Automated infant hearing screening using the ABR: development and validation. American Journal of Audiology 4, 6–14.

Joint Committee on Infant Hearing. (2007). Year 2007 Position Statement: Principles and guidelines for early hearing detection and intervention programs. Pediatrics, 120 (4), 898–921.

Kemp, D. T. (1978). Stimulated acoustic emissions from the human auditory system. Journal of the Acoustical Society of America, 64, 1386–1391.

Kemp, D. T., and Ryan, S. (1993). The use of transient evoked otoacoustic emissions in neonatal hearing screening programs. Seminars in Hearing, 14, 30–44.

Lonsbury-Martin, B. L., and Martin, G. K. (1990). The clinical utility of distortion product otoacoustic emissions. Ear and Hearing, 11, 144–150.

Mason, J. A., and Herrmann, K. R. (1998). Universal infant hearing screening by automated auditory brainstem response measurement. Pediatrics, 101, 221–228.

Maternal and Child Health Bureau. (2002). National core and performance outcome measures. 205.153.240.79/search/core/cormenu.asp. Last accessed April 27, 2007.

Mehl, A. L., and Thomson, V. (1998). Newborn hearing screening: the great omission. Pediatrics, 101, E4

Moeller, M. P. (2000). Early intervention and language development in children who are deaf and hard of hearing. Pediatrics, 106, E43.

National Center for Hearing Assessment and Management (NCHAM). (2007a). Universal newborn hearing screening: summary statistics of UNHS in the United States. www.infanthearing.org/status/unhsstate.html. Last accessed April 27, 2007.

National Center for Hearing Assessment and Management (NCHAM). (2007b). Policy Statements Regarding Newborn Hearing Screening. www.infanthearing.org/policystatements/index.html. Last accessed April 27, 2007.

National Institutes of Health. (1993). Early identification of hearing impairment in infants and younger children. Rockville: National Institutes of Health.

Olusanya, B., McPherson, B., Swanepoel, de W., Shrivastav, R., and Chapchap, M. (2006). Globalization of infant hearing screening: the next challenge before JCIH? Journal of the American Academy of Audiology, 17, 293–295.

Paradise, J. L. (1999). Universal newborn hearing screening: should we leap before we look? Pediatrics, 103, 670–672.

Toward Equality. (1988). A report to the Congress of the United States: toward equality—Commission on Education of the Deaf. Washington, DC: U.S. Government Printing Office.

Tueller, S. J. (2006). Maternal worry about infant health, maternal anxiety, and maternal perceptions of child vulnerability associated with newborn hearing screen results. Master's Thesis, Utah State University, Logan, UT.

U.S. Department of Health and Human Services (HHS). (1990). Healthy People 2000: national health promotion and disease prevention objectives. Washington, DC: Public Health Service.

U.S Preventive Services Task Force. (1996). Screening for hearing impairment. In: US preventive services task force guide to clinical preventive services (pp. 393–405) 2nd ed. Baltimore: Williams & Wilkins.

Vohr, B. R., Carty, L. M., Moore, P. E., and Letourneau, K. (1998). The Rhode Island Hearing Assessment Program: experience with statewide hearing screening (1993–1996). Journal of Pediatrics, 133, 353–357.

White, K. R. (1997). Universal newborn hearing screening: issues and evidence. www.infanthearing.org/summary/prevalence.html. Last accessed April 27, 2007.

White, K. R. (2003). The current status of EHDI programs in the United States. Mental Retardation and Developmental Disabilities Research Reviews, 9, 79–88.

White, K. R., and Behrens, T. R. (Eds.). (1993). The Rhode Island Hearing Assessment Project: implications for universal newborn hearing screening. Seminars in Hearing, 14, 1–22.

Yoshinaga–Itano, C., Sedey, A. L., Coulter, D. K., and Mehl, A. L. (1998). Language of early- and later-identified children with hearing loss. Pediatrics, 102, 1161–1171

Part II

Diagnosing Hearing Disorders in Infants and Children

Chapter 5

Hearing Test Protocols for Children

Jane R. Madell and Carol Flexer

- ♦ **The Cross-Check Principle for Test Batteries**
- ♦ **Pediatric Audiologic Test Protocols**
- ♦ **Why Behavioral Audiologic Tests Need to Be Included in the Evaluation of All Infants and Children**
- ♦ **Steps To Take before Initiating Behavioral Audiologic Testing of Infants and Children**

  Selecting the Appropriate Test Protocol
  Setting Up the Test Room

- ♦ **Obtaining a Case History**

  Collecting Case History Information
  Topics to Be Covered in a Case History
  Summary

- ♦ **Functional Auditory Assessments**

Key Points

- Pediatric audiologic assessments involve the selection of developmentally appropriate protocols that include the cross-check principle.

- Before beginning testing, the child's cognitive age and physical status must be determined.

- A case history contributes valuable diagnostic information, provides an opportunity to observe the child, and allows a rapport to be established between the audiologist and the family.

- Functional auditory assessments, in the form of paper and pencil surveys, can assist in monitoring the baby's or child's auditory progress over time.

♦ The Cross-Check Principle for Test Batteries

There are four main purposes for a pediatric audiologic assessment: (1) to obtain a measure of peripheral hearing sensitivity that rules out or confirms hearing loss as a cause of the baby's or child's problem; (2) to confirm the status of the baby's or child's middle ear; (3) to assess auditory functioning using speech perception measures when possible; and (4) to observe and interpret the baby's or child's auditory behaviors.

To this end, a test battery approach employing the "cross-check" principle is standard. The cross-check principle, originally described by Jerger and Hayes (1976), posits that several appropriate behavioral and electrophysiologic tests must be used to determine the extent of a child's auditory function (Stach, 1998). A test battery approach furnishes detailed information, avoids drawing conclusions from a single test, allows for the identification of multiple pathologies, and provides a comprehensive foundation for observing a child's auditory behaviors. **Table 5–1** summarizes each test in the pediatric threshold test battery and discusses when each is appropriate.

The purpose of this chapter is to discuss the audiologic tests in the various pediatric test protocols, to emphasize the need for behavioral audiologic assessments for all infants and children, to detail the steps in administering a test protocol including selecting the appropriate protocol, to describe obtaining pediatric case histories and, finally, to summarize functional auditory assessments.

♦ Pediatric Audiologic Test Protocols

The American Speech-Language-Hearing Association (ASHA) (2004) recommends the following test protocols according to the chronological/developmental age of the child:

1. Birth through months of age (age is adjusted for prematurity). When infants are very young or experiencing severe

Table 5–1   A Summary of Tests Used in Pediatric Assessments

Test	Expected Infant/ Child Response	Cognitive Age Range	Benefit	Challenges
Behavioral Observation Audiometry (BOA)	Change in sucking in response to auditory stimulus; other behavioral changes are not accepted because they usually indicate suprathreshold responses.	Birth–6 months	Enables the audiologist to obtain valuable behavioral responses in infants; part of the cross-check principle. Testing can be conducted in soundfield, with earphones, with bone oscillator, hearing aids, or cochlear implants. Enables accurate fitting of technology because minimal response levels (MRLS) can be obtained	Requires careful observation of infant sucking on the part of the audiologist. Cannot be used with infants who do not suck, e.g., Infants who use feeding tubes. Testing can be performed only when the infant is in a calm awake, or light sleep state. BOA has not been generally accepted in the audiology community because audiologists typically have not been trained to use a sucking response paradigm.
Visual Reinforcement Audiometry (VRA)	Conditioned head turn to a visual reinforcer; usually a lighted animated toy.	5–36 months	Enables the audiologist to obtain valuable behavioral responses in infants and young children; part of the cross-check principle. Because responses are conditioned, more responses can be obtained in one test session. Testing can be conducted in soundfield, with earphones, with bone oscillator, hearing aids, or cochlear implants. Enables accurate fitting of technology because MRL can be obtained. The state of the infant or child is less problematic because the child can be more easily involved in the task.	Some children will not accept earphones so obtaining individual ear information can be challenging.
Conditioned Play Audiometry (CPA)	Child performs a motor act in response to hearing a sound (e.g., the listen and drop task)	30 months to 5 years.	Accurate responses can be obtained at threshold level. Testing can be conducted in soundfield, with earphones, with bone oscillator, hearing aids, or cochlear implants.	Keeping the child entertained and involved long enough to obtain all the necessary information can be challenging.
Immittance	None	All	Provides information about middle ear functioning and about intactness of the auditory system reflex arc.	The child must sit still, not speaking or moving during the test battery.
Transient Otoacoustic Emissions (TOAE)	None	All	Measures outer hair cell function. Presence of emissions indicates no greater than a mild hearing loss. Contributes to evaluation of the overall function of the auditory system.	The infant or child must sit still, not speaking during testing. Cannot rule out mild hearing loss.
Distortion Product Otoacoustic Emissions (DPOAE)	None	All	Measures outer hair cell function. Presence of emissions indicates no greater than moderate hearing loss. Contributes to evaluation of the overall function of the auditory system.	The infant or child must sit still, not speaking during testing. Cannot rule out moderate hearing loss.
Auditory Brainstem Response Testing (ABR)	None	All	Tonal ABR provides frequency specific threshold information. Click ABR provides information about the intactness of the auditory pathways, including measures contributing to the diagnosis of auditory neuropathy.	The infant or child must be asleep, sedated or very still for the duration of testing. ABR testing is not a direct measure of hearing and is not a substitute for behavioral audiologic testing.

developmental disabilities, ASHA recommends that the testing of infants or children should rely primarily on physiologic measures of auditory function, such as auditory brainstem responses (ABRs) using frequency-specific stimuli to estimate the audiogram. In addition, otoacoustic emissions (OAEs) and acoustic immittance measures should be used to supplement ABR results. Case history, parent/caregiver report, behavioral observation of the infant's responses to a variety of sounds, developmental screening, and functional auditory assessments should also be performed.

Pearl

- The authors of this book propose a primary role for behavioral audiologic assessments, even for this very young population. See Chapter 6 and the DVD.

---

2. Five through 24 months of age   At these ages, ASHA (2004) suggests that behavioral assessments should be performed first, with VRA (visual reinforcement audiometry) being the behavioral test of choice. OAEs and ABRs should be assessed only when behavioral audiometric tests are unreliable, ear-specific thresholds cannot be obtained, behavioral results are inconclusive, or auditory neuropathy is suspected. Developmental screening and functional auditory assessments also should be performed; please refer to **Table 5–4** at the end of the chapter for a summary of functional auditory assessments. See Chapter 7 for detailed information about VRA.

3. Twenty-five through 60 months of age: ASHA (2004) suggests that behavioral tests (VRA or CPA [conditioned play audiometry]) and acoustic immittance tests are usually sufficient. Speech perception tests should also be performed in combination with developmental screening and functional auditory assessments.

The expected outcomes of pediatric audiologic protocols are extensive and include: (1) identification of hearing loss; (2) identification of auditory neuropathy, if present, or of a potential central auditory processing/language disorder; (3) quantification of hearing status based on behavioral and electrophysiologic tests; (4) development of a comprehensive report of historical, physical, and audiologic findings, and recommendations for treatment and management; (5) implementation of a plan for monitoring, surveillance, and habilitation of hearing loss; and (6) provision of family-centered counseling and education.

♦ Why Behavioral Audiologic Tests Need to Be Included in the Evaluation of All Infants and Children

The *Guidelines for the Audiologic Assessment of Children from Birth to 5 Years of Age* (2004) suggests that behavioral testing is not the preferred method for evaluating hearing in in-fants birth to 4 months of age for identifying hearing loss and selecting hearing aids because of (1) the prolonged cooperation required from the child; (2) excessive test time needed; (3) poor frequency resolution; and (4) poor test-retest reliability. There is no doubt that evaluating hearing in infants and young children is time consuming and can require prolonged cooperation. However, these challenges should not lead to the conclusion that behavioral testing should not be conducted. If we believe that the information obtained from behavioral testing is valuable, if not critical, our goal should be to develop procedures that will permit us to obtain reliable behavioral test results. It would not occur to any of us to make a determination about auditory function or to fit amplification on a normally developing 5-year-old without a good behavioral audiogram, and for good reason. The behavioral audiogram provides valuable information, and within certain limits, it should be possible to obtain good quality behavioral evaluations on infants and children of any age or developmental status.

Chapters 6 to 10 describe in detail the techniques for the behavioral evaluation of infants and children. In addition, the DVD that accompanies this book will demonstrate these behavioral test techniques. We hope that the text and DVD together will assist the audiologist in learning the necessary skills to optimize behavioral test results. The DVD may also be helpful to the experienced clinician who wishes to update skills.

♦ Steps to Take before Initiating Behavioral Audiologic Testing of Infants and Children

Selecting the Appropriate Test Protocol

A pivotal factor in obtaining reliable test results is the selection of the appropriate test protocol. To do so, it is essential to know the child's cognitive level and physical abilities. Knowledge of what tasks the child is capable of performing *before* initiating testing is critical.

Cognitive Age

There are three behavioral techniques, each of which is appropriate for children at different developmental levels, allowing for some flexibility at upper and lower age limits: behavioral observation audiometry (BOA) is the appropriate behavioral technique for infants from birth to 6 months cognitive age; VRA is appropriate for infants from 5 months to 36 months cognitive age; and conditioned play audiometry (CPA) is the appropriate technique for children whose cognitive age is 30 to 36 months and older. Knowing the child's cognitive age allows the audiologist to select the appropriate test method, which is essential. For example, it would not be a good idea to ask a 2-month-old to raise her hand when she heard a sound. Doing so would lead to the conclusion that every 2-month-old child is deaf.

Unfortunately, it is not always possible to rely solely on chronological age to determine cognitive level. Although many children function at the same levels cognitively and chronologically, not all do. Much of the information obtained from the case history will be helpful in determining cognitive level. If speech and language skills are at or close to age level, one can assume that chronological and cognitive ages are the same or relatively close. Unfortunately, many children undergo audiologic evaluations because they are not developing speech and language skills, so other information is needed to determine cognitive level. Motor development can be a useful marker. If a child's motor skills are at age level, the child is usually cognitively close to chronological level, at least for the purpose of the tasks that are necessary for testing hearing.

Reports from other clinicians, including speech-language pathologists and pediatricians, can provide very useful information about developmental level. A variety of scales used by pediatricians can give the audiologist an idea about developmental level. Experience spending time with young children also will assist the audiology student in developing an "intuition" that will support the selection of the appropriate test protocol.

It is not a good idea to use the trial-and-error method to choose a test protocol; this method may work some, but not all, of the time. If a child's cognitive and chronological levels are too far apart, using an inappropriate test may give the false appearance of hearing loss, or yield inaccurate thresholds because the child will not respond appropriately to the test stimulus.

Physical Status

Once a child's cognitive level has been established, her physical condition needs to be evaluated to be certain that the child is capable of performing the test tasks. For BOA, we are primarily looking for changes in sucking, which is relatively easy to discern. Does the child suck? If yes, the audiologist can implement the BOA procedure. An infant may have an eating problem and receive food through feeding tubes, but if she uses a pacifier, sucking still can be observed. However, if the infant does not suck, it is probably not possible to obtain reliable observation audiometry responses. (See Chapter 9, Evaluation of Hearing in the Special Needs Child, for alternative test techniques.)

VRA uses a conditioned head turn in response to presentation of a sound stimulus, which requires the child to have vision good enough to see the reinforcing toy, and neck control sufficient to turn and look for the reinforcing toy. This task is most often performed with the child sitting either in a highchair or on someone's lap. A child who cannot sit can be placed in an adaptive supported position such as an infant seat that will still allow a conditioned head turn to be made. If the child cannot make a head turn, it will not be possible to use VRA. If the child is blind or for some other reason cannot see the reinforcer, it will not be possible to use standard VRA protocols. A creative audiologist may be able to generate some adaptive protocols. (See Chapter 9.)

Play audiometry requires that the child perform a motor task in response to the presentation of a sound. The ability to accomplish this task is limited only by the creativity of the audiologist. If the child cannot hold a toy and drop it in a bucket, she may be able to blink, move a finger, or push a button, for example. Specific test information about the various behavior protocols is discussed in the following chapters.

Setting Up the Test Room

Using a Two-Room Setup

There are several ways to set up a test room for evaluation of hearing in infants and young children. The most common is a two-room setup with an audiologist and audiometer in one room and the child, parent, and test assistant in the other. When using this setup, the audiologist and the test assistant must have a full view of the child. The audiologist, who is presenting the test stimuli, needs to be able to observe the child's behavioral state to know when and when not to present stimuli (e.g., do not present a stimulus if the child is fidgeting or trying to get out of the chair), and both testers need to be able to judge the presence or absence of a response.

It is also important that the two testers be able to communicate. If possible, the test assistant should have an earphone to hear directions or suggestions from the audiologist in the control room. An FM system also can work well for clinician-to-clinician communication. It is important that the test assistant knows when the stimulus is being presented so that she can determine whether or not to reinforce a child's response. For example, if a child looks toward the VRA toy when a sound has been presented, the test assistant will be enthusiastic, clapping and laughing. If the child looks toward the toy when there has been no test stimulus, the test assistant does not reinforce the response. If the test assistant does not have earphones or an FM system, the tester and test assistant must develop visual cues to ensure that they are communicating.

Using a One-Room Setup

Some audiologists use a one-room test setup, either for all testing or for selected testing. The advantage of a one-room

Table 5–2 Steps That Need to Be Taken before Beginning the Pediatric Assessment

1. Determine the child's cognitive age from:
   Case history
   Reports from other evaluations
   Infant developmental screening scales
2. Evaluate the child's physical status in terms of:
   Upper-torso control
   Head and neck control
   Vision
   Ability to manipulate toys
3. Choose the test room setup:
   1 room with 1 audiologist
   2 rooms with 2 audiologists, or 1 audiologist and 1 test assistant
   2 rooms with 1 audiologist and 1 parent who also functions as a test assistant

test setup is that testing can be accomplished with only one audiologist, who now performs both the tester and test assistant roles, thus having more control of the test situation. To accomplish this type of testing, the audiologist places the audiometer in the test room where the child will be. The setup should be arranged so that the child cannot see the audiometer controls and does not know when the interrupter switch is being pressed. The controls for the reinforcer toy for VRA also need to be located in a place not visible to the child. The audiologist can sit in front of the child and provide the stimulus, test assistance as needed (such as handing the child toys for play audiometry or distracting the child for VRA), and reinforcement as needed (either social or VRA). Even in centers where a two-room test setup is the norm, there are times when it is convenient to have the tester and child in the same room.

Experimenting with a variety of test setups will assist the audiologist in finding the one that is most comfortable for each test situation. See **Table 5–2** for a summary of steps that need to be taken before the actual pediatric assessment is initiated.

♦ Obtaining a Case History

A good case history is a valuable tool and an often overlooked part of an audiologic evaluation (Ehrlich, 1983). All diagnosticians recognize the need to obtain some information before beginning testing, and the amount needed will vary according to the reason for the evaluation. If the evaluation is a presurgical or postsurgical evaluation because a child is scheduled for insertion of pressure equalization tubes, it may not be necessary to obtain an extensive history. If, however, the child is being seen for evaluation because of concern about hearing, speech and language development, developmental delay, or problems in school, an extensive history is needed. Failure to obtain sufficient history information may reduce the quantity and quality of data obtained from the evaluation and diminish the role of

both the assessment and the audiologist to a technical one rather than a professional and diagnostic one.

Taking a case history obviously provides information necessary to learn about a child's development and health. A case history also provides an opportunity to observe the child and to become acquainted with the family and caregivers to understand their concerns and needs and to assess their objectivity. If different family members have dissimilar viewpoints, this difference of opinion frequently emerges during the interview process. The time spent obtaining a history also provides an opportunity to observe the child and his interactions with family members and others, and may uncover differences of opinion or interpretation between the audiologist's observations and those of the family members. Finally, taking a case history provides an excellent opportunity to develop rapport with and insights into the family, which may increase their willingness to accept your assessment results and subsequent recommendations for management.

By the end of the interview, the audiologist should have a good picture of the child's cognitive and developmental status as well as an initial estimate of the child's auditory skills.

Collecting Case History Information

Some clinics mail out questionnaires in advance of the appointment and have families complete them before coming in for the evaluation. This method allows the family to think about answers, to check with other family members or clinicians if needed, and to find addresses of health-care providers and schools, for example. Advance information is especially helpful if the child is brought to the evaluation by someone other than the parents (e.g., older sibling, grandparents, or foster parents). If the child is a foster child, mailing out the questionnaires in advance allows the responsible social service agency to provide the necessary information. However, not all families will complete forms even if they are received in advance.

Pearl

- Obtaining a case history permits the audiologist to learn about the child and to understand the parents' concerns and assessment expectations. History taking also facilitates the development of a rapport between the audiologist and the family that will be invaluable when counseling about test results.

Some programs give families questionnaires to complete when they arrive at the center just before being seen for evaluation. Although this method limits the time for completing the form and for thinking about the answers and does not permit obtaining information that is not easily recalled, it ensures that some information will be obtained.

Even when history forms are completed in advance by the family, the audiologist still needs to ask questions and spend time reviewing the information before initiating testing. This review will frequently reveal incomplete answers that will need to be finished before testing can begin. Some audiologists prefer to collect history information by asking all the questions themselves. Although this method allows the audiologist to direct specific questions as needed and expand or delete questions in certain areas, it extends the time scheduled for an evaluation because all information must be obtained at the time of the audiologic assessment.

Some basic areas should be reviewed in any history. Other questions will present themselves as the interviewer learns more about the child and the concerns of the parents or caregivers. A printed history form is frequently useful because it provides basic information; however, it is important not to let the form limit the questions.

Topics to Be Covered in a Case History

A complete history covers several content areas, and depending on the reason for the evaluation, emphasizes different segments of information. For example, if this evaluation is an initial one or if the child has not been seen recently, the obvious first question is, "Why have you brought your child here today?" By determining the reason for the visit, the audiologist can find out what the parent's or caregiver's concerns are and begin to get a picture of the goals of the evaluation. (Asking an older child why he is here today helps the audiologist understand what the child thinks is happening.) The next step is obtaining specific information. See **Table 5–3** for a list of case history topics.

Summary

Obtaining a history takes time but provides valuable information. At the very least, by the end of obtaining a history, the audiologist should have a very good sense of:

Caution

- The case history form should be viewed simply as a guide to the interview process.

Table 5–3   List of Information to Be Obtained in Case History Items

Birth and Prenatal History	Communication History: Hearing
Previous pregnancies	Parents thoughts of child's hearing?
Illnesses during the pregnancy, including the week of pregnancy an illness occurred	Sounds to which child responds
	Does the child distinguish between sounds (phone, doorbell)?
RH Incompatibility, ABO Blood incompatibility	Does the child want TV/CD/DVD/computer loud?
Medications, drugs (legal and illegal) taken during the pregnancy	Does hearing fluctuate? Under what conditions?
Complications during the pregnancy	Are sounds uncomfortable? What sounds? Under what conditions?
Length of the pregnancy	**Amplification history:**
Delivery: cesarean section or vaginal	Does the child wear a hearing aid and/or a cochlear implant? Name and model number of the instrument(s)? Which ears?
Birth weight	Does the child wear an FM system? Name and model number of the instrument? Which ears?
Complications at birth: anoxia, jaundice, APGAR scores, breech, other	Who recommended the devices?
Length of hospitalization	When were they acquired?
	When does the child wear them? E.g., All day? Only at school?
Health History	**Communication History: Speech and Language**
Colds, allergy, ear infections	Age of babbling, first word, phrases, sentences
High fevers	Does the child understand verbal requests with, without visual cues?
Immunizations	
Meningitis	How does the child communicate his/her needs? Voice, gesture, sign?
Other viruses (mumps, cytomegalovirus)	
Immunization history; reaction to immunizations	Has there been a change in the child's speech and language?
Drugs taken regularly and drug reactions	Did the child speak and then stop?
Feeding or swallowing problems	
Seizures	
Head injury	
Developmental History	**Social History**
Motor milestones: sitting, crawling, walking	When did the child feed himself? Dress himself?
Age of visual response to parents	Does she play with other children?
Is walking clumsy? Does the child fall a lot?	What toys or objects does the child like to play with?

Feeding and eating history
Age of toilet training

Educational History
Current school
Type of educational program
Previous school placements
Reasons for change in school placement
Special services received in school
Describe educational problems or concerns

Special Services
What special services does the child receive in school? Outside of school?
Speech-language therapy
Hearing (auditory) therapy
Occupational therapy
Physical therapy
Psychological services
Educational tutoring
Other

Other Evaluations
What other evaluations has the child had (evaluator, dates, and results)?
Audiologic
Speech-language
Hearing (auditory) therapy
Occupational therapy
Physical therapy
Psychological
Educational
Pediatric
Otolaryngologic
Neurologic
Psychiatric

Does the child have any behavior problems?
How does the child get along with other children? Adults? Family?
Have there been any changes in the child's behavior?
Does the child respond to others? Make eye contact?

♦ the child's cognitive status and motor abilities, which are critical for selecting the appropriate behavioral test protocol (BOA, VRA, or CPA)

♦ the child's speech, language, and developmental levels, which are important in selecting test materials for speech perception testing

During the audiologic evaluation, the audiologist determines if her initial impressions were accurate or not. It may be helpful to try to estimate the audiogram from history information and from observation of the child before beginning the test. Doing so over a period of time will improve the audiologist's ability to take a history and make accurate observations of a child's auditory status.

♦ Functional Auditory Assessments

An important part of a basic test battery for an infant or child of any age is an evaluation of auditory function. Numerous tests and surveys have been developed for this purpose. Functional auditory assessments are typically accomplished by having the teacher, student, or parent complete a questionnaire before and after the use of a hearing aid, cochlear implant, personal FM, or sound field system or the delivery of therapy or educational services. Most important, functional auditory assessments can monitor the child's auditory progress over time. **Table 5–4** displays a summary of functional auditory assessment tools.

Discussion Questions

1. Discuss the factors that need to be taken into consideration before beginning the actual pediatric assessment.

2. Identify five reasons for taking a case history.

3. Detail some of the reasons for performing functional auditory assessments, and summarize four tools.

4. Discuss the tests that are included in a pediatric test battery for a typical 12-month-old baby; include the concept of the cross-check principle.

Table 5–4   Functional Auditory Assessment Tools for Infants and Young Children

Measurement Tool	Authors	Age Range	Purpose
Auditory Behavior in Everyday Life (ABEL) (2002)	Purdy, et al., 2002	Children 2–12 years	Twenty-four-item questionnaire with 3 subscales (aural-oral, auditory awareness, social/conversational skills) which evaluates auditory behavior in everyday life
Children's Home Inventory for Listening Difficulties (CHILD) (2000)	Anderson & Smaldino, 1998, 2000	Children 3–12 years	Parent and self-report versions that assess listening skills in 15 natural situations
Children's Outcome Worksheet (C.O.W.) (2003)	Williams	Children 4–12 years	Teacher, parent, and child rating scales of classroom and home listening situations with amplification device; to specify 5 situations where improved hearing is desired
Early Listening Function (E.L.F.) (2000)	Anderson, 1989, 2000	Infants and toddlers; 5–months, 3 years	Parent observational rating scale of structured listening activities conducted over time to record distance learning
Functional Auditory Performance Indicators (F.A.P.I.) (2003)	Stredler-Brown & Johnson, 2001–2003	Infants through school-age	Parent or interventionist assessment of functional auditory skills over time
Infant-Toddler Meaningful Auditory Integration Scale (IT-MAIS) (1997)	Robbins, Renshaw, & Berry, 1991	Infant-toddler and older child versions	Structured parent interview scale designed to assess spontaneous auditory behaviors in everyday listening situations
Listening Inventories for Education (L.I.F.E.) (1998)	Anderson & Smaldino, 1998, 2000	6 years and above	Student and teacher rating scales designed to assess listening difficulty in the classroom
Little Ears (2003)	Kuhn-Inacker, et al. 2003	Birth and up	Questionnaire for the parent with 35 age-dependent questions that assess auditory development
Meaningful Auditory Integration Scale (MAIS) (1991)	McKonkey Robbins, et al.	Children 3 to 4 years and up	Parental interview with 10 questions that evaluates meaningful use of sound in everyday situations; attachment with hearing instrument, ability to alert to sound, ability to attach meaning to sound
Parent's Evaluation of Aural/Oral Performance of Children (PEACH) (2000)	Ching, Hill, & Psarros, 2006	Preschool to 7 years	Interview with parent with 15 questions targeting the child's everyday environment. Includes scoring for 5 subscales (use, quiet, noise, telephone, environment)
Preschool Screening Instrument For Targeting Educational Risk (Pre-school SIFTER) (1996)	Anderson & Matkin, 1996	3 to 6 years	Questionnaire with 15 items completed by the teacher that identifies children at risk for educational failure; has 5 subscales (academics, attention, communication, class participation, behavior)
Screening Inventory for Targeting Educational Risk (SIFTER) (1989)	Anderson, 1989, 2000	6 years through secondary school	Teacher questionnaire designed to target academic risk behaviors in children with hearing problems; has 5 subscales (academics, attention, communication, class participation, behavior)
Teacher's Evaluation of Aural/Oral Performance of Children (TEACH) (2000)	Ching, Hill, & Psarros, 2006	Preschool to 7 years	Interview with teacher having 13 questions targeting the child's everyday environment. Includes scoring for 5 subscales (use, quiet, noise, telephone, environment)

References

American Speech-Language-Hearing Association. (2004). Guidelines for the Audiologic Assessment of Children from Birth to 5 Years of Age. www.asha.org/members/deskref-journals/deskref/default.

Anderson, K. (1989). Screening Instrument for Targeting Educational Risk (SIFTER). Tampa: Educational Audiology Association. www.hear2learn.com.

Anderson, K. (2000). Early Listening Function (ELF). www.hear2learn.com.

Anderson, K., and Matkin, N. (1996). Screening Instrument for Targeting Educational Risk in Preschool Children (Age 3-Kindergarten) (Preschool SIFTER). www.hear2learn.com.

Anderson, K., and Smaldino, J. (1998). The Listening Inventory for Education: An Efficacy Tool. (LIFE). www.hear2learn.com.

Anderson, K., and Smaldino, J. (2000). Children's home inventory for listening difficulties. (CHILD). www.hear2learn.com.

Ching, T. C., Hill, M., and Psarros, C. (2000). Strategies for Evaluation of Hearing Aid Fitting for Children (PEACH and TEACH). Paper presented at the International Hearing Aid Research Conference, August 23, Lake Tahoe, NV. www.nal.gov.au.

Ehrlich, C. (1983). A case history for children, in Handbook of clinical audiology (3rd ed., pp. 607–620). Jack Katz (Ed.). Baltimore: Williams and Wilkins.

Jerger, J. F., and Hayes, D. (1976). The cross-check principle in pediatric audiology. Archives of Otolaryngology, 102, 614–620.

Kuhn-Inacker, H., Weichbold, V., Tsiakpini, L., Coninx, S., and D'Haese, P. (2003). Little ears: Auditory questionnaire, Innsbruck, Austria: MED-EL.

Purdy, S. C., Farrington, D.R., Moran,C.A., Chard, L. L., and Hodgson, S. A. (2002). ABEL: Auditory behavior in everyday life. American Journal of Audiology, 11, 72–82.

Robbins, A. M., Renshaw, J. J ., and Berry, S. W. (1991). Evaluating meaningful integration in profoundly hearing impaired children (MAIS). American Journal of Otolaryngology, 12, 144–150.

Stach, B. A. (1998). Clinical audiology: An introduction. San Diego: Singular Publishing Group.

Stredler-Brown, A., and Johnson, D. C. (2001-2003). Functional Auditory Performance Indicators: An Integrated Approach to Auditory Development. www.arlenestredlerbrown.com

Williams, C. (2003). The Children's Outcome Worksheets (COW): An Outcome Measure Focusing on Children's Needs (ages 4-12). News from Oticon, January 2005, www.oticon.com.

Chapter 6

Using Behavioral Observation Audiometry to Evaluate Hearing in Infants from Birth to 6 Months

Jane R. Madell

♦ **The History of Behavioral Testing of Infants**

Noisemakers

Early Infant Hearing Screening Programs

Infant Thresholds

The Need for Behavioral Testing of Infants

♦ **Diagnostic Audiologic Evaluation of Neonates**

The Basics of Behavioral Observation Audiometry

Testing Protocol of Behavioral Observation Audiometry

Other Factors That Influence Behavioral Observation Audiometry Test Results with Infants

Adding Objectivity to Behavioral Observation Audiometry

Key Points

- Auditory brainstem response (ABR), auditory steady state response (ASSR), and otoacoustic emission (OAE) testing provide critical information about the status of the auditory pathways, but are not direct measures of hearing.

- Only behavioral testing can provide a direct measure of hearing.

- When carefully performed, using appropriate criteria (including changes in sucking as an indication of a response), behavioral observation audiometry (BOA) can accurately measure thresholds in infants younger than 6 months.

Nonbehavioral tests such as ABR testing, ASSR testing, and OAEs are frequently used to assist in estimating peripheral hearing in infants (ASHA 2004). Although these tests are an important part of the audiology practice, they are, in fact, not tests of hearing. The only true test of hearing is behavioral assessment. ABR, ASSR, and OAE measures provide information about the integrity of specific sites within the auditory system (Delaroche, Thiebaut, and Dauman, 2004; Gravel, 2000; Hicks, Tharpe, and Ashmead, 2000; Sininger, 1993). Only behavioral testing truly tests hearing, since it measures the response of the entire auditory system from the outer ear through the cerebral cortex. Behavioral tests permit measurement of what an infant actually perceives; so they are measures of functional hearing abilities.

Numerous authors have posited the necessity for cross-checking physiological results with behavioral data by using a battery of tests to determine hearing sensitivity (Bess and Humes, 2003; Gravel, 2000; Hicks, Tharpe, and Ashmead, 2000; Jerger and Hayes, 1976; Madell, 1998; Northern and Downs, 2002). Behavioral testing of infants 6 months and older is a well documented part of the clinical practice of audiology (ASHA 2004). Behavioral evaluation of infants younger than 6 months is more difficult to achieve and less well documented. This chapter will describe a behavioral technique that can be used to successfully evaluate hearing in infants younger than 6 months.

♦ The History of Behavioral Testing of Infants

As early as the 1940s, attempts were made to develop behavioral techniques to assess hearing in infants (Ewing and Ewing, 1940, 1944; Froeschels and Beebe, 1946). Sir Alexander and Lady Ewing used percussion sounds and pitch pipes to elicit aural reflex responses (eye blinks). Wedenberg began infant screening in Sweden in 1956 using pure tones to elicit the auro-palpebral reflex. Froding continued Wedenberg's work using a small gong and mallet. Some clinicians used the infant's ability to turn toward the sound to assess hearing. Frisina (1963) reported that between 2 to 4 months of age infants could turn toward a sound. However, Northern and Downs (1974) reported that head turning does not occur before the age of 6 months, and Gerber (1977) reported the average age of head turn to be at 7 $^1/_2$ months.

Noisemakers

Noisemakers were the most common sound source employed for early hearing tests. They were selected for testing because they were readily available, simple and inexpensive, and could be used in any setting (a sound room was not required) and it was believed that infants would respond more reliably to noisemakers than to pure tone stimuli. The difficulty with noisemakers is that they usually have very broad frequency responses. Furthermore, their intensity is not easy to control even with practice exerting the pressure necessary to make the sound, and stabilizing the distance from the infant's ear. Bove and Flugrath (1973), and Poblano et al. (2000) analyzed different noisemakers to determine their frequency responses so that responses to noisemakers could provide more useful information. Even if noisemakers cannot provide sufficient information to be used to assess hearing, they can provide some gross information about how an infant responds to sound. Specifically, noisemakers can provide some evidence of an infant's ability to alert to sound and localize to the source (Northern and Downs, 2002).

Before using any noisemakers, information should be obtained about the auditory signals they emit, including their frequency response and intensity. Results of noisemaker tests must be viewed with caution. For example, a noisemaker may have the bulk of its energy in the 2000 to 4000 Hz range, but also have energy at 500 Hz at 30 to 40 dB less intensity than the high frequencies. What can be surmised about the infant's response to this stimulus? It is possible that the infant hears the high frequency component of the stimulus, but it is also possible that the infant has a high frequency hearing loss, does not hear the high frequency part of the signal, and is responding to the low frequency component.

Early Infant Hearing Screening Programs

The first large-scale infant hearing screening program in the United States was a citywide hearing screening project in Denver, conducted by Marion Downs and Graham Sterritt in 1964. They used a handheld noise generator that emitted a 90 dB SPL noise centered at 3000 Hz. Downs and Sterritt (1964, 1967), Northern and Downs (1991), and Werner and Gillenwater (1990) attempted to develop a standardized procedure to assess an infant's behavioral arousal, but a significant number of false-positive test results made the testing unreliable. Several authors have described techniques for assessing behavioral responses in infants, including observation of eye widening, quieting, eye shifting, head orienting, limb movement, and changes in respiration. Attempts have been made to calibrate the observer (Mencher et al, 1977; Weber, 1969), to assess the state of the infant (Eisenberg, 1969), and to precisely calibrate the signal (Thompson and Thompson, 1972.) A major problem with using the auropalpebral reflex, the Moro reflex, or changes in limb movement or respiration is that these behaviors are not elicited to threshold stimuli, but rather are responses to suprathreshold stimuli. Although some infants with hearing loss were

identified using these methods, many with less than severe to profound hearing losses were missed. In spite of all attempts to improve test protocols, BOA continued to be considered "unreliable."

Infant Thresholds

Because behavioral test protocols frequently did not reveal threshold responses, some audiologists proposed that responses at 60 to 70 dB SPL be interpreted as normal hearing for very young infants (McConnell and Ward, 1967, Northern and Downs, 1984). However, others demonstrated that infants hear at essentially adult levels (Berg and Smith, 1983; Eisele, Berry, and Shriner 1975; Madell, 1995a, 1998; Olsho, 1984; Olsho et al 1988; Spetner, and Olsho 1990; Werner and Gillenwater, 1990). Olsho et al (1984) Olsho et al, (1987b, 1988), and Nozza (2006), reported that average behavioral thresholds of 3-month-olds were worse than thresholds for young adults by 15 to 20 dB between 250 and 4000 Hz, and by about 30 dB at 8000 Hz. By 6 months of age, hearing sensitivity in the high frequencies improves but thresholds at 250 Hz remain elevated by about 15 dB. Thresholds improved by 20 dB between 3 and 6 months. Olsho et al (1988) discussed that the audibility curve of younger infants may differ in shape compared with the curve of older infants and adults. It was assumed that this audibility curve difference was, at least in part, due to the characteristics of the external and middle ears in infants. Arlington (2000) and Olsho et al (1988) postulated that some of the threshold differences may be related to sensory immaturity.

Gravel (2000); Hicks, Tharpe, and Ashmead (2000); and Olsho et al (1987a,b, 1988,) use an observer-based procedure developed by Olsho to reduce tester bias in evaluating hearing in infants as young as 2 to 5 weeks. In this method, a trial consists of a sound or a no-sound interval. One or two trained observers watch the infant and make a determination as to whether the interval contained a sound, or no sound, based on the infant's response. The observer receives feedback as to whether a sound is present. Once the observer demonstrates a false-positive rate of less than 25% reliable, testing begins. Hicks, Tharpe, and Ashmead (2000) used this technique with two observers testing 2 - and 4-month-old infants. They successfully obtained thresholds for 4-montholds, but were not successful in obtaining thresholds for 2-month-olds. Several authors evaluating hearing in infants report that results could be optimized by enhancing the test conditions. This enhancement included reducing visual distractions (Muir, Clifton, and Clarkson, 1989), using a salient auditory stimulus (Thompson and Thompson, 1972), reinforcing desired behaviors (Olsho et al, 1987a, 1988), and using changes in sucking as the response criteria (Delaroche Thiebaut, and Dauman, 2004; Madell, 1995a, 1998). Because of the critical need to obtain reliable test results on infants, research in this area will need to continue.

The Need for Behavioral Testing of Infants

Over time, the demand for infant hearing screening has increased significantly, so that many states have mandated newborn hearing screening requirements. (See Chapter 4 for a complete discussion of newborn hearing screening.) As more infants survive and as hearing screening becomes more universal, audiologists are being asked to assess hearing in very young infants who have failed newborn screening and to manage hearing loss when it is identified. One of the first steps in hearing loss management is the selection and fitting of appropriate amplification. Hearing aid fitting requires an accurate assessment of the degree and type of hearing loss, with both ear and frequency specific information obtained by air and bone conduction.

Many audiologists feel comfortable testing hearing in infants older than 6 months using visual reinforcement audiometry (VRA), but do not feel comfortable testing younger infants, developmentally delayed infants, or critically ill infants. If an infant fails a hearing screening at birth, hearing aids should be fit within a few weeks. Work by Apuzzo and Yoshinaga-Itana (1995); Yoshinaga-Itana, Couter, and Thomson (2001), and others have demonstrated that infants who are fit with appropriate technology before they are 6 months old can develop speech and language skills commensurate with their normal hearing peers, and that infants fit with technology older than 6 months, do not catch up to those fit earlier. Sharma, Dorman, and Spahr (2002) have demonstrated that infants who receive auditory stimulation at a sufficiently early age have evoked potential latencies similar to normal hearing peers, but infants who do not have sufficiently early access do not.

Behavioral testing allows the parents to participate in testing by allowing them to assist in determining when the infant is responding to a sound. If parents are provided with information about what to observe, they can be active participants in testing, facilitating acceptance, and understanding of hearing loss (Gravel and McCaughey, 2004). Electrophysiologic testing, on the other hand, provides little for a family to observe. It is clear that we must develop test techniques for evaluating very young infants that will provide the ear and frequency specific information necessary for the evaluation, selection, and fitting of amplification. Real-ear measures provide good information about how much sound is reaching the eardrum, but this information is difficult to interpret without good information about the status of the infant's unaided hearing. Tonal ABR and ASSR measures provide some of this information but thresholds obtained may vary by ± 15 dB. BOA techniques can assist in obtaining ear and frequency specific information and can provide confirmation of information obtained from electrophysiologic tests.

♦ Diagnostic Audiologic Evaluation of Neonates

The goal of an audiologic evaluation of an infant is usually to determine if the child has sufficient hearing to develop speech and language. A complete diagnostic evaluation of infants should include immittance testing to assess middle ear status, and a test technique that will provide frequency and ear specific information, ideally for both air and bone conduction. The most common test protocols for evaluating

neonates include immittance testing with a high-frequency probe tone, auditory brainstem response testing (ABR), auditory steady state evoked potential (ASSEP) and/or OAE.

Immittance testing assesses middle ear status, but does not provide information about hearing. ABR and ASSEP provide information about the auditory system's ability to receive sound, but are not direct measures of hearing. OAEs assess function of the outer hair cells of the cochlea but, again, are not a direct measure of hearing. Information about an infant's ability to hear and attend to auditory stimuli can be obtained only with behavioral testing. For that reason, no at-risk infant or child should be released from audiologic follow-up until behavioral test results are obtained. (See Chapter 13 for a discussion of immittance testing, Chapter 14 for a discussion of OAE testing, and Chapter 15 for a discussion of ABR and ASSEP testing.)

Pearl

- Although ABR, ASSR, and OAE testing provides important information about the status of the auditory system, only behavioral testing directly tests hearing. For this reason, it is critical that audiologists have a behavioral technique that is accurate for assessing hearing in infants younger than 6 months.

The Basics of Behavioral Observation Audiometry

What Is Being Observed?

Historically, many behaviors have been used to assess hearing in infants (arousal, limb movement, respiration changes, eye blink), but these behaviors have not proven to be sufficiently repeatable, and more importantly, they have not been good indicators of threshold. The behavior most likely to provide threshold responses is a change in sucking (Delaroche, Thiebaut, and Dauman, 2004; Madell, 1988, 1995a, 1998; Widen and Keener, 2003). Arousal responses, limb movements, and eye blinks frequently reveal suprathreshold level responses, but rarely threshold, since these behaviors typically are elicited to louder stimuli. Sucking responses, however, although present at suprathreshold levels, are frequently observed at, or close to, threshold. Either initiation or cessation of sucking is an acceptable response. Some infants will start sucking when a sound is presented, others will cease sucking, and some will do both.

Pearl

- Cessation or initiation of sucking is the only reliable response for obtaining behavioral thresholds in infants younger than 6 months.

Maximizing Observation of the Sucking Response

Sucking can be observed with a bottle, nursing at the breast, or with a pacifier. The family should be instructed to bring the infant to the evaluation session hungry so that he will be ready to suck. The infant needs to be as comfortable as possible during testing, so, if the infant normally drinks from a bottle, the family should bring one. If the infant normally nurses, it would be best if the infant is nursed during testing. For this test procedure to succeed, the mother has to be comfortable being observed nursing, and some women are not. If the mother understands the reason for the intrusion on her privacy, she usually acquiesces. If the infant uses a pacifier, the family should bring one along. After the infant is finished eating, testing can frequently continue by observing sucking with a pacifier. If an infant is very hungry, it is best to allow him a little time to eat to enable him to get over that initial extreme hunger before beginning testing.

As soon as the baby settles down, testing can begin. The best way to observe the sucking response is to be able to see the infant's mouth close-up. A good view of the mouth can easily be obtained by having a video camera in the test room that can be adjusted from the control room. By using the zoom on the camera, it is possible to focus directly on the infant's mouth, which will enable the audiologist to have an excellent view of sucking. If a camera is not available, the audiologist needs to be certain that she can clearly see changes in sucking to use this technique.

How Does One Know That the Sucking Is a Response to a Sound Stimulus?

As with all other behavioral responses, timing is the key factor. When using play audiometry with a child, we question the validity of the child's response if it comes a long time after presentation of the stimulus. With any test protocol, (behavioral or electrophysiologic) responses can be accepted only if they fall within a reasonable time window after presentation of the stimulus. Infants are fairly consistent, internally. Some respond to the "on" of the stimulus and others respond to the "off." The timing of the response is also usually consistent. Infants respond at about the same number of seconds after presentation of the stimulus each time, with the response time slightly shorter for louder stimuli (Madell, 1998; Northern and Downs, 2002; Thompson and Weber, 1974; Widen and Keener, 2003).

Positioning the Infant

The necessity of appropriately positioning the infant cannot be overstated. Positioning may, in fact, be the most important factor in obtaining accurate test results with behavioral observation audiometry. To obtain reliable test results, the infant needs to be resting in a comfortable position with full support of the head and torso, and must be visible to the testers. If the child is nursing, the mother will be holding the child in her arms. If the child is using a bottle or a pacifier, the child may be held in someone's arms or placed in an infant seat (**see Fig. 6–1A–C**). The advantage of an infant seat is that the infant will not be receiving any "signals" from the mother when he hears the sound. Involuntary movements such as stiffening by the mother in response to sound or movement of the breast or bottle can be transmitted to the infant; therefore, changes in sucking may

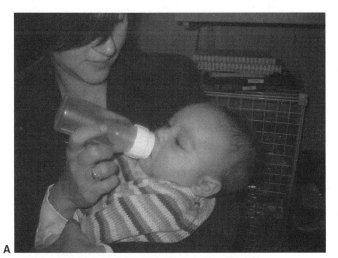

A

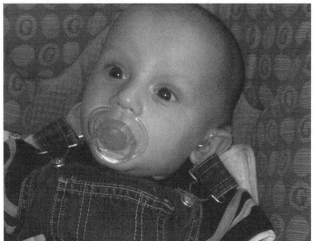

B

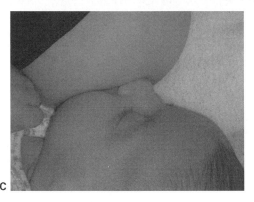

C

Figure 6–1   Positioning the infant for testing: (**A**) using a bottle, (**B**) using a pacifier, and (**C**) nursing at the breast.

occur that are not related to the auditory stimuli. If the infant is being held, the mother or other person holding the infant should be very carefully instructed about the need to remain silent and still throughout testing to eliminate interfering with test results. It is sometimes useful to have the mother wear earphones to prevent her from hearing and being influenced by the sound; however, many mothers prefer not to wear earphones because they want to hear what their baby is hearing.

The Role of the Test Assistant

BOA is best accomplished by using two or more observers. One is the audiologist controlling the test equipment, usually outside of the room where the infant is placed. The second observer typically is sitting next to the infant. Positioning of all players needs to be carefully orchestrated to be certain that both testers can easily see the infant.

The test assistant has several responsibilities. He must constantly be monitoring the infant to be certain that the baby's head and torso are comfortably balanced to minimize or preclude fussing and straining. If the infant becomes fussy, testing will need to stop until the infant can be made comfortable (Madell, 1998). For older infants, or infants using a bottle or a pacifier, the test assistant must keep the infant focused at the midline, again so that the infant is comfortable and not distracted. It is sometimes helpful to hold a colorful toy (Madell, 1998) or an LED (light emitting diode, usually a small red light) (Hicks, Tharpe, and Ashmead, 2000; Olsho, 1987a) in front of the infant in a position that allows the infant's head to be centered. The toy should not be held above the infant's head so he needs to move his neck to see it. Visual distractions need to be kept to a minimum (Muir, Clifton, and Clarkson, 1989) to be certain that extraneous stimuli are not interfering with observation of responses. It is important that the person holding the toy or LED make no change in the movement of the toy when the sound is presented. Any change in movement can confound the interpretation of whether the infant is responding to the sound or to the change in the distracter. If the infant is in an infant seat, the test assistant may be the one holding the bottle or pacifier and holding the visual distracters. Finally, the test assistant will be one of the observers who judges whether or not the infant responded to the sound presentation by changing his or her sucking behavior.

The Role of the Parents

The parents cannot be relied on as observers. Their stakes are too high, they are not experienced in the task, and they may not understand exactly what constitutes an acceptable response. Parents are, however, very valuable in helping the testers to understand the baby and assisting in making the baby comfortable. At least one parent needs to be in the test room to assist in understanding the test protocols and test results. If both parents are present, the other parent can observe from the control room. The audiologist in the control room can point out responses during testing to assist in the parent's understanding of the tests. Their observation of how the baby does or does not respond will be helpful when interpreting the final test results and presenting subsequent follow-up recommendations (Flasher and Fogel, 2004).

Testing Protocol of Behavioral Observation Audiometry

Soundfield versus Earphone Testing

A complete audiogram includes air and bone conduction thresholds in each ear at frequencies of 250 to 8000 Hz. However, infants will provide only a limited number of responses in one test session, so testing protocols need to be designed to obtain the most information with the fewest responses. The goal of the initial audiologic evaluation of an infant is usually to be certain that the infant has sufficient hearing to develop speech and language. It may not be necessary to obtain ear specific information at the first visit. (Occasionally, a child is referred to a pediatric audiologist because of a medical condition that requires ear-specific information immediately, but this is more frequently the exception rather than the rule. When detailed information is required during the first test session, the test protocol will obviously have to change.) Ear specific information is important and must be obtained prior to releasing an infant from audiologic follow-up, but the more important question at the time of the initial evaluation is, Does the infant hear enough to learn language? Should the initial audiologic evaluation indicate that hearing is normal in at least one ear utilizing soundfield testing, it may not be critical to obtain information about each ear separately at that visit. However, if the initial testing indicates that hearing is not within normal limits in the soundfield, then ear-specific information is critical so that management can proceed. No infant should be released from audiologic follow-up until ear-specific information is obtained.

Under most conditions, testing should begin in soundfield. Soundfield testing is less stressful for the infant and allows two ears to be stimulated at the same time. This ensures testing of the best hearing ear. It also permits parents to hear the sounds; this can be very useful in their understanding of the test results. Earphone testing can follow later in the initial test session, or in a subsequent test session. When earphone testing is being attempted, insert earphones are the earphones of choice for infants. Insert earphones **(Fig. 6–2)** will remain appropriately seated in the ear canal and will provide the most accurate results in tiny ears. Circumaural earphones are frequently too large and are very difficult to keep in place.

If testing indicates thresholds at lower than normal hearing levels, bone conduction testing is essential. The bone vibrator should be held in place with either a pediatric sized headband, or a fabric one that goes around the head and across the forehead using Velcro to secure it in place. If a metal headband is used, soft material such as foam or other padding should be used for comfort and to keep the headband from moving. If a hearing loss is confirmed, the same test protocols can be used to assess functional gain with amplification in soundfield.

Test Stimuli

When planning the test session, it is important to keep in mind that infants will provide only a limited number of responses; and so each stimulus presentation must be considered carefully. The goal of the testing is to obtain frequency-specific test results. Warble tones or narrow bands of noise

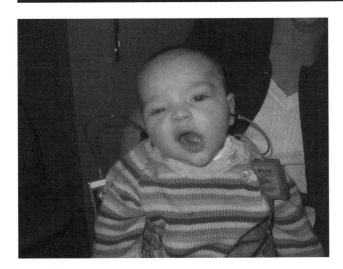

Figure 6–2   Infant with insert earphones.

will provide this information. Broadband stimuli such as music, conversational speech, or white noise will not. Narrow bands of noise are frequently easier for an infant to respond to (Gravel, 2000; Madell 1998), and may provide thresholds that are 5 to 10 dB softer than those obtained with warble tones.

Speech awareness thresholds to low (ba), mid-high (sh), and high (s) frequency speech stimuli can be used to confirm warble tone/noise band thresholds. The threshold for "ba" should be close to the threshold obtained at 500 Hz, "sh" should be close to the threshold obtained at 2000 Hz, and "s" should be close to the threshold obtained at 3000 to 4000 Hz (Ling, 2002; Madell, 1995b, 1998).

Presentation of Test Stimuli

Many normal hearing infants respond better to high-frequency stimuli, so it is reasonable to begin at a high frequency, usually 2000 Hz. To explain, if there is concern about middle ear pathology, low-frequency hearing could be compromised, so it may be better to begin with a high-frequency stimulus (2000 Hz). On the other hand, if a significant sensorineural hearing loss is suspected, hearing may be better at low frequencies, so testing should begin with 500 Hz. After obtaining thresholds at 500 and 2000 Hz, make a determination about what is the next most important piece of information to have. For example, if thresholds at both 500 and 2000 Hz are normal, it would be more important to obtain a threshold at 4000 Hz than at 1000 Hz, since hearing is likely also to be normal at 1000 Hz. However, if hearing at 500 Hz is at 30 dB HL and hearing at 2000 Hz is at 70 dB HL, it would be very important to know what hearing is at 1000 Hz.

Several indications can clue the audiologist about which frequencies and intensities should be used to begin testing:

♦ Observe the infant's responses to noisemakers.

♦ Observe the infant's responses to voice and environmental sounds.

♦ Question the parents about the infant's response to sound before testing.

Presentation of stimuli should begin at a soft level slightly above where you expect the infant to respond, and then be increased in 10-dB steps until a response is observed. The initial stimulus should not be so loud as to startle the infant. If the initial stimulus is much louder than threshold, it may be difficult to regain the infant's attention to threshold-level stimuli. When the infant responds, decrease intensity in 10-dB steps, decreasing stimuli in 5-dB steps when close to estimated threshold, and then increase intensity in 5- or 10-dB steps as would be done with any other population. Especially with infants, no response should be recorded until it is observed at the same level three times.

Timing is critical. If stimuli are presented too quickly, the infant will ignore them. A sound that comes out of silence is more likely to elicit a response. To obtain reliable responses, it is important to observe the infant carefully. If an infant startles to a sound, it is probably significantly above threshold. The way the baby responds when the stimulus is loud will provide clues about the type of response and latency that can be expected. This information can be used to interpret responses when the stimulus intensity decreases **(Table 6–1)**.

Table 6–1   Behavioral Observation Audiometry Test Protocol

1. Bring infant into test room in hungry state.
2. Seat infant so torso is supported and infant is not fidgety, and so tester(s) can easily see mouth.
3. Monitor infant state during testing and stop if infant becomes fidgety.
4. Instruct parents not to respond to test stimuli or responses from the child.
5. Test assistant will keep infant centered, observe responses, and monitor parents' behavior.
6. Begin testing in soundfield.
7. Begin testing with a stimulus that is slightly above estimated threshold.
8. Test one low (500 Hz) and one high (2000 Hz) frequency initially and select additional frequencies to test depending on initial responses.
9. Reduce thresholds in 10-dB steps and increase in 5- to 10-dB steps to bracket threshold. Record a response after three reversals.
10. Take breaks as needed to calm the infant and increase usable test time.
11. If soundfield testing indicates a hearing loss, test bone conduction.
12. If infant is still responding, or at the next test session, test with insert earphones.
13. Test with technology as needed.

Other Factors That Influence Behavioral Observation Audiometry Test Results with Infants

The audiologist must know something about the infant to obtain reliable test results. Spending a little time with the infant before beginning testing will increase the likelihood of obtaining reliable test results. It is important to have a good estimate of the infant's developmental, neurologic, and behavioral status. Can the infant do whatever is required for testing? If we are looking for sucking changes, we need to know that the infant sucks steadily. Some infants take a few sucks and stop, then start again. When an infant has an irregular sucking pattern, it becomes very difficult to use sucking to assess hearing. Some infants, because of serious medical conditions, will be fed with a gastrointestinal tube. If the infant uses a pacifier, it may still be possible to test hearing by measuring nonnutritive sucking responses. However, if the infant does not use a pacifier, it will not be possible to measure hearing using a sucking technique.

Are there concerns about the infant's neurologic status that could affect testing? For example, is the child alert to the environment? A baby may indicate visual and tactile awareness by making postural changes and meaningful eye-gaze to people and environmental events. In a visually alert baby, lack of response to sound is strongly suggestive of a true hearing loss. However, if the infant is not alert to visual or tactile stimuli, an inability to respond to auditory stimuli may not be an indication of hearing loss.

Adding Objectivity to Behavioral Observation Audiometry

The Test Setting

Infant State and Positioning

Monitor the infant's state to increase the likelihood that it will be possible to accurately observe responses. State refers to the infant's level of arousal, from deep sleep to hysterical crying (**Fig. 6–3**).

Movement of Test Assistant and Parent/Caregiver

Everyone in the test room with the child must

- be still and nonresponsive to the test stimuli
- keep the infant focused at midline
- be reminded not to respond to the stimulus by altering the movement of the toy or facial expressions

Test Stimuli and Response

The most critical element in obtaining reliable responses is to predetermine what will constitute a response (Flexer and Gans, 1986; Madell, 1998; Widen, 1993). If it has been decided that sucking is the acceptable response, the audiologist should not then also accept eye widening or a head turn

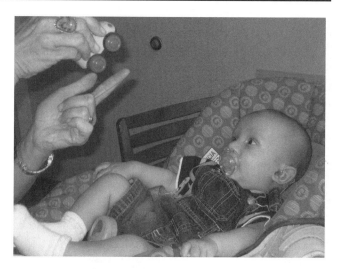

Figure 6–3 Position of infant for observation audiometry.

as a response. Changing response criteria during testing runs the risk of accepting behaviors as responses that are not actually responses. The response must be time-locked to the presentation of the stimulus. All of the infant's responses must be repeatable. The use of multiple observers to determine if a response is present also will increase reliability, as will the use of silent controls (Gravel and McCaughey, 2004).

Comparison of Behavioral Observation Audiometry Thresholds to VRA, CPA, and ABR

By carefully following the sucking test protocols detailed in this chapter, and observed on the accompanying DVD, observation responses can be used to obtain reliable thresholds. **Figs. 6–4A–D** are typical of many multiple audiograms which demonstrate that thresholds can be obtained accurately by using BOA. These audiograms make the best possible case for the reliability of the BOA sucking technique by comparing thresholds obtained with BOA, VRA, and play audiometry over several years on four children. Work is currently being conducted at our center on infants referred for hearing evaluation after failing newborn hearing screening or referred by parents because of family history or concern about the infants' responses to sound. Results indicate that BOA, appropriately conducted, using the sucking paradigm discussed in this chapter, can accurately identify hearing levels in infants when compared to ABR thresholds.

Developing Comfort Using Behavioral Observation Audiometry

Clinicians who are comfortable using ABR to assess infants may want to add BOA to their protocol to gain experience with the technique before making behavioral testing a regular part of clinical practice. As with most other skills, it

PURE TONE AUDIOMETRY (RE ANSI - 1969) / FREQUENCY IN Hz

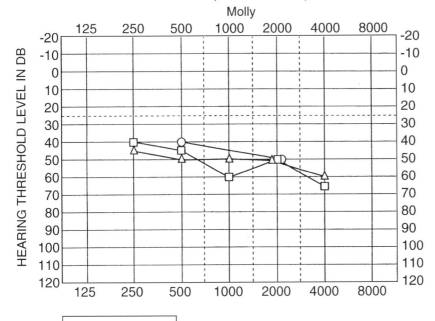

A

PURE TONE AUDIOMETRY (RE ANSI - 1969) / FREQUENCY IN Hz

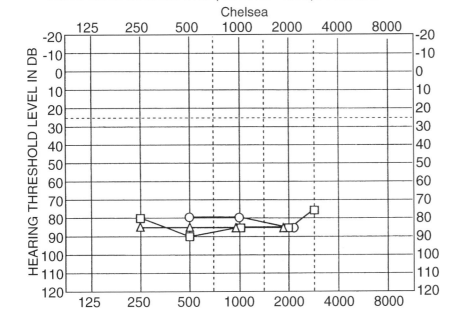

B

Figure 6–4 (A–D) Comparison of thresholds with behavioral observation (BOA), visual reinforcement (VRA), and play audiometry.

(Continued)

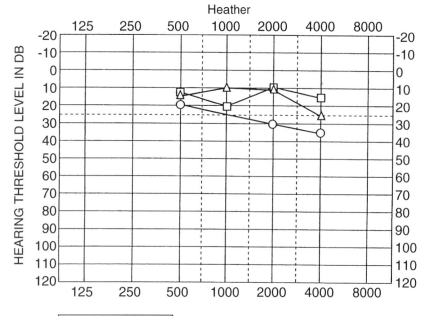

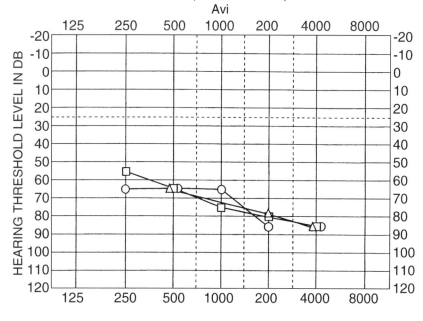

Figure 6–4 *(Continued)* **(A–D)**

takes experience to become a competent tester when using the BOA sucking paradigm detailed in this chapter. It is important to be certain that the test situation is appropriately organized so as to maximize the ability to observe changes in sucking. The clinicians should have good communication with each other to enable them to share information during testing. All infant responses should be repeatable. Viewing the DVD that accompanies this book will be helpful in developing the necessary BOA skills.

Discussion Topics

1. Discuss why behavioral observation audiometry has not been considered a good clinical tool in the past.

2. Discuss why sucking is a more reliable threshold response when testing infants.

3. Discuss ways to maximize objectivity in BOA.

References

Apuzzo, M. L., and Yoshinaga-Itana, C. (1995). Early identification of infants with significant hearing loss and the Minnesota Child Development Inventory. Seminars in Hearing, 16, 124–139.

American Speech-Language-Hearing Association. (2004). Guidelines for the Audiologic Assessment of Children from Birth to 5 Years of Age. www.asha.org/members/deskref-journals/deskref/default.

Berg, K. M., and Smith, M. C. (1983). Behavioral thresholds of tones during infancy. Journal of Experimental Child Psychology, 35, 409–425.

Bess, F. H., and Humes, L. E. (2003). Audiology: the fundamentals. 3rd ed. Philadelphia: Lippincott Williams & Wilkins.

Bove, C., and Flugrath, J. M. (1973). Frequency components of noisemakers for use in pediatric audiological evaluations. Volta Review 75, 551–556.

Delaroche, M., Thiebaut, R., and Dauman, R. (2004). Behavioral audiometry: protocols for measuring hearing thresholds in babies aged 4–18 months. International Journal of Pediatric Otorhinolaryngology, 68, 1233–1243.

Downs, M. P., and Sterritt, G. M. (1964). Identification audiometry for neonates: a preliminary report. Journal of Auditory Research, 4, 69–80.

Downs, M. P., and Sterritt, G. M. (1967). A guide to newborn and infants hearing screening. Archives of Otolaryngology, 85, 15–22.

Eisele, W. A., Berry, R. C., and Shriner, T. H. (1975). Infant sucking response patterns as a conjugate function of change in the sound pressure level of auditory stimuli. Journal of Speech and Hearing Research 18, 296–307.

Eisenberg, R. B. (1969). Auditory behavior in the human neonate: functional properties of sound and their ontogenetic implications. International Audiology, 8, 34–45.

Ewing, J. R., and Ewing, A. W. G. (1940). Discussion on audiometric tests and the capacity to hear speech. Journal of Laryngology and Otology, 55, 339–355.

Ewing, J. R., and Ewing, A. W. G. (1944). The ascertainment of deafness in infancy and early childhood. Journal of Laryngology and Otology, 54, 309–333.

Flasher, L. V., and Fogel, P. T. (2004). Counseling skills for speech-language pathologists and audiologists. Clifton Park, NY: Delmar Learning.

Flexer, C., and Gans, D. P. (1986). Distribution of auditory response behaviors in normal infants and profoundly multihandicapped children. Journal of Speech and Hearing Research, 29, 425–429.

Frisina, R. (1963), Measurement of hearing in children. In J.F. Jerger, (Ed.), Modern developments in audiology, New York: Academic.

Froeschels, E., and Beebe, H. (1946). Testing the hearing of the newborn. Archives of Otolaryngology, 44, 710–714.

Gerber, S. E. (1977). *Audiometry in Infancy*. New York: Grune and Stratton.

Gravel, J. (2000) Audiologic assessment for the fitting of hearing instruments: big challenges from tiny ears. In R. Seewald (Ed) A sound foundation through early amplification. Proceedings of an International Conference, Vanderbilt-Bill Wilkerson Press, Phonak, AG, Nashville, TN, 2000, pp. 33–46.

Gravel, J. S., and McCaughey, C. C. (2004). Family-centered audiologic assessment for infants and young children with hearing loss. Seminars in Hearing, 25, 309–317.

Hicks, C. B., Tharpe, A. M., and Ashmead, D. H. (2000). Behavioral auditory assessment of young infants: methodological limitations or natural lack of auditory responsiveness? American Journal of Audiology, 9, 124–130.

Jerger, J. F., and Hayes, D. (1976). The cross-check principle in pediatric audiometry. Archives of Otolaryngology, 102, 614–620.

Ling, D. (2002). Speech and the hearing impaired child. (2nd ed.) Washington, DC: Alexander Graham Bell Association of the Deaf and Hard of Hearing.

Madell, J. R. (1988). Identification and treatment of very young children with hearing loss. Infants and Young Children, 1, 20–30.

Madell, J. R. (1995a). Behavioral evaluation of infants after hearing screening: Can it be done? Hearing Instruments, 12, 4–8.

Madell, J. R. (1995b). Speech audiometry for children. In S.E. Gerber (Ed.) Pediatric audiology (pp. 84–103). Washington, DC: Gallaudet University Press.

Madell, J. R. (1998). Behavioral evaluation of hearing in infants and young children. New York: Thieme.

McConnell, F., and Ward, P. (1967). Deafness in childhood. Nashville: Vanderbilt University Press.

Mencher, G. T., McCullouch, B., Derbyshire, A.J ., and Dethlefs, R. (1977). Observer bias as a factor in neonatal hearing screening. Journal of Speech and Hearing Research, 20, 27–34.

Muir, D. W., Clifton, R. K, and Clarkson, M. G. (1989). The development of a human auditory localization response: a U-shaped function. Canadian Journal of Psychology, 43, 199–216.

Northern, J., and Downs, M. (1974). Hearing in children. Baltimore: Williams and Wilkins.

Northern J., and Downs, M. (1984). Hearing in children. Baltimore: Williams and Wilkins.

Northern, J., and Downs, M. (1991). Hearing in children. 4th ed. Baltimore: Williams and Wilkins.

Northern, J. L., and Downs, M. P. (2002). Hearing in children. 5th ed. Baltimore: Lippincott Williams & Wilkins.

Nozza, R. (2006). Developmental psychoacoustics: auditory function in infants and children. Paper presented at the 4th Widex Congress of Paediatric Audiology, Ottawa, Canada, May 19–21, 2006.

Olsho, L. W. (1984). Infant frequency discrimination. Infant Behavior and Development, 7, 27–35.

Olsho, L. W., Koch, E. G, Halpin, C. F., and Carter, E.A. (1987a). An observer-based psychoacoustic procedure for use with young infants. Developmental Psychology, 23, 627–640.

Olsho, L. W., Koch, E. G., and Halpin, C. F. (1987b). Level and age effects in infant frequency discrimination. Journal of the Acoustical Society of America, 82, 454–464.

Olsho, L. W., Koch, E. G., Carter, E. A., Halpin, C. F., and Spetner, N. B. (1988). Pure tone sensitivity of human infants. Journal of the Acoustical Society of America, 84, 1316–1324.

Poblano, A., Chayo, I., Ibarra, J., and Reuda, E. (2000). Electrophysiological and behavioral methods in early detection of hearing impairment. Archives of Medical Research, 31, 75–80.

Sharma, A., Dorman, M. F., and Spahr, A. J. (2002). A sensitive period for the development of the central auditory system in children with cochlear implants: implications for age of implantation. Ear and Hearing, 23, 532–539.

Sininger, Y. S. (1993). Evaluation of hearing in the neonate using the auditory brainstem response. Consensus Development Conference on Early Identification of Hearing impairment in Infants and Young Children, (pp. 95–97). Bethesda: National Institutes of Health.

Thompson, M., and Thompson, F. (1972). Response of infants and young children as a function of auditory stimuli and test method. Journal of Speech and Hearing Research, 15, 699-707.

Weber, B. A. (1969). Validation of observer judgments in behavioral observation audiometry. Journal of Speech and Hearing Research, 34, 350–355.

Wedenberg, E. (1956). Auditory tests on newborn infants. Acta Otolaryngologica, 46, 446–461.

Werner, L., and Gillenwater, J. (1990). Pure tone sensitivity of 2-5 week old infants. Infant Behavior and Development, 13, 355–375.

White, K. R., Maxon, A. B., Behrens, T. B., Blackwell, P. M., and Vohr, B. R. (1992). Neonatal screening using evoked otoacoustic emissions: the Rhode Island hearing assessment project. In F. H. Bess and J. W. Hall III (Eds). Screening children for auditory function. Nashville: Bill Wilkerson Center Press.

White, K. R., Vohr, B. R., and Behrens, T. B. (1993). Universal newborn screening using transient evoked otoacoustic emissions: results of the Rhode Island hearing assessment project. Seminars in Hearing, 14, 18–29.

Widen, J. E. (1993). Adding objectivity to infant behavioral audiometry. Ear and Hearing, 14, 49–57.

Widen, J. E., and Keener, S. (2003) Diagnostic testing for hearing loss in infants and young children. Mental Retardation and Developmental Disabilities Research Reviews, 9, 220–224.

Yoshinaga-Itana, C, Couter, D., and Thomson, V. (2001) Developmental outcomes of children with hearing loss born in Colorado hospitals with and without universal newborn hearing screening programs. Seminars in Neonatology, 6, 521–529.

Chapter 7

Using Visual Reinforcement Audiometry to Evaluate Hearing in Infants from 5 to 36 Months

Jane R. Madell

♦ **Test Protocols**

    Visual Reinforcement Audiometry

    Conditioning Orienting Response Audiometry

♦ **Visual Reinforcers**

♦ **Positioning the Infant or Child**

♦ **Distractors**

♦ **The Test Assistant**

♦ **Training and Conditioning the Response**

♦ **Testing**

    Test Room Setup

    Positioning

    Beginning Testing

    Conditioning Children with Very Profound Hearing Loss

    Frequency of Reinforcing the Response

    Test Stimuli

    Test Conditions

    Test Order

    Frequency-Specific Stimuli

    Enticing a Child to Wear Earphones

    Stimuli Presentation

    What Is Normal Hearing?

♦ **Summary of Factors That Affect Test Results**

Key Points

- Once infants reach 5 to 6 months of age, most can be conditioned to make a head turn response to the presence of an auditory stimulus.

- Positioning is critical. The infant should be seated to maximize torso control. If the child is having a problem sitting upright and balancing, it will be difficult to make a head turn.

- Reinforcement should be provided only when it is certain that the child is responding to the stimulus. Turning on the reinforcing toy when the child has not heard the sound will decrease the reliability of conditioning.

- Visual reinforcement audiometry (VRA) can be used to test children using earphones, the bone conduction transducer, hearing aids, cochlear implants, and FM systems.

Behavioral methods are the first choice for diagnostic testing of auditory function because they provide the most information about an infant's ability to use hearing. Once infants reach 5 to 6 months of age, behavioral testing becomes much easier to accomplish because infants can be conditioned to respond to sound (ASHA 2004). The most common test techniques involve training the infant to make a conditioned head turn in response to a test stimulus. Infants only a few months of age will naturally turn toward a sound source. Most infants will turn toward the sound source a few times, but the head turning behavior will habituate to repeated stimuli. Fortunately, this head turning behavior can be shaped using an operant discrimination procedure that permits obtaining numerous responses to auditory stimuli. The sound stimulus is used to cue the child to seek the visual reinforcement. Use of a positive reinforcement such as a lighted toy or short video clip will increase the number of responses. Conditioned responses have the advantage of being more repeatable then unconditioned responses, and more responses usually can be obtained during one sitting.

Several visual conditioning techniques have been used. VRA (Linden and Kankkunen, 1969) and conditioned orienting response (COR) (Suzuki and Ogiba, 1960) are the most commonly used protocols. VRA uses a conditioned head turn reinforced by a lighted toy. COR requires that the infant localize the sound source before reinforcement with a lighted toy, and reinforcement is provided only if the child turns toward the correct side.

to the correct side. Standard hearing testing requires only the ability to identify if a sound is present. It does not require that the listener identify where the sound is coming from. Young babies may have a difficult time determining which way to turn, but older babies and children will be able to do the task. The ability to localize a sound close to threshold can be difficult for anybody.

♦ Test Protocols

Visual Reinforcement Audiometry

VRA is the most commonly used reinforcement procedure. It is used to evaluate hearing in children who are cognitively between 5 to 6 months and 36 months of age. It uses a conditioned head turning response that is shaped by the examiner's control of a stimulus-reinforcement paradigm. The foundation for VRA was laid by Suzuki and Ogiba in work published in 1960. The term was first used by Liden and Kankkunen in 1969. The technique was refined by Wilson and Thomson (1984), and Moore, Wilson, and Thompson (1975, 1977 and in numerous other publications between 1977 and 1984. The audiologist presents a stimulus. If the child detects the stimulus, she will turn toward it. The audiologist then activates a reinforcer. After a few repetitions, the child learns to seek the reinforcer when she hears the sound (Primus and Thompson, 1985; Primus, 1987).

Conditioning Orienting Response Audiometry

COR testing, originally described by Suzuki and Ogiba (1960) uses the same conditioning techniques as VRA. Sound may be presented from either the right or left loudspeakers, but the child will be reinforced only when turning

♦ Visual Reinforcers

A variety of toys are available for use as reinforcers. Moore, Thompson, and Thompson (1975) investigated use of different reinforcers and their effect on responses. They compared no reinforcement, social reinforcement, blinking lights, and complex visual reinforcement, and concluded that the complex reinforcement resulted in significantly more localizations than did simple reinforcers. The best reinforcers are novel and interesting. Mechanical toys that are brightly illuminated such as clowns that play drums, dogs that bark, or elephants that eat ice cream cones are excellent.

The reinforcer should be enclosed in a cloudy lucite box so it is not easily observable until it is turned on. Stacking two or three toys on top of each other in individual lucite boxes permits the audiologist to vary the reinforcer and increase the novelty, thereby increasing the length of time a child will attend to the task (**Fig. 7–1**). Most VRA systems permit turning on the sound and lights separately or together. This on-off switch is particularly useful when a child is frightened by the noise made by the reinforcing toy. Occasionally, children react negatively to the reinforcers. Some children are frightened by the sound or the movement. If the sound is the problem, it can be turned off and the lights can be used alone. If the movement is a problem, the toy can be held still and a light can be flashed on and off as a reinforcer. If the

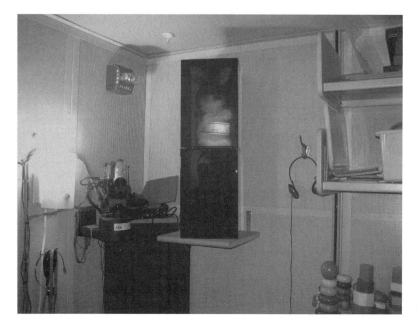

Figure 7–1   VRA toys.

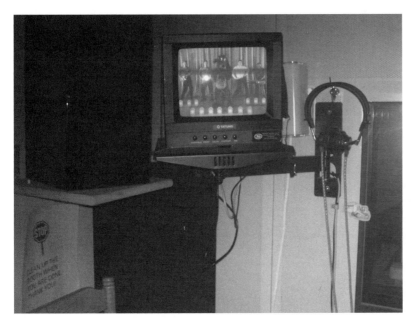

Figure 7–2   Video VRA.

child is disturbed by the toys regardless of whether or not they are making noise, there are two alternatives. One is to use video clips as the reinforcer using a small TV and a DVD player, and the second is to darken the tests room and shine a flashlight through the test room window as a reinforcer. The light can either flash on and off or can be waved around in circles. A head turn toward the tester's window will be used to determine a response. (If this protocol is going to be used, the test room will usually need to be reorganized so the child is seated facing away from the test room window.)

For older children, or children who are no longer interested in the VRA toys, a cartoon video works particularly well as a reinforcer (**Fig. 7–2**). The TV sound should be off so as not to interfere with test stimuli. Because the video is constantly changing, it will be of ongoing interest. A small TV monitor can be placed above the loudspeaker with the VCR or DVD player on the tester's side of the booth. The audiologist can activate the video in the same way as a mechanical toy.

◆ Positioning the Infant or Child

A critical factor for obtaining reliable VRA thresholds is the ability to keep the infant's or child's attention focused at midline in a position that easily permits a head turn. Proper positioning is critical. The child needs to be seated comfortably so that the upper body is steady and allows the infant or child to turn easily to look at the toy. The child should not be leaning over trying to get something from the floor, trying to maintain balance, or looking for something or someone seated behind. Older children with very good body control may be able to make a head turn of 180 degrees to look for the reinforcer, but a young or neurologically impaired child will not. For these children, a head turn of more than 90 degrees is very difficult and may

significantly reduce their ability to respond, and so it is critical that the children be carefully focused at midline (**Fig. 7–3**).

An infant who does not yet have good upper body control because of young age or neurologic or developmental concerns, and does not sit comfortably, will have difficulty making a head turning response. Positioning for these children will be especially critical. A child without good upper body control should be seated leaning back in a reclining seat or leaning against a parent so that she does not need to struggle to maintain position. This position will leave the infant with enough energy to make a head turn toward the reinforcer.

> **Pearl**
>
> - Positioning is critical. The infant needs to be seated so that she can easily make a conditioned head turn. If the child does not sit up easily, she should be positioned in a reclining position, leaning back against someone or in a reclining chair, so she does not need energy to control her torso.

◆ Distractors

A variety of toys can be useful as distractors. They should be quiet, simple, and interesting but not engrossing. Colorful toys, puppets, finger games, stacking toys, toys with pieces that connect, magnets on a magnet board or on the test room wall, or making funny faces will keep the infant focused straight ahead so that a clear head turn can be observed. Young children should view the toys being manipulated by the test assistant but should not manipulate

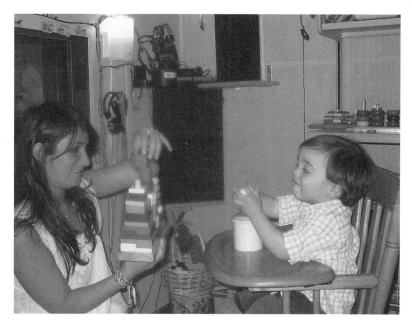

Figure 7–3 Positioning for VRA.

them, since this will likely be too distracting. Older children may be able to manipulate some toys as long as they are not too interesting or require too much concentration. Edible distractions are frequently very useful, provided they are not too noisy. (Crunchy food will interfere with listening, and food that takes too long to swallow can significantly extend test time and interfere with the flow of testing.)

◆ The Test Assistant

Accurate VRA depends on the ability of the examiner or test assistant to keep the child attentive. An audiologist, test assistant, or parent needs to be responsible for keeping the infant facing forward. The test room should not be cluttered. Toys that are not being used should be out of view so that the infant will not be distracted by anything except the adult who is keeping the child focused. (See Chapter 12 for more information about the test assistant's responsibilities.)

The test assistant may be an audiologist, an audiology student, or an audiology assistant. An experienced test assistant will make testing most efficient. When a test assistant is not available, parents or caregivers can often be very good at this task. With limited instruction they can frequently do this job very well, especially with typically developing children. They know their children well and know how to entertain them. If a parent is going to have the responsibility of distracting the child, she needs to be told to be relatively quiet so as not to interfere with presentation of test stimuli. Even more critical, she must understand that she must not react to the sound in any way that might cue the child. Instructions for the parent or the test assistant should include:

- Don't respond to the sound.
- Don't look at the reinforcement toy until after the child does.
- Don't change your body language when the sound is presented.
- Don't alter the way you are playing with the toys when the sound is presented.
- Act "deaf" to the sound.

◆ Training and Conditioning the Response

The VRA procedure involves two distinct phases. The first is the training/conditioning phase, where the baby or toddler is conditioned to respond to the visual reinforcer. The second is the testing phase, during which thresholds are obtained once the baby is conditioned.

Operant behavior is willful behavior elicited by a stimulus and controlled by the behavior that is increased or decreased by changes in the environment (Diefendorf and Gravel, 1996; Gravel, 2000). In VRA or COR the head turning response is increased by the positive reinforcement of the reinforcing toy. There are two approaches to training the response. The first is to pair the stimulus with the reinforcer, turning both on at the same time. The child will frequently turn to the reinforcing toy and learn the task. If the child looks up but does not turn, the audiologist can attract the child's attention to the reinforcer. The second is to begin by observing the child's response and then providing a reinforcer when the child naturally turns to the sound. During the training/conditioning phase, the stimulus should always be presented at an intensity that the audiologist is sure the child can hear, and every correct head turn should be reinforced. If the reinforcer is activated when there is no stimulus or when the child cannot hear the stimulus, the infant will not be able to make the association between the sound and the reinforcer and will only be confused. If there is any question at all about whether or not the child heard the stimulus, the reinforcer should not be activated. Training/conditioning is considered complete when the infant consistently turns when a stimulus is presented, and when there are very few random head turns.

◆ Testing

Once the infant or child is conditioned to the visual reinforcer, the testing phase can begin.

Test Room Setup

It is usually best to begin testing in soundfield. Inserting earphones may be stressful to the child and reduce cooperation. Beginning testing in soundfield will provide basic information about hearing, and once that is obtained, testing can proceed with earphones or with the bone vibrator. By then the child will be more comfortable in the test situation and may be more willing to accept earphones.

To perform soundfield testing, the test room needs to be large enough to be able to have loudspeakers set up at a sufficient angle and distance from the infant to permit an obvious head turn. If the room is too small, the loudspeakers and reinforcing toy may be within the child's line of sight, making it difficult to see a change in head position. Since the response we are seeking is a conditioned head turn, the child should be seated at no less than a 45-degree angle from the loudspeakers and reinforcer, and preferably at 90 degrees (**see Fig. 7–3** and **Fig. 7–4**). The reinforcing toy should not be in the child's line of sight when she is facing forward. The test setup needs to be such that there is no doubt as to whether or not the infant made a head turn, rather than a casual gaze toward the toy. When performing VRA, the sound is usually presented from one loudspeaker, and the reinforcing toys are on the side of the loudspeaker. No matter whether the child hears the sound in the right or left ears, she will turn toward the same toy.

Positioning

Ideally the child should be seated in a highchair and not on a parent's lap. If the child is on someone's lap, the adult may respond to the sound and inadvertently give a cue to the child. If the child must sit on an adult's lap because she will not sit alone or does not have sufficient torso control to sit alone, the adult needs to be instructed not to respond in any way to the presentation of the sound stimulus. Noise-canceling earphones can be used to keep the adult from responding to the sound stimulus. However, the use of earphones may make it very difficult for the adult to interact with the infant, which may make both the infant and the adult uncomfortable. Most parents are capable of sitting still and not responding when the reason is made clear to them. In addition, parents usually prefer to hear what their child is hearing so that they can better understand the test results.

Beginning Testing

If a child has anything less than severe or profound hearing loss, it should be relatively easy to get an initial response. The child should be seated in the high chair or on a parent's lap and facing forward. The room does not need to be silent, but it should be relatively quiet. The audiologist begins by presenting stimuli at a level at which the child is expected to respond. If the child hears the sound, she will likely look up from the toy and search for the sound source. If there is no response, the audiologist increases the intensity until there is a response. Once a response is obtained, the reinforcer is turned on. If the infant looks up but does not turn to the reinforcer, the test assistant should attract the child's attention to the reinforcer. When this has been done a few times, the infant will usually have learned the task and testing can begin. Before attracting the child's attention to the reinforcer, it is *essential* that the audiologist be absolutely certain that the child heard the sound. **Figure 7–4** shows a child making a conditioned head turn to the VRA toy.

Conditioning Children with Very Profound Hearing Loss

Children with severe to profound hearing loss, or with auditory attention or auditory processing problems, may not have the ability to localize to sound. For these children in particular, it will be necessary to pair the stimulus with the sound and teach the child to seek the reinforcer. If the child does not respond to even very loud sounds, it may be useful to train the child to respond to a tactile stimulus, since even a child with no usable hearing will be able to feel the bone vibrator. Place a bone vibrator in the child's hand or on the knee and have the test assistant or parent hold it in place. The sound or vibration is then paired with the reinforcer and the child is conditioned to that stimulus. After the child responds consistently to a tactile stimulus, return to an air-conducted stimulus in soundfield or under earphones and try again. Sometimes pairing the tactile stimulus with an auditory stimulus will assist in training the response. If the reason for lack of response is severity of hearing loss, it is essential that the infant accept earphones because earphone signals can almost always be presented at a louder intensity than those from loudspeakers (**Fig. 7–5**).

The intensity of the initial test stimuli is important. Ideally the stimulus should be presented slightly above threshold but not too much above threshold. Several researchers (Eilers et al, 1991; Gravel, 2000; Tharpe and Ashmead, 1993) have demonstrated that the starting level influences false responses. The louder the starting intensity, the greater the false response rate. Wilson and Moore (1978) and Wilson, Moore, and Thompson (1976) demonstrated that once a child is conditioned for VRA, responses do not vary as a

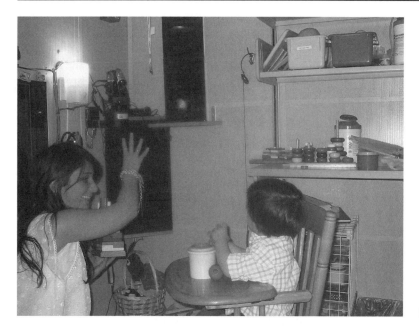

Figure 7–4   Turning toward reinforcer.

function of age. Data from 6- to 7-month-olds and 11- to 13-month-olds indicated that thresholds did not vary by age.

Frequency of Reinforcing the Response

The tendency of most testers is to reinforce every response the child makes in the effort to be sure to condition the response. The anxiety to be sure to reinforce every appropriate response can occasionally result in the audiologist providing reinforcement when, in fact, the infant has not really provided a head turn and may not have heard the stimulus. This will confuse the child and reduce response reliability. In addition, frequent reinforcement will cause more rapid habituation of the response. Research on behavioral conditioning has demonstrated that intermittent reinforcement is more reliable than constant reinforcement and provides more responses. The best reinforcement schedule begins with 100% reinforcement, and decreases to less frequent

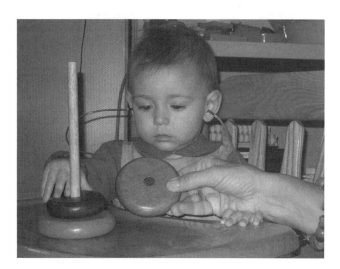

Figure 7–5   Infant with insert earphones.

reinforcement. Occasionally failing to reinforce the response will increase the total number of responses the infant is likely to provide in any individual test session. If there is any question about whether or not the child heard the stimulus, the reinforcer should not be activated. The rule is "If in doubt, don't." Nothing is lost by failing to reinforce when a stimulus is present, but a great deal may be lost by reinforcing when the infant does not hear a stimulus.

Pitfall

- If in doubt—don't. It is critical that the reinforcer be turned on only when the child has made an appropriate head turn. If the reinforcer is turned on when the child has not heard a sound, the child becomes confused and response reliability is decreased.

Test Stimuli

Any test stimulus used in behavioral testing can be used with VRA or COR. Speech stimuli are frequently used as the initial test stimulus with children because they are familiar and are likely to get their attention. Any speech stimulus can be used to obtain a speech awareness threshold. To obtain frequency specific speech information, it will be necessary to use low, mid-high, and highfrequency stimuli (such as *ba*, *sh*, and *s*), which will be in agreement with pure tone thresholds at low, mid-high, and highfrequency stimuli. Using a broad band stimulus such as music or running speech (e.g., Hello Jody, how are you today?) will provide a threshold that is in agreement with the softest pure tone threshold, (See Chapter 10 for more information about speech audiometry with children.)

To obtain a complete audiogram, thresholds are needed at several if not all frequencies. Although pure tones are usually the stimulus of choice, other stimuli are also very useful and may be helpful in obtaining a complete audiogram. Narrow band noise may be more interesting to infants and young children and may hold their attention longer than pure tones. Alternating between pure tones, warble tones, and narrow noise bands may also increase interest and the number of repeatable responses. Narrow band noise stimuli are easier for young infants to respond to than to warble tone or pure tone stimuli (Gravel, 2000). Noise band thresholds may be 5 to 10 dB softer than those obtained with pure tones; this needs to be taken into consideration when evaluating the responses. For soundfield testing, noise bands or warbled pure tones are the stimuli of choice.

Test Conditions

Visual reinforcement audiometry can be reliably used in all test conditions required for the evaluation of hearing in infants and young children. Testing can be accomplished in soundfield, with insert earphones, with circumaural earphones, with a bone vibrator, and with technology (hearing aids, cochlear implants, or FM systems). These conditions will permit us to obtain almost all required audiologic information.

Test Order

Some audiologists begin every evaluation with immittance testing. Although there is no doubt about the usefulness of this procedure, it is important to take the child into consideration when selecting tests and test order. An infant who is frightened of the test facility or the tester may be very distressed by having a stranger come up to him to place an immittance probe in the ear at the beginning of the evaluation. If you proceed to do the test and the child becomes very distressed, the rest of the testing may be difficult or impossible to accomplish. If the child seems distressed or even wary, it may be better to wait until the end of the session for immittance testing.

The same case can be made for the decision as to whether to begin testing using earphones or soundfield. No doubt earphone testing is the goal, but it may be better to get some information in soundfield before presenting earphones. When testing very young children, it is useful to assume that each response may be the last one obtained. Therefore, it is very important to think carefully about the order of testing. If earphones are tried first and the child becomes upset and gives

only one reliable response, very little information is obtained. However, if the child is kept happy by starting in soundfield and thresholds are obtained at 500 and 2000 Hz, something is known about her hearing even if testing has to stop at that point. Day et al (2000) tested typically developing infants both in soundfield and with insert earphones and demonstrated that significantly more responses were obtained for soundfield testing than for insert earphone testing.

Frequency-Specific Stimuli

Using the theory that each threshold obtained may be the last requires good planning when testing. After beginning at 500 Hz or 2000 Hz, depending on whether there is concern about conductive hearing loss (CHL) or sensorineural hearing loss (SNHL), a decision must be made about how to proceed. If the concern is for CHL, begin testing at 2000 Hz in each ear, and then go to 500 Hz since for most patients with CHL hearing will be better at high frequencies, facilitating conditioning. If the concern is that the infant or child may have SNHL, begin at 500 Hz, then proceed directly to 2000 Hz, since for most patients with SNHL, hearing is better in the low frequencies. Depending on the contour of the partial audiogram and the cooperativeness of the child, decide if it would be better to proceed with 4000 Hz, 1000 Hz, 250 Hz, bone conduction, or earphones. If there is a significant difference between the thresholds at 500 and 2000 Hz, it will be critical to test 1000 Hz before proceeding to other frequencies to obtain a good picture of the audiometric contour. If the audiogram is fairly flat, the 1000 Hz threshold may be left to last and can frequently be estimated from the rest of the thresholds if time is limited or the child stops cooperating. If soundfield testing indicates hearing loss, bone conduction testing might be selected as the next test procedure to determine whether hearing loss is conductive or sensorineural. If it is not possible to obtain bone conduction thresholds, either because the child can no longer attend or because it is not possible to get the child to accept the bone oscillator, immittance may provide sufficient information to begin a plan of treatment. If the child is still cooperative, earphone testing should be attempted. No child should be dismissed from audiologic follow-up until earphone testing has been accomplished (**see Table 7–1**).

Table 7–1   Protocol for Visual Reinforcement Audiometry

1. Seat child in high chair, in a child's chair, or on a parent's lap
2. The test assistant or parent keeps child's attention focused front using quiet toys
3. The auditory stimulus is presented at comfortably loud level above expected threshold. The conditioning/reinforcing toy is turned on and, if the child does not turn, the test assistant calls attention to the toy. The auditory stimulus and the conditioning toy are kept on together for 3–4 seconds
4. Step 3 is repeated until the child consistently turns to the auditory stimulus.
5. When the child is conditioned to respond, the auditory stimulus is presented without turning on the conditioning/reinforcing toy. If the child turns toward the sound, the reinforcing toy is turned on and conditioning is complete.
6. Testing proceeds obtaining thresholds for one low (500 Hz) and one high (2000 Hz) frequency stimulus. The stimulus is decreased until the child stops responding, and is then increased to bracket threshold.
7. Additional frequencies to be tested will be determined by the responses to the initial frequencies tested.
8. Testing proceeds using insert earphones, bone vibrator, and technology (hearing aids, cochlear implants, and FM systems.)
9. The reinforcing toy is turned on only when the child make a conditioned head turn in response to a sound. When in doubt, do not turn on the reinforcer.

Enticing a Child to Wear Earphones

Enticing a young child to wear earphones can be a little tricky, but is usually possible. Start by having the test assistant wear the earphones, then the parents, and then offer them to the child. If the child refuses at first, let everyone have another turn, and then offer the earphones to the child once more. If she stills refuses, it is important to make a judgment about how serious the refusal is. If the protest is minimal, try pushing the matter. Someone needs to keep the child occupied with a toy while someone else puts the earphones on. Frequently, once the child hears a sound or music and can observe the reinforcer, the resistance will stop or at least be reduced to a low enough level to permit testing to proceed. If it doesn't, and the child starts to become very upset, it may be better to hold off and try again at a later date, or try different earphones (inserts versus circumaural), or try a handheld circumaural earphone at the child's ear. Circumaural earphones are easy to put on and can frequently be put in place in a couple of seconds. However, they can be heavy for a little head, making it difficult for the baby or toddler to turn toward the reinforcer, and they can fall off with movement. In addition, positioning of the headphones is critical for obtaining accurate thresholds, especially in high frequencies. Insert earphones are more comfortable to wear because they are very lightweight and, because they are always well positioned, may provide more accurate thresholds, but they take more effort to insert. If after really trying, the child will not accept earphones, ask the parents to try to persuade the child to accept earphones at home. It is sometimes easy to persuade a child to accept earphones by having the parents plug earphones into the TV at home, and not allowing the child to watch videos or TV without wearing the earphones. In a few days the child will be wearing them consistently at home, and once she wears them at home there should be no problem persuading him to wear them in the clinic.

If testing can be performed using a combination of loudspeakers, earphones, and bone conduction transducers, consider testing different frequencies with each transducer. The combination of information can provide a fairly complete picture of the child's hearing (**Fig. 7–6**).

Stimuli Presentation

When testing children, audiologists frequently feel the need to obtain many responses at one intensity before recording thresholds. This is understandable, but may significantly reduce the total number of thresholds obtained. Infants and young children will respond for only a limited time. Each presentation needs to be carefully considered. Eilers et al (1991) and Gravel (2000) used computer simulation to test

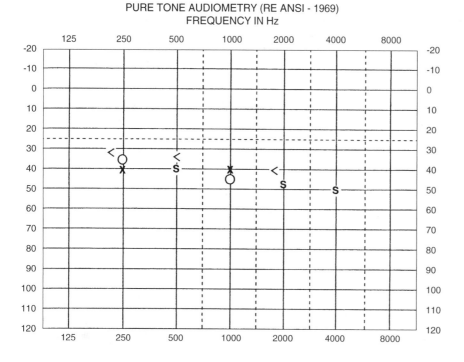

Figure 7–6 Audiogram with different information from different transducers.

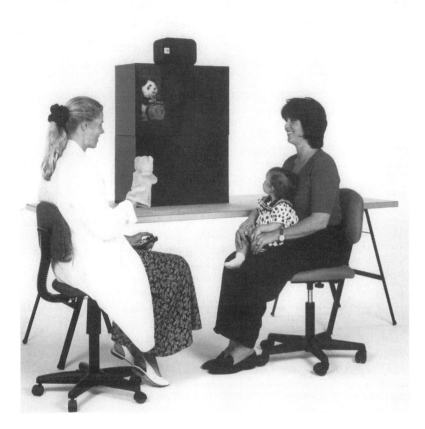

Figure 7–7   IVRA (From Intelligent Hearing Systems, Miami, FL. Reprinted with permission.)

infants and determined that more than three reversals were not useful in obtaining thresholds. There was less than a 3-dB difference when more than three reversals were obtained. So, bite the bullet and trust the responses that are observed.

A mistake that is frequently made when testing young children is related to timing of presentation of the stimulus. When testing infants, test time is limited, so there is a tendency to present stimuli too quickly. If a child is asked to make a conditioned head turn frequently, both the stimulus and the reinforcer will become uninteresting and the child will stop responding. Taking time and presenting stimuli after a longer period of silence will increase the likelihood that the stimulus is interesting, causing the child to look up. On the other hand, having a very extended "off" period can also have a negative effect. The correct timing will vary from child to child.

In the attempt to eliminate tester bias in recording responses, a computer-controlled test protocol was developed by Widen (1984; 1990). The technique uses only one examiner who is in the test room with the child. When the examiner determines that the child is centered, a button is pushed, which calls for a trial. The examiner votes as to whether the child makes a head turn during the predetermined response interval. The software determines if a sound is present during the interval. If a sound

is present and the examiner records a response, the software provides the reinforcement. The determination about signal level and type is determined by the software (**Fig. 7–7**).

What Is Normal Hearing?

There has been much discussion about what is considered normal hearing in infants. Early data (Primus, 1991) indicated that normally hearing infants did not respond to sound until it was at about 60 dBHL. Several other studies (Berg and Smith, 1983; Diefendorf and Gravel, 1996; Gravel, 2000, Madell, 1995, 1998; Sinnott, Pisoni, and Aslin, 1983; Widen et al, 2000, Wilson et al, 1976, 1978; Nozza and Wilson, 1984; Olsho et al, 1988) demonstrated that infants with normal hearing respond to sound at only slightly higher than adult levels. Infant responses should be no more than 15 to 20 dB HL and by 1 year of age, children should be responding at adult levels. Widen et al (2000) demonstrated that 94% of high-risk infants have essentially normal hearing sensitivity (20 dB HL) at 1000, 2000, and 4000 Hz in both ears.

The concept of minimal response level (MRL) is useful when evaluating children. The responses we obtain may not be threshold in the way we think of thresholds for adults, but they are repeatable and reliable and may be close to true threshold.

◆ Summary of Factors That Affect Test Results

Many factors affect the reliability of test results.

- ◆ Developmental age is critical. As mentioned before, it is essential to know the child's developmental age to select the appropriate test protocol.

- ◆ Neurologic status is also critical. The child must be capable of attending and of making the appropriate physical response (in this case, a conditioned head turn.) If the child's neurologic status will not permit a head turn, the test will not be valid.

- ◆ Behavioral status is also important. If a child is very fussy or uncomfortable, it may not be possible to elicit the best results. It may be worth it to take the time to make the child comfortable (change diapers, provide food, and comfort) before proceeding with the test.

- ◆ Positioning is very important. If the child is seated in such a way as to reduce upper body control, there is very little chance that he will be able to make reliable conditioned head turns. If the neurologic status is a concern, the range of the required head turn may be limited. Requiring a head turn of more than 90 degrees will likely not be successful with many children with neurologic concerns (see Chapter 9 for a discussion of evaluating children with special needs.)

- ◆ Distractors must be interesting but not too engrossing.

- ◆ Reinforcers must be interesting and attractive.

- ◆ Parents and other adults in the test room must be careful not to be distracting and not to clue the infant as to the presence of an auditory stimulus.

- ◆ The test stimuli should be varied to keep the child's attention.

- ◆ Presentation timing of stimuli should be varied so as to be unpredictable.

For a new tester this sounds like a great deal to keep in mind, and initially it is. But with experience, controlling these factors becomes second nature. However, during any evaluation even the most experienced testers should stop when test problems arise, review what they are doing and try and think about what might be changed to improve test results. Behavioral testing is both a science and an art.

Discussion Topics

1. Describe the conditioning paradigm.

2. Discuss factors to consider in keeping a child's attention and increasing test time.

3. Discuss the reliability of VRA for obtaining audiometric thresholds

---

References

American Speech-Language-Hearing Association. (2004). Guidelines for the Audiologic Assessment of Children from Birth to 5 Years of Age. www.asha.org/members/deskref-journals/deskref/default.

Berg, K. M., and Smith, M. D. (1983). Behavioral thresholds for tones during infancy. Journal of Experimental Child Psychology, 35, 409–425.

Day, J., Bamford, J., Parry, G., Shepherd, M., and Quigley, A. (2000). Evidence of the efficacy of insert earphone and soundfield VRA with young infants. British Journal of Audiology 34:329–334.

Diefendorf, A. O., and Gravel, J. S. (1996). Behavioral Observation and Visual Reinforcement Audiometry. In Gerber, S. (Ed.), Pediatric Audiology. Washington, D.C.: Gallaudet University Press.

Eilers, R. E., Miskiel, E., Ozdamar, O., Urbano, R., and Widen, J. E. (1991). Optimization of automated hearing test algorithms: simulations using an infant response model. Ear and Hearing, 12, 191–198.

Gravel, J. S. (2000). Behavioral audiologic assessment for hearing aid fitting: big challenges from tiny ears. In R. Seewald (Ed.), A Sound Foundation through Early Amplification. Proceedings of an International Conference, Vanderbilt-Bill Wilkerson Press, Phonak, AG, Nashville, TN, 33–46.

Liden, G., and Kankkunen, A. (1969). Visual reinforcement audiometry, Acta oto-Laryngologica 67, 281–292.

Madell, J. R. (1995). Behavioral evaluation of infants after hearing screening: Can it be done? Hearing Instruments, December 4–8.

Madell, J. R. (1998). Behavioral Evaluation of Hearing in Infants and Young Children. New York: Thieme.

Moore, J. M., Thompson, G., and Thompson, M. (1975). Auditory localization of infants as a function of reinforcement conditions. Journal of Speech and Hearing Disorders, 40, 29–34.

Moore, J. M., Wilson, W.R., and Thompson, G. (1977). Visual reinforcement of head-turn responses in infants under 12 months of age. Journal of Speech and Hearing Disorders, 42, 328–334.

Nozza, R. J., and Wilson W. R. (1984). Masked and unmasked pure-tone thresholds of infants and adults: development of auditory frequency selectivity and sensitivity. Journal of Speech and Hearing Research, 27, 613–622.

Olsho, L. W., Koch, E. G., Carter, E. A., Halpin, C. F., and Spentner, N. B. (1988). Pure tone sensitivity of human infants. Journal of the Acoustical Society of America, 84, 1316–1324.

Primus, M. A., and Thompson, G. (1985). Response strength of young children in operant audiometry. Journal of Speech and Hearing Research, 28, 539–547.

Primus, M. A. (1987). Response and reinforcement in operant audiometry. Journal of Speech and Hearing Disorders, 52, 294–299.

Primus, M. A., (1991). Repeated infant thresholds in operant and nonoperant audiometric procedures. Ear and Hearing, 12, 119–122.

Sinnott, J. M., Pisoni, D. B., and Aslin, R. N. (1983.) A comparison of pure tone auditory thresholds in human infants and adults. Infant Behavior and Development 6, 3–17.

Suzuki, T., and Ogiba, Y. (1960). A technique of pure-tone audiometry for children under three years of age: conditioned orientation reflex (COR) audiometry. Revue do Laryngologie, Otologie, Rhinologie, 8, 33–45.

Tharpe, A. M., and Ashmead, D. H. (1993). Computer simulation technique for assessing pediatric auditory test protocols. Journal of the American Academy of Audiology, 4, 80–90.

Widen, J.E. (1984). Application of visual reinforcement audiometry (VRA) to high risk infants. Paper presented to Audiology Update. Pediatric Audiology, Newport, RI.

Widen, J.E. (1990). Behavioral screening of high risk infants using visual reinforcement audiometry. Seminars in Hearing, 11, 342–356.

Widen, J. E., Folsom, R. C., Cone-Wesson, B., et al. (2000). Identification of neonatal hearing impairment: hearing status at 8 to 12 months corrected age using a visual reinforcement audiometry protocol. Ear and Hearing, 21, 5, 471–488.

Wilson, W. R., and Moore J. M. (1978). Pure-tone earphone thresholds of infants utilizing visual reinforcement audiometry (VRA). Paper presented at American Speech and Hearing Association Convention, San Francisco.

Wilson, W. R., Moore, J. M., and Thompson, G. (1976). Sound-field auditory thresholds of infants utilizing visual reinforcement audiometry (VRA). Paper presented at American Speech and Hearing Association Convention, Houston, TX, 1976.

Wilson, W. R., and Thompson, G. (1984). Behavioral audiometry. In Jerger, J. (Ed.), Pediatric Audiology. San Diego: College Hill Press.

Chapter 8

Using Conditioned Play Audiometry to Test Hearing in Children Older than 2 $^1/_2$ Years

Jane R. Madell

Key Points

- Play audiometry can be successfully accomplished with children once they reach a cognitive age of about 30 months.

- By being creative, the pediatric audiologist can find tasks that keep the young child interested and sufficiently cooperative to obtain necessary testing information.

- The audiologist needs to own the responsibility for obtaining test results. If testing is not completed, the audiologist must take responsibility and say "on this day, I cannot test this child."

Play audiometry was first described by Lowell et al in 1956. Their technique provided valuable guidance for the audiologic evaluation of very young children. Audiologists have been following their protocol, with slight modifications, since that time.

As has been known for decades, once children reach a cognitive age of about 30 months they can begin to voluntarily cooperate in hearing testing. By this age, children can be taught to drop a toy in a bucket or put a ring on a ring stand when they hear a sound. If the child can be enticed to cooperate, a great deal can be learned about his hearing. The challenging task for the pediatric audiologist is to find ways to keep the young child entertained for a long enough time to complete the hearing test.

♦ Assessing the Child's Cognitive Age

As with all other behavioral test techniques, the first task is to determine the child's cognitive age. Regardless of the child's chronologic age, behavioral testing requires that the child's cognitive age be determined. Play audiometry will be easily accomplished with children who are cognitively older than 3 years, and will not be easily accomplished for children younger than $2^1/_2$ years. Some children around 2 years of age will be able to perform play tasks but many will not, and those who can do it may not be able to perform the task for a sufficiently long time to complete an audiogram. Selecting the wrong test procedure means that one may be unable to obtain any thresholds, may obtain very few thresholds, or may obtain inaccurate thresholds (Diefendorf, 2002; Madell, 1998; Martin, 1996; Thomson et al, 1989).

Cognitive information can be obtained in several ways. A good case history will provide some information. If the child's motor development is within normal limits and he has no other significant developmental issues such as autism or pervasive development disorder (PDD), she should be able to perform the play task. If speech and language development are grossly within normal limits (as determined by observation and discussion with parents (Linden et al, 1985), cognitive levels can be assumed to be close to normal as well. If a child has other developmental disabilities, cognitive levels will be harder to ascertain and results of specific developmental tests may be required. Once it is determined that a child is cognitively older than 30 months, play audiometry can be attempted. Children who have frequent hearing tests, such as those with hearing loss or recurrent otitis media, are likely to learn the "listen and drop" task earlier. Visual reinforcement audiometry (VRA) often becomes boring after repeated test sessions, so when a child becomes familiar with the audiologist and the test environment, he may be willing to try the play task at a younger age.

◆ Training a Child for Play Audiometry

When conditioning a child to play audiometry, it is critical that the child actually hears the stimulus used to train the response. If the child does not hear the sound, the audiologist will be conditioning the child to silence, causing a great deal of confusion and inaccurate test results. After obtaining a case history and interacting with the child during the interview, the audiologist should have some idea about the loudness level at which to begin presenting stimuli. If the child responds to speech at a normal conversational level, testing can probably begin by presenting test stimuli at 40 to 50 dB HL. If the child does not respond to speech at a normal conversational level but seems to be developing normally in other ways (motor development and play activities), it is possible that the child has significant hearing loss and a loud stimulus will be needed.

Training the Task

The play audiometry task requires that the child hold a toy up to his ear and perform a motor task (drop the toy in the bucket, etc.) when the sound is presented. The toy is held up to the ear for two reasons: (1) as a specific signal that the child is ready to listen; and (2) as a clear indication of the motor act of dropping the toy in the bucket. To explain, if the child is playing with the toy, or holding it right above the bucket, it is not clear when the toy goes into the bucket whether the drop was truly a response to the sound, or whether the child just decided to drop the toy at that moment. When training the listen and drop task, begin with an easy play activity, such as dropping a block in a bucket. Do not start with a task that requires good dexterity such as slipping a chip into a slot or fitting a small peg into a hole (**Fig. 8–1**).

> **Pearl**
>
> • Having a variety of interesting toys will increase the probability of keeping the child's attention long enough to get the information needed for testing.

There are several ways to begin the training. The test assistant can begin by demonstrating the task. He holds the toy to his ear, and when the sound is presented says "I hear that" and drops the toy in the bucket. If the child seems

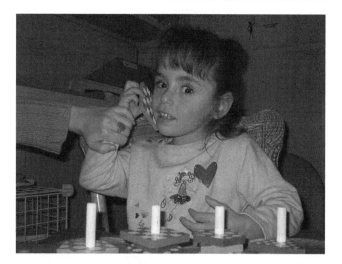

Figure 8–1   Helping a child get ready to listen for play audiometry.

hesitant, allow the parent to try for one or two sound presentations. Then hand the child the toy, hold his hand up to his ear, and when the sound is presented say "We heard that" and, hand over hand, with the tester's hand over the child's hand, move the child's hand to drop the toy in the bucket. After a few tries, the tester should feel the child's hand start to move when the sound is presented. That is the clue to let the child carry out the task alone. If the child seems hesitant and you are certain that he hears the sound, give his hand a little nudge to help him get going. If he still needs assistance, try demonstrating the task again saying "Okay, it's my turn." Doing the task together, with both the tester and the child holding a toy and dropping it in the bucket when the sound is presented may help. It is important to be careful that the child is not simply imitating the motor task or dropping the block when the test assistant does, but is, in fact, responding to a sound stimulus. After several attempts, the child will need to do the listen and drop task himself. Say "It's your turn" and let the child do the task. If the child looks up when the sound is presented but is hesitant about putting the toy in the bucket, it is all right to say, "You heard that, put it in." If the child continues to look to the test assistant for approval before putting the toy in the bucket, the test assistant should look at the floor or at the bucket to signal to the child that he is on his own. If the child is still unable to execute the task, start over again and retrain the task.

If there is uncertainty as to whether the child has heard the sound even at loud levels, try conditioning the child with the bone vibrator from the audiometer. Even a child with no hearing will feel the tactile stimulation of the bone vibrator at 250 Hz at maximum output. Place the vibrator on the mastoid with a headband, or in the child's hand or on the knee and hold his hand closed with your own. Use your other hand to help the child hold the toy up to his ear, and then place it in the bucket when the vibrator is turned on. Once the child learns the task with the vibrator, return to an air-conducted stimulus and try again.

✦ Test Protocol

Choosing the Test Stimulus

If a child responds to speech (e.g., if he answers when called), it may be best to begin with a speech stimulus. The easiest speech utterance may be the command "Put it in." The child will understand the verbal command and learn the task easily. Use of a speech stimulus will provide a speech awareness threshold, but will not give any frequency-specific information. Once the child is conditioned to the listen and drop task, change the stimulus to tones or narrow band noise to obtain an audiogram.

If the child displays some developmental concerns such as autism, PDD, or multisystem developmental delay, he may not respond to speech stimuli. In that case, testing should begin with tones, noise bands, or music. (See Chapter 9, Evaluation of Hearing in the Special Needs Child).

Test Order

Test protocol needs to take into consideration the fact that 2-, 3-, and 4-year-olds are not always very cooperative. Testing should begin with the tasks that require the least cooperation and move on to more difficult tasks as the child becomes more comfortable. It is easiest to begin testing in soundfield, since many children initially object to earphones. If a child has anything less than profound hearing loss, there should be no problem hearing a stimulus in soundfield. If conductive hearing loss (CHL) is the concern, begin with a high-frequency stimulus, which should be more easily heard. If the concern is that the child might have a sensorineural hearing loss (SNHL), begin with a low-frequency stimulus, since hearing is likely to be better in the low frequencies.

After obtaining at least one low- and one high-frequency threshold, a decision has to be made about which test information is most crucial and about how likely the child is to accept earphones. If CHL is the concern and a decision needs to be made about insertion of PE tubes, discrete ear information and bone conduction thresholds can be critical. If the concern is SNHL, separate ear information is still important, but it may be more important to obtain an idea of the contour of the audiogram before trying earphones on the child. Remember, once earphones are used, twice as many thresholds are required. That is, twice as many responses from the child are necessary to obtain an audiogram because each frequency needs to be tested for both ears.

When the audiologist is ready to try earphone testing, a decision needs to be made about whether to begin with circumaural headphones or with insert earphones. Circumaural headphones are easy to put in place quickly. However, they can be heavy for a small head and even little children are amazingly quick at removing them or pushing them out of position; circumaural headphones need to be positioned directly over the ear canal. Insert earphones will definitely be in the right place (directly in the ear canal), but they require more effort to insert, and poking at the child's ears may be distressful to the child. Nevertheless, whenever possible, it is best to attempt to persuade the child to accept insert earphones because they will provide the best test results.

Regardless of the type of hearing loss suspected, an attempt should be made to obtain bone conduction thresholds. Once the child accepts the bone vibrator, thresholds are usually easy to obtain. If time or attention is a problem, two to three thresholds should be sufficient. For CHL, the most critical thresholds to obtain by bone conduction are probably 250, 500, and 2000 Hz. If hearing loss is sensorineural, 500, 2000, and 4000 Hz are probably the most critical frequencies to test by bone conduction. It is not unusual with SNHL to have bone conduction thresholds at levels that are better than air conduction thresholds in the low frequencies, probably due to a tactile (not auditory) response. If a standard metal bone-conduction headband used, a piece of foam should be used to make it more comfortable and to improve fit. A Velcro headband can also be used; this is often more comfortable for little heads. (**See Fig. 8–2A,B** for different bone-conduction headbands.)

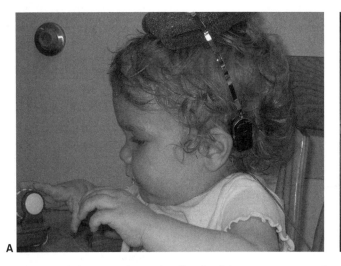

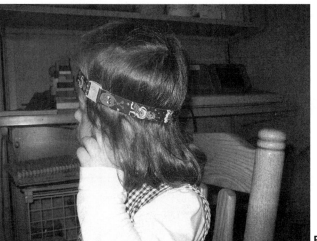

A   B

Figure 8–2   **(A)** Bone conduction headband with foam to improve comfort. **(B)** Bone conduction headband held in place with Velcro.

Test Room Setup

For many children, testing is most easily accomplished using two testers in a two-room test setup. One audiologist will present test stimuli from the control room, and the test assistant will work with the child in the test room. This two-room test procedure is especially important for soundfield testing.

When earphone testing is being performed, it is possible to have one tester sit next to the child in the sound room, and act as both tester and test assistant. In a one-tester situation, it difficult to test hearing in soundfield. If there is only one tester, and if there is concern that the child will not accept earphones immediately, it is possible to train the child to perform the listen and drop task before the earphones are placed on her head. Put the earphones on the test table near the child and set the signal to a loud level that the child can be expected to hear based on previous observations. Then train the child to perform the play audiometry task. Once the child is responding reliably, place the earphones on her head and proceed in the usual way. Some test set-ups allow for the audiometer in the test room to be attached to loudspeakers so that all testing can be performed in a one-room setup. This has its benefits in that it does not require two audiologists to test a child, but the audiologist may sometimes feel the need for more than two hands to accomplish everything smoothly, especially with a difficult-to-test child.

Testing Children with Hearing Loss

Children with mild or moderate hearing loss or with CHL do not require any special test adaptation, except that the audiologist may need to be creative in keeping the child entertained and cooperative through repeat testing. However, children with severe and profound hearing loss may need some test adaptations. If the child does not respond to soundfield stimuli at the audiometric limits, it may be possible to obtain a response using a bone vibrator either held in her hand, on the knee, or on the mastoid. No matter how severe a child's hearing loss, he will feel the vibrator at 250 Hz since this is a tactile stimulus, not an auditory one. Once the child responds consistently to the tactile stimulus, begin testing with earphones at 250 or 500 Hz. Insert earphones are usually preferable if the child will accept them. (For more information, see Chapter 9, Evaluation of Hearing in the Special Needs Child.)

◆ Special Test Techniques

Tangible Reinforced Operant Conditioning Audiometry

Tangible reinforced operant conditioning audiometry (TROCA) was developed for use with special populations (Lloyd, 1966; Lloyd, Spradin, and Reid, 1968; Martin and Coombes, 1976; Northern and Downs, 2002). TROCA uses food or tokens as reinforcers instead a movable toy. A clown or other toy is frequently used to dispense the reinforcer when the child pulls the arm, head, etc.

TROCA can be useful for children with developmental disabilities, for children who are not interested in the visual reinforcer, or for children with visual disabilities who cannot see a reinforcer that is a few feet away. Very small pieces of food are used to prolong the length of time the child will respond. The food selected needs to be something that will be quickly swallowed so that the test can proceed in a timely fashion. Cheerios are a useful reinforcer. Candy has been used and is reinforcing for children, but many parents are not happy about having their children fed sugar. Once the child is no longer interested in the food, testing will need to end. (See Chapter 9, Evaluation of Special Needs Children.)

◆ Computer-Assisted Reinforcement

A computer-assisted reinforcement procedure uses a laptop computer that is placed in the sound room with the child, parent, and test assistant. On the computer screen is an interesting PowerPoint program that is controlled by a remote mouse operated by the audiologist in the control room. Every click of the mouse adds a feature to a picture on the screen; e.g., completing a clown face. The child has a mouse or other apparatus that is not actually connected to the computer. The child is conditioned to click his mouse every time he hears a sound. Of course, his mouse does not do anything, but the child does not know that. If the child pushes his mouse when a sound is presented, the audiologist uses his remote mouse to add a feature to the picture

Table 8–1   Test Protocol for Conditioned Play Audiometry

1. Sit the child in a highchair or at a children's table so he is comfortably seated
2. Select a toy that will be enjoyable for the child and within his skill range.
3. Begin using a test stimulus that you expect the child to be able to hear.
4. Begin by demonstrating the task. The test assistant holds the toy to his ear. When he hears the sound he says "I hear that" and drops the toy into the bucket.
5. After a few presentations, the child is given the toy and the test assistant holds the toy to the child's ear. When the sound is heard the test assistant helps the child drop the toy into the bucket.
6. Care must be taken to encourage the child to drop the toy in the bucket ONLY when you are certain the child heard the sound.
7. This is repeated until the child is able to do the task without assistance.
8. Once the child is conditioned and performing reliably, testing can begin.
9. If the child seems to be bored, change toys to increase interest.
10. Testing can be accomplished by air and bone conduction, with hearing aids, cochlear implants, and FM system.

on the screen. If the child clicks his mouse when a sound is not presented, no feature is added to the picture. Computer pictures or games can be changed as needed, to maintain the child's interest.

◆ What to Do if the Child Will Not Cooperate

A child is a child. Especially with a very young child, the audiologist, not the child, should be in control. If testing cannot be accomplished, the audiologist needs to accept responsibility and say, "I was not able to test this child," rather than "This child is not testable." Owning responsibility for a test failure encourages the audiologist to try many procedures before giving up. There are some children from whom it is not possible to obtain good cooperation. However, there should be very few children for whom little or no information is available at the end of a test session.

The answer to the question of what to do if the child will not cooperate really starts with what *not* to do. First, do not offer choices that are not bona fide choices. For example, do not ask the child if he wants to have a hearing test or if he wants to put on earphones when there actually is no choice about the matter. Genuine choices can be offered about which of two games the child wants to play, or whether he wants to start testing with words or beeps. Those are realistic choices that can permit the child to feel that he has some control over the situation. Next, do not give up. If cooperation is difficult to obtain, try taking a short rest. Have the child go for a walk or take a drink from the water fountain and then try again. Try some new toys. Try a new test assistant. Perhaps a parent would be a better test assistant for a particular child. Try using different test stimuli to make the game more interesting; children need to be entertained. Try a different test room, a different chair, or allow the child to sit on a parent's lap.

Do *not* try to use a different test technique if that technique is not appropriate. For example, if a child is cognitively at 3 to 4 years of age, do not try to use visual reinforcement audiometry. Although the child may make a few responses using VRA, the older child will quickly become bored. Moreover, it will not be possible to obtain more than a few responses, and it will be difficult to determine if the responses were really at threshold. However, VRA reinforcers may be used to support the play task. Tell the uncooperative child that if he cooperates, the toy will be turned on.

Other "bribes" may also be useful. Promises such as "after we are finished you can have . . ." work very well. Possible rewards include stickers, stamps, food, and candy. Sometimes it is useful to offer the treat during testing. Providing occasional reinforcement during the test session if the child seems to be fading (such as a piece of a cookie, fruit, raisins, cheerios, or candy) may prolong the child's cooperation. As with all other promises, when a child is told that something will or will not occur, the promise should be fulfilled. For example, if a sticker is promised after putting five blocks in the box, be sure to provide the sticker after exactly five blocks. If the child is told that he cannot leave until the game is finished, that promise too, needs to be kept. In other words, think about what is promised to children before the words are spoken, and be prepared to carry out any promises that are made.

Giving some indication about how long the task will take is very useful. The audiologist can say something like, "when all of these marbles are put in the jar, we will be finished." Children have no idea how long an audiometric test will take unless a concrete referent is provided for them.

◆ Parents in the Test Room

Under most circumstances, parents should be involved in test situations. Their role will be limited, but they are a source of comfort for the child. In addition, seeing how the child performs, and hearing what the child can and cannot hear is very helpful when counseling about test results. When two parents accompany a child, one can sit with the child and the other can observe from the control room. Having a parent on the control room side permits the audiologist to point out events and behaviors that are happening during testing that will assist in later counseling. For example, pointing out that a child is having increased difficulty hearing the soft speech signal may help the parent understand the effect of hearing loss.

On the other hand, for some children, having a parent in the test room reduces cooperation. Some parents have a parenting style that does not require the child to carry out tasks that he does not want to complete. For some parents, if the child becomes distressed or frustrated, the parent will remove the child from the situation rather than have the child be distressed. If that is the case, it may be best to have the parent leave the room and watch from the control room. As a last resort, and one that should be used only very, very rarely, it is sometimes necessary to tell children that if they do not cooperate, the parent will have to wait outside. Sending the parent out for a short time may increase the child's cooperation. Removing parents is not a procedure that should be tried on a first visit, but it may be considered at a reevaluation if testing cannot be accomplished because of the child's uncooperative behavior.

Pitfall

- When a child is not cooperating, it is tempting to try a different test protocol such as moving from play audiometry to VRA. This is almost always a bad choice. If the child is cognitively old enough to do play, testing with VRA will give inaccurate test results, and may suggest hearing loss that is not present.

♦ Summary

With a little creativity, play audiometry is easy to accomplish with children. The following tips are useful to consider:

♦ Keep the test room orderly to avoid distracting the child.

♦ Be prepared to change toys frequently to maintain the child's attention.

♦ Offer only choices that are genuine; for example, do not ask a child if he wants a hearing test when that is not a bone fide choice.

♦ Include parents in testing to assist them in understanding the results.

♦ CPA can be performed in all necessary conditions including using earphones or technology (hearing aids, cochlear implants, and FM systems).

Discussion Questions

1. What are some techniques for persuading a child to cooperate when he is not interested in doing so?

2. What are the steps in deciding what frequencies to test in what order for a child with suspected SNHL; for a child with suspected CHL?

References

Diefendorf, A. O. (2002). Detection and assessment of hearing loss in infants and children. In Katz, J. (Ed.), Handbook of clinical audiology, 5th edition. Baltimore: Lippincott Williams & Wilkins.

Linden, G., and Harford, E. R. (1985). The pediatric audiologist: from magician to clinician. Ear and Hearing, 6, 6–9.

Lloyd, L. (1996). Behavioral audiometry viewed as an operant procedure. Journal of Speech and Hearing Disorders, 31, 128–135.

Lloyd, L. L., Spradin, J. E., and Reid, M. J. (1968). An operant audiometric procedure for difficult to test patients. Journal of Speech and Hearing Disorders, 33, 236–245.

Lowell, E., Rushford, G., Hoversten, G., and Stoner, M. (1956). Evaluation of pure-tone audiometry with pre-school age children. Journal of Speech and Hearing Disorders, 21, 292–302.

Madell, J. R. (1998). Behavioral evaluation of hearing in infants and young children. New York: Thieme.

Martin, F. N., and Clark, J. G. (1996). Behavioral Hearing Tests with Children. In Martin, F.N. and Clark, J.G. (Eds.), Hearing care for children. Needman Heights, MA: Allyn & Bacon.

Martin, F. N and Coombes, S. (1976). A tangibly reinforced speech reception threshold procedure for use in small children. Journal of Speech and Hearing Disorders, 41, 333–338.

Northern, J. L., and Downs, M. P. (2002). Hearing in children. 5th ed. Baltimore: Lippincott Williams & Wilkins.

Thompson, M., Thompson, G., and Vethivelu, S. (1989). A comparison of audiometric test methods for 2-year-old children. Journal of Speech and Hearing Disorders, 54, 174–179.

Chapter 9

Evaluation of Hearing in Children with Special Needs

Jane R. Madell

Key Points

- By appropriately controlling the test environment and using the appropriate test protocols, almost any child can be tested using behavioral techniques.

- If a child cannot be tested, the audiologist needs to take ownership for the inability to test and say "I was unable to test this child" rather than "this child is untestable."

Testing an infant or child with special needs demands unique skills from the audiologist in all areas, from taking a case history to modifying test protocols and tasks. Frequently, parents bring a child for evaluation because they have concerns about her development. If a child is not speaking, the first question is "Does she hear?" The audiologist is often the first person to evaluate a child, especially if the disability has not been identified in the newborn nursery. To begin with, when taking a case history, a parent may report that the child has been diagnosed with autism, pervasive developmental disorder (PDD), Down syndrome, etc.

It is the audiologist's responsibility to find out about the particular disorder so that she can more effectively test and be an effective participant on the team.

The audiologist must be familiar with multiple disorders that can either cause hearing loss or interfere with a child's using hearing to learn. These disorders include autism, PDD, Down syndrome, CHARGE, and other developmental disorders. Although the audiologist is not the professional who diagnoses these disorders, she should be able to recognize them and understand their effect on hearing. Doing so will enable her to select test protocols, make referrals for additional evaluations, and arrange for management.

Many developmental disabilities do not result in hearing loss—that is, when appropriately tested the children have normal audiograms. However, because of other contributing factors, they may have problems learning language and responding to sound. It is frequently a difficult task to make the appropriate diagnosis, but doing so will improve the likelihood that the child will be directed toward appropriate follow-up.

A very old textbook (Myklebust, 1954) provides wonderful descriptions of various auditory disorders. Although the terminology is outdated and the book is now out of print, it has a lot of useful information, and for clinicians interested in becoming pediatric audiologists, it is well worth the effort to search out and read the book. It can be found in many audiology libraries as well as on the Internet.

◆ Testing Hearing in Infants and Children with Severe and Profound Hearing Loss

Children with severe and profound hearing loss who are developing normally should be able to be taught auditory test tasks in the same way as their normally hearing peers, except that the sound will need to be much louder. Since children with severe and profound hearing loss frequently do not hear sounds, they may not know how to attend to auditory signals. Therefore, it may take more than the usual number of presentations for the child to learn to respond to the conditioning task. It is critical that the audiologist be absolutely certain that the child hears the sound before either turning on the visual reinforcer when using VRA, or signaling to the child to "listen and drop" for play audiometry.

Pearl

- Children with severe and profound hearing loss can be very visually alert. It is important that the audiologist be certain not to provide any visual cues when testing that might suggest to the child that she should respond (either by looking toward the VRA reinforcer or by dropping a toy in the bucket). It is essential that the audiologist provide no reinforcement unless she is absolutely sure that the child heard the sound to avoid reinforcing random behavior.

For very young children, testing usually begins in soundfield. If the room is quiet and activities are kept to a minimum, it should be fairly easy to see if the child responds to a loud stimulus. Begin with low-frequency stimuli, since children with hearing loss commonly hear low frequency signals better than high frequencies. If the child does not respond, it will be useful to encourage him to accept earphones, since most audiometers can present an earphone signal at a greater intensity than can be obtained in soundfield. (Centers that see large numbers of children with severe and profound hearing loss may want to consider installing power amplifiers and loudspeakers to permit soundfield testing of more intense signals.)

If the child is not responding to an auditory stimulus, it may be possible to obtain a response using a tactile stimulus. Condition the child to a tactile stimulus by placing a bone vibrator in the child's hand, on the knee, or on the mastoid. Even if the child cannot hear the stimulus, she will feel it and should easily become conditioned to the task. Once the child is conditioned, it is useful to pair the tactile

and auditory stimuli, then fade the tactile stimulus and see if the child continues to respond. It may take several attempts, but unless the child has no measurable hearing, it should be possible to teach her to respond to an auditory signal using this tactile technique.

Because children with hearing loss are evaluated frequently, they are likely to grow tired of hearing testing. A great deal of creativity will be demanded of the audiologist to keep the child interested. Using multiple VRA toys could maintain the child's interest for a little while longer, but creative toys alone may be insufficient. Using a TV with cartoons as a reinforcer may be more interesting for a 2-year-old child than are standard VRA toys. Children with hearing loss frequently learn the listen and drop task of play audiometry earlier than their normal hearing peers because they are tested so often. An interesting and enthusiastic audiologist with many good toys may be able to keep a child's attention long enough to obtain a sufficient number of thresholds using either visual reinforcement audiometry (VRA) or play audiometry (Madell, 1998).

It is not reasonable to expect that any young child will be able to attend long enough to obtain air conduction thresholds in each ear, bone conduction thresholds, speech audiometry measures, and assessment of performance with technology (monaurally and binaurally) in one test session. Parents need to be advised in advance that it is not likely that all the necessary information will be obtained in one test session and that, depending on the child, it may take two or three test sessions to complete each evaluation. When parents understand that the audiologist is trying to maximize the child's functioning, they are usually understanding about the need for repeat visits.

◆ Testing Hearing in Infants and Children with Developmental Delay

Unfortunately, having one disability does not prevent a child from having another. Many children with developmental disabilities have also been identified with hearing loss. Some of the syndromes and disorders associated with developmental disabilities (e.g., Down syndrome, CHARGE, cytomegalovirus, premature birth) are also associated with impaired hearing. Abilities of these children vary greatly. Some have mild delays and others have significant ones. Some of these children have structurally deformities of the ear and many have significant middle ear disease (Shoup and Roeser, 2007). As a result, every child identified with any developmental disability or delay should be followed audiologically until ear and frequency-specific information is obtained. If no hearing loss is identified, and if the disorder is not a progressive one, the infant can be discharged from follow-up. However, if the disorder has the potential for being progressive (e.g., cytomegalovirus, central nervous system dysfunction) or fluctuating (e.g., conductive hearing loss in Down syndrome), children should be monitored on a regular basis. It is very helpful for the audiologist to learn as much as possible about the disorders that frequently present in the audiology clinic, and the specific disorder that any one child may express.

Understanding a disorder will help the clinician understand what kind of behavior may be expected from the child, what types of auditory disorders are expected, and the prognosis for development of speech, language, and hearing. However, it is important to remember that every disorder presents in variable ways. The developmental delay may be mild or severe, and the auditory disorder may be mild or severe. Information about the disorder is a starting place for effective audiologic assessment, but only a start.

When evaluating normally developing children, assumptions are made about developmental age that cannot be made when evaluating children with developmental disabilities. With all children, and especially with special needs infants and children, it is critical to know the cognitive age to select the appropriate test protocol. Flexer and Gans (1985) demonstrated that by carefully assessing the developmental age of children with profound multiple disabilities, thresholds were obtained at the same levels as with normally developing children of the same developmental age. This confirms that children with developmental delay can be accurately evaluated for hearing loss if their developmental age is correctly determined. If the child is in an early intervention or educational program, the staff at the program should be able to provide information about her developmental age. The pediatrician may also be able to provide this information. With experience evaluating children, most pediatric audiologists will develop the necessary intuition to determine enough about cognitive level to select the appropriate test protocol. It is most important to look at motor and play skills. Language, especially for a child with hearing loss who has not had sufficient auditory input, is not likely to be a good indicator of cognitive age. Once the child's cognitive age is known, it is possible to select the appropriate test protocol: BOA, VRA, or CPA (Kile, 1996).

Positioning

The specific test protocols described in Chapters 6, 7, and 8 (BOA, VRA, and CPA), emphasize that positioning of the child is critical. The infant needs to be situated so that she is comfortable, not straining, and can attend to auditory stimuli. A great deal of care needs to be taken to keep a child with any neurologic disorder centered. A child with a neurologic disorder and for whom motor activity is difficult will have trouble making a significant head turn. She must be focused straight forward with the visual reinforcer at 45 degrees and no more than 90 degrees from midline. If the child does not have good trunk control, she needs to be seated in a chair that will provide trunk stabilization. Infants will be able to use standard infant seats or will lean against a parent. Older children will need adaptive chairs or strollers that can offer the necessary support to facilitate head, trunk, and neck control. Many children will be able to turn toward a reinforcement toy if seated in a chair that affords trunk and neck stabilization.

For children who are engaged in play audiometry, positioning needs to permit optimum range of motion of arms and hands. Some children may need to be held upright to make available the upper body support that allows them to use their arms and hands for the play activity. Play tasks should be carefully selected to be within the child's skill range. Putting pegs into a pegboard may be too difficult, but throwing pegs into a basket may be a motor skill that the child can accomplish (Madell, 1998). TROCA (Lloyd, Spradin, and Reid, 1969) is a play audiometry task that was designed to assist in testing children with developmental disabilities. For more information about TROCA, see Chapter 8.

Timing of Test Stimulus Presentation

Delivery of the test signal may require a little more consideration with this population. Because motor control is an issue for many children with neurologic disorders, the audiologist needs to carefully observe the child to be certain she is stabilized and comfortable before presenting a stimulus. If the child is squirming and trying to attain a stabilized position, she may not be able to respond to a stimulus. In that case, absence of response is not an indication of inability to hear the stimulus.

Difficulties in Obtaining Responses

There are several issues to be considered in obtaining and interpreting reliable responses from children with developmental disabilities. First, the response the child makes may be qualitatively different than that obtained from normally developing children. For example, it may take her longer to focus on a reinforcer and to refocus on the distraction toy. There may be a longer latency between presentation of the test stimulus and the response. In some cases, the child may demonstrate a very short latency, turning almost as soon as the stimulus is presented. An extremely rapid response may be an indication of sound sensitivities. More commonly however, motor responses may be slower than with normally developing children. The audiologist will need to be sensitive to this latency differential and change the timing of stimulus presentation accordingly.

Children with developmental delays may fatigue more quickly and may habituate more rapidly to test stimuli and reinforcers. The child may fixate on the visual reinforcer and thus require a great deal of effort from the test assistant to refocus the child's attention after each stimulus presentation. To maximize test results, the test assistant needs to be very alert to the child's mood and change distractors, reinforcers, and play toys quickly to keep her interested and alert. Social reinforcers are frequently very helpful.

Some children with neurologic disorders may react negatively to the visual reinforcer toys; they may become fearful and anxious. When this happens, the audiologist needs to react quickly. Most VRA systems allow the audiologist to set the reinforcement toy so that it can be presented with a light only, or with light, motion, and sound. Obviously, if the sound is frightening for the child, the audiologist needs to turn off the sound and use only the light, or light and motion with no sound. Using TV with cartoons as the reinforcers may also be very helpful.

Special Test Procedures

Several test protocols have been developed for use with children who experience developmental delay when standard test protocols do not work. One such procedure is a tactile-auditory conditioning procedure (Friedlander, Silva, and Knight, 1973; Verpoorten and Emmen, 1995) in which a child is conditioned by pairing a tactile stimulus with an auditory one and gradually withdrawing the tactile stimulus as the child learns the task. This procedure can be implemented using a bone vibrator held in the child's hand or placing her hand on the loudspeaker membrane. The child may remove her hand when the stimulus stops or may make an active response (as in play audiometry) and put her hand on the loudspeaker when the stimulus is presented. As the child learns the task, the tactile stimulus is faded. Another procedure (Lancioni, Coninx, and Smeets, 1989; Lancioni and Coninx, 1995) uses an air puff that is paired with an auditory stimulus. The air puff can be directed to the child's face, eyes, hand, or neck, and will evoke defensive responses such as eye blinking or head turning. An air cylinder or earmold blower is used to supply the air puff.

◆ Testing Hearing in Infants and Children with Physical Challenges

Children with cerebral palsy or other physical challenges can be tested audiologically as long as consideration is made for their specific motor needs. Some children with physical challenges have cognitive issues and others do not, so it is not accurate to make an assumption about a child's cognitive age when selecting a test protocol. Children with special needs are usually tested often, so psychological testing data may be available that can provide useful information for determining cognitive level and selecting the appropriate test protocol.

It is important to be sure that the child is positioned to keep the upper body steady, facilitating a head turn for VRA or use of arms and hands for CPA. The audiologist must be flexible in selecting test tasks. When using play, it is important to select toys that are easy enough for the child to manipulate so she can do the "listen and drop" task. Some children will have such severe motor delays that it may be necessary to rely on something like an eye blink to demonstrate that the child has heard the sound. Motor skills may make it difficult for a child to push a button to identify that she has heard the sound. In that case, using play audiometry when the child is older may be appropriate. Speech audiometry may be difficult to accomplish, because many children with physical disabilities are not able to repeat words clearly enough to measure speech perception. When that is the case, testing will be limited to closed-set tests (Madell, 1998; Shoup and Roeser, 2007). See Chapter 10 for more information about speech perception tests.

◆ Testing Hearing in Infants and Children with Autistic Spectrum Disorder and Pervasive Developmental Disability

Children with auditory attention disorders such as those associated with autism, pervasive developmental disorder (PDD), multisystem developmental delay, or regulatory disorders tend to have normal hearing sensitivity (Downs, Schmidt, and Stephens, 2005; Gravel et al, 2006) but they may be unable to attend consistently to auditory stimuli, which is frequently typical of their difficulties in responding to a variety of other sensory stimuli (Davis et al, 2005). However, with a little extra effort these children can be reliably tested. These populations of children frequently fail to make eye contact, they may find tactile stimuli aversive, and they may demonstrate repetitive behaviors such as hand flapping and inability to communicate verbally. (For more information about autism, see Egelhoff et al, 2005 and Greenspan 1995, 1998).

For this population, the test setup should be very well controlled. The child needs to be seated in a position that does not permit her to easily walk away from the test situation. A strong wooden highchair is ideal and can hold children as old as 7 or 8. The audiologist needs to know if the child has an aversion to tactile stimuli and, if she does, be very careful to limit touching.

Pearl

- Testing should definitely begin in soundfield for a child with tactile sensitivity because touching the child to place earphones may be so distressing that the audiologic evaluation will not be able to be completed.

As with any population, it is important to identify cognitive age so that the suitable test protocol can be selected. VRA is usually the appropriate test protocol for children from 5 to 36 months; however, children with autistic spectrum disorder (ASD) frequently continue to respond appropriately, using VRA for several more years.

Because children with ASD and PPD may "tune out" voices, it is usually best to avoid speech stimuli, at least initially, and to have the test room as quiet as possible. Music such as the *Sesame Street* theme, the theme from a favorite TV show, or familiar recorded children's songs played through the loudspeaker will often attract the child's attention. Once the child has sought out the stimulus, the visual reinforcer can be activated. Timing of test stimuli is very important with children in this population, because they frequently habituate to stimuli quickly. Stimuli should not be presented too close together. When a child seems to have "tuned out," it is useful to try different stimuli (noise bands or warble tones), to change the reinforcer toy, or to present very loud stimuli, which may attract the child's attention again and redirect it to the test stimulus.

For behavioral testing, it is important to have the child focused forward but not too involved with the toys. Finding an appropriate distraction toy that will keep a child interested but not too involved can be a problem with this population of children. If the child is more visually than auditorally attentive (which is frequently the case), a toy that is too interesting may cause the child to "tune out" to auditory stimuli. Finding the right type of distraction toy for the individual child requires some creativity, because this group of children can be difficult to entertain.

Many of these children are sensitive to loud sounds (Gomet et al, 2002). Their parents report that they have difficulty tolerating sound in the environment and will cry, hit, or demonstrate other negative behavior if there is a loud sound, for example, when the family gathers for a party, and everyone sings "Happy Birthday," or when certain household appliances are turned on. Others will "shut down" if there is too much auditory stimulation, so it is important that loud stimuli be carefully controlled to keep the child tuned in but not frightened. Stimuli should be presented at low levels and intensity increased gradually. Some children with these disorders ignore sound and almost appear "deaf." For these children, the use of a loud stimulus sometimes helps them to "tune in" when their attention has been decreased. Presenting a loud stimulus sometimes makes the child alert, after which it is possible to persuade her to respond to less intense stimuli.

When taking a case history, it is important to obtain a very clear description of the sounds that cause problems for the child. Some parents will report that all sounds are a problem, and others will describe specific sounds such as the vacuum cleaner or the microwave that cause distress. It is not unusual for a parent to report, for example, that crying babies cause the child to be distressed but other loud sounds do not. Distress to the sound of a baby crying, with no other complaints of sound tolerance problems, is almost always *not* an auditory problem. By obtaining uncomfortable loudness thresholds (UCLs) and demonstrating that the child does not have a problem with very loud sounds when playing with toys, parents can be helped to understand that the problem is not auditory but a response to something in the environment, and that a desensitization activity may help reduce the negative response.

Obtaining UCL thresholds should be attempted only after other testing is completed, because the loud stimuli may be distressing to the child. To obtain UCLs, the test assistant should engage the child's attention using a toy. If the child is involved with a toy, a more realistic response to loud sounds can be observed. UCL testing is usually performed in soundfield with narrow band noise stimuli, beginning with a low-intensity stimulus so as not to startle the child and then, keeping the signal on, gradually increasing it from below threshold to high intensity with a limit of 85 to 90 dB HL. (Momentary exposure at loud levels will not cause threshold shift.) Testing should proceed from 500 Hz through 6000 Hz. If children can tolerate loud sounds in the test room, the negative responses to sounds outside the test room are most likely not indicative of an auditory problem but may be a response elicited by an unfamiliar sound. Because these children frequently "tune out" stimuli, a high-intensity sound captures their attention and may startle them and be considered aversive.

For a child who demonstrates problems tolerating loud sounds, a desensitization program needs to be developed by her clinicians. For some children sounds are uncomfortable and cause distress at softer than expected levels. For these children, the sounds in the environment should be carefully controlled. Sometimes recommendations for ear protectors or noise-canceling earphones are made to enable the child to comfortably attend school or social events; however, use of these devices does not allow the child to learn to tolerate environmental sounds and further separates the child from her peers.

◆ Testing Hearing in Children with Attention Deficit/Hyperactivity Disorder

A child with attention deficit/hyperactivity disorder (ADHD) comes into the clinic with a great deal of energy. He has a difficult time attending and sitting still; as a result, testing may take longer than expected. If he enters the test room before the audiologist, he may start opening drawers and cabinets and dissecting headphones. When he selects a toy, he may leave it and go to another, and even with direction, he has difficulty stopping and putting away toys he is no longer using. Such a child is frequently talking; he interrupts others and has difficulty listening to the audiologist and following directions (Shoup and Roeser, 2007; Madell, 1998). To successfully accomplish the audiologic evaluation, the test room must be carefully organized. A structured test environment includes seating the child in a highchair or at a table with the chair pulled in close to encourage him to stay seated, and so his feet are firmly placed on the floor or on a stool. If feet are hanging loosely, the child is likely to fidget. The audiologist needs to remind the child constantly to attend, and should change toys frequently to keep interest. Stimuli should be presented only when the child is attending. If the child becomes bored, it may be possible to gain more test time by taking a small break, by doing jumping jacks in the test room, or by taking a walk to the water fountain.

◆ Testing Hearing in Infants and Children with Visual Impairment

Testing children with visual impairment with VRA is obviously difficult. If the child cannot see the reinforcer, he cannot respond to it. If the child has limited vision, he can be moved closer to the reinforcer or the reinforcer can be moved closer to the child to make it easier for the child to see. If this modification is not sufficient, an alternative is to darken the test room and use a bright flashlight close to his face. If the child does not have sufficient vision to see the bright light, a tactile stimulus such as a bone vibrator may be successful. The bone vibrator can be used as the reinforcer by moving the child's hand to the vibrator when the sound is presented. If the child likes the vibrator, he will make the association and reach for it when he hears the sound. The air-puff technique described above for children with developmental delay may be useful

(Friedlander, Silva, and Knight, 1973; Lancioni, Coninx, and Smeets, 1989; Lancioni and Coninx, 1995; Verpoorten and Emmen, 1995). Children who are blind and who function at the 3-year-old level and higher should be able to perform play audiometry tasks by selecting toys that do not require difficult manipulation.

◆ Testing Hearing in Graduates of the Neonatal Intensive Care Unit

Neonatal intensive care unit (NICU) graduates need to be evaluated in the same way as other infants. Research by Smith et al (1992) indicates that as many as 35% of NICU graduates may have hearing loss, which makes it clear that hearing testing of this population is critical. Testing should be delayed until the infant is stable, and is frequently delayed until a few days before hospital discharge. However, if the infant is to be hospitalized for several months, it is necessary to test earlier than discharge so that if there is hearing loss, she will not be functioning without auditory stimulation during critical developmental months. It is very important that every attempt be made to identify hearing loss if present and to fit the infant with appropriate amplification so that he is not left without auditory stimulation for an extended period of time. ABR and OAE will be the first tests for this population, but behavioral testing should also be considered.

Although NICU graduates are evaluated in the same way as other infants, there may be some additional testing difficulties. As with other infants, it is critical to obtain an accurate developmental age and use the appropriate test protocol. Some NICU graduates function like children with developmental delays, even after age is corrected for prematurity, and will need the same considerations as are suggested for that population. Many have feeding problems and may not suck. If that is the case, it will be very difficult to accomplish BOA, but air-puff audiometry may be possible (Friedlander, Silva, and Knight, 1973; Lancioni, Coninx, and Smeets, 1989; Lancioni and Coninx, 1995; Verpoorten and Emmen, 1995). NICU babies live in a very noisy environment and, as a result, may not attend to sound. The audiologist who works with NICU patients may be able to assist in monitoring the auditory environment and in helping to control noise levels.

◆ Testing Hearing in Children with Functional Hearing Loss

It is not unusual for children between the ages of 8 and 12 years to occasionally demonstrate functional hearing loss (Burk et al, 1958, Shoup and Roeser, 2007). Functional hearing loss, sometimes called malingering or faking, occurs when a child knowingly exaggerates hearing thresholds. The typical scenario is that a child fails a hearing screening either in school or in the pediatrician's office and is referred to an audiologist for a complete evaluation. The audiologist may suspect that hearing loss is functional if the following are present: (1) test results do not agree with the child's ability to communicate (i.e., the child seems to understand with no difficulty although thresholds indicate moderately severe hearing loss, or he has a great deal of difficulty communicating when thresholds are near normal); (2) speech recognition thresholds are much better or worse than pure tone thresholds; (3) responses to speech stimuli are unusual (e.g., consistently saying only half the spondee word); (4) test results are not repeatable; or (5) unmasked bone conduction thresholds are much poorer in one ear than in the other.

If functional hearing loss is suspected, try first to reinstruct the child. It may be helpful to suggest to the child, "Maybe you did not understand the directions. This is hard to do. You need to raise your hand even if the sound is very, very soft." Alternatively, the audiologist can suggest that there may be something wrong with the equipment, which is causing the problem. "There must be something wrong with this equipment. It is making it seem that you have much worse hearing than I know you have. Let's go into a different test room and try again." You are not exactly telling the child that you think he is faking hearing loss, but you are making it clear that you know the results are not accurate.

If cooperative test results are not obtained on the second try, it will be necessary to rely on alternative techniques to get results. It is very helpful to use a portable audiometer and have the child seated next to you so that you can make eye contact. It is much more difficult for a child to say she does not hear a sound when looking you in your eye.

If the child's responses still are not providing accurate results, have him "count the beeps." Tell the child that he will hear one, two, or three beeps and to tell you how many he hears. Start at a level that the child admits to hearing. For example, if the child admits to hearing at 40 dB HL, present two beeps at 40 dB HL and when the child says "two," present two beeps at 40 dB HL and one beep at 35 dB HL. If the child responds, "three," you know that the child heard three beeps at both 35 dB HL and 40 dB HL. Continue in this fashion until consistent thresholds are obtained.

Obtaining the audiogram is actually the easy part. Now the audiologist needs to explain test results to both the child and the parent. One could simply say that the child has normal hearing and send him home, but that may be begging the issue. Why did the child feel the need to simulate hearing loss?

If the audiologic evaluation takes this "crutch" away, will the child substitute something else? It is probably useful to tell the child that he has normal hearing. However, it is important to discuss with the parents or caregivers that the child may have difficulties that are causing stress and suggest that they find out if anything is bothering the child. It is possible that simply being aware that the child is under stress will help the parents provide the necessary support. If not, telling them about the child's behavior during testing can alert them to seek help.

◆ Conclusion

Children with all types of developmental, behavioral, and auditory disorders are testable using behavioral procedures. A review of the literature and the experience of many pediatric audiologists clearly indicate that reliable test results can be obtained on almost any child. The audiologist has to believe that she can test the child and be creative in finding ways to accomplish the task. If test results cannot be obtained, the audiologist needs to take ownership of the problem and assume responsibility for the unfavorable outcome. It is not the child's fault that testing could not be completed. The audiologist needs to say (at least to herself) "I was unable to test this child." On another day, testing may be more successful, especially if the audiologist can identify the problems that were apparent during the failed testing and make changes to improve results. The reward of accurately assessing the hearing of a child who is difficult to evaluate is well worth the effort.

Discussion Questions

1. How is testing different when evaluating a child with autism compared with a typically developing child?

2. What special protocols would be used to test children with significant motor impairments?

3. What kind of evaluation protocol should be used to test children who are diagnosed with ADHD?

References

Berk, R. L., and Feldman, A. S. (1958). Functional hearing loss in children. New England Journal of Medicine, 259, 214–216.

Davis, R., and Stiegler, L. N. (2005). Toward more effective audiologic assessment of children with autism spectrum disorders. Seminars in Hearing, 26, 241–252.

Downs, D., Schmidt, B., and Stephens, T. J. (2005). Auditory behaviors of children and adolescents with pervasive developmental disorders. Seminars in Hearing, 26, 226–240.

Egelhoff, K., Whitelaw, G., and Rabidoux, P. (2005). What audiologists need to know about autism spectrum disorders. Seminars in Hearing, 26, 4:202–209.

Flexer, C., and Gans, D. P. (1985). Comparative evaluation of the auditory responsiveness of normal infants and profoundly multihandicapped children. Journal of Speech and Hearing Research, 28, 163–168.

Friedlander, B. Z., Silva, D. A., and Knight, M. S. (1973) Selective responses to auditory and auditory-vibratory stimuli by severely retarded dearblind children, Journal of Auditory Research, 13, 105–111.

Gomot, M., Giard, M., Adrien, J., Barthelemy, C., and Bruneu, N. (2002). Hypersensitivity to acoustic change in children with autism: electrophysiological evidence for left frontal cortex dysfunctioning. Psychophysiology, 39, 577–584.

Gravel, J. S., Dunn, M., Lee, W. W., and Ellis, M. A. (2006). Peripheral audition of children on the autistic spectrum, Ear and Hearing, 27, 299–312.

Greenspan, S. (1995). The challenging child. Reading, MA, Addison-Wesley.

Greenspan, S., and Weider, S. (1998) The child with special needs. Reading, MA, Perseus Books.

Greenspan, S. (2005). Early identification of autistic spectrum disorder. Journal of Developmental Learning Disorders, 25: 138–149.

Kile, J. E. (1996). Audiologic assessment of children with Down syndrome. American Journal of Audiology, 5, 44–52.

Lancioni, G. E., Coninx, F., and Smeets, P. M. (1989). A classical conditioning procedure for the hearing assessment of multihandicapped persons. Journal of Speech and Hearing Research, 54, 88–93.

Lancioni, G. E., and Coninx, F. (1995). A classical condition procedure for auditory testing: air puff audiometry. Scandinavian Audiology, 24, 43–48.

Lloyd, L. L., Spradin, J. E., and Reid, M. J. (1968). An operant audiometric procedure for difficult to test patients. Journal of Speech and Hearing Disorders, 33, 236–245.

Madell, J. R. (1998). *Behavioral Evaluation of Hearing in Infants and Young Children*. New York: Thieme Medical Publishers.

Myklebust, H. (1954). Auditory disorders in children, a manual for differential diagnosis. New York: Grune and Stratton.

Shoup, A. G., and Roeser, R. (2007). Audiologic evaluation of special populations in audiology. In *Audiology Diagnosis*, Roesser, R. J, Valente, M., and Hosford-Dunn, H (Eds.) New York: Thieme Medical Publishers, 314–334.

Smith, R. J. H., Zimmerman, B., Connolly, P. K., Jerger, S. W., and Yelich, A. (1992). Screening audiometry using the high-risk register in a level III nursery. Archives of Otolaryngology—Head and Neck Surgery, 118, 1306–1311.

Verpoorten, R. A., and Emmen, J. G. (1995). A tactile-auditory conditioning procedure for the hearing assessment of persons with autism and mental retardation. Scandinavian Audiology. 24, 49–50.

Chapter 10

Evaluation of Speech Perception in Infants and Children

Jane R. Madell

Key Points

- Speech perception testing is a critical part of the audiologic test battery. It provides information about how a child can be expected to function in daily listening situations.

- Selecting a test at the appropriate language level is critical.

- Testing should be conducted with and without technology (hearing aids, cochlear implants, and FM systems).

- Testing should be conducted at normal and soft conversational levels in quiet and with competing noise.

♦ Speech Perception Testing

Purpose of Speech Perception Testing

Speech audiometry, appropriately used, can be an extremely valuable part of the clinical audiology test battery, particularly for evaluating and monitoring auditory function in children. Pure tone testing provides information about degree and type of hearing loss, but does not provide information about auditory function. How a person is able to use hearing for the perception of speech is critical for the development of language and accurate speech production. Speech perception testing is the only part of the audiologic test battery that assesses how a child hears speech (Madell, 2007; Van Vliet, 2006).

Pearl

- Speech perception testing is the only part of the audiology test battery that functionally assesses auditory performance. Speech perception information can be used to determine how a child is functioning with and without technology, in quiet, and with competing noise. Speech perception information should be used to plan remediation including suggesting modifications in technology and in selecting and managing educational placement.

Evaluating speech perception skills can be very helpful in determining the kind of auditory difficulties a child may be having, and in planning remediation. For example, word recognition scores that are poorer than expected compared with pure tone thresholds at normal and soft conversational levels can be strong indicators for aggressive treatment—medical, audiologic, or educational. Testing at soft conversational levels and in the presence of competing noise can effectively demonstrate the need for technology, the need to change technology, the need for an FM system in the classroom, or the need for auditory therapy.

Information available from the evaluation of large numbers of adults and children (Boothroyd, Hanin, and Hnath, 1985; Boothroyd, 2004) indicates that word recognition ability decreases as the degree of hearing loss increases. However, the effect of hearing loss is much more significant for children than for adults because of the impact that even mild hearing loss can have on the development of speech and language (Clopton and Silverman, 1977; McKay, Chapter 31 in this text; Ross and Giolas, 1978; Wallace et al., 1988). Word recognition testing evaluates the extent to which a child's hearing loss has adversely affected speech perception and put development of speech and language at risk.

For children who have identified hearing losses or auditory processing disorders, word recognition testing is useful in monitoring progress during treatment. Almost everyone agrees that regardless of the mode of communication families choose to educate their children who experience hearing loss, all children should be given the opportunity to maximize their auditory skills. Providing appropriate technology is a necessary but incomplete step toward this goal. Children must be taught to use residual hearing for perception of speech and language. Even young children with profound hearing losses can be taught, with the proper technology, to use audition for the reception of speech and language. The use of audition will positively affect language growth and improve speech production.

The audiologist who evaluates a child annually, semiannually, or quarterly may be in a better position to evaluate auditory progress than the therapist or teacher who sees the child several times a week. If a therapy program is successful, the child's word recognition should continue to improve and, over time, the child should be able to perform more difficult auditory tasks. During routine evaluations the audiologist can monitor the child's progress and assist teachers and therapists in modifying treatment goals to improve the child's auditory functioning.

Pearl

- The audiologist who sees a child less frequently is in a better position to monitor changes in performance than teachers and other clinicians who see him daily or weekly.

How Speech Perception Is Evaluated

The goal of speech audiometry is to obtain as much information as possible about a child's speech perception abilities. There are several ways to evaluate speech perception, and each procedure provides different information. Erber's classic work (1976, 1979) describes an auditory skills matrix that is a useful way to think about the different components of speech perception testing and auditory listening tasks. Four response tasks can be used to assess performance:

1. *Detection* is the ability to tell when a stimulus is present. Detection is assessed using threshold tests (speech awareness threshold).

2. *Discrimination* is the ability to determine if two stimuli are the same or different. Discrimination is tested in tasks like the visually reinforced infants speech detection (VRISD), when an infant is asked to identify when the stimulus changes (Ba ba ba ba ba sh sh).

3. *Identification* is the ability to recognize the stimulus being presented and to identify it by repeating, pointing, or writing. Identification is assessed during word recognition testing.

4. *Comprehension* is the ability to understand what the stimulus means. The child may point to a picture and indicate that he also comprehends the stimulus, or may simply repeat back the words without understanding, which indicates identification.

The most common task to assess speech perception skills in English uses a monosyllabic word as the stimulus. Results can be scored by recording the number of words identified correctly and/or by scoring the number of phonemes repeated correctly. Phoneme testing is the most difficult task in the stimulus hierarchy because it is the least redundant and provides the fewest cues; however, phoneme scoring provides valuable information about exactly what is perceived. Connected discourse, on the other hand, is easiest to understand, since the listener may acceptably extrapolate words he does not correctly perceive from contextual cues. Unfortunately, connected discourse provides very little information about which specific phonemes are being misperceived and are causing perception difficulties. As a result, connected discourse testing is not usually performed during audiologic testing, but is more frequently used during therapy to improve auditory skills.

What Speech Perception Testing Measures

Speech perception testing can help determine how a child is functioning in everyday listening situations with and without technology, and can assist in making decisions about management. Children who are hearing well at normal and soft conversational levels in quiet, and in noise, should be able to hear well in the classroom. Children who can hear well at normal conversational levels in quiet, but who do not hear soft speech well, or cannot hear well in noise will have a difficult time hearing in a typical classroom. They may be able to hear the teacher with the FM, but will not hear other children. Children who cannot understand speech, even at normal conversational levels, will not be able to rely on audition to learn in the classroom. Knowing what a child can hear with and without technology, will help the educational team determine if a technology is appropriate or needs to be modified, and will assist in identifying appropriate classroom placement and the need for ancillary services.

Speech perception testing can

♦ demonstrate benefit with technology (hearing aids, cochlear implants, and FM systems)

♦ demonstrate improvement in auditory functioning over time

♦ identify problems that develop over time including

  ♦ reduction in auditory functioning

  ♦ equipment deterioration or failure

♦ identify specific-speech perception errors that require remediation

♦ demonstrate habilitation and rehabilitation needs

♦ assist in selecting the appropriate educational environment

Goal of the Audiologic Evaluation

In addition to the basic audiologic assessment of degree and type of hearing loss, a critical part of the evaluation of children is the measurement of the actual use of hearing in daily listening situations (in quiet and with competing noise), including assessment with technology if it is used. Although audiologists routinely evaluate speech perception under earphones during basic hearing testing, speech perception testing is not always measured in soundfield (unaided) to assess functional auditory skills, and is not always assessed with technology.

Asking a child, parents, or for that matter, an adult with hearing loss, if he is "doing well" with technology will not provide enough information about auditory function. Some users have low expectations about what is possible with technology and do not expect to understand speech in difficult listening situations; others may expect to hear better then normal hearing peers when using technology. Observing the child's communication skills during casual conversation will provide some information but cannot lead to an accurate evaluation of auditory functioning because the listener will be using general knowledge to "fill in the blanks" for what is not heard. Without speech perception testing, it is not possible to predict

♦ what the child hears

♦ what the child does not hear

♦ if there has been a change in auditory perception

♦ if something can be done to improve auditory functioning

When Should Speech Perception Be Measured?

Speech perception should be measured: when hearing loss is identified, at every reevaluation, when selecting or changing technology, when changing technology settings, or at any time that concern develops about auditory functioning. For young children with hearing loss, speech perception should be reevaluated about four times per year. Older children should be evaluated twice yearly, and adults, who ought to be better able to monitor their own functioning, should be evaluated annually (Madell, 2002).

♦ Speech Threshold Tests

Speech threshold information is very useful in

♦ providing basic information about auditory status

♦ confirming pure tone thresholds

♦ determining the level to begin speech perception testing

Speech Awareness or Speech Detection Thresholds

The speech awareness threshold (SAT) or speech detection threshold (SDT) is a test that uses speech stimuli to determine threshold—the lowest level at which a person can detect the presence of the stimulus 50% of the time. SATs are usually used only when more complex speech stimuli cannot be used, such as when testing a very young child who does not have the vocabulary for other speech testing or when testing a person with extremely poor or no word recognition ability—as may be seen in some children with profound hearing loss.

Using voice (running conversation) or music will provide general information that sound is being heard. However, because both are very broadband stimuli, a threshold obtained with conversational speech or music does not offer frequency specific information. A threshold to music at 40 dB HL tells us that at some frequency the person is hearing at 40 dB HL; it does not tell us if that is a low or high frequency or if the person is hearing throughout the frequency range required for speech.

More useful information is obtained by using individual phonemes such as in the Ling Six Sound Test (Ling, 2002). The test items are selected to provide frequency specific information to low, mid-high, and high- frequency stimuli and include a/i/u/sh/m/ and /s/. The vowels /a/, and /u/ and the consonant /m/ assess perception of low-frequency stimuli, /i/ includes both low- and mid- to high-frequency information, /sh/ assesses perception of mid- to high-frequency information, and /s/ assesses perception of high-frequency information.

A shorter version of the Ling 6 Sound test (Madell, 1998, 2007) uses three sounds: /ba/ for assessing low-frequency information, /sh/ for assessing mid- to high-frequency information, and /s/ for assessing high-frequency information. Although it takes slightly longer to obtain these three thresholds than to obtain one, the information is much more valuable than that obtained using a single broad-frequency stimulus. The information is frequency specific and provides information about how a person can be expected to perceive stimuli across the frequency range needed for speech. In addition, since the test is frequency specific, it can be more directly compared with pure tone thresholds.

Speech Reception Threshold

The speech reception threshold (SRT) determines the lowest level at which a person can identify speech stimuli 50% of the time. It differs from detection tasks, which require only that the person be aware of the presence of speech, not identify the stimulus. The test materials selected will depend on the individual being tested. When possible, it is desirable to use test materials and procedures that are standardized on adults so that results are comparable across patients. Older children with good language skills will be able to perform well on the standard tests that were developed for adults. Young children may not have the vocabulary or may be too shy to repeat back what the tester has said. For these children, a task that requires pointing to pictures, objects, or body parts will be easier and will produce useful results (Madell, 1998, 2007; Ramkissoon, 2001).

The test procedure for SRTs requires that the person be familiar with the material being presented. Familiarity will make testing easier and result in a threshold at a softer level than that obtained from a test in which any vocabulary word might be used. Standard testing uses spondee words (two syllable words with equal stress on both syllables.) With children who can perform this task, the audiologist reads the list of words at a comfortably loud level, permitting speech reading if necessary, with the child repeating the word to verify that the word is correctly identified. Once the child is familiar with the words, the audiologist begins testing using audition alone, and reduces the intensity until the child begins making errors. The audiologist then ascends and descends, establishing the level at which the child can correctly repeat the words 50% of the time. ASHA guidelines for speech reception threshold testing (1988) describe a complex procedure which, while resulting in an accurate threshold, may be too time consuming for use with some children. Cramer and Erber (1974) found that best results were obtained by asking the child to say the word and point at the same time. This combined task may increase the child's attention to the task and results in improved scores. Litovsky (2003, 2004a, 2004b, 2005) has developed the Crisp and Crisp, Jr. (Children's Realistic Index for Speech Perception) closed set spondee tests which can be performed with a picture book or on a computer. The tests are designed to be used with or without competing noise. When used without competing noise, they are threshold tests.

◆ Infant Speech Discrimination Tests

Bertoncini and Berger (2004) describe a protocol based on the Visual Reinforcement Infant Speech Discrimination procedure, which can be used to test discrimination of speech contrasts and to categorize various speech stimuli. The original protocol was described by Werker, Shi, and Desjardins (1998), and uses a task in which an infant is asked to identify a change in the speech stimulus. For example, the phoneme /a/ may be presented and contrasted with /sh/ as follows: a a a a a a sh sh sh a a a. Infants are trained to make a conditioned head turn to the new stimulus, and the standard VRA procedure can be used as reinforcement. Older children can use other tasks to indicate that they have heard the change in stimulus.

◆ Children's Speech Perception Testing

Speech perception tests are designed to evaluate a child's ability to understand speech under different listening conditions. Unlike threshold testing, word recognition testing is performed at suprathreshold levels. Testing may be conducted at different intensities and under varying conditions of competing noise. The selection of test materials and test conditions will depend on the child's vocabulary level and the child's ability to cooperate. Scoring requires accurate perception of all the phonemes in any word to obtain a correct score. By modifying the response task and types of reinforcement, it is possible to learn a great deal about a child's speech perception skills. Several factors affect speech perception test results.

Selecting the Appropriate Test

Vocabulary Level

It is essential that the audiologist know the child's vocabulary level to select the appropriate test. The child's vocabulary age may be determined by using a standardized vocabulary test, by obtaining information from testing at another evaluation, or from the reports of parents, speech-language pathologists, or teachers. When the previous alternatives are not available, it will be necessary for the audiologist to make a determination about vocabulary level through conversation with the child. Selecting test materials which contain vocabulary words that are not in the child's lexicon will result in a score that is not an accurate reflection of his speech perception abilities.

Degree of Hearing Loss

Degree of hearing loss should not be a factor in selecting tests of speech perception. Tests should be selected based on the individual child's abilities. It is unfair to the child to make assumptions about how he will be able to perform based on the pure tone audiogram alone. Many children with profound hearing losses are capable of using residual hearing for reception of auditory information (especially with the availability of cochlear implants). However, it is undoubtedly true that profound hearing loss makes it more difficult to receive information using the auditory channel. For children who have not had the advantage of early intervention, who have not been trained in a program that emphasizes the use of audition, or who do not have the ability to use audition, special tests have been developed that make speech perception testing possible. (See Tests for Severe and Profound Hearing Loss in this chapter.)

Closed-Set versus Open-Set Testing

Word recognition tests can be divided into two categories: closed-set tests and open-set tests. In closed-set testing, the number of possible items is restricted. Items might be numbers, body parts, pictures, or alphabet letters to which the child will point. The child being tested understands what all the possible test stimuli are and will select his response from that limited number of potential items. By simply guessing and pointing to a picture, a child has some chance of attaining a correct score.

Open-set testing, on the other hand, offers no clues. The child is asked to repeat what he hears without any indicators. Any word in the child's vocabulary is a possibility. In some cases, the child may be asked to repeat what he hears even if it is not a word (e.g., nonsense syllables). Open-set testing is much more difficult than closed-set testing, and it will frequently result in lower scores. However, open-set paradigms will provide a more realistic picture of speech perception capabilities in conversation. As soon a child is capable of the task, open-set testing should be used, since it will provide a more accurate representation of how the child is performing when compared with children of the same age. By the time a child reaches kindergarten, open-set testing should be attempted.

Recorded versus Monitored Live Voice Testing

Recorded testing has the advantage of being more easily comparable from test session to test session and from one audiologist to another. It avoids the possibility of the tester modifying his voice either intentionally or unintentionally, to assist the child in obtaining a higher score. On the other hand, recorded testing is more time consuming, and prevents the audiologist from making the adaptations that are sometimes needed when testing young children. A child may require

- more off-time between stimuli than the recording permits to be able to attend

- that an item be repeated if he becomes distracted or begins to talk to a parent or the test assistant

- time-out for encouragement

It is certainly possible to stop a tape or CD player and rewind, but this is often difficult to accomplish efficiently. Experienced pediatric audiologists, who are aware of the

Table 10–1 Word Recognition Testing for an 8-Year-Old Using Monitored Live Voice and Recorded Testing Demonstrating Different Results

PBK	Monitored Live Voice	Recorded
50 dB	100%	100%
35 dB	100%	95%
50 dB +5 SNR	100%	50%
50 dB 0 SNR	100%	50%
35 dB 0 SNR	88%	32%

Abbreviations: dB, decibels; SNR, signal to noise ratio.

pitfalls, can obtain accurate results using monitored live voice (MLV) testing.

Table 10–1 shows speech perception scores for an 8-year-old with normal hearing who was tested with MLV and then tested with recorded stimuli. It is clear that the monitored live voice testing can overestimate the child's auditory functioning. The recorded testing was in agreement with the parent's and school's description of the child's functioning and made a case for referring the child for an auditory processing evaluation.

Pearl

- MLV testing, because it is easier for children than recorded testing, and because it may be easier for the audiologist as well, will frequently show higher scores than recorded testing and thus overestimate the child's actual auditory abilities. Therefore, it is important to use recorded tests whenever the child is capable of doing the task. Recorded testing will provide a more accurate representation of auditory performance.

Phoneme-Scoring versus Whole-Word Scoring

Most of the tests that we use to evaluate speech perception are scored according to whether or not the person correctly identifies the whole word. If the person makes an error on one phoneme, the entire word is scored as wrong. The whole word method of scoring may be depriving us of useful information.

Arthur Boothroyd has written extensively about phoneme scoring and its advantages; he has developed tests that rely on phoneme scoring (1968, 1984, 1988). Actually, phoneme scoring can be used with any test. By recording the phoneme errors that a child makes during any speech perception test, we can learn what parts of the auditory spectrum are not being appropriately perceived. For example, vowel errors indicate insufficient low frequency information. Inability to correctly perceive sibilants indicates insufficient high frequency information or possible upward spread of masking caused by too much low-frequency amplification. Knowing the exact spectral bands of the phonemes that are misperceived will provide even more specific information. Such information may permit us to make changes in the frequency response of the child's hearing aids or cochlear implants, to make earmold modifications, and to make suggestions about auditory training goals.

Half-List versus Full-List

The issue of using only a half list of words in a test versus using the entire or full list has been debated in the field of audiology for years. Obviously, using a full 50-word list reduces the chance of scoring error. However, when working with young children, several additional factors need to be considered. With young children time is of the essence. It is necessary to acquire a great deal of information in a short period of time, and it may not be possible to obtain test results in all the necessary test conditions if too much time is spent on any one test. However, the necessity for speed does not permit using less than the required number of stimuli to obtain reliable results. Short lists should be used only when a short-list protocol has been validated. The number of words used must be sufficient to obtain all the information necessary to assess the child's speech perception abilities. This assessment can usually be achieved with 25 words on most tests, but not with only 10 words. Except in rare cases like the Isophonemic Word Lists (Boothroyd, 1968), which have been standardized as 10-word (30-phoneme) lists, 10 words will not provide a sufficient number or variety of stimuli to obtain an accurate score.

Use of a Carrier Phrase

Most word recognition tasks were designed to be used with a carrier phrase. The carrier phrase alerts the child to attend and places the word in a sentence context that more accurately represents its use in normal conversation. The carrier phrase usually ends with a vowel so that the carrier phrase does not influence the word. Common carrier phrases are "you will say," "show me the," "where is the," or "tell me."

♦ Description of Children's Speech Perception Tests

Closed-Set Tests

The most frequently used closed-set tests for very young children are NU-CHIPS [Northwestern University Children's Hearing in Pictures] (Elliot and Katz, 1980), and the WIPI [Word Intelligibility by Picture Identification] (Ross and Lerman, 1970). The NU-CHIPS is a four-item test with vocabulary appropriate for children aged 3 to 5 years, and the WIPI is a six-item test with vocabulary appropriate for children aged 4 to 6 years. The foils in the WIPI are more similar to each other requiring finer auditory skills, which, along with the fact that it has six items, make the test more difficult.

The Alphabet Test (Ross and Randolph, 1990) asks the child to point to one or two alphabet letters. The errors are scored according to how phonemically close to correct the answer is. For example, if the stimulus is /p/ and the child points to /b/ the answer is wrong by only one distinctive feature (voicing). If the child had pointed to /z/ the response would have been off by three distinctive features (voicing, manner, and place), indicating a much more significant problem in auditory perception, and the child would have received a lower score.

The Auditory Numbers Test (ANT) (Erber, 1980), is a fun way to test number perception. There are pictures of one, two, three, or more ants on cards. The tester says a number and the child selects the appropriate card. The same information can be obtained by having the child repeat the number spoken by the tester. Number identification requires only vowel perception, so scores obtained with numbers are measuring only low frequency perception.

The CRISP and CRISP Jr. (Children's Realistic Inventory of Speech Perception) (Litovsky, 2003, 2004a, 2004b, 2005) are closed-set, four-item forced choice tests that use spondee words and different levels of competing noise. The noise level at which a child can identify spondees accurately is determined. The test can be performed using either a computer or a book format with the child pointing to the selected picture.

When standardized tests cannot be used, body parts or names of familiar objects can be substituted as test stimuli. However, if a very small set of stimuli are used, the results must be interpreted with caution.

Open-Set Tests

Word Tests

Open-set testing, because it does not have a limited set from which the listener selects an answer, is more difficult than closed-set testing. The response is limited only by the vocabulary of the person being tested.

The NU-CHIPS and WIPI word lists can be used without the pictures, making the task open-set rather than closed-set. These tests are useful because vocabulary level can be easily identified.

The Phonetically Balanced Kindergarten (PBK) test (Haskins, 1949) is an open-set test with kindergarten-level vocabulary.

The Isophonemic Words Lists (Mackersie, Boothroyd and Minnear, 2001) use 10-item CNC word lists with school-age vocabulary and is scored for phonemes and whole words correct.

The Minimal Pairs Test (Robbins, et al., 1988) was designed for use with cochlear implant patients. The listener is shown two pictures with words that differ by only one phoneme (e.g., bear and pear). For each pair, the difference is one phonologic contrast (e.g., place, manner, or voicing). During the course of the test manner, place and voicing are tested for consonant discrimination, and vowel place and height are tested for vowel discrimination.

The Lexical Neighborhood Test (LNT) and Modified Lexical Neighborhood Test (MLNT) (Kirk, Pisoni, and Osberger, 1995) were designed for cochlear implant evaluations and use words that do not have similar words or confusions. This makes these tests easier than some of the other open-set tests. There are a limited number of test lists of comparable difficulty, reducing the number of conditions that can be tested.

Older children and adults can be tested using the more familiar Consonant Nucleus Consonant Test [CNC] (Peterson and Lehiste, 1962) or NU 6 (Tillman and Carhart, 1966) word lists. As a child's vocabulary increases and skills improve, the more difficult tests should be used, since they provide a measure of performance that can better be compared with scores obtained for typically hearing peers.

Sentence Tests

Sentence tests provide beneficial information about how a person communicates in general conversation; they provide clues about the ability of the child to "fill in the blanks" when he receives only part of the message. Even though sentence tests are useful, they are not a substitute for monosyllabic word tests that provide more specific information and are more helpful in planning remediation.

The most frequently used sentence tests are the Hearing in Noise Test (HINT) (Nilsson, Soli, and Sullivan, 1994), the Hearing in Noise Test for Children [HINT-C] (Nilsson, Soli, and Gelnett, 1996), and the CUNY (City University of New York) sentences (Boothroyd, Hanin, and Hnath, 1985).

The Matrix Test (Tyler and Holstad, 1987) is intended for children 4 to 6 years of age. It uses a closed-set format and has two levels of difficulty of materials. The child has a test plate with several pictures. The child is presented with a sentence composed of one word from each column. The child can either repeat the sentence or point to two correct pictures.

Tests for Special Populations

Tests for Very Young Children

Because young children have limited vocabularies, tests need to be selected with care to be certain that testing is assessing auditory perception and not vocabulary knowledge. Possible test stimuli for very young children include body parts and familiar toys or objects.

Standardized tests include Early Speech Perception Test [ESP] (Moog and Geers, 1990), which has a low verbal version that uses objects, for very young children, and a standard version that uses pictures. Subtest 1 assess syllabification (monosyllabic [shoe], bisyllabic [two syllables with unequal stress—baby], spondee [equal stress on both syllables—airplane], or trochee [three syllables—ice cream cone]). Subtest 2 is a spondee test. Subtest 3 assesses perception of monosyllabic words using primarily vowel perception.

The Potato Head Task (Robbins, 1994) uses the familiar Potato Head game to assess perception by asking the child, for example, to "give Potato Head the blue shoes."

Tests for Children with Profound Hearing Loss

Tests for children with profound hearing loss are based on the assumption that a such a child will not be able to perform on the more common standardized tests. Limited speech perception ability may be true for some patients, but with cochlear implants, expectations are changing. Tests for children with profound hearing loss should be used only when the child cannot perform on standard tests.

The tests most commonly used for children with profound hearing loss are closed-set tests. These include the ANT (Erber, 1980), the ESP, (Moog and Geers, 1990), the Potato Head Task (Robbins, 1994), and the Alphabet Test (Ross and Randolph, 1990). Other tests are the Minimal Auditory Capabilities Test (MAC) (Owens et al., 1981), and the Test of Auditory Comprehension (TAC) (Los Angeles County, 1980).

♦ Selecting the Appropriate Test Protocol

It is clearly important to select the appropriate test protocol. The first step in selecting the appropriate test is to know the child's auditory language age—the language the child has developed through listening.

Caution

- A child may have a sign language vocabulary or a lipreading vocabulary at a 9-year-old level, but have only a preschool-age vocabulary when using listening alone without visual cues.

Because audiologic speech perception tests are performed using listening alone, it is important that the test we select is based on auditory skill level. **Figure 10–1** describes the protocol for beginning testing. If a child's auditory language level is lower than 2 years, the ESP is the initial test, and if the auditory language age is 9 years, testing will begin with the NU 6 or CNC.

Figure 10–2 describes the general concept of proceeding through the tests. If the child does extremely well, it is possible that a test has been selected that is too easy. The subsequent step should be to proceed to the next more difficult test and repeat testing. For example, if a child obtains a score of 80% on the NU CHIPS, that test is too easy. The test can be made more difficult by

- testing in more difficult conditions, such as moving to open-set testing at 50 dB HL

- continuing using closed set-testing at soft conversational speech levels (at 35 dB HL)

- presenting speech in noise (50 dB HL +5 SNR)

- if vocabulary permits, testing can move to a more difficult test

In this example, testing could proceed to the WIPI, the PBK, or the CNC or NU-6 tests, depending on the child's vocabulary level.

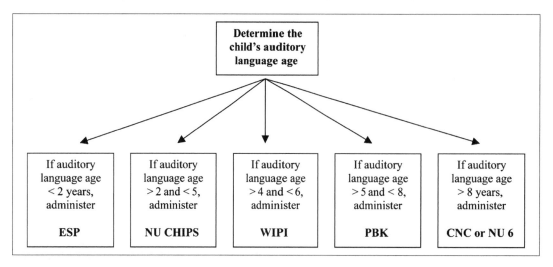

Figure 10–1 Speech perception test protocol. Determining appropriate start level.

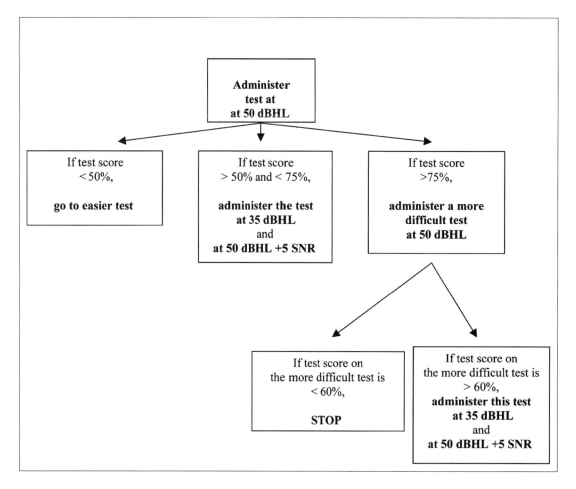

Figure 10–2 Speech perception test protocol. Determining steps in selecting test conditions.

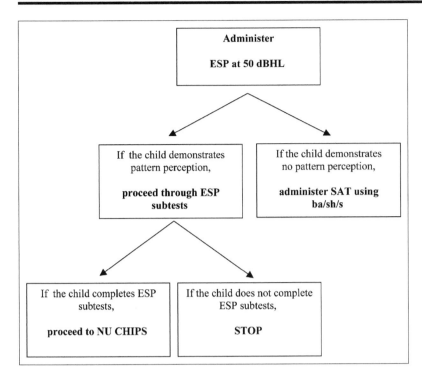

Figure 10–3 Speech perception test protocol. Test sequence when using the ESP for children with an auditory language age younger than 2 years.

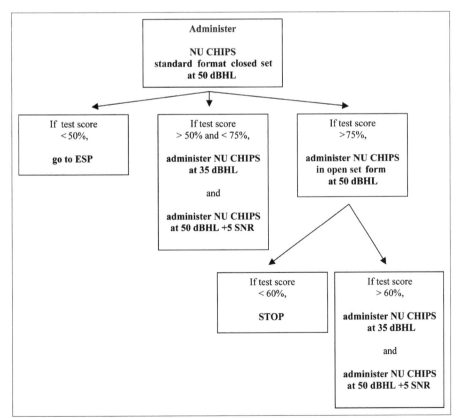

Figure 10–4 Speech perception test protocol. Test sequence when using the NU CHIPS for children with an auditory language age between 2 and 5 years.

Figure 10–3, Fig. 10–4, Fig. 10–5, Fig. 10–6, and Fig. 10–7 describe the protocol to use when starting with specific tests. Testing in soundfield should always begin at a normal conversational level of 50 dB HL. If the child does well at that level, testing continues at a soft speech level of 35 dB HL and then in noise, at a normal conversational level of 50 dB +5 SNR. If a child does well at this noise level, additional testing should be performed at 50 dB at 0 SNR and at 35 dB at 0 SNR.

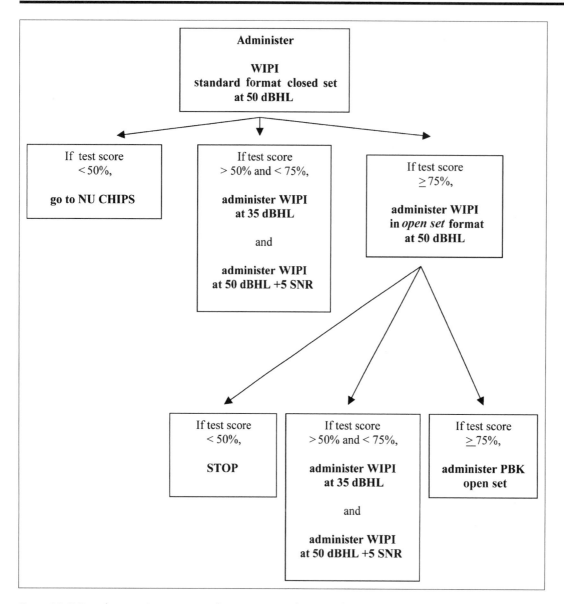

Figure 10–5 Speech perception test protocol: Test sequence when using the WIPI for children with an auditory language age between 4 and 6 years.

◆ Evaluating Functional Listening

Testing speech perception skills under earphones reveals important information about the functioning of individual ears, but it does not provide information about performance in daily listening. Standard audiologic test protocol suggests testing speech perception at 40 dB louder than the speech threshold (40 dB SL). A significant body of research has indicated that testing at this level is likely to provide the best word recognition scores for people with normal hearing. If the child has normal hearing, this level may be close to the typical conversational level of 50 dB HL. However, if the child's speech threshold is 30 dB HL, and speech perception is tested at 70 dB HL, we are not seeing a realistic picture of

how the child hears normal conversation in daily listening situations. To obtain a more realistic picture of how a child is performing in day-to-day situations, it is useful to assess speech perception at normal (50 dB HL) and soft (35 dB HL) conversational levels in quiet.

It is also necessary to assess hearing in the presence of competing noise, since the child must hear in noisy environments at school and at home. It is useful to test normal conversational levels at +5 and 0 dB signal to noise ratio (SNR), and soft speech at 0 dB SNR. Speech noise or white noise will provide the easiest competing noise condition since it is not confused with speech and is relatively easy to ignore. Single talker babble poses a very difficult listening task, because it is easy to understand what the distracting person is saying and therefore will be difficult to tune-out.

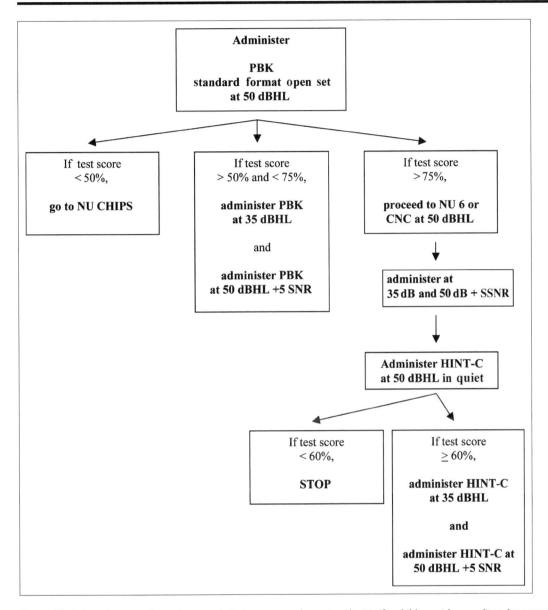

Figure 10–6 Speech perception test protocol. Test sequence when using the PBK for children with an auditory language age between 5 and 8 years.

Multitalker babble with numerous talkers (10 to 12 talkers) is easier to tune out than four talker babble because the number of talkers makes it difficult to identify individual words. Four talker babble is a relatively difficult stimulus, since it is possible to understand some of what is said and therefore, adds to the confusion when listening to the primary signal. For this reason, four talker babble is a good stimulus to use since it is difficult, but realistic.

By testing in more difficult conditions, the audiologist will be able to identify children who may have auditory processing problems and who require additional testing. Children with otitis media who are experiencing problems that indicate difficulty hearing in a classroom may also be identified (Rosenfeld, Madell, and McMahon (1997).

◆ Evaluating the Use of Technology

When evaluating the benefit that the child receives from technology, it is important to assess

◆ each piece of equipment, individually

◆ each ear, separately

◆ both ears, together and with the FM system to be certain it is providing the expected benefit.

Without doing this precise testing, it will not be possible to identify problems with individual pieces of equipment. If,

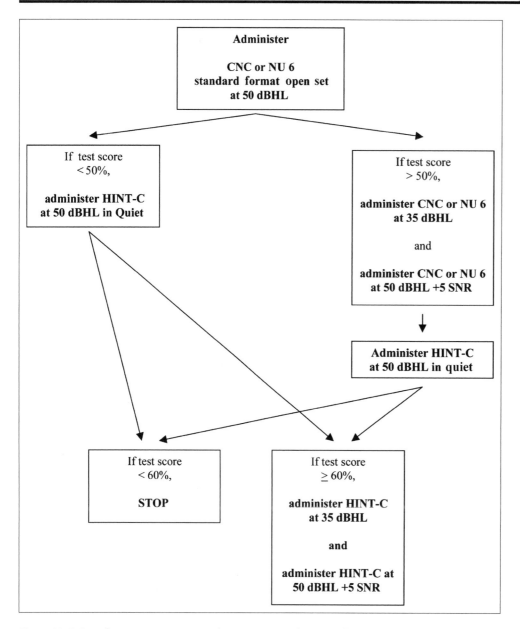

Figure 10–7 Speech perception test protocol. Test sequence when using the NU 6 or CNC test for children with an auditory language age older than 8 years.

for example, one hearing aid is providing insufficient gain, or if speech perception with one hearing aid is significantly poorer than with the other hearing aid, binaural testing will not identify the problem and the audiologist will not know there is a discrepancy that requires attention (**see Fig. 10–8**).

Figure 10–8 shows test results for a child who has poorer word recognition in the left ear that is resulting in poor binaural word recognition. If testing had been performed binaurally only, the audiologist would not know that the child has good speech perception in the right ear. Since aided gain is the same for both ears, speech perception discrepancies may indicate that there is some distortion in the left hearing aid, or that the child has poor auditory skills in the left ear and needs auditory training work on the left ear alone.

♦ Developing a Speech Perception Test Protocol

The first thing to consider when developing a test protocol is the purpose of the test. Is the test being performed to obtain the best possible score? If that is the case, it would be best to select very easy test materials on which the person can be expected to do very well. On the other hand, if the purpose is to see how the person compares to normal hearing peers, testing must be conducted with tests that would be used to test normal hearing peers. If the purpose is to monitor technology or technology settings, testing should be performed

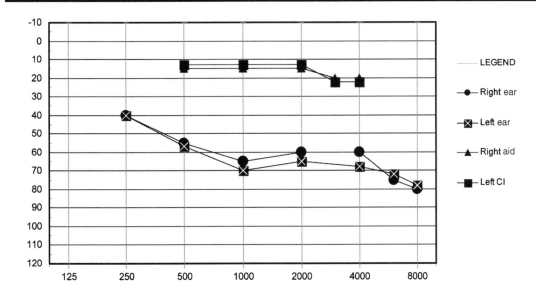

NU 6	Right aid	Left aid	Binaural	+ FM
50 dB	88%	67%	67%	100%
35 dB			67%	88%
70 dB			73%	DNT
50 dB +5SNR			35%	75%

Figure 10–8 Binaural speech perception is poorer than the best monaural speech perception.

with each piece of equipment alone, and also in whatever combinations the equipment is used on a daily basis. If the purpose is to assess areas needing habilitation/rehabilitation and to plan for educational placement, it will be important to monitor performance in difficult listening situations and to score appropriate vocabulary-level tests using both whole word and phoneme scoring.

Test Materials

Test materials must be linguistically appropriate, neither too easy nor too difficult.

It may be necessary to select different tests for each ear if the two ears function differently **(see Fig. 10–9)**. The evaluation report must be clear about what tests were used in which condition so they can be appropriately interpreted. Level of complexity of the test material must be considered. To obtain a complete picture of a person's auditory abilities,

it may be useful to test monosyllabic words, nonsense syllables, and sentences, all of which can be scored for number of words and phonemes correctly identified.

Test Conditions

When testing speech perception using earphones, it is standard practice to test at 40 dB SL (louder than the pure tone average), or 40 dB above the SRT. When testing with technology, test at levels that will provide a good indication of how the person functions in a variety of daily listening situations **(see Table 10–2)**. With technology, test monaurally, binaurally, and with FM system.

Test Modality

Testing in the auditory-only mode will provide information about how the child is using auditory information. Audi-

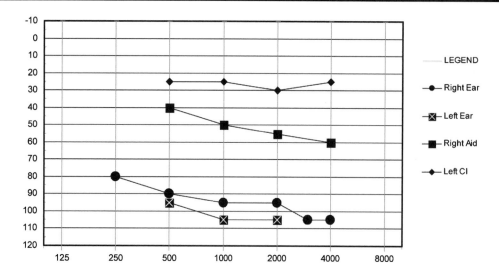

		Right aid	Left CI	Binaural
50 dB HL	NuChips – closed set	64%	96%	
	NuChips – open set		88%	88%
35 dB HL	NuChips – open set		66%	74%
50 dB HL + 5 SNR	NuChips – open set		78%	86%

Figure 10–9 Using different tests for different ears. CI, cochlear implant.

tory-only testing is critical for monitoring technology to determine if adjustments need to be made to the technology, and to understand how the person functions when visual cues are not available. Testing in the visual-only mode will provide information about how the child is using visual information, primarily speech reading. Testing in the auditory-visual mode will provide information about a combination of auditory and visual skills.

Audiological emphasis on testing in the auditory-only mode does not imply that a child will be asked to ignore

Table 10–2 Suggested Test Conditions for Speech Perception Testing in Soundfield, with and without Technology

Testing in quiet
Normal conversation 50 dB HL
Soft conversation 35 dB HL

Testing in competing noise (4 talker babble)
Normal conversation 50 dB HL at +5 SNR
Normal conversation 50 dB HL at 0 SNR
Soft conversation 35 dB HL at 0 SNR

Abbreviations: dB, decibels; HL, hearing level; SNR, signal to noise ratio.

visual cues in daily communication. Auditory-only testing is simply the best way to obtain information about auditory skills and necessary audiological modifications to improve communication. Information about auditory perceptual skills is critical no matter what communication approach the child uses.

Stimulus Presentation

Recorded testing is the preferred test method because it is most repeatable. This makes it easy to compare test results over time. Some young children, who cannot sit still and attend consistently, may require that testing be adaptable. For these children, MLV testing is easier to use. When MLV testing is used, the audiologist must monitor the voice level using a VU meter to be certain that the level is well controlled. When using MLV testing, rate of presentation should be close to that of the recorded test. If an adaptive test protocol is used (if test stimuli are eliminated or words are repeated), this must be noted and taken into account when describing test results. As children age and skills improve, testing should advance to using recorded stimuli.

Test Format

Closed-set tests are easier for the child to perform because the possible choices are limited, and all targets are present for the child to select. Open-set format is the preferred method because it is a more realistic estimate of everyday performance.

◆ Items to Consider when Reviewing the Report of an Audiologic Evaluation

When reviewing a report of an audiologic evaluation, it is important to know how testing was accomplished. Was testing accomplished in open- or closed-set? Was testing performed recorded or MLV? How loud was the test signal? Was each ear tested separately with technology? Even though closed-set, MLV testing may be appropriate for a three-year-old, but it is not the appropriate test protocol for a 10-year-old in a mainstream setting. The *NU CHIPS* (Elliot and Katz, 1980) is an appropriate test for a preschool child or a child with a preschool vocabulary, but it is no longer appropriate for a mainstreamed third grader who should have a vocabulary significantly above the preschool level.

Pitfall

- Assessing a child's speech perception capabilities with a test that is too easy will result in an inflated test score that will not provide an accurate estimate of the child's daily functioning.

If a child performs well binaurally at a normal conversional level, but does not do well at a soft speech level or with competing noise, he will have problems hearing at school or at home. The audiologist will then need to try to improve the child's ability to hear soft speech and to hear in noise. With a hearing aid, it may be possible to increase gain. With a cochlear implant, it may be possible to increase the sensitivity. If the technology cannot be adjusted, it indicates the need for a change in technology or for the use of an FM system in many listening situations for auditory access.

By recording and evaluating phoneme scoring, it is feasible to determine which phonemes are not being heard. It is then possible to extrapolate the frequencies that the child cannot access. For example, if a child is not hearing /s/, it is likely that there is insufficient gain between 4000 Hz and 6000 Hz. Knowing this specific frequency information will assist the audiologist in determining how to change technology settings and in suggesting to the auditory therapist what needs to be emphasized during auditory therapy.

Pearl

- Recording phoneme errors can assist in identifying specific areas of the frequency spectrum that may be able to be accessed by changing hearing aid or cochlear implant settings to improve auditory performance.

◆ Conclusion

It is critical that everyone working with a child who has hearing loss have high expectations for what the child is capable of achieving and what the technology is capable of

Table 10–3 Speech Perception Evaluation Form

	Right Unaided	Left Unaided	Soundfield, No Technology	Right Technology	Left Technology	Binaural Technology	FM + Technology
Words							
50 dB HL word score							
phonemes							
35 dB HL word score							
phonemes							
50 dB HL +5 SNR							
Word score							
phonemes							
50 dB HL 0 SNR							
Word score							
phonemes							
35 dB HL 0 SNR							
Word score							
phonemes							
Sentences							
50 dB HL							
35 dB HL							
50 dB HL +5 SNR							

Abbreviations: dB, decibels; FM, frequency modulated; HL, hearing level; SNR, signal to noise ratio.

providing. If the child cannot hear some sounds, audiologists need to modify the technology settings. If the child is using the best possible hearing aid and cannot hear a portion of the speech signal, it may be time to consider moving to cochlear implants. The goal of audiologic management is to have the child hear as much as possible to maximize auditory learning. By fully evaluating auditory skills, the audiologist can go a long way to improving auditory functioning.

When a child performs well at normal conversational levels (50 dBHL) but poorly for soft speech (35 dBHL) and in competing noise (50 dBHL +5 SNR), it is very easy to demonstrate the need for an FM system in school and in other difficult listening situations (ballet class, sports, the car, restaurants) by comparing test results under several conditions with and without the FM system. Children who perform well at loud levels but poorly at normal and soft levels will have difficulty hearing everyday speech at home and in school. This difficulty may indicate the need for a change in technology or technology settings, the need to use an FM on a full-time basis, or that it may be time to consider a move from hearing aids to cochlear implants.

Table 10–3 is an example of a test form that can be used to record test scores. At first look it appears to be daunting,

but the more boxes that are completed, the more information the audiologist has by which to make treatment decisions. Although not all boxes will be completed at each evaluation, the more boxes that are filled in, the more information the audiologist has at his fingertips.

Speech perception testing offers the best opportunity for the audiologist to learn about a child's auditory performance and to make critical modifications in technology and recommendations for management. Although it may be time consuming, its value is well worth the effort. In the long run, it may be one of the most important services we can offer the children we have the privilege to work with.

Discussion Questions

1. Which factors need to be considered in developing a test battery for a three-year-old with a severe hearing loss?

2. Which factors need to be considered in developing a test battery for a 15-year-old with a mild hearing loss?

3. What are the considerations in selecting test levels?

References

Bertoncini, J., and Berger, B. (2004). Assess speech perception capacities in young children with cochlear implants: a psycholinguistic approach. International Congress Series, 1273, 296–299.

Boothroyd, A., Hanin L., and Hnath, T. (1985). A sentence test of speech perception: reliability, set equivalence, and short term learning (internal report RCI 10). New York: City University of New York.

Boothroyd, A. (1988) Amplitude compression and profound hearing loss. Journal of Speech and Hearing Research, 31:362–376.

Boothroyd, A (1984) Auditory perception of speech contrasts by subjects with sensorineural hearing loss. Journal of Speech and Hearing Research, 27, 134–144.

Boothroyd, A. (1968) Developments in speech audiometry. Sound 2:3–10.

Boothroyd, A. (2004). Measuring auditory speech perception capacity in very young children. International Congress Series, 1273, 292–295.

Clopton, B. M. and Silverman, M. S. (1977). Plasticity of binaural interaction, II: Critical period and changes in midline response. Journal of Neurophysiology, 40, 1275–1280.

Cramer, K. D. and Erber, N. P. (1974) A spondee recognition test for hearing impaired children. Journal of Speech and Hearing Disorders, 39: 304–311.

Elliot, L., and Katz, D. (1980). Development of a new children's test of speech discrimination. St Louis, Auditec.

Erber, N. P. (1979) An approach to evaluating auditory speech perception ability. Volta Review 81:16–24.

Erber, N. P. (1980). Use of the Auditory Numbers Test to evaluate speech perception abilities of hearing impaired children. Journal of Speech and Hearing Disorders, 45, 527–532

Erber, N. P. and Alencewicz, C. M. (1976) Audiologic evaluation of deaf children. Journal of Speech and Hearing Disorders, 41:256–267.

Haskins, H. (1949). A phonetically balanced test of speech discrimination for children. Master's Thesis, Northwestern University, Evanston, IL.

Kirk, K. I., Pisoni, D.B., and Osberger, M.J. (1995). Lexical effects on spoken word recognition by pediatric cochlear implant users. Ear and Hearing, 16, 470–481.

Litovsky, R. Y. (2003). Method and system for rapid and reliable testing of speech intelligibility in children. U.S. Patent No. 6,584,440.

Litovsky, R. Y., Johnston, P., Parkinson, A., Peters, R., and Lake, J. (2004a). Bilateral cochlear implants in children: effect of experience. In R. Miyamoto (Ed.) International congress series. Vol. 1273. Elsevier, p. 451–454.

Litovsky, R. Y., Parkinson, A., Arcaroli, J., Peters, R., Lake, J., Johnstone, P., and Yu, G. (2004b). Bilateral cochlear implants in adults and children. Archives of Otolaryngogy—Head and Neck Surgery, 130, 648–655.

Litovsky, R. Y. (2005). Speech intelligibility and spatial release from masking in young children. Journal of the Acoustical Society of America, 117, 3091–3099.

Los Angeles County, Office of the Los Angeles County Superintendent of Schools, Audiology Services, and Southwest School for the Hearing Impaired (1980). Test of Auditory Comprehension. North Hollywood: Forworks.

Mackersie, C. L., Boothroyd, A., and Minnear, D. (2001). Evaluation of the Computer-Assisted Speech Perception Test (CASPA). Journal of the American Academy of Audiology, 27, 134–144.

Madell, J. (1998). Behavioral evaluation of hearing in infants and young children, New York: Thieme.

Madell, J. (2002). Speech Audiometry for Children. In S Gerber (Ed.) The handbook of pediatric audiology. Washington, DC: Gallaudet University Press.

Madell. J. (2007). Using speech perception to maximize auditory performance, Volta Voices, March–April, 16–20.

Moog, J., and Geers, A. (1990). Early speech perception test for profoundly hearing-impaired children. St Louis: Central Institute for the Deaf.

Nilsson, M., Soli S. D., and Sullivan, J.A. (1994). Development of the Hearing in Noise Test for the measurement of speech reception thresholds in quiet and in noise. Journal of the Acoustical Society of America, 95, 1085–1099.

Nilsson, M., Soli, S.D., and Gelnett, D.J. (1996). Development of the Hearing in Noise Test for Children (HINT-C). Los Angeles: House Ear Institute.

Owens, E., Kessler, D. K., Telleen, C. C., and Schubert, E.D. (1981). The minimal auditory capabilities (MAC) battery. Hearing Aid Journal, 34, 9–34.

Peterson, G. E, and Lehiste, I. (1962). Revised CNC lists for auditory tests. Journal of Speech and Hearing Disorders, 27, 62–70.

Ramkissoon, I. (2001). Speech recognition thresholds for multilingual populations. Communication Disorders Quarterly, 22, 158–162.

Robbins, A. M., Renshaw, J. J., Miyamoto, R. T., Osberger, M. J., and Pope, M. L. (1988). Minimal Pairs Test. Indianapolis, IN: Indiana University School of Medicine.

Robbins, A. M. (1994). The Mr Potato Head Task. Indianapolis, IN, Indiana University School of Medicine.

Rosenfeld, R. M., Madell, J. R., and McMahon, A. (1997). Auditory function in normal hearing children with middle ear effusion. In D. J. Lim, et al. (Eds.), Proceedings of the Sixth International Symposium on Recent Advances in Otitis Media. Ontario, BC: Decker Periodicals, 354–356.

Ross, M and Giolas, T. G. (1978) Auditory Management of Hearing Impaired Children: Principals and Prerequisites for Intervention. Baltimore, University Park Press.

Ross, M., and Lerman, J. (1970). A picture identification test for hearing impaired children. Journal of Speech and Hearing Research, 13, 44–53.

Ross, M., and Randolph, K. (1990). A test of the auditory perception of alphabet letters for hearing impaired children: the APAL test. Volta Review, 92, 237–244.

Tillman, T. W., and Carhart, R. (1966). An expanded test for speech discrimination utilizing CNC monosyllabic words (N.U. Auditory Test No 6). Technical Report SAM-TR-66-55. Brooks Air Force Base, TX, USAF School of Aerospace Medicine.

Tyler, R. S., and Holstad, B. (1987) A closed set speech perception test for hearing-impaired children. Iowa City, University of Iowa.

Wallace, I. F., Gravei, J. S., McCarton, C. M. and Ruben, R. J. (1988) Otitis media and language development at 1 year of age. Journal of Speech and Hearing Disorders, 54:245–251.

Werker, J. F., Shi, R., and Desjardins, R. (1998). Three methods for testing infants speech perception. In A. Slater (Ed.), Perceptual Development: Visual, Auditory, and Speech Perception in Infancy, East Sussex. UK: Psychology Press.

Van Vliet, D. (2006). When it comes to audibility, don't assume, measure. Hearing Journal 86.

Chapter 11

Screening, Evaluation, and Management of Hearing Loss in the School-Aged Child

Rebecca Kooper

♦ **Hearing Screening**

Who Should Be Screened for Hearing Loss?

Who Should Be Screened for Middle Ear Disorders?

Where Will the Screening Take Place?

What Tests Are Recommended?

What Are the Testing Protocols?

Who Will Administer the Screening?

What Is the Follow-up Protocol?

Screening the Difficult-to-Test Child

♦ **Audiologic Evaluation**

The Responsibilities of the Educational Audiologist

Frequency Modulation Evaluation

Report Writing

Monitoring Amplification

In-Service Workshops

Collaborating with School Personnel

♦ **Summary**

Key Points

- Screening programs should be designed to separate children who are at risk for hearing loss or middle ear disorders from children with normal hearing.

- Audiologists must develop screening protocols to meet the needs of their specific populations.

- Assessment of the hearing status of school-aged children is similar to the assessment of adults, with added emphasis on speech audiometry to determine how the hearing loss is affecting the development of speech and language skills.

- Educational audiologists play an integral role in the assessment and management of hearing loss in the school-aged child.

♦ Hearing Screening

The goal of a hearing screening program is to identify children who may have hearing loss and therefore require further testing. It is important to identify these children as early as possible, since hearing loss can adversely affect educational performance. The early identification and subsequent management of hearing loss in children can help improve academic achievement (Apuzzo and Yoshinaga-Itano, 1995; Bess, Dodd-Murphy, and Parker, 1998). Fortunately, the acceptance of Universal Newborn Hearing Screening in most states has lowered the age of identification of congenital hearing loss. However, there remains a need to screen the school-aged child because later-onset hearing loss may occur.

Later-onset and progressive hearing loss can occur in children for a variety of reasons, including

- syndromes such as Usher or Hunter syndrome (Sprintzen, 2001)

- disorders such as enlarged vestibular aqueduct

- genetic disorders such as connexin 26 mutations

- nonsyndromic progressive sensorineural hearing loss

- infectious diseases such as meningitis or measles

- ototoxicity from chemotherapy (Berg, Spitzer, and Gavin, 1999)

- exposure to high intensity levels of noise and music (Brookhouser, Worthington, and Kelly, 1992)

Fluctuating conductive hearing loss resulting from otitis media can also disrupt the learning process. Therefore, screening children for middle ear disorders is an important step in minimizing the negative effects of chronic otitis media (Gravel et al, 2006; Rosenfeld, Madell, and McMahon, 1997).

When developing a screening program for school districts, audiologists need to consider the following issues:

+ Who should be screened?

+ How often should children be screened?

+ Where will the screening take place?

+ Should the screening program be limited to identifying those at risk for hearing loss or should it also identify those at risk for middle ear disorders?

+ What tests should be included in the screening program?

+ Who will perform the tests?

+ What is the follow-up protocol for those who fail the screening tests?

The Individuals with Disabilities Education Act (IDEA) is a federal law that requires states to identify children with disabilities, including children with hearing loss. Therefore, many states have promulgated legal regulations to identify these children. Screening protocols vary from state to state, and audiologists must contact their state agencies to determine if there is a mandated screening protocol.

Who Should Be Screened for Hearing Loss?

State regulations dictate who should be included in a hearing screening program. Audiologists may also consider guidelines offered by the American Speech-Language-Hearing Association (ASHA) (1996) when developing a screening program. These guidelines suggest screening

+ all children upon entry to school

+ annually, all children from kindergarten to third grade

+ all children in the seventh grade

+ all children in the 11th grade

+ children who were absent for previous screenings

+ new entrants to school who do not have records of passing a hearing screening

+ children who have failed a grade

+ children who are entering a special education program for the first time

+ children with the following risk factors:

  ◇ a family history of late onset or hereditary hearing loss

  ◇ otitis media for more than 3 months

  ◇ craniofacial anomalies

  ◇ stigmata or other findings associated with a syndrome that includes hearing loss

  ◇ head trauma with loss of consciousness

  ◇ exposure to excessively high noise levels

  ◇ exposure to ototoxic drugs

  ◇ parents or school personnel suspect a hearing loss

Parents or school personnel can complete screening checklists such as the Screening Instrument for Targeting Educational Risk (SIFTER) (Anderson, 1989), Fisher's Auditory Problems Checklist (Fisher, 1985) or Children's Auditory Processing Performance Scale (CHAPPS) (Smoski, 1990), or they can alert school personnel of the need for screening.

Who Should Be Screened for Middle Ear Disorders?

A decision must be made whether to include a screening for middle ear disorders as part of the hearing screening program. Since chronic middle ear dysfunction and subsequent fluctuating hearing loss can adversely affect academic performance, screening for these disorders may be recommended for children who are at risk for middle ear problems. The American Academy of Audiology (1997) includes the following children in the "at risk" category:

+ with craniofacial anomalies

+ of Native American heritage

+ with known histories of chronic otitis media

+ have had middle ear effusion that persists for 4/3 months

+ diagnosed with learning disabilities

+ diagnosed with speech and language delays

+ diagnosed with sensorineural hearing loss

+ have failed the pure tone screening

Where Will the Screening Take Place?

Screening must take place in a quiet environment. It must be quiet enough for a student with normal hearing to be able to hear the test frequencies at 20 dB hearing level (HL). If ambient noise levels are too high to hear test signals at 20 dB, it is not acceptable to raise the intensity level of the stimuli. Rather, it is recommended that the environment be modified to improve the acoustics. These acoustic recommendations may include installing carpeting or acoustic ceiling tiles. Selecting a test room that is away from known noise sources such as heating systems, gymnasiums, cafeterias, and playgrounds is essential.

What Tests Are Recommended?

Pure tone screening is the basic component of a hearing screening program. Immittance testing may be added to screen for middle ear disorders. The decision to include immittance testing would be based on the population in the school. It would be wise to include it in kindergarten centers or special education school programs. Tympanometry is the most common immittance measure used in schools. If tympanometry is to be included in the screening protocol, it must be preceded by an otoscopic evaluation of the external ear canal to ensure that the ear canal is free from obstructions such as debris and cerumen. The presence of pressure equalizing (PE) tubes should be noted at this time.

Even though ASHA (1996) does not recommend using otoacoustic emissions (OAEs) as a screening tool for the school-aged population, some audiologists continue to investigate their use. However, pure tone tests continue to be the most effective screening tool (Krueger and Ferguson, 2002).

What Are the Testing Protocols?

A hearing screening should be performed at the frequencies 1000, 2000, and 4000 Hz at 20 dB HL. A child must respond to all frequencies in both ears to pass the screening. Testing can be performed using routine test procedures or conditioned play audiometry if needed. Referral for a rescreening is recommended if the child fails to respond to any frequency in either ear. The rescreening should take place as soon as possible, preferably within 24 to 48 hours. Children who fail the rescreening should be referred for a complete audiologic evaluation.

More comprehensive screening protocols may be instituted. The Colorado Department of Education (2004) recommends including 500 Hz for children from preschool through fifth grade if tympanometry is not available.

Some studies have noted the increased prevalence of noise-induced hearing loss in children. To identify these children, it has been suggested that screening frequencies include 6000 and 8000 Hz, because these frequencies are sensitive to noise-induced hearing loss (Montgomery and Fujikawa, 1992).

Controversial Point

• With the increase of noise-induced hearing loss in younger children, should the more comprehensive screening protocols that include frequencies higher than 4000 Hz become the accepted procedure for all to use?

If tympanometry is performed, a rescreen is recommended for children 7 years and older if peak admittance is less than 0.4 mmho or tympanometric width is greater than 400 daPa. Children 6 years and younger should be rescreened if they exhibit static admittance less than 0.3 mmho or tympanometric width greater than 200 daPa. Rescreening should take place within 4 to 6 weeks. If the child fails the screening again, a medical referral is warranted (ASHA, 1996).

To identify those at risk for tympanic membrane perforation, refer immediately if tympanometric volume is greater than 1.0 cm^3 and is accompanied by a flat (type B) tympanogram. However, do not refer if PE tubes can be visualized through otoscopy.

Acoustic reflex tests and tympanometric peak pressure are not considered appropriate screening procedures.

Who Will Administer the Screening?

Personnel conducting the screenings usually include audiologists, speech-language pathologists, and school nurses. Individual state regulations may allow additional people to be placed on this list. All who are conducting the hearing screenings should have knowledge of the following topics:

♦ Goal of hearing screenings

♦ Familiarity with audiologic equipment

♦ Requirements for an appropriate test environment

♦ How to instruct students on screening procedures

♦ Criteria for passing and failing the hearing screening

♦ How to report results

♦ How to follow up with parents and school personnel

♦ How to test the very young or difficult-to-test child.

What Is the Follow-up Protocol?

Parents should be notified about the results of the screening and the need for further evaluation. Children who are referred for a complete audiologic evaluation should be seen within 3 months of the referral. It is important for personnel to follow up to ensure that the audiologic diagnostic evaluation was performed. The strength of a screening program is only as good as its follow-up procedures. If children who fail the screening are not seen for a full audiologic evaluation, the screening program has failed. Diligent follow-up procedures need to be in place as part of the program.

Screening the Difficult-to-Test Child

Some children cannot be tested with standard pure tone screening methods. These children may have significant developmental delays or substantial physical problems that prevent them from being able to physically respond to the test stimulus. Some of these children respond well to conditioned play audiometry. Others are unable to perform that technique. A notation of "CNT" (cannot test) on the screening form does not mean that the screening requirement has been fulfilled. Merely "trying" to administer the test is not sufficient. Other screening tools such as OAEs may be used (Lyons, Kei, and Driscoll, 2004). If other screening tests are not available, a complete audiologic evaluation must be recommended. Follow-up protocols need to ensure that every child is screened with some test measure that concludes with a definitive statement regarding hearing status.

Pearl

• No matter how difficult it is to test a child, it is possible to screen everyone. Audiologists need to diligently identify the correct screening tool to meet each individual child's specific needs.

◆ Audiologic Evaluation

The standard audiologic evaluation typically includes case history, otoscopy, immittance measures (tympanometry, static immittance, and acoustic reflexes), pure tone air and bone conduction thresholds, speech audiometry, and OAEs. This evaluation is usually completed by the child's pediatric audiologist. However, once children enter the public school arena, they may receive audiologic services provided by the school district. To qualify to receive these services, they must be included in the child's Individualized Education Plan (IEP). (For more information on IEP development, see Chapter 23) The following services may be included in the IEP:

◆ A complete unaided audiologic evaluation and aided evaluation with the child's hearing aid or cochlear implant and frequency modulation (FM) system

◆ Provision and use of an FM system in the classroom

◆ Management plan for monitoring personal and classroom amplification

◆ In-service workshops for school staff

The Responsibilities of the Educational Audiologist

(For Specific information on audiological procedures, see Chapter 7–10.)

The Audiologic Evaluation

Educational audiologists provide audiologic services in the school district. They have a unique perspective as they can observe the child in their school environment and collaborate with school staff. While the audiologic assessment usually includes the standard battery stated above, educational audiologists often expand their assessment to include a more in-depth evaluation of speech recognition skills.

Speech audiometry provides information about how a child functions in the real world. Although the degree of hearing loss has a significant impact on speech scores, hearing sensitivity is not the sole determinate of speech reception skills. Some children with good access to the auditory signal, as indicated by pure tone testing, may have great difficulty following conversational speech. Conversely, children with hearing loss may have excellent speech reception skills. Speech audiometry includes speech reception thresholds (SRTs), speech detection thresholds (SDTs), and speech recognition testing. An evaluation of speech in noise is essential to determine how the child will function in the classroom. (For a complete discussion of speech audiometry, see chapter 10.) Sometimes an educational audiologist can administer an evaluation in the classroom to provide information about how the child performs in his daily environment. The Functional Listening Evaluation (Johnson and Von Almen, 1997) is performed in the classroom and demonstrates how noise and distance may have an adverse effect on the speech recognition abilities of students with hearing loss.

Pearl

◆ When sharing test results with school personnel, it is especially important to perform a speech recognition test at conversational levels (50 dBHL) to help the teacher understand how the child is performing in the classroom

Some educational audiologists administer assessments of auditory skills that are components of an auditory training curriculum. Curriculums such as the Developmental Approach to Successful Listening II (DASL II) (Stout and Windle, 1994) or Speech Perception Instructional Curriculum and Evaluation (SPICE) (Moog, Biedenstein, and Davidson, 1995) include these assessments. Other tests such as the Test of Auditory Comprehension (Trammel, 1981) provide information on auditory memory, speech in noise and auditory comprehension. This information could help the teacher of the deaf or SLP develop appropriate auditory training goals.

Frequency Modulation Evaluation

FM systems are assistive listening devices that have become commonly used in the schools. Children with various auditory needs have benefited from the use of FM in the classroom. With the advent of different types and models, it is essential to evaluate the child to ensure that maximum benefit is derived from the device. For more information on FM systems, see chapter 20.

Report Writing

When writing audiologic reports, clinical audiologists often use terminology that is unfamiliar to school personnel. To help teachers meet the needs of the child with hearing loss, educational audiologists create reports that will explain how hearing loss will affect communication. Reports should include information such as: "With hearing aids, the student will not detect the softer speech sounds such as /s/, /sh/, /f/ and therefore may have difficulty understanding concepts of plurals and possessives" or "The student will have difficulty understanding speech at a distance of 6 ft or more from the speaker."

Plotting audiologic results on a familiar sounds audiogram is also helpful. This graphically depicts the sounds that are inaudible to the student and may help the educational staff understand the effects of the hearing loss on communication **(Fig. 11–1).**

Monitoring Amplification

Plans for the monitoring and maintenance of personal and classroom amplification should be created for each child. This plan should include a statement of who will provide the amplification check, how often it will be done, and what steps will be taken when equipment malfunctions.

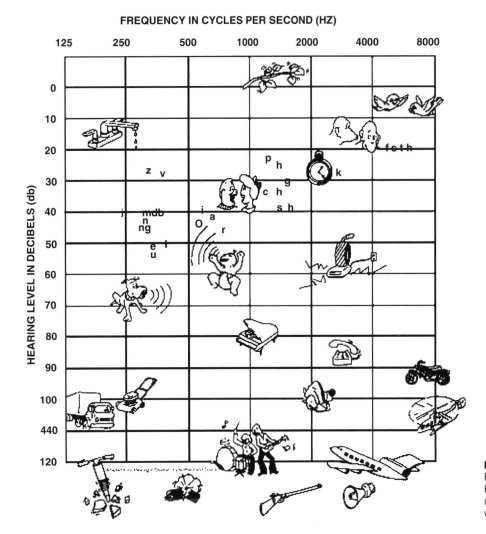

Figure 11–1 Speech sounds audiogram. From Northern, J., and Downs, M. (2002). Hearing in children (5th Ed., p. 18). Baltimore: Lippincott Williams & Wilkins. Used with permission.

In-Service Workshops

Educational audiologists should provide in-service workshops to school personnel. Topics of these workshops should include

♦ Hearing loss. How hearing loss affects learning, communication, and language development in the classroom. Tapes or CDs that simulate hearing loss are especially useful to help school personnel understand the effect of hearing loss on communication. Techniques to maximize communication in the classroom should be reviewed as well as techniques to minimize noise in the classroom. The student's audiologic report should be reviewed and interpreted to staff.

♦ Hearing aids and cochlear implants. How a hearing aid or cochlear implant works should be reviewed. A description on how to perform a daily listening check should be detailed.

♦ FM systems

◊ Reasons an FM needed in the classroom. This topic includes a review of classroom acoustics and the limitations of personal amplification in the classroom

◊ How an FM works. It is helpful when reviewing how an FM works to provide the teachers with an opportunity to listen through an FM system.

◊ Effective use of FM in the classroom. It is important to review when to use an FM and when not to use an FM. Proper microphone placement should be demonstrated at this time.

◊ Daily listening check of FM and troubleshooting techniques

Collaborating with School Personnel

Educational audiologists must collaborate with school personnel to design a program of services that best suits each child's specific needs. The teacher of the deaf and the speech language pathologist are two people who often have the greatest contact with the student. If equipment malfunctions, it is important that these staff members know who to call to help reduce equipment down time.

♦ Summary

Since hearing loss can negatively affect a child's academic performance, a complete audiologic evaluation needs to be performed on all children who fail a hearing screening or on all children for whom hearing loss is suspected. The accuracy of the assessment depends on the evaluation and comparison of various test procedures. When evaluating the school-aged child, it is important to determine her auditory and speech perception skills with tests that can be performed in the sound booth and in the classroom. Educational audiologists work with school personnel to ensure that the child's auditory needs are met and to maximize her access to audition in the classroom. Proper assessment and management can increase the child's chances of success, academically and socially.

Discussion Questions

1. What would be the screening recommendations for a class of kindergarten children and for a class of high school students?

2. Excessively high noise levels in the room where hearing screening is performed may cause school personnel to want to raise the intensity of the test stimulus. They come to you, the audiologist, for advice. How do you solve this problem?

3. A second-grade student is doing poorly in school. The speech-language pathologist notes that this child seems to have great difficulty hearing in noise. The child passes the hearing screening test. What is the next recommendation?

4. A first-grade student with a moderate sensorineural hearing loss is entering public school for the first time. What steps should the educational audiologist take to help this child have a successful school year?

References

Apuzzo, M. L., and Yoshinaga-Itano, C. (1995). Early identification of infants with significant hearing loss and the Minnesota Child Development Inventory. Seminars in Hearing, 16, 124–139.

American Academy of Audiology. (1997). Identification of hearing loss and middle-ear dysfunction in preschool and school-age children. Maclean: American Academy of Audiology.

American Speech-Language-Hearing Association. (1996). Guidelines for audiologic screening. Rockville: ASHA.

Anderson, K. (1989). Screening instrument for targeting educational risk (S.I.F.T.E.R.). Tampa: Educational Audiology Association.

Berg, A. L., Spitzer, J., and Gavin, J. Jr. (1999). Ototoxic impact of cisplatin in pediatric oncology patients. Laryngoscope, 109, 1806–1814.

Bess, F. H., Dodd-Murphy, J., and Parker, R. A. (1998). Children with minimal sensorineural hearing loss: prevalence, educational performance, and functional status. Ear & Hearing, 19, 339–354.

Brookhouser, P. E., Worthington, D. W., and Kelly, W. J. (1992). Noise induced hearing loss in children. Laryngoscope, 102, 645–655.

Colorado Department of Education. (2004) Standards of Practice for Audiology Services in the Schools.

Fisher, L. I. (1985). Learning disabilities and auditory processing. In R. J. Van Hattam (Ed.), Administration of speech language services in schools: a manual (pp. 231–290). San Diego: College-Hill Press.

Gravel, J. S., Roberts J., Rousch, J., et al. (2006). Early otitis media with effusion, hearing loss, and auditory processes at school age. Ear & Hearing, 27, 353–368.

Individuals with Disability Education Act. (IDEA), PL 101-476. (October 30, 1990). Title 20, U.S.C. 1400 et seq: US Statutes at Large, 104, 1103–1151.

Johnson, C., and Van Almen P. (1997). The function listening evaluation. In C. Johnson, P. Benson, and J. Seaton (Eds.) Educational audiology handbook (pp. 336–339). San Diego: Singular Publishing Group.

Krueger, W. W., and Ferguson, L. (2002). A comparison of screening methods in school-aged children Otolaryngology Head Neck Surgery, 127, 516–519.

Lyons, A., Kei, J., and Driscoll, C. (2004). Distortion product otoacoustic emissions in children at school entry: a comparison with pure-tone screening and tympanometry results. Journal of the American Academy of Audiology, 15, 702–715.

Montgomery, J. K., and Fujikawa, S. (1992). Hearing thresholds of students in the second, eighth and twelfth grades. Language, Speech, and Hearing Services in Schools, 23, 61–63.

Moog, J., Biedenstein, J., and Davidson, L. (1995). The SPICE, St Louis: Central Institute for the Deaf.

Smoski, W. (1990). Use of CHAPPS in a children's audiology clinic. Ear and Hearing, 11, 53S–56S.

Sprintzen, R. (2001). Syndrome identification for audiology, San Diego: Singular Publishing.

Stout, G., and Windle, J. (1994) Developmental approach to successful listening II. Englewood: Resource Point, Inc.

Tillman, R., and Carhart, R. (1966). An expanded test for speech discrimination utilizing CNC monosyllabic words. Northwestern University test no. 4. Technical report no SAM-TDR-62-135, San Antonio: USAF School of Aerospace Medicine, Brooks Air Force Base.

Trammel, J. (1981) Test of Auditory Comprehension (TAC). North Hollywood: Foreworks.

Chapter 12

The Role of the Test Assistant in Assessing Hearing in Children

Jane R. Madell

♦ Working with Parents
♦ Behavioral Observation Audiometry
♦ Visual Reinforcement Audiometry
♦ Conditioned Play Audiometry

♦ Speech Audiometry
♦ Keeping Order in the Test Room
♦ Conclusion

Key Points

- The test assistant is responsible for engaging the infant or child, keeping the child interested and attentive, and keeping family members at ease so they can cooperate with test protocols.

- In behavioral observation audiometry (BOA), the test assistant is responsible for monitoring the positioning of the child, observing responses, and monitoring parent/caregiver's behavior.

- In visual reinforcement audiometry (VRA), the test assistant's first responsibility is to assist in training the child to the task and then keeping the child focused at midline so she can make a conditioned head turn.

- With conditioned play audiometry (CPA), the test assistant teaches the child the listen and drop task, and then assists the child in completing the test activities.

- An important responsibility for the test assistant is keeping the test room in order.

When evaluating infants and young children, testing is frequently more easily and accurately accomplished with two examiners. Both examiners may be audiologists, or one may be an audiologist and the other a communication assistant or a parent. If there are two audiologists, they can alternate roles; one behind the audiometer and one interacting with the child. If the test assistant is not an audiologist, alternating roles will not be possible.

Whether one or two audiologists are participating in testing, only one is in charge and "calling the shots." The "managing audiologist" (for want of a better term) will determine the test protocol, presentation mode, order of testing, and timing of presentations. The managing audiologist usually sits in front of the audiometer. Sometimes, with a difficult-to-test child, the person working with the child may manage the session and give directions to the second audiologist, who is sitting behind the audiometer and presenting test stimuli.

The purpose of this chapter is to describe the critical role of the test assistant during various pediatric tests. Please refer to Chapters 6 through 8 for detailed information about behavioral assessment of infants and children.

♦ Working with Parents

The test assistant is responsible for engaging the infant or child, keeping him interested and attentive, and keeping family members at ease so they can cooperate with test protocols. The test assistant needs first to be certain that family members understand exactly what is being tested, how testing is accomplished, and what their role will be. The child may be seated on a parent's lap or in an infant seat, highchair, or in a chair at a test table. The parent may be seated next to or slightly behind the child to be able to observe but not distract him. In other cases, especially if the child is uncomfortable with strangers, the parent may be the best person to play with him, with direction from the audiologist.

The first responsibility of the test assistant is to explain the test protocol to the family. The test assistant should describe what testing will consist of, what will be expected of the child, and what will be expected of the family. Family members need to understand that they must appear interested, but must not respond to any test stimuli before the child responds, to be certain that the responses obtained are measures of the child's hearing and not his ability to receive cues from the parents. It is frequently difficult for parents to sit still and not react when the child does not seem to be responding to the presentation of test stimuli. Parents may need to be instructed not to say "Did you hear that?" to look expectantly when sounds are presented, to look at the reinforcing toy during VRA, or to suggest that the child put the toy in the bucket when the parent hears the sound. When speech stimuli are used, the parents may need to be reminded that they cannot repeat the tester's stimuli for the child (e.g., she said "baseball," say baseball) when the child fails to respond. If the child is looking to the parent or test assistant for encouragement, it may be best to look away from the child. Look at the toy, the loudspeaker, or the floor so the child understands that he will not receive cues from adults in the room about when to respond.

Once family members understand that their distracting behaviors may make it difficult to obtain reliable results, they are usually willing to do whatever is needed to obtain an accurate test. The use of noise-canceling earphones may be effective in reducing extraneous behaviors from family members. Some parents, however, prefer to be able to hear the precise sounds that the child can and cannot respond to; this is frequently very helpful when they receive counseling about test results.

◆ Behavioral Observation Audiometry

For BOA, both the managing audiologist and the test assistant need to have a good view of the infant so both can judge if a response was made. If the infant is in an infant seat, either the test assistant or the parent may be holding the bottle, because, as detailed in Chapter 6, sucking is the primary reliably observed behavior. If the infant is being nursed or is not comfortable in an infant seat, he will be in a parent's arms. If the parent is holding the infant or the bottle, the test assistant needs to be certain that the parent is not changing the way she is holding the bottle or breast, or moving it in or out of the infant's mouth when sound stimuli are presented.

The test assistant needs to be certain that the infant is seated comfortably and not fidgeting. If may be helpful for the test assistant to hold and manipulate a bright toy or a light-emitting diode (LED) display in front of the infant to keep him focused straight ahead and to reduce fidgeting. If the test assistant is using a toy or light to distract the infant, the object should be placed so that he does not have to move his head up or down to see it.

When a sound is presented, both the test assistant and the managing audiologist need to judge the response. The test assistant needs to be careful about how she informs the managing audiologist about the observation. The testers need to work out a signal system such as a minor head nod indicating yes or no, or finger movement (one for yes, two for no). If the test assistant repeatedly says "No, I didn't see anything," his speech compromises the quiet test environment and is likely to be very disturbing to the family. Because the test assistant is right next to the baby, he will be able to make suggestions about when a rest or repositioning may be needed.

Pearl

- Before testing, audiologists should work out a way to communicate with each other without communicating to the family. A system to signal observation of responses or changes needed during testing might consist of head nods or finger taps.

◆ Visual Reinforcement Audiometry

In VRA, the test assistant's first responsibility is to help train the child to the task, and then keep the child focused at midline so the child can make a conditioned head turn. Positioning is especially important for young children and for children with neurological or developmental delays. The test assistant needs to be certain that the child is comfortably seated, has sufficient neck support if needed, and is facing forward. If the child is turned toward one side and sound stimuli are being presented and reinforced from the other side, it may be difficult for him to make a sufficient head turn to be counted as a response. Focusing the child at midline will be most easily accomplished if the test assistant is seated in front of the child but in a position that permits the managing audiologist to also see the child. The distraction toys the test assistant selects should be easily manipulated, bright, and entertaining. As soon as the child starts to lose interest and look away, a new toy should be presented.

When training the child to the VRA task, the test assistant will keep the child's attention focused front. If the child does not turn and look on his own when the VRA toy is turned on, the test assistant will attract him to the reinforcing toy by waving at the toy or taping the lucite box holding the toy to get the child's attention to the toy. Once the child is trained for the task, the test assistant is responsible for keeping him focused forward and away from the reinforcing toy. The child should be observing (not manipulating) the distracting toys, since physical play may be too engrossing, especially for young children and children with developmental issues. Older children may be able to play with some simple toys and still respond to sound. The test assistant needs to be alert and aware of how the child is responding and whether playing with a toy is interfering with attention. If it is, the tester will need to take the toys away from the child.

◆ Conditioned Play Audiometry

With CPA, the test assistant teaches the child the listen and drop task and assists him in completing the test activities. The test assistant must make a judgment about the child's motor skills so he can select toys that the child is capable of using, and must note when the child's interest is flagging and determine when a new toy is needed. For children who do not wish to cooperate, the test assistant will need to present a "firm but kind" attitude to increase cooperation. When the child is not cooperating, the test assistant will need to determine when it would be good to involve the parent in obtaining cooperation and when it is best to leave the parent out. As with VRA, the amount of interaction the tester and child will have will depend partly on the personality of the tester and partly on the child. However, because children who are able to do CPA are older, more interaction with the test assistant is to be expected.

♦ Speech Audiometry

The use of a test assistant can be critical for speech audiometry. If a closed-set task is being used, the test assistant will be responsible for turning pages and being certain that the managing audiologist knows how the child responded. If an open-set format is being used and the child is repeating the test stimulus, the test assistant may need to be the audiologist's "ears," especially if the child is responding in a very soft voice that is typical of many young children. The test assistant needs to find a way to let the audiologist know if the child's response was correct and if not, what the error was so that the audiologist can accurately score the response, especially when using phoneme scoring. It is important that the test assistant provide response accuracy information without making the child feel as if he is doing poorly at the task. The assistant can employ several strategies. The test assistant can simply repeat what the child says in a sufficiently loud voice for the audiologist to hear, or just repeat the error words. For example, if the stimulus item is "Say the word mouth." and the child says "mouse," the test assistant can say "mouse" or "mouse, good job." The audiologist will know that an error was made, will be able to record what the error was, and the child will not feel that he is failing at the task.

♦ Keeping Order in the Test Room

The test room does not have to be silent during testing, but it should be quiet. Conversations should be at a minimum. The amount of interaction between the tester and child will depend partly on the personality of the tester and partly on the child. For some children, smiling, clapping, and enthusiastic comments of "hurrah" will encourage longer attention to the VRA task. For other children, "cheerleading" will be intrusive and better results will be obtained if the test assistant is quieter or even silent. A silent test assistant is frequently valuable with a child with PDD or other developmental disorders. The test assistant will need to observe the child and determine what behavior produces the best results.

An important responsibility for the test assistant is keeping the test room in order. When a child is brought into a test room, most of the toys should be out of sight.

However, one or two toys could be visible to entice the child to enter the room and to sit in the test chair. Bringing a young child, especially a difficult-to-evaluate child, into a room that has toys all over the floor will make it difficult to seat the child and have him focus on the task. When toys are put away, they should be sorted appropriately. All parts of each toy should be placed in the correct box to facilitate moving quickly from one activity to the next. Using a peg board or a puzzle with a missing piece may result in annoyance or frustration for the child. Having toy cars mixed up with Lego pieces also can be problematic. Toy confusions often waste time while the child discusses what is missing and why things are in the wrong place. Some children need to examine each piece before using it to determine what it is and where it belongs. For some children, disorganization and missing pieces can interfere with testing.

♦ Conclusion

The test assistant is critical to obtaining accurate results in a timely manner. An enthusiastic, cheerful test assistant who enjoys children is likely to elicit good results.

When the test assistant and the managing audiologist disagree or are not communicating well, it is probably best if they take a moment to leave the test room and discuss how they want to proceed out of earshot of the family. It hardly encourages confidence if the testers cannot agree about what to do.

Pitfall
• Audiologists should not disagree in front of families. It can be distressing to the family and reduce trust about test results.

Communication between the audiologist and test assistant can be accomplished using a talk back system with the audiometer in which the tester uses the audiometer microphone and the test assistant uses earphones. If the audiometer does not have a talk back system, communication can be accomplished by using an FM system; the tester wears the microphone, and the test assistant wears the receiver. An experienced and professional team will make testing infants and children fun, and allow results to be obtained efficiently and accurately.

Discussion Questions

1. What are some ways the audiologist and test assistant can communicate during testing?

2. What are the responsibilities of the test assistant during BOA, VRA, and play?

Chapter 13

Middle-Ear Measurement in Infants and Children

M. Patrick Feeney and Chris A. Sanford

- ♦ **Overview**
- ♦ **The Role of the Middle Ear and Developmental Aspects**
- ♦ **Some Basic Principles of Middle Ear Measurement**
- ♦ **Infant Tympanometry**

- ♦ **Conducting Middle Ear Measurements**
  - Otoscopic Examination
  - Tympanometry
  - Acoustic Stapedius Reflex Testing

Key Points

- Development of the external and middle ear over the first 6 months of life results in tympanometric results that may not reflect middle-ear function when using a 226 Hz probe tone.

- Evidence is mounting to suggest that 1000 Hz tympanometry may provide greater sensitivity to middle ear disorders in neonates and young infants.

- Otoscopy should be conducted before the admittance evaluation to ensure that the test can be conducted safely, and to gather information for test interpretation.

- If published normative data are used for middle-ear assessment, ensure that measurements are obtained using the same test parameters (e.g., probe frequency, pump speed) as the published studies, or collect local norms.

- The results of the middle-ear test battery should be cross-checked with other behavioral and physiologic test results.

- A quantitative description of the tympanogram is desirable in addition to a description of its shape.

- The measurement of infant acoustic stapedius reflexes should be conducted with a high-frequency probe tone. A broad-band probe signal may also prove useful as this becomes available.

- Acoustic reflex activator stimuli for insert phones are calibrated in a 2-cm^3 cavity and may be reported in dB hearing level (HL). This calibration is not appropriate for infant ears and likely underestimates the level of the reflex activator in the infant ear canal.

♦ Overview

Middle ear measurement is a fundamental component of the audiologic test battery, and its importance is nowhere more evident than in pediatric assessment. Tympanometry and acoustic reflex testing are the basic components of the middle ear test battery, which provides information about the middle ear, cochlea, auditory nerve, auditory brainstem, and cranial nerve VII. Therefore, the middle ear test battery is useful as a cross-check with other physiological and behavioral tests (see Chapter 5). However, because of the anatomic development of the conductive mechanism of the peripheral ear over the first 6 months of life, tests that we can readily use to detect middle-ear status in older infants and children with a 226 Hz probe tone provide little useful information in young infants. A new approach to this problem using 1000 Hz tympanometry will be discussed. This chapter will also focus on when and how to conduct middle ear testing in children and the interpretation of test results. Although a brief overview will be provided here, it is assumed that the reader has a basic knowledge of the principles of acoustics and aural acoustic immittance, which form the foundation for current middle-ear measurement (see Keefe and Feeney, in press; Margolis and Hunter, 1999; Wiley and Fowler, 1997).

♦ The Role of the Middle Ear and Developmental Aspects

The middle ear contains the tympanic membrane, ossicles, ligaments, muscles, and an air space. This system serves to transfer acoustic vibrations in air to the fluid-filled cochlea. If the middle ear were removed from this process, a 60-dB hearing loss would result. Sounds at more intense levels would reach the cochlea through skull vibration. The gain in sound transfer to the cochlea is provided in part by two simple machines. The area difference between the tympanic membrane and the oval window of the stapes increases the force per unit area on the stapes footplate, much like a thumbtack allows us to puncture wood with our thumb. The second simple machine is a lever provided by the size and orientation of the malleus and incus, which also boosts sound energy at the stapes footplate. These two factors combine for as much as a 30-dB gain in sound transfer to the cochlea. If the middle ear were missing entirely, sound would strike the oval and round windows of the cochlea approximately in phase, causing an additional reduction in the efficiency of sound transfer to the cochlea and leading to the maximal conductive hearing loss of 60 dB.

The acoustic stapedius reflex (ASR) is a response of the auditory system to high levels of sound. It is detected clinically by noting a small change in acoustic middle ear function as the stapedius muscle contracts to pull on the stapes and stiffen the annular ligament in the oval window. The ASR, a bilateral effect, involves activation of fibers in the auditory nerve and brainstem which trigger a response from the motor nucleus of the seventh (facial) nerve to activate the facial nerve and contract the stapedius muscle. For this cascade of events to occur, each station along the way must be functional. Thus, the reflex may be absent because of a lesion anywhere along the pathway. By examining the pattern of ASR responses for ipsilateral and contralateral stimulation, the audiologist derives a wealth of knowledge about the function of the peripheral auditory system from the middle ear to the brainstem. It has been demonstrated that infants with auditory dys-synchrony may pass a newborn hearing screening with otoacoustic emissions (OAEs), a preneural phenomenon, even though the auditory brainstem response (ABR) and ASR are absent (Hood, 1999). This suggests a role for the ASR as a tool for newborn hearing screening when paired with OAE screening. Both tests could be conducted with the same probe; more costly ABR screening should not be needed.

There are significant changes in the human external and middle ear over the first postnatal months of life that likely affect its sound conduction properties (Ruah et al, 1991; Saunders, Kaltenbach, and Relkin, 1983). These changes include: (1) a growth of the bony portion of the ear canal wall and resulting decrease in the length of the cartilaginous portion of the canal; (2) an increase in the overall size of the ear canal; (3) a decrease in the density of the ossicles over the first 6 months of life caused by ossification and absorption of residual mesenchyme (Eby and Nadol, 1986); (4) changes in the orientation of the tympanic membrane to be more vertical (Ikui, Sando, and Fujita 1997); and (5) progressive stiffening of the ossicular joints (Saunders, Kaltenbach, and Relkin, 1983). Studies by Keefe et al (1993) and Sanford and Feeney (2007) used wideband energy reflectance, an emerging tool for middle ear assessment, to suggest that the acoustic properties of the infant ear change markedly over the first 6 months of life.

◆ Some Basic Principles of Middle Ear Measurement

During traditional tympanometry a tone is presented to the hermetically sealed ear canal and its level is monitored using a microphone. The level of the tone is held constant by using an automatic gain control circuit while the static pressure in the ear canal is varied using an air pump (**Fig. 13–1**). The frequency of the probe tone is specified as 226 Hz at a level equal to or less than 90 dB sound pressure level (American National Standards Institute [ANSI] S3.39, 1987). The ease of energy flow through the ear, its acoustic admittance as a function of frequency, Y_a, is equal to the ratio of total acoustic volume velocity of the source, u, to the total sound pressure, p,

$$Y_a = \frac{u}{p}.$$ **(Equation 13–1)**

The u is the rate at which the acoustic displacement over a surface such as a speaker cone varies with time. Assuming a constant u source in clinical admittance systems, the voltage to the probe-tone amplifier required to keep the tone at a fixed sound-pressure level is directly proportional to the Y_a.

The term *acoustic immittance* refers to both acoustic admittance and its inverse acoustic impedance

$$(Y_a = \frac{1}{Z_a})$$ **(Equation 13–2)**.

The discussion in this chapter is limited to admittance measurements. Y_a can be represented in the complex plane as a vector composed of two components, acoustic conductance G_a and acoustic susceptance B_a, which can be plotted in Cartesian coordinates (**Fig. 13–2**). We can solve for the admittance magnitude $|Y_a|$ by using the Pythagorean theorem:

$$|Y_a| = \sqrt{G_a^2 + B_a^2}$$ **(Equation 13–3)**

G_a on the horizontal axis is the portion of Y_a directly related to energy transfer through the ear and ranges from zero, no energy transfer, to positive values to the right. The conductance is positive for the middle ear, in which frictional

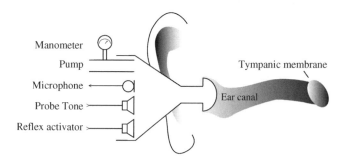

Figure 13–1 The basic components of a tympanometer. One receiver is used for the presentation of the probe tone, which is monitored by the microphone. The second receiver is used for the presentation of an ipsilateral acoustic stapedius reflex activator. The pump varies the air pressure in the ear canal.

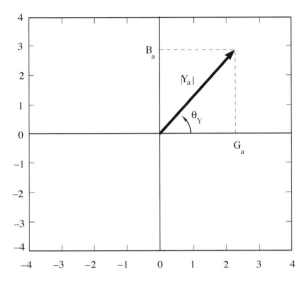

Figure 13–2 Cartesian plot of the acoustic admittance vector. $|Y_a|$ represents the magnitude of the admittance vector. The acoustic susceptance B_a has both compliant (+) and mass (−) components. The acoustic conductance G_a is in phase with flow of energy through the system. The symbol θ_Y represents the admittance phase angle.

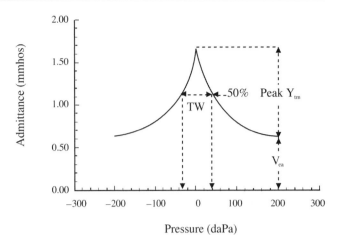

Figure 13–3 Measurements made with a tympanogram include V_{ea}, which is the equivalent volume in cm^3; *peak Y_{tm}*, which is the peak-compensated static acoustic admittance in millimhos (mmhos); and *TW*, the tympanometric width, which is the width of the tympanogram in daPa measured at one half its height.

forces are responsible for dissipating energy. This causes the admittance vector to lie in the right half of the complex plane (**Fig. 13–2**). A condition of G_a near zero might occur in the measurement of a fluid-filled middle ear with little or no acoustic energy transfer to the middle ear. B_a is the portion of Y_a related to energy storage in the system, which is composed of two opposing forces, compliant susceptance (positive) and mass susceptance (negative).

The value B_a for a 1 cm^3 volume of air at 226 Hz at sea level is approximately equal to 1 mmho, the unit of admittance, making it straightforward to calibrate admittance instruments using this probe frequency. In a calibration cavity there would be no energy transfer, so that $G_a = 0$. When a system such as the ear is at its resonance frequency (around 1000 Hz for adults), the positive and negative values of B_a cancel, leaving G_a to dominate energy flow through the system. In this case the phase angle, θ_Y, between the admittance vector and the conductance would be 0°. The opposite situation occurs in the case of measurement in a calibration cavity where $G_a = 0$, and $\theta_Y = +90°$, a pure compliant susceptance. If the system were mass dominated, θ_Y would be negative and the admittance vector would be pointed down in the bottom right quadrant (**Fig. 13–2**).

To circumvent the problem of trying to measure the middle ear admittance with the added admittance of the ear canal as measured at the plane of the probe tip, we can use vector tympanometry, a measurement of Y_a as a function of ear canal pressure (**Fig. 13–3**). In theory, the middle ear admittance is reduced to near zero with high positive or negative air pressure in the ear canal. What is left is the admittance of ear canal space, Y_{ec}. We can then subtract Y_{ec} from the total admittance measured at the tympanometric peak to arrive at the admittance of the middle ear Y_{me}, also referred to as peak-compensated static acoustic admittance, *peak Y_m* (ANSI S3.39, 1987). Another clinically useful measurement

of the vector tympanogram is its width (TW) in daPa measured at half the height of *peak Y_m* calculated from the positive tail (**Fig. 13–3**).

Another useful quantity, the equivalent volume (V_{ea}), may be calculated in terms of the susceptance as:

$$V_{ea} = \frac{\rho c^2 B_a}{2\pi f} \qquad \textbf{(Equation 13–4)}$$

where ρ (rho) represents the density of air, and *c* equals the speed of sound. V_{ea} varies with frequency, and when measured in adult ear canals is positive at low frequencies and becomes negative at high frequencies. V_{ea} for a low-frequency probe tone is useful for determining such things as the patency of pressure equalization (PE) tubes or the possibility of a tympanic membrane perforation.

Several studies have recently shown that wideband measurement of the power transfer to the middle ear may be useful in pediatric assessment (Allen, Jeng, and Levitt, 2005; Feeney and Sanford, 2005; Keefe et al, 2000; Keefe and Sanford 2003). A discussion of this technology is beyond the scope of the chapter. However, see Keefe and Feeney (in press) for a review of the method and pediatric applications.

◆ Infant Tympanometry

Based on results from several studies, low-frequency tympanometry measurements are generally considered valid and reliable predictors of middle ear function by about 7 months of age (Cantekin et al, 1980; Hunter and Margolis, 1992; Keefe et al, 1996; Roush et al, 1995). Several studies have investigated the developmental changes in traditional immittance measurements in infants to elucidate this issue (De Chicchis et al, 2000; Holte and Margolis, 1991; Meyer, Jardine, and Deverson, 1997; Roush et al, 1995).

Two studies of infants and children ranging in age from 6 months to 4 years reported a small, but statistically significant increase in static acoustic admittance and a decrease in tympanometric width as a function of age (De Chicchis et al, 2000; Roush et al, 1995). Holte and Margolis (1991) conducted a longitudinal study of multifrequency tympanometry in newborn infants through 4 months of age. They reported that admittance magnitude stayed approximately the same across age for a 226-Hz probe tone, but increased with age at higher frequencies (400 to 900 Hz). However, at all frequencies above 226 Hz, irregular tympanometric patterns were observed that were inconsistent with the Vanhuyse model, which explains the progression of tympanogram shapes with increasing probe frequency in multifrequency tympanometry (Hunter and Margolis, 1992). Holte and Margolis (1991) showed that by 4 months of age tympanograms followed the Vanhuyse model fairly consistently up to 900 Hz. They also reported that although general changes in development of Y_{tm} and θ_Y were observed, these responses were characterized by substantial intersubject variability.

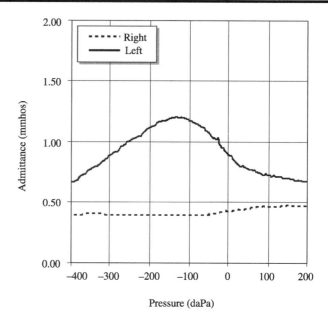

Figure 13–4 The Y_a 1000 Hz tympanograms for a neonate who failed his newborn hearing screening for the right ear (dashed line) and passed on the left ear (solid line). The *peak* Y_{tm} on the right was 0.53 mmhos with +200 daPa compensation.

Pearl

- Are you unsure about the Vanhuyse model? A good reading of Hunter and Margolis (1992) will go a long way toward improving your understanding of this model and demonstrate just how important it is in interpreting tympanometry results.

To investigate suggestions that pressure-induced changes in the external ear canal influenced middle ear measurements, Holte and Margolis (1991) introduced positive and negative pressure pulses in the ear canal and used video monitoring to determine a percent change in ear canal diameter relative to resting diameter. They found that the pressure-induced change in ear canal diameter steadily decreased as a function of age, dropping from an 18% change at 1 to 7 days to no change at 4 months of age. They also reported that in some cases, where no ear canal wall motion was observed, there were still multiple peaks in the 226-Hz tympanograms. Correlations that were computed to assess the relationship between the complexities of tympanometric patterns and the amount of wall distention failed to reach significance. Based on this result, the authors suggested that ear canal wall mobility and tympanometric patterns are not related.

Meyer, Jardine, and Deverson (1997) documented changes in Y_a tympanograms for a single infant using 226- and 1000-Hz probe frequencies. They reported results similar to Holte and Margolis (1991), in that change in resonant frequency progressed from low to high frequency with age. This was evidenced by the more complex tympanometric shapes observed with the 226 Hz probe tone at younger ages. Results for the 226-Hz probe tone showed gradual change from complex to simple tympanometric shapes with

age, indicating a shift from a mass to stiffness-dominated middle ear system with age. The opposite effect was observed for tympanometric results for the 1000-Hz probe tone; tympanograms gradually changed from simple to more complex with age. In addition, Meyer, Jardine, and Deverson (1997) reported a flat 1000-Hz tympanogram in conjunction with a normal 226-Hz tympanogram during a period of time when the infant presented with middle ear pathology.

The Y_a 1000-Hz tympanograms of a neonate who was referred for failing a newborn hearing screening for the right ear with distortion product OAEs, as well as a secondary ABR screening with a click stimulus at 30 dB nHL, is shown **(Fig. 13–4)**. The infant passed both screening tests for the left ear. The right tympanogram is essentially flat, and the left tympanogram shows a relatively normal shape. The infant is being followed for right conductive hearing loss, which is expected to be transient. This example illustrates the utility of 1000-Hz-probe-tone tympanometry for young infants. Similar case reports have been presented by Margolis et al (2003).

Special Consideration

- A comprehensive set of normative 1000-Hz infant tympanometry data has yet to be established. See Calandruccio, Fitzgerald, and Prieve (2006), Kei et al (2003), and Margolis et al (2003) for suggested guidelines and limited data for selected ages.

◆ Conducting Middle Ear Measurements

Otoscopic Examination

An otoscopic examination is essential before the admittance evaluation is undertaken. For young children and infants, it is often helpful if the child sits on the parent's lap during otoscopy and subsequent admittance testing. The parent should be advised that if little hands make a grab for the ear, the parent should intercept. Before otoscopic examination, a child is often comforted to be shown that the clinician is holding a "flashlight" and that she can see the light shining on her. A cursory look into the parent's ears by the audiologist may also be reassuring for the child. It is best not to ask permission of the child to look in her ear; rather, just go about your business in a confident and comforting manner letting her know what you are doing. If the child is reluctant to let you perform otoscopy, you may be able to complete the task with the help of an assistant who can distract the child momentarily with an interesting toy, similar to the role of a toy waiver in behavioral testing. This toy distraction technique may also be useful during tympanometry and ASR testing.

The appropriately sized speculum should be selected based on an observation of the child's external ear. The best view will be obtained with a speculum tip slightly smaller than the ear canal diameter, allowing it to be inserted into the canal while allowing the maximum lumen for viewing purposes. It is important to create a bridge between the scope and the patient's head with the pinky or ring fingers of the hand holding the scope. This bridge will allow your hand to move with sudden movements of the patient's head rather than dislodging the speculum or pushing it uncomfortably against the canal wall. The other hand may be used to straighten the ear canal by gently pulling horizontally backward on the pinna. This last step should be undertaken with great care, especially if there is a history of ear pain.

Once the speculum is positioned in the canal, you may move your eye close to the scope to view the canal. As you may have only a quick look with some pediatric patients, it is important to see if the ear canal is: (1) clear enough to allow the insertion of an admittance probe tip; (2) free from excessive cerumen; (3) free from other obstructions like PE tubes that have been extruded from the tympanic membrane; and (4) not draining excessively such that the probe would be plugged. It is also important in this quick look to see if: (1) the normal landmarks of the tympanic membrane can be seen (light reflex, umbo, and short process of malleus); (2) the tympanic membrane appears normal or is inflamed or perforated; (3) a PE tube appears to be in place or not; and (4) there is any scarring or tympanosclerosis of the tympanic membrane, which could lead to abnormal tympanometry.

Tympanometry

Preparing to Test

Daily calibration of the tympanometer with the included calibration cavities ensures valid test data. It is also helpful to check that instrument defaults are to your liking when you work with other audiologists. A self-administered tympanogram is also useful in that it provides a biological check and ensures that the system has not developed an internal pressure leak. For pediatric assessment, one should have an admittance instrument capable of multiple probe frequencies and the calibration of each should be checked per the manufacturer's recommendations. The standard 226-Hz probe tone specified in ANSI S3.39 (1987) may be used from age 7 months to adulthood, but higher frequency probe tones are required to test young infants, as discussed above.

Many tympanometers allow the examiner to adjust other test parameters in addition to probe frequency. A rapid pressure sweep rate, often available in a screening-test mode, may be useful in obtaining data quickly in children. Some systems offer a rapid sweep rate such as 600 daPa/s except near the tympanogram peak, where the rate slows to 200 daPa/s. Care must be taken to duplicate the probe frequency and sweep rate if test results are compared with published normative data. For example, *peak Y_{tm}* increases with pressure sweep rate (Shanks and Wilson, 1986). Otherwise, locally collected age-specific normative data are preferable. Many commercial systems offer a standard ear canal pressure range (e.g., + 200 to -300 daPa) and an extended pressure range (e.g., +300 to -600 daPa). The extended range is useful in detecting a tympanogram peak in cases of extreme negative middle ear pressure where rising admittance is often noted with increasing negative pressure in the standard pressure range, but the pressure limit is reached before the tympanogram peak is observed. Extreme negative middle ear pressure could help to explain normal hearing in an ear with a flat tympanogram obtained within the standard pressure range. However, the extended pressure range should be used judiciously, as the standard range is sufficient for most ears and is more comfortable for the patient, which increases the likelihood that both ears will be tested.

Obtaining a Seal

The otoscopic examination provides an opportunity to judge the size of the probe tip appropriate for the patient. A standard admittance probe tip will be inserted in the ear canal to obtain a hermetic seal, and thus should be large enough to afford a snug fit. If using a screening tip, this will be held against the canal during the test and should be larger than the canal opening, but smaller than the concha bowl for a good fit. With some devices the tympanometer is a handheld device, which is used with a screening probe tip held against the opening of the ear canal. As with otoscopy, gently pulling horizontally back on the pinna straightens the ear canal and makes it less likely to collapse when the probe tip is inserted. Although beginning clinicians often have difficulty obtaining a hermetic seal to complete the test and may be notified repeatedly that there is a leak, the art of consistently obtaining an appropriate seal comes with practice. However, on occasion the most seasoned clinician will have difficulty obtaining a seal for tympanometry. If selecting a different probe tip does not solve the problem, re-examine the ear with the otoscope to make sure you have the correct angle on the ear canal when inserting the probe tip. An ear with a patent PE tube or a perforation may register a very large equivalent volume including the ear canal, middle ear, and mastoid air spaces. This volume may exceed the measurable limit on some equipment, causing the instrument to register a leak. It is important to know if this is a limitation for your equipment, and what the upper limit of measurable equivalent volume is. Many instruments will be able to collect the data and record a large volume as long as the pressure is not actually leaking.

Most systems default to a starting pressure of +200 daPa and then sweep pressure from a positive to negative direction. However, the difficulty in obtaining a seal may be increased by starting the sweep with positive air pressure, as this may act to push the probe out of the ear canal. When having difficulty maintaining a seal, changing to a negative starting pressure may allow a tympanogram to be obtained because in this case the starting pressure is not acting to push the probe out of the ear. However, negative-to-positive pressure sweeps may result in increased complexity of tympanogram shape (Shanks and Wilson, 1986).

Interpretation

Single-frequency 226 Hz admittance-vector tympanometry is universally used in clinical assessment for adults and children. This was initially interpreted qualitatively in terms of pressure continua (Jerger, 1970). A tympanogram with normal single-peaked shape, normal amplitude, and normal peak pressure is a Jerger Type A. Type B is flat, indicative of ears with effusion or tympanic membrane perforation; Type C displays a peak with excessive negative pressure. Other subtypes were used to describe various conditions such as Type A_S, normal pressure peak but abnormally shallow amplitude, often seen in otosclerosis. Many audiologists and physicians continue to refer to tympanograms using this system. However, in addition to describing the shape of the tympanogram, most audiologists provide a quantitative assessment made possible with the advent of calibrated admittance instruments and ANSI S3.39 (1987). This allows for a quantitative assessment of *peak Y_{tm}*, *TW*, *V_{ea}*, and tympanometric peak pressure (TPP).

The next step is to determine if the tympanogram is within normal limits. Some general guidelines will be provided, but normative data collected with your preferred instrumentation settings are ideal. For all ages, flat tympanograms (where Y_{tm} is 0) are abnormal, with the caveat that a flat tympanogram with a standard pressure range may be masking an ear with extreme negative pressure. Flat tympanograms with large equivalent volumes ($V_{ea} \geq 1$ cm^3) are suggestive of a patent PE tube or a perforation, and if pre- and post-PE-tube insertion measurement are available, a change in V_{ea} ≥ 0.4 cm^3 suggests that the tube is patent (Shanks et al, 1992). These criteria were obtained with insert-type probe tips with a 226 Hz probe tone as measured at +200 daPa in children ranging from infancy to 7 years. A large V_{ea} in an ear without a tube is suggestive of a tympanic membrane perforation, and thus a medical referral is indicated.

A flat tympanogram with normal ear canal volume and a tympanogram with an abnormally low *peak Y_{tm}* or abnormally wide *TW* are suggestive of middle ear effusion (MEE).

For ages 6 to 30 months a value of *peak Yt_m* <0.2 mmhos is suggestive of MEE. This is also the case for ears with *peak Y_{tm}* ≥ 0.3 mmhos, but *TW* >235 daPa (Roush et al, 1995). These criteria were obtained with an automatic tympanometer with a 226 Hz probe tone and a +200 daPa compensation. The Amercan Speech-Language-Hearing Association (1997) screening criteria suggest that for ages 1 year to school-age, children should be referred for retest if *peak Y_{tm}* <0.3 mmhos with a +200 daPa compensation or with TW .200 daPa (see also Margolis and Hunter, 1999).

TPP is an indicator of middle ear pressure and should be reported. However, efforts to use TPP as a screening tool and basis for referral have not been successful (see Margolis and Hunter, 1999 for a review).

Acoustic Stapedius Reflex Testing

ASR testing typically follows tympanometry using the same equipment and probe placement; ear canal pressure is adjusted to peak tympanometric pressure for maximum sensitivity. For screening purposes, many systems offer an automated search for a reflex at several levels, stopping when a criterion admittance shift is obtained (typically 0.02 or 0.03 mmhos for a 226-Hz probe tone). There are two important caveats related to ASR testing in young infants. A 226-Hz probe tone results in absent reflexes in the majority of neonates, whereas with a 1000 Hz probe tone nearly all neonates have a measurable reflex. Second, ipsilateral ASR activator signals are typically calibrated in a 2-cm^3 coupler to establish a dB HL value. This calibration is not appropriate for infant ears and underestimates the level of the reflex activator in the infant ear canal. Otherwise, it has been shown that ASR thresholds for children are similar to adults.

Pitfall
• To avoid confusion, when reporting contralateral ASR results, it is helpful to specify which ear received the activator stimulus (e.g., with the probe in the left ear and activator in the right ear ASR results were within normal limits).

When an ASR occurs there is a frequency-dependent shift in admittance. In adults, the reflex causes a decrease in admittance at frequencies below about 700 Hz and an increase in admittance above this frequency with a positive peak admittance shift around 1000 Hz (Feeney, Keefe, and Marryott, 2003) **(Fig. 13–5)**. This shift as a function of frequency is age dependent, although the time-course for the development of an adult-like ASR shift is not known. We recently showed that for 6-week-old infants there was a maximal negative shift in admittance at 1000 Hz during a contralateral ASR reflex compared with the maximal positive shift for adults **(Fig. 13–5)**. Although the time course is not known, the zero-crossing point will shift down in frequency with development and at some point would occur near 1000 Hz, presumably making the reflex difficult to detect with a 1000-Hz probe tone. It is suggested that a wideband

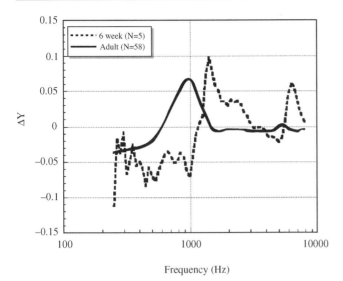

Figure 13–5 The average shift in admittance as a function of frequency during the contralateral ASR for five infants from Feeney (2005) and 58 ears for 34 adults from Feeney and Sanford (2003). The reflex shifts were normalized by dividing the shift by the baseline admittance ($\Delta Y = [|Y|$ activator $- |Y|$ baseline$] / |Y|$ baseline). At 1000 Hz there was a maximal positive shift in admittance for the adults and a maximal negative shift in admittance for the infants.

probe signal such as a chirp or click would be more successful in detecting a reflex across development in infants than a single frequency. More data are needed on acoustic reflexes in infants across the first 6 months of life when the middle ear is undergoing significant change (Keefe et al, 1993; Sanford and Feeney, 2007).

References

Allen, J. B., Jeng, P. S., and Levitt, H. J. (2005). Evaluation of human middle ear function via an acoustic power assessment. Journal of Rehabilitation Research and Development, 42, 63–78.

American National Standards Institute. (1987). Specifications for instruments to measure aural acoustic impedance and admittance (aural acoustic immittance) (ANSI S3.39-1987). New York: ANSI.

American Speech-Language-Hearing Association. (1997). Guidelines for audiologic screening. Rockville: ASHA.

Calandruccio, L., Fitzgerald, T. S., and Prieve, B. A. (2006). Normative multifrequency tympanometry in infants and toddlers. Journal of the American Academy of Audiology, 17, 470–480.

Cantekin, E. I., Bluestone, C. D., Fria, T. J., Stool, S. E., Beery, Q. C., and Sabo, D. L. (1980). Identification of otitis media with effusion in children. Annals of Otology, Rhinology & Laryngology, 89, 190–195.

De Chicchis, A. R., Todd, N. W., and Nozza, R. J. (2000). Developmental changes in aural acoustic admittance measurements. Journal of the American Academy of Audiology, 11, 97–102.

Eby, T. L., and Nadol, J. B. Jr. (1986). Postnatal growth of the human temporal bone: implications for cochlear implants in children. Annals of Otology, Rhinology & Laryngology, 95, 356–364.

Feeney, M. P., Keefe, D. H., and Marryott, L. P. (2003). Contralateral acoustic reflex thresholds for tonal activators using wideband reflectance and admittance measurements. Journal of Speech, Language, and Hearing Research, 46, 128–136.

Feeney, M. P., and Sanford, C. A. (2005). Detection of the acoustic stapedius reflex in infants using wideband energy reflectance and admittance. Journal of the American Academy of Audiology, 16, 278–290.

Holte, L., Margolis, R. H., and Cavanaugh, R. M. Jr. (1991). Developmental changes in multifrequency tympanograms. Audiology, 30, 1–24.

Hood L. J. (1999). A review of objective methods of evaluating auditory neural pathways. Laryngoscope, 109, 1745–1748.

Hunter, L. L., and Margolis, R. H. (1992). Multifrequency tympanometry: current clinical application. American Journal of Audiology, 1, 33–43.

Ikui, A., Sando, I., and Fujita, S. (1997). Postnatal change in angle between the tympanic annulus and surrounding structures: computer-aided three-dimensional reconstruction study. Annals of Otology, Rhinology & Laryngology, 106, 33–36.

Keefe, D. H., Bulen, J. C., Arehart, K. H., and Burns, E. M. (1993). Ear-canal impedance and reflection coefficient in human infants and adults. Journal of the Acoustical Society of America, 94, 2617–2638.

Keefe, D. H., and Feeney, M. P. (In press). Principles of acoustic immittance and acoustic transfer functions. In J. Katz, Handbook of clinical audiology (6th ed.). Baltimore: Lippincott, Williams and Wilkins.

Keefe, D. H., Folsom, R. C., Gorga, M. P., Vohr, B. R., Bulen, J. C., and Norton, S. J. (2000). Identification of neonatal hearing impairment: ear-canal measurements of acoustic admittance and reflectance in neonates. Ear and Hearing, 21, 443–461.

Keefe, D. H., and Levi, E. (1996). Maturation of the middle and external ears: acoustic power-based responses and reflectance tympanometry. Ear and Hearing, 17, 361–373.

Keefe, D. H., and Simmons, J. L. (2003). Energy transmittance predicts conductive hearing loss in older children and adults. Journal of the Acoustical Society of America, 114, 3217–3238.

Discussion Questions

1. What components comprise a vector tympanogram, and how do they relate to the function of the middle ear?

2. What quantitative and qualitative descriptors should be used to report on the results of vector tympanometry?

3. Is there a reason to obtain special middle ear measurement equipment for pediatric assessment? Why or why not?

4. You are seeing a five-year-old child who recently had PE tubes inserted. Her hearing has improved in one ear, but she continues to have a conductive hearing loss in the other ear. The otoscopic examination reveals that the tubes appear to be in place in both ears. What can admittance measurement contribute to the assessment of this child?

5. An 18-month-old is referred to you for a hearing evaluation by his pediatrician because of parental concern that she has not started to talk. You are unable to condition the child for VRA, but you obtain normal 226-Hz tympanograms and normal otoacoustic emissions. In addition to rescheduling the child for repeat behavioral assessment, what tests should be conducted or scheduled?

Acknowledgments The authors thank Monica Feeney for preparing the figures.

Kei, J., Allison-Levick, J., Dockray, J., et al. (2003). High-frequency (1000 Hz) tympanometry in normal neonates. Journal of the American Academy of Audiology, 14, 20–28.

Margolis, R. H., Bass-Ringdahl, S., Hanks, W. D., Holte, L., and Zapala, D. A. (2003). Tympanometry in newborn infants—1 kHz norms. Journal of the American Academy of Audiology, 14, 383–392.

Margolis R. H., and Hunter L. L. (1999). Tympanometry: basic principles and clinical applications. In Musiek, F. E., and Rintelmann, W. F. (Eds.), Contemporary perspectives in hearing assessment (pp. 89–130). Boston: Allyn and Bacon.

Meyer, S. E., Jardine, C. A., and Deverson, W. (1997). Developmental changes in tympanometry: a case study. British Journal of Audiology, 31, 189–195.

Roush, J., Bryant, K., Mundy, M., Zeisel, S., and Roberts, J. (1995). Developmental changes in static admittance and tympanometric width in infants and toddlers. Journal of the American Academy of Audiology, 6, 334–338.

Ruah, C. B., Schachern, P. A., Zelterman, D., Paparella, M. M., and Yoon, T. H. (1991). Age related morphologic changes in the human tympanic membrane, Archives of Otolaryngology—Head & Neck Surgery, 117, 627–634.

Sanford, C. A., and Feeney, M. P. (2007). Energy reflectance tympanometry in infants. Poster session presented at the midwinter meeting of the Association for Research in Otolaryngology, Denver, CO.

Saunders, J. C., Kaltenbach, J. A., and Relkin, E. M. (1983). The structural and functional development of the outer and middle ear. In Romand, R. (Ed.), Development of auditory and vestibular systems. New York: Academic Press.

Shanks, J. E., Stelmachowicz, P. G., Beauchaine, K. L., and Schulte, L. (1992). Equivalent ear canal volumes in children pre- and post-tympanostomy tube insertion. Journal of Speech, and Hearing Research, 35, 936–941.

Shanks, J. E., and Wilson, R. H. (1986). Effects of direction and rate of ear-canal pressure changes on tympanometric measures. Journal of Speech, and Hearing Research, 29, 11–19.

Wiley, T. L., and Fowler, C. G. (1997). Acoustic immittance measures in clinical audiology. San Diego: Singular Publishing.

Chapter 14

Otoacoustic Emissions in Infants and Children

Beth A. Prieve

♦ **Important Background Information**

♦ **Screening**

Newborns

♦ **Children**

♦ **Final Note**

Key Points

- Otoacoustic emissions (OAEs) are excellent screening tools for detecting hearing loss in newborns.

- OAEs are an integral part of the pediatric diagnostic test battery. They can help determine site-of-lesion and can be used as cross-checks against other results from the test battery.

- Published literature is available to guide us in using OAEs in screening and diagnostic test batteries.

Pearl

- Do you want more in-depth knowledge about OAEs? A good starting point is to read *Otoacoustic Emissions: Clinical Applications*, 3rd ed. (Robinette and Glattke, 2007).

♦ Important Background Information

Three essential areas of background information are needed for clinicians to use OAEs effectively in the clinic. First, it is critical to have a basic understanding of the generation of OAEs so that hearing loss can be properly diagnosed. OAEs are linked to the normal functioning of the outer hair cells (OHCs) and are believed to be a by-product of cochlear amplifier processing. They reflect mechanical rather than neural cochlear responses. OAEs are considered preneural. Two examples supporting this thinking are that they can be generated even when the eighth nerve has been severed (Siegel and Kim, 1982) and that OAEs reverse polarity along with the stimulus. Because most hearing loss involves OHC loss, OAEs are reduced or absent in persons with cochlear loss. Although mjost hearing loss involves OHC loss and can be detected by OAE testing, some etiologies of hearing loss, such as auditory neuropathy/auditory dys-synchrony, involve dysfunction of neural pathways and not the cochlea (see Chapter 32 for more information about auditory neuropathy). Consequently, OAEs are particularly useful for diagnosing the location of auditory lesions.

The mechanical source for the cochlear amplifier and OAEs is under investigation. Currently, two main hypotheses are being considered. One hypothesis is that somatic motility, which is the rapid changes in OHC length and shape with electrical stimulation, is linked with OAEs

Kemp's (1978) description of OAEs has significantly changed our understanding of cochlear processing and has influenced clinical audiology. OAE measurements are now a standard part of the pediatric test battery, helping us in the identification and diagnosis of hearing loss and assisting in choosing appropriate (re)habilitation. OAE measurements are noninvasive and quick to perform; essential attributes for pediatric patients. Audiologists can obtain ear-specific information when it cannot be obtained through pure-tone audiometry.

The focus of this chapter is to provide basic information about how clinicians can use measures of OAEs in infants and children for identification and diagnosis of hearing loss. Toward this goal, supporting articles have been chosen that illustrate certain points and offer current, pertinent literature for infants and children. This chapter is not meant to be an exhaustive source describing OAEs and their clinical use. There are hundreds of excellent publications about basic properties of OAEs and their clinical use, but reviewing such an extensive bibliography is beyond the scope of this chapter.

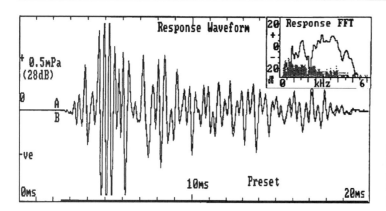

Figure 14–1 The large panel illustrates a TEOAE plotted as a function of time for an infant aged two months. The inset shows TEOAE level (open area) and noise level (shaded areas) as a function of frequency. The TEOAE was evoked by an 80 dB pSPL click.

(Liberman et al, 2002). The second hypothesis is that the source of the cochlear amplifier and OAEs is in the nonlinearity of the OHCl stereocilia bundle (for overview, see Ricci, 2003). It is possible that both OHC somatic motility and stereocilia contribute to the production of OAEs in mammals, and that the contributions of these mechanisms change depending on the stimulus level (Liberman, Zuo, and Guinan, 2004).

Second, although OAEs can be evoked with virtually any auditory stimuli, OAEs evoked by clicks (referred to as transient-evoked OAEs–TEOAE), and two sinusoids (distortion product OAEs) are used clinically. When measuring a TEOAE, a click is presented to the ear at a fixed rate. The OAE occurs in the time period following the click. Responses are averaged to reduce the noise. A typical click level is 75 to 80 dB pSPL and often, a specialized stimulus presentation paradigm and subtraction process is used to eliminate possible artifact caused by the transducers and middle ear. Two separate waveforms are collected in tandem, which allows determination of whether an OAE is present by analyzing how similar the two responses are to each other. **Figure 14–1** illustrates the time waveform of a TEOAE in the large panel and the corresponding frequency response in the inset panel.

When using TEAOEs to identify or diagnose hearing loss, the broadband TEAOE in the frequency domain is analyzed into smaller bands, such as half-octave bands. Three response attributes in each band can be used to assess whether the response is an OAE: (1) the absolute level; (2) the emission level compared with the noise level (emission-to-noise ratio, or ENR); and (3) the reproducibility between the two waveforms.

Distortion product OAEs (DPOAEs) are the other type of OAE used clinically. To record DPOAEs, two sinusoids (called primaries) are presented to the ear at the same time. The lower frequency primary is referred to as f1, and the higher frequency primary is f2. When two primaries are presented to a healthy ear, it will produce intermodulation distortion products that are mathematically related to the frequencies of the primaries. The distortion product at the frequency 2f1-f2 is the one used clinically. A typical frequency ratio (f2:f1) to evoke the DPOAE is 1.22. Common primary levels for f2 and f1 are 55 dB SPL and 65 dB SPL, respectively, because research has shown that the midlevel stimuli are better at identifying hearing loss than high-level stimuli

(e.g., Stover et al, 1996). Usually pairs of primaries with a fixed ratio and level difference between f1 and f2 are presented sequentially at frequencies matched to those used on the audiogram. Stimuli are presented and DPOAEs averaged for a pair of stimuli before presentation of the next pair of stimuli. DPOAE level at 2f1-f2 is plotted as a function of f2 frequency by the solid line and the corresponding noise is represented by a dashed line in **Fig. 14–2**.

This type of recording and display of DPOAEs is often referred to as a DP-gram. To decide whether a DPOAE is present, absolute DPOAE level is used or the DPOAE level compared with the noise (ENR). In most clinical equipment, the noise is the average level in a few frequency bands lower and higher in frequency than the DPOAE frequency.

Finally, it is essential for clinicians to understand that OAEs change level and frequency content as the child develops. TEOAE and DPOAE levels are higher in newborns than in adults (for review, see Prieve, 2007). Moreover, TEAOE and DPOAE levels in infants are higher than in older children and young adults, and children aged 1 to 5 years have higher OAE levels than older children and adults. The changes in OAE levels across age are frequency dependent, with no significant decrease for frequencies 1500 Hz and higher (Prieve et al., 1997a; 1997b). Among preterm infants, DPOAE and TEOAE levels increase with postconceptional age (Smurzynski, 1994). In addition, TEOAE levels increase between birth and 4 weeks of age (Hancur, 1999; Welch et al, 1996).

Pitfall

- Although there are differences in TEOAE and DPOAE levels with age, there are few age-dependent norms for clinical use.

◆ Screening

Newborns

DPOAEs and TEOAEs, as well as screening auditory brainstem response (SABR), are recommended by the Joint Committee on Infant Hearing (2000) as screening tools in

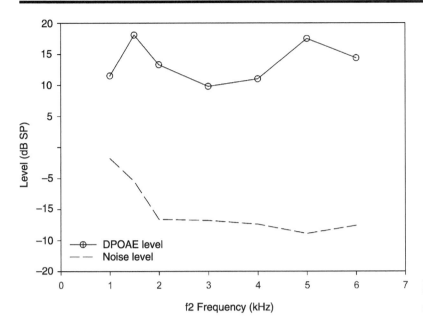

Figure 14–2 DP-gram from an infant aged six months. The solid line illustrates DPOAE level as a function of frequency and the dashed line is the corresponding noise.

universal newborn hearing screening programs. Numerous articles have been published about screening programs that have used OAEs, either alone or in combination with SABR. Data from screening programs with large numbers of babies demonstrate that OAE is a feasible screening tool; 90 to 96% of babies pass screening criteria. Factors affecting the percentages of babies passing include the use of different pass criteria, length of training of personnel, ambient noise, and age of babies at time of test (Prieve, 2007). Most important to consider, however, is how well TEOAEs and DPOAEs actually identify hearing loss.

To determine how well a test identifies hearing loss, all infants, whether or not they pass a hearing screening, must have their screening outcome compared with their hearing status (normal hearing or hearing loss) using a gold standard. The National Institutes of Health (NIH) funded a large-scale, multicenter study that used this research design to determine which screening tool, TEOAEs, DPOAEs, or SABR, identified hearing loss with the greatest accuracy. A total of 7170 infants were enrolled in the study, which included 4478 infants that were cared for in the NICU. The remaining babies were cared for in the well-baby nursery and included 353 well babies with risk indicators for hearing loss (JCIH, 1994). TEOAEs were evoked by 80-dB peak sound pressure level (pSPL) clicks, DPOAEs were evoked using two pairs of primaries at different levels (f2 level = 50 dB SPL and f1 level = 65 dB SPL; f1 and f2 levels both 75 dB SPL), and SABRs were evoked by click levels of 30 dB normal hearing level (nHL). A computerized test program was used that randomized the order of tests in both ears. Details for passing criteria, stopping rules, noise or artifact rejection, and response filtering can be found in Gorga at al, 2000, Norton et al, 2000a, and Sininger et al, 2000.

Of the total number of infants, about 3100 had their hearing tested behaviorally using visual reinforcement audiometry with insert earphones when they were 8 to 10 months of age. Minimal response levels (MRLs) were measured to pulsed, frequency modulated tones presented at 1000 Hz,

2000 Hz and 4000 Hz, and to speech presented monitored-live voice to obtain a speech awareness threshold (SAT). The lowest level at which stimuli were presented was 20 dB HL and the intensity step-size was 10 dB (Widen et al, 2000). MRLs lower than 30dB HL were considered to be consistent with normal hearing sensitivity. MRLs 30 dB HL or higher were considered to be indicative of hearing loss. The MRLs were used as the gold standard against which screening results were compared. Relative operating characteristic (ROC) curves were constructed for TEOAEs and DPOAEs by comparing different OAE ENRs at 1, 2, or 4 kHz to the MRL of the corresponding frequency. The best ENR at any of the three frequencies was compared against the SAT MRL. For construction of SABR ROC curves, different Fsp values, which are an ABR equivalent of signal-to-noise ratio, were compared with MRLs obtained using each of the four stimuli (for a description of Fsp, refer to Sininger et al, 2000). The area under the ROC curve is an indication of how well the screening test identified normally hearing and hearing-impaired ears; 1.0 indicates that hearing status was identified perfectly. The areas under the ROC curves for the screening tools ranged from 0.70 to 0.92 when infants suspected of having progressive hearing loss and middle ear pathology were excluded.

Based on these ROC areas, several important conclusions can be made. First of all, none of the areas were 1.0, indicating that no screening test identified hearing loss with 100% accuracy. Second, TEOAEs, DPOAEs, and SABR all identified hearing loss with approximately the same accuracy, although some small differences were noted. DPOAEs evoked by mid-level primaries (f1 level = 65 dB SPL and f2 level = 50 dB SPL) identified hearing loss better those evoked by primaries presented at 75 dB SPL. TEOAEs and DPOAEs evoked by midlevel stimuli outperformed SABR slightly at identification of hearing loss at 2000 Hz and 4000 Hz, SAT and pure tone average (PTA) based on hearing loss at 2000 Hz and 4000 Hz. Screening ABR outperformed TEOAEs and DPOAEs at identification of hearing loss at 1000 Hz and was

Table 14–1 Calculated Lower and Upper Range and Percentiles of TEOAE and DPOAE ENR Collected Using a Newborn Screening Procedure.

	DPOAE, ENR (dB)		TEOAE, ENR (dB)	
	NH	HL	NH	HL
Bottom of Range	−8	−28	−5	−30
25th percentile	3	−18	7	−18
50th percentile	5	−10	10	−9
75th percentile	10	−7	15	−5
Top of range	22	8	28	11

Source: Values were calculated from Fig. 5 in Norton et al (2000b). (For abbreviations, see below.)

slightly better at identifying hearing loss using a PTA that included 1000 Hz. All of the screening tools identified almost 100% of moderate, severe, and profound hearing loss, but mild hearing loss was only identified at rate of about 50%. Another important finding from the NIH study was that the percentage of infant passes was similar for SABRs, TEOAEs and DPOAEs using the midlevel primaries (Norton et al, 2000b).

Based on the NIH study, the question arises: "Are there recommended criteria to use for identification of hearing loss?" **Table 14–1** lists the calculated top and bottom of the range of OAE ENRs, as well as the 25th, 50th, and 75th percentiles of the best DPOAE and TEOAE ENRs at 2000 Hz and 4000 Hz from infants having normal hearing and hearing loss based on PTAs, including 2000 Hz and 4000 Hz.

The table indicates that the range of ENRs is different for both types of OAEs in infants with normal hearing and in those with hearing loss; however, there is no one criterion that screening programs can use that will identify hearing loss but pass infants with normal hearing. For example, some infants who had normal PTAs did not have measurable DPOAEs or TEOAEs, given that the bottom of the range has ENRs of negative numbers. Although the 75th percentile of ENRs for infants with hearing loss indicates that no OAE was present, some infants with hearing loss had DPOAEs and TEOAEs that were between the 50th and 75th percentile of ENRs for infants with normal hearing.

> **Pearl**
>
> • Even though no criterion identifies hearing loss perfectly, clinicians should keep in mind that OAEs do detect most moderate, severe, and profound hearing loss.

Knowledge of the results from screening programs using particular pass criteria will allow clinicians to make informed judgments about the characteristics of their own universal newborn hearing screening program. The stimuli and pass criteria for TEOAEs and the DPOAE measures that were used by the NIH study are provided in **Table 14–2**. Other programs have used different pass criteria; however, in these studies the results of screening were not compared with behavioral hearing in all children. One large-scale study has used 75% reproducibility in frequency bands at 2000, 3000, and 4000 Hz, rather than ENR (Vohr et al, 1998) and many other programs use OAEs in combination with SABR (e.g., Prieve and Stevens, 2000; Wessex Universal Neonatal Hearing Screening Trial Group, 1998;) to identify hearing loss.

> **Pearl**
>
> • The description and results of the entire NIH newborn hearing screening study can be found in the October 2000 issue of the journal *Ear and Hearing*.

♦ Children

There are few reports of using OAEs as screening tools in older children. Large-scale studies in school-aged children have concluded that traditional behavioral screening is preferred over OAE screening (Krueger and Ferguson, 2002; Sabo, Winston, and Macias, 2000; Taylor and Brooks, 2000). Infants, toddlers, and preschool children are more difficult

Table 14–2 Pass Criteria for TEAOEs and DPOAEs Used in the NIH Study.

	Stimulus		Pass Criteria
	Type	Levels	
TEOAE[a]	Customized click	80 dB pSPL	SNR in 4 out of 5, $^1/_2$-octave bands 3dB SNR at 1.0 and 1.5 kHz 6dB SNR at 2, 3, and 4.1 kHz
DPOAE[b]	f2 = 1.0, 1.5, 2.0, 3.0 4.0 kHz f2/f1 ratio = 1.22	f1 = 65 dB SPL f2 = 50 dB SPL	SNR at $^4/_5$, f2 frequencies 3 dB higher than 2 standard deviations above the mean noise

[a]Norton, et al, 2000a

[b]Gorga et al, 2000

Abbreviations: DPOAE, distortion product otoacoustic emission; SNR, signal-to-noise ratio; TEOAE, transient evoked otoacoustic emission.

to test, and the American-Speech-Language-Hearing Association (1997) recommended that audiologists perform the testing. One study was conducted in Japan in which TEOAE results were compared with pure-tone screening results in children aged 2.5 to 3.5 years. The authors concluded that TEOAEs were useful for screening in this population if an audiologist was not available (Beppu, Hattori, and Yanagita, 1997).

Otoacoustic Emissions in the Diagnostic Test Battery

The uses of TEOAEs and DPOAEs are different in the diagnostic test battery than they are for newborn hearing screening. For hearing screening, the goal is to identify hearing loss. In the diagnostic test battery, OAEs are used to provide ear- and frequency-specific information that can assist with site-of-lesion determination and serve as a cross-check against other results of the test battery.

Once again, the question arises, "What are the best criteria to use as part of a diagnostic test battery for infants and children?" In starting to address this question, clinicians should consider applying more stringent criteria for test battery use than they employ in their newborn hearing screening programs. The prevalence of hearing loss is higher in the population of patients that come to an audiology clinic than in general populations of newborns or children. Infants and children are brought to the audiology clinic because there is a concern about their hearing, which is a risk indicator for hearing loss (JCIH, 2000). Second, when infants and children are being tested at an audiology clinic, the recording conditions are likely to be more optimal than they are in a screening setting. Although there are no clear OAE criteria to be used for infants and children in a diagnostic setting, there are studies that can guide us in choosing reasonable OAE criteria and lead us in developing our own norms. Numerous studies have been published about OAEs in ears with hearing loss, but only a few selected studies are presented in this chapter. These studies included ears with normal hearing and ears with hearing loss, as it is important to know the range for OAEs in ears with normal hearing as well as whether OAEs from ears with hearing loss fall within that normal range. Furthermore, these studies used measures obtainable from the equipment and finally, the population of ears under study were conducted on or included children.

A template that included DPOAEs from ears with normal hearing and hearing loss, which could be used clinically, was pioneered by Gorga and colleagues (1997). In the study, DPOAEs were measured in 1267 ears from 806 participants ranging in age from 1.3 to 96.5 years. The f2:f1 ratio was 1.22 and the level of f2 was 55 dB SPL and the f1 level was 65 dB SPL. Rules based on ENR, minimum absolute DPOAE level and test time were used in data collection. Templates were constructed for both DPOAE level and ENR, with a replica of the template for DPOAE level presented in the left panel of **Fig. 14–3**.

The technique for making this type of template was adopted by Nicholson (2003) and Nicholson and Widen (2004) for TEAOEs measured with the ILO88 equipment in both FullScreen and QuickScreen modes (see Robinette and Glattke, 2007 for detailed information on these two types of stimulus/recording paradigms). The template for the FullScreen (middle panel) was based on OAEs measured from 240 ears of 135 participants aged 3.1 to 29.1 years. The template for the QuickScreen data was based on 84 ears of 49 participants aged 1.0 to 17.5 years. In both TEAOE templates, ENR ratio in half-octave bands, rather than TEOAE level, is plotted. For both of these templates, the stimulus was a click presented at 80 dB _/_ 3 dB pSPL, and stimulus presentation and recording were done in the nonlinear mode. In addition, there had to be a minimum of 50 averages contributing to the final OAE.

On each of these templates, four solid lines on the graphs depict percentiles for populations of ears where

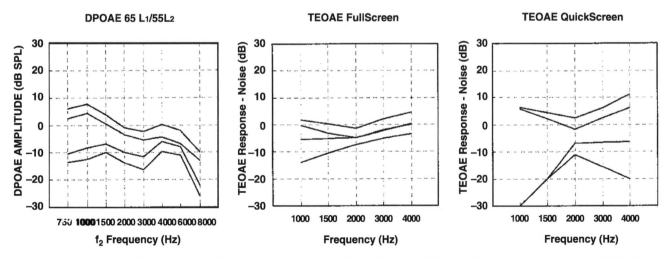

Figure 14–3 Examples of clinical templates for DPOAEs (left panel), TEOAEs using the FullScreen option (middle panel) and TEOAEs using the QuickScreen option (right panel). Please see text for details. (From Nicholson, N., and Widen, J.E. (2007). Evoked otoacoustic emission in the evaluation of children. In Robinette, M., and Glattke, T. (2007). Otoacoustic emissions: Clinical applications, 3rd ed. New York: Thieme, pp. 360–394. Reprinted with permission.)

normal hearing was defined as a behavioral threshold of 20 or lower dB HL at the frequencies listed on the x-axis. The top solid line and the second solid line in each panel represent the 95th and 90th percentiles, respectively, of DPOAE level (left panel) or TEAOE ENR (middle and right panels) from populations of ears with hearing loss. If you are testing a patient, and that patient's response is higher than the 95th percentile of OAE responses from ears with hearing loss, there is reasonable confidence that the ear has normal hearing. The third and fourth solid lines from the top of the graph represent the 10th and 5th percentiles (respectively) of DPOAE levels (left panel) or TEOAE ENR (middle and right panels) from populations of ears with normal hearing. If you are testing a patient and that patient's response falls below the 5th percentile of responses from normally hearing ears, you can be reasonably confident that the ear has hearing loss. The most difficult interpretation of hearing status is if an individual's data fall between the second and third lines from the top. This area is below the 90th percentile of responses from ears with hearing loss and higher than the 10th percentile of responses from ears with normal hearing. Said another way, the OAE response is within the overlapping range of response values from ears with hearing loss and those with normal hearing. In this case, you cannot be certain whether the ear has normal hearing or hearing loss, although there are examples of individual data with OAE responses in this range that have mild hearing loss (Gorga et al, 2005; Nicholson and Widen, 2007).

Although these templates are extremely useful for clinicians to determine whether an OAE is likely associated with normal hearing or hearing loss, care must be taken to make sure that the stimulus and recording parameters of use and patient population are similar to those used to construct the template. In addition, the equipment may vary. There are currently no standards for acceptable equipment characteristics. Clinical equipment varies greatly in the frequency response of the probes, how the probes are calibrated, how responses are averaged, and how noise is defined. In addition, the ages and characteristics of the population on which the template was based must be similar to the patients in the clinician's practice. An example of how normative responses differ among two studies is shown in **Fig. 14–4**.

Fig. 14–4 illustrates cumulative distributions of DPOAE level for patients whose hearing thresholds were classified as normal based on behavioral (Gorga et al, 1997) or ABR (Prieve et al, 2006) threshold testing. The black lines depict data from Gorga et al (1997), in which the pre-cursor of the Bio-Logic Scout(r) was used to collect data from more than 1200 ears in patients 1 to 96 years old. The gray lines depict data collected using the Otodynamics equipment in 45 ears of infants aged 3 to 35 weeks (median = 10 weeks) (Prieve et al, 2006). The three line types represent data for three f2 frequencies. For every f2 frequency, the DPOAE levels from the mixed population of children and adults are lower than those for the population composed only of infants. A horizontal line is drawn at the 10th percentile, demonstrating that it is quite different for the two populations. For example, at 2000 Hz, the 10th percentile from the study by Gorga et al (1997) is approximately -10 dB SPL, and that for the study by Prieve et al (2006) is about 4 dB SPL. Were an infant who had a DPOAE level of -8 dB SPL at 2000 Hz to be tested, that response would fall squarely within the region of "unknown" on the template shown in **Fig. 14–3**, but actually falls below the 5th percentile of DPOAE levels from normally hearing ears if compared with infants of her own age. The important point from this graph is that although the use of published templates is an excellent way to analyze individual clinical data, care must be taken to validate that the template is appropriate for your clinical population and equipment.

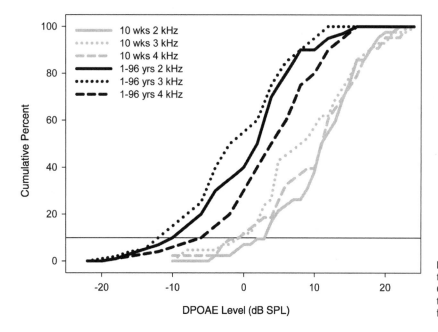

Figure 14–4 Comparison of cumulative distributions of DPOAE levels from two studies. Data from Gorga et al. (1997) are depicted by black lines and those from Prieve et al. (2006) in gray lines. See text for details.

A few final, important points are worth noting. The accuracy of identifying hearing loss is best from 2000 Hz to 4000 Hz, whether using TEOAEs (Hussain et al, 1998; Prieve et al, 1993; Norton et al, 2000b; Nicholson, 2003) or DPOAEs (Gorga et al, 1993; 1997; 2000; 2005). At lower frequencies (750 Hz and 1000 Hz) as well as at higher frequencies (6000 Hz and 8000 Hz), identification of hearing loss is poorer. The identification of hearing loss at these frequencies can be improved by performing a multivariate statistical technique such as logit or discriminant function analyses. These techniques allow inclusion of OAE and noise levels for multiple frequencies to predict hearing loss at a single, chosen frequency (e.g., Dorn et al, 1999; Nicholson, 2003). Gorga et al (2005) provides weights and equations to calculate the logit function output for identification of hearing loss at a given frequency by DPOAEs. These weights and equations calculated from a large clinical study (Gorga et al, 1997) were successfully applied to a smaller, clinical population using the Biologic Scout(r) DPOAE system. Finally, it has also been shown that requiring DPOAEs or TEOAEs to meet criteria at more than one frequency (e.g., 4 of 5 f2 test frequencies) improves identification of hearing loss (Gorga et al, 1999; 2005).

Can the Middle Ear Affect Otoacoustic Emissions?

Because the stimulus used to evoke OAEs must pass through the middle ear to go to the cochlea, and the OAE must travel back through the middle ear to be recorded in the ear canal, even minor pathologies can alter OAEs. Therefore, it is important to test middle ear function or determine the possibility of a conductive hearing loss if OAEs are absent in a diagnostic evaluation. TEOAE and DPOAE levels are reduced, but not usually to the point that they are absent, in infants and children having negative tympanometric peak pressure (measured from a tympanogram) (Type C). (Choi, Pafitis, and Zalzal, 1999; Hof et al, 2005a; 2005b; Lonsbury-Martin et al, 1994; Koike and Wetmore, 1999; Koivunen et al, 2000; Prieve et al, submitted). The amount of OAE level reduction does not appear to be related to the severity of the negative pressure (Koike and Wetmore, 1999; Trine, Hirsch, and Margolis, 1993; Prieve et al, submitted). A within-infant study found that the mean TEOAE reduction was about 4 dB across frequency bands for mean changes in tympanometric peak pressure of -169 daPa (Prieve et al, submitted). Although this was a significant change, it did not significantly change whether the infants passed a criterion of 6 dB ENR ratio in all bands centered at 2000, 3000, and 4000 Hz. Small reductions in pass rate have been reported for children as well (Hof et al, 2005b; Koike and

Wetmore, 1999). Although a reduction in OAE levels caused by slight middle ear alteration is not a major problem for children undergoing a diagnostic test battery, middle ear status significantly affects the pass rates of newborn hearing screening programs (e.g., Chang et al, 1993; Doyle et al, 2000; Keefe et al, 2003).

TEOAEs measured when tympanograms have no discernable peak pressure (flat or Type B) are dramatically reduced in amplitude and often are not measurable (Choi, Pafitis, and Zalzal, 1999; Lonsbury-Martin et al, 1994; Koike and Wetmore, 1999; Koivunen et al, 2000). For children with otitis media, the two middle ear factors most closely associated with absent TEOAEs are viscosity (Amedee, 1995) and quantity of effusion (Koivunen et al, 2000). The clinician must realize that OAEs can still be present in infants and children with negative middle ear pressure, and sometimes even in those with flat tympanograms. Having negative tympanometric peak pressure on a tympanogram or a flat tympanogram should not preclude the audiologist from measuring OAEs as part of the test battery.

How To Obtain Good Recordings

A proper probe fit is essential for good OAE recordings. A good probe fit keeps out unwanted room noise from the ear canal, maintains the proper stimulus level, and prevents reductions in measured OAE level. Measuring OAEs in a sound-treated booth is optimal, but testing can easily be performed in a quiet room if the probe fit is good. The probe needs to be placed firmly into the ear, which can be done by grasping the back of the pinna while the probe is inserted. The probe assembly can be clipped to the child's shoulder; however, it is often helpful to clip the assembly to the parent if the child is sitting on the parent's lap, or to the chair if the child is sitting quietly in the chair. You can coax a child to sit quietly by reading a book with a low-level voice or having a video playing. Because identification of hearing loss is not as good below 1500 Hz and children are noisier than adults, recording time can be reduced by not testing low frequencies. The equipment should be calibrated according to the manufacturer's suggestions, and often, a test run in a standard cavity is done every day to ensure there are no equipment artifacts that would affect OAE measurement. Finally, most equipment has a measure to determine the stability of the stimulus while the test is being conducted, which indicates whether the probe is moving in the ear canal. A high stability measure (e.g., higher than 75%) as well as an acceptably low noise level, should be assessed to ensure that the OAE test was properly conducted. If the child is somewhat noisy, additional averaging may be needed to reduce the noise floor.

◆ Final Note

OAEs are excellent tools for use in identifying hearing loss in a screening situation, and as site-of-lesion and cross-check measures in a diagnostic setting. Abnormal OAE measures, together with normal middle ear measures and hearing loss, lead us to suspect that there is OHC loss. In this case, it is reasonable to suspect that the cochlear amplifier is compromised and hearing aids are an appropriate rehabilitation strategy. Management is more difficult if the OAEs are robust, but pure-tone and speech audiometry indicates hearing loss. These test outcomes, along with acoustic reflex and ABR test results, may be consistent with the diagnosis of auditory neuropathy/auditory dys-synchrony. If the child has this diagnosis, the approach to (re)habilitation is not as clear, and may include cochlear implants (e.g., Peterson et al, 2003).

Controversial Point

- Despite widespread clinical use for identification of hearing loss, researchers are investigating whether OAEs show change before behavioral thresholds change, especially with noise exposure and ototoxic drugs. This issue is not resolved for general and clinical populations.

Discussion Questions

1. What are the possible sources for changes in OAEs with development?

2. At what point in your diagnostic test battery should you measure OAEs? At the beginning? At the end? Before you measure tympanograms? And, does it depend on age of the child?

3. Speculate as to why OAEs are better at detecting mid- and high-frequency hearing loss than low-frequency hearing loss.

4. Patient scenario: You are performing a hearing screening for a child going through diagnostic testing for speech and language delay. You have measured minimal response levels in soundfield at 15 dB HL at 500, 1000, and 2000 Hz in a child aged 18 months. You also measure TEOAEs in both ears that have ENRs of 15 dB at bands centered at 2000, 3000, and 4000 Hz using the Otodynamics QuickScreen mode. Does this child have hearing sensitivity within normal limits? Do you need to perform more testing on this child?

References

Amedee, R. G. (1995). The effects of chronic otitis media with effusion on the measurement of transiently evoked otoacoustic emissions. Laryngoscope, 105, 589–595.

American Speech-Language-Hearing Association. (1997). Guidelines for audiologic screening. Rockville: ASHA.

Beppu, R., Hattori, T., and Yanagita, N. (1997). Comparison of TEOAE with play audiometry for screening hearing problems in children. Auris Nasus Larynx, 24, 367–371.

Chang, K. W., Vohr, B. R., Norton, S. J., et al. (1993). External and middle ear status related to evoked otoacoustic emission in neonates. Archives of Otolaryngology–Head and Neck Surgery, 119, 276–282.

Choi, S. S., Pafitis, I. A., and Zalzal, G. H. (1999). Clinical applications of the transiently evoked acoustic emissions in the pediatric population. Annals of Otolology, Rhinology and Laryngology, 108, 132–138.

Dorn, P. A., Piskorski, P., Gorga, M. P., et al. (1999). Predicting audiometric status from distortion product otoacoustic emissions using multivariate analyses. Ear and Hearing, 20, 149–163.

Doyle, K. J., Rodgers, P., Fujikawa, S., and Newman, E. (2000). External and middle ear effects on infant hearing screening tests. Otolaryngology–Head and Neck Surgery, 122, 477–481.

Gorga, M. P., Dierking, D. M., Johnson, T.A., et al. (2005). A validation and potential clinical application of multivariate analyses of distortion-product otoacoustic emission data. Ear and Hearing, 26, 593–607.

Gorga, M. P., Neely, S. T., and Dorn, P. A. (1999). DPOAE test performance for a priori criteria and for multifrequency audiometric standards. Ear and Hearing, 20, 345–362.

Gorga, M. P., Neely, S. T., Ohlrich, B., et al. (1997). From laboratory to clinic: a large scale study of distortion product otoacoustic emissions in ears with normal hearing and ears with hearing loss. Ear and Hearing, 18, 440–455.

Gorga, M. P., Norton, S. J., Sininger, Y. S., et al. (2000). Identification of neonatal hearing impairment: distortion product otoacoustic emissions during the perinatal period. Ear and Hearing, 21, 400–424.

Hancur, C. (1999). Transient-evoked otoacoustic emissions in the neonatal period. Master's thesis, Syracuse University.

Hof, J. R., Anteunis, L. J. C., Chenault, M. N., and Van Dijk, P. (2005a). Otoacoustic emissions at compensated middle ear pressure in children. International Journal of Audiology, 44, 317–320.

Hof, J. R., van Dijk, P., Chenault, M. N., and Anteunis, L. J. C. (2005b). A two-step scenario for hearing assessment with otoacoustic emissions at compensated middle ear pressure (in children 1–7 years old). International Journal of Pediatric Otorhinolaryngology, 69, 649–655.

Hussain, D. M., Gorga, M. P., Neely, S. T., Keefe, D. H., and Peters, J. (1998) Transient evoked otoacoustic emissions in patients with normal hearing and in patients with hearing loss. Ear and Hearing, 19, 434–449.

Joint Committee on Infant Hearing. (1994). Position statement. American Speech-Hearing-Language Association, 36, 38–41.

Joint Committee on Infant Hearing. (2000). Year 2000 position statement: principles and guidelines for early hearing detection. Pediatrics, 106, 798–817.

Keefe, D. H., Gorga, M. P., Neely, S. T., and Zhao, F. (2003). Ear-canal acoustic admittance and reflectance measurements in human neonates, II: Predictions of middle-ear dysfunction and sensorineural hearing loss. Journal of the Acoustical Society of America, 113, 407–422.

Kemp, D. T. (1978). Stimulated acoustic emissions from the human auditory system. Journal of the Acoustical Society of America, 64, 1386–91

Koike, K. J., and Wetmore, S. J. (1999). Interactive effects of the middle ear pathology and the associated hearing loss on transient-evoked otoacoustic emission measures. Otolaryngology–Head and Neck Surgery, 121, 238–244.

Koivunen, P., Uhari, M., Laitakari, K., et al. (2000). Otoacoustic emissions and tympanometry in children with otitis media. Ear and Hearing, 21, 212–217.

Krueger, W. W., and Ferguson, L. (2002). A comparison of screening methods in school-aged children. Otolaryngology–Head and Neck Surgery, 127, 516–519.

Liberman, M. C., Gao, J., He, D. Z., et al. (2002). Prestin is required for electromotility of the outer hair cell and for the cochlear amplifier. Nature, 419, 300–304.

Liberman, M. C., Zuo, J., and Guinan, J. J. (2004). Otoacoustic emissions without somatic motility: can stereocilia mechanics drive the mammalian cochlea? Journal Acoustical Society of America, 116, 1649–1655.

Lonsbury-Martin, B. L., Martin, G. K., McCoy, M. J., and Whitehead, M. L. (1994). Otoacoustic emissions testing in young children: middle-ear influence. The American Journal of Otology, 15, 13–20.

Nicholson, N. (2003). Transient evoked otoacoustic emissions in relation to hearing loss: univariate and multivariate analyses. Dissertation Abstracts International, 64, 5432.

Nicholson, N., and Widen, J. E. (2004). Templates for diagnostic interpretation of TEOAEs. Poster presented at the 16th Annual American Academy of Audiology convention, Salt Lake City, UT.

Nicholson, N., and Widen, J. E. (2007). Evoked otoacoustic emissions in the evaluation of children. In M. Robinette, , and T. Glattke (Eds.), Otoacoustic emissions: clinical application (3rd Ed.). New York: Thieme.

Norton, S. J., Gorga, M. P., Widen, J. E., et al. (2000a). Identification of neonatal hearing impairment: transient evoked otoacoustic emissions during the perinatal period. Ear and Hearing, 21, 425–442.

Norton, S. J., Gorga, M. P., Widen, J. E., et al. (2000b). Identification of neonatal hearing impairment: evaluation of transient evoked otoacoustic emission, distortion product otoacoustic emission, and auditory brain stem response test performance. Ear and Hearing, 21, 508–528.

Owens, J. J., McCoy, M. J., Lonsbury-Martin, B. L., et al. (1993). Otoacoustic emissions in children with normal ears, middle ear dysfunction, and ventilating tubes. American Journal of Otology, 14, 34–40.

Peterson, A., Shallop, J., Driscoll, C., et al. (2003). Outcomes of cochlear implantation in children with auditory neuropathy. Journal of the American Academy of Audiology, 14, 188–201.

Prieve, B. A. (2007). Otoacoustic emissions in neonatal hearing screening. In: Robinette, M., and Glattke, T. (Eds.), Otoacoustic emissions: clinical application (3rd Ed.). New York: Thieme.

Prieve, B. A., Calandruccio, L., Georgantas, L. M., Mazevski, A., and Fitzgerald, T. S. (submitted). Changes in transient-evoked otoacoustic emissions with negative tympanometric peak pressure in infants and toddlers.

Prieve, B. A., Fitzgerald, T. S., and Schulte, L. E. (1997a). Basic characteristics of COAEs in infants and children. Journal of the Acoustical Society of America, 102, 2860–2870.

Prieve, B. A., Fitzgerald, T. S., Schulte, L. E., et al. (1997b). Basic characteristics of DPOAEs in infants and children. Journal of the Acoustical Society of America, 102, 2871–2879.

Prieve, B. A., Gorga, M. P., Schmidt A.L., et al. (1993). Analysis of transient-evoked otoacoustic emissions in normal-hearing and hearing-impaired ears. Journal of the Acoustical Society of America, 93, 3308–3319.

Prieve, B. A., and Stevens, F. (2000). The New York State Universal Newborn Hearing Screening Demonstration Project: introduction and overview. Ear and Hearing, 21, 85–91.

Prieve, B. A., Vander Werff, K., and Georgantas, L. (2006). Toneburst ABR, OAE and middle ear measures in sleeping infants. Poster presented at the 18th Annual American Academy of Audiology convention, Minneapolis, MN.

Ricci, A. (2003). Active hair bundle movements and the cochlear amplifier. Journal of the American Academy of Audiology, 14, 325–338.

Robinette, M., and Glattke, T. (Eds.). (2007). Otoacoustic emissions: clinical application. New York: Thieme.

Sabo, M. P., Winston, R., and Macias, J. D. (2000). Comparison of pure tone and transient otoacoustic emissions screening in a grade-school population. American Journal of Otology, 21, 88–91.

Siegel, J. H., and Kim, D. O. (1982). Cochlear biomechanics: vulnerability to acoustic trauma and other alterations as seen in neural responses and ear-canal sound pressure. In D. Hamernik, D. Henderson, and R. Salvi (Eds.), New perspectives on noise-induced hearing loss. New York: Raven Press, pp. 137–151.

Sininger, Y. S., Cone-Wesson, B., Folsom, R.C., et al. (2000). Identification of neonatal hearing impairment: auditory brain stem responses in the perinatal period. Ear and Hearing, 21, 383–399.

Smurzynski, J. (1994). Longitudinal measurements of distortion-product and click-evoked otoacoustic emissions of preterm infants: preliminary results. Ear and Hearing 15, 210–223.

Stover, L., Gorga, M. P., Neely, S. T., et al. (1996). Toward optimizing the clinical utility of distortion product otoacoustic emission measurements. Journal of the Acoustical Society of America, 100, 956–967.

Taylor, C. L., and Brooks, R. P. (2000). Screening for hearing loss and middle-ear disorders in children using TEOAEs. American Journal of Audiology, 9, 50–55.

Trine, M. B., Hirsch, J., and Margolis, R. (1993). The effect of middle ear pressure on transient evoked otoacoustic emissions. Ear and Hearing, 14, 401–407.

Vohr, B. R., Carty, L. M., Moore, P. E., et al. (1998). The Rhode Island Hearing Assessment Program: experience with statewide hearing screening (1993–1996). Journal of Pediatrics, 133, 353–358.

Welch, D., Greville, K. A., Thorne, P. R., et al. (1996). Influence of acquisition parameters on the measurement of click evoked otoacoustic emissions in neonates in a hospital environment. Audiology, 35, 143–157.

Wessex Universal Neonatal Hearing Screening Trial Group (1998). Controlled trial of universal neonatal screening for early identification of permanent childhood hearing impairment. Lancet, 352, 1957–1964.

Widen, J. E., Folsom, R. C., Cone-Wesson, B., et al. (2000). Identification of neonatal hearing impairment: hearing status at eight to 12 months corrected age using a visual reinforcement audiometry protocol. Ear and Hearing, 21, 471–487.

Chapter 15

Auditory Evoked Response Testing in Infants and Children

Suzanne C. Purdy and Andrea S. Kelly

♦ **What Are Auditory Evoked Responses and How Are They Recorded?**

♦ **Auditory Brainstem Response**

Neuromaturation and Response Generators

Choice of Stimulus for Auditory Brainstem Response Recordings

Choice of Stimulus Polarity

Tone Burst Auditory Brainstem Response

Neurological Applications of Auditory Brainstem Response

Bone Conduction Auditory Brainstem Response

♦ **Auditory Steady State Response**

♦ **Middle Latency Response**

♦ **Cortical Auditory Evoked Potentials**

♦ **Transducers and Stimulus Calibration**

Key Points

- For auditory brainstem response (ABR) and auditory steady state response (ASSR) testing, infants need to be well settled in a deep sleep for good quality recordings.

- Electrode contacts need to be good (low impedances) and the environment should be free of electrical noise to obtain quality evoked response recordings.

- Frequency specific testing is easy to do and is essential for fitting of hearing aids for children whose hearing loss has been detected via universal newborn screening.

- Clinicians do not need to wait for confirmation of evoked response testing with behavioral data — hearing thresholds can be reliably estimated using evoked responses.

- Bone conduction ABR should be performed when a hearing loss is identified using ABR or ASSR, to determine if there is a conductive component to the hearing loss.

- Cortical evoked responses show great promise for validating hearing aid fitting in young infants who are not able to provide reliable behavioral responses to sound.

♦ What Are Auditory Evoked Responses and How Are They Recorded?

The auditory brainstem response (ABR) and the auditory steady state response (ASSR) are the auditory evoked responses most commonly recorded in infants and children. Other less commonly recorded responses that also have clinical utility in pediatric audiology are the middle latency response (MLR), the electrocochleogram (ECoG), and cortical auditory evoked potentials (CAEPs) [also referred to as the late latency response (LLR) or the slow vertex response (SVR)]. These responses differ in terms of where they are generated in the auditory system and consequently occur at different times after presentation of an auditory stimulus. Optimal stimulus and recording parameters also differ. This chapter focuses on the evoked responses that are used most widely in pediatric audiology, the ABR and, to a lesser extent, ASSR. Clinical applications of CAEP, MLR, and ECoG are also discussed briefly.

All evoked responses represent summed auditory neural activity, usually recorded using sensors (electrodes) attached to the surface of the scalp or head. Each evoked response has a characteristic appearance and is usually described in terms of the timing (latency) and amplitude of particular peaks in the evoked response waveform.

Table 15–1 Characteristics of Auditory Evoked Responses Used Clinically for Testing Children and Clinical Applications of these Responses

Evoked Response	Latency Range	Clinical Applications	Stimuli Typically Used
ABR	0–15 milliseconds	Newborn hearing screening	Click
		Diagnosis of AD/AN	Click
		Oto-neurological investigation of retrocochlear pathology	Click
		Objective estimation of pure tone hearing thresholds	Short duration tone bursts
ASSR	0–15 milliseconds	Objective estimation of pure tone hearing thresholds	Frequency and/or amplitude modulated continuous tones
ECoG	0–3 milliseconds	Diagnosis of AD/AN; Objective estimation of pure tone hearing thresholds	Clicks and tone bursts
MLR	15–50 milliseconds	Assessment of central auditory function	Clicks
CAEP	50–400 milliseconds	Objective evaluation of hearing aids	Speech sounds and long duration tone bursts
		Objective evaluation of hearing in cases where ABR may be inaccurate because of neurological damage	

Abbreviations: ABR, auditory brainstem response; AD/AN, auditory neuropathy/auditory dys-synchrony; ASSR, auditory steady-state response; CAEP, cortical auditory evoked potentials; ECoG, electrocochleogram; MLR, middle latency response

Table 15–1 summarizes typical latencies and clinical applications of the evoked responses discussed here. **Fig. 15–1** shows a schematic diagram of an evoked response recording system.

With the exception of ASSR and screening ABR, most clinical evoked response recording systems enable clinicians to view a "time waveform" of the response (**see example in Fig. 15–2**). The time waveform is a plot of evoked response amplitude (voltage) as a function of time after stimulus presentation. **Fig. 15–2** shows a tone burst ABR recorded from a 4-month-old infant in response to a 4000-Hz tone burst. The infant has mild to severe hearing loss thought to be caused by oxygen deprivation at birth. The time waveforms contain electrical noise plus the evoked response. The ABR peaks at 8 to 10 milliseconds, referred to as "wave V," can be seen at levels down to 90 dB, but is not present at 80 dB normal hearing level (nHL). As the stimulus presentation level reduces, wave V amplitude reduces and latency increases slightly. This effect of stimulus level on response

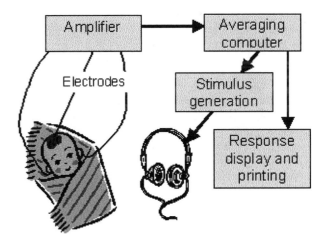

Figure 15–1 Schematic diagram of evoked response recording equipment. Stimuli can be delivered to a range of transducers such as insert earphones, supraaural earphones, a bone conductor, or a loudspeaker.

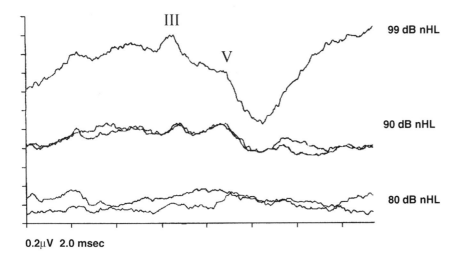

0.2μV   2.0 msec

Figure 15–2 Example of 4000 Hz tone burst ABR responses recorded to stimuli at reducing presentation levels in a 4 month old infant with severe high frequency hearing loss. At stimulus levels of 90 and 80 dB nHL, repeat recordings are overlaid.

amplitude and latency is characteristic of all neural auditory evoked responses. At near-threshold levels repeat recordings were obtained to verify the presence or absence of an evoked response and the two waveforms were overlaid.

Because auditory evoked responses are very small compared with background electrical "noise," stimuli are presented multiple times and computer averaging is used to extract the response. The "noise" could be other brain or cardiac electrical activity generated by the child or it could be electrical noise in the environment generated by equipment or the power supply to the room. In the ABR example in **Fig. 15–2** the "baseline" recording at 80 dB nHL contains no repeatable ABR waveform, but does contain electrical noise.

◆ Auditory Brainstem Response

Neuromaturation and Response Generators

In older children and adults the ABR to a high-level click stimulus consists of a series of positive and negative peaks occurring at 1.5 to 6 milliseconds (with each peak separated by about 1 millisecond), labeled as waves I, II, III, IV, V, and VI (Jewett and Williston, 1971). Waves IV and V are often merged and hence may appear as a "IV/V complex." Wave V is the most robust component in the ABR waveform and may be the only identifiable peak, particularly at near-threshold levels. The lower panel in **Fig. 15–3** shows an adult-like ABR recorded to high level click stimuli from a school-aged child.

Because of the complexity of ipsilateral and contralateral central auditory connections in the brainstem, a simple serial model of successive ABR peaks generated by successive brainstem nuclei is unlikely to be valid.

Pearl

- Current evidence indicates that ABR peaks represent summed activity of the auditory nerve, and multiple fiber tracts and brainstem nuclei.

Waves I and II arise from the distal (i.e., close to the cochlea) and proximal (i.e., close to the brainstem) ends of the auditory nerve, and it is probable that wave III is largely from the cochlear nucleus, wave IV is from the superior olivary complex, wave V is from the lateral lemniscus fiber tract, and the negativity following wave V (SN_{10}) is from the contralateral inferior colliculus (Moller, 2007).

Differences in the normal click ABR waveform of infants versus children are illustrated in **Fig. 15–3,** which shows the ABR evoked by 80 dB nHL clicks in a 3-month-old infant versus a 7-year-old child. The two overlaid waveforms show the stimulus artifact right at the beginning of the trace for both infant and child. For the infant the cochlear microphonic (CM) is very evident before wave I. The CM waveform originates in the cochlea rather than in the nerve, as it inverts when the stimulus polarity reverses from rarefaction to condensation (Dallos, 1973). CM is present in infants with normal hearing (Starr et al, 2001) but is abnormally large and may be present in the absence of other ABR peaks in infants with auditory neuropathy/auditory dys-synchrony (AD/AN) (Berlin et al, 1998). The ABR recording from the child may contain CM before wave I, but this is difficult to determine because the ABR was recorded with only one click polarity (rarefaction). Ipsilateral and contralateral recordings are shown, recorded with

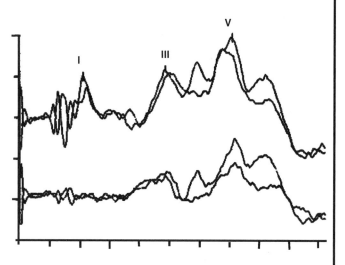
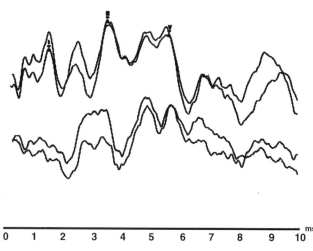

Figure 15–3 Click-evoked (80 dB nHL, 17.1/s) ABR recordings for a 3-month-old infant (left) and a 7-year-old child (right), both of whom have normal hearing. For the infant the overlaid waveforms are separate recordings for rarefaction and condensation clicks. For the child the overlaid waveforms are repeat recordings for rarefaction clicks. In each case two ABR channels were used to record both ipsilateral and contralateral waveforms. Ipsilateral recordings are shown above and contralateral recordings are shown below.

the noninverting (positive, "active") electrode on the vertex, and the inverting (negative, reference) electrode on the same or opposite ear relative to the stimulus ear (ipsilateral versus contralateral). Later peaks are typically more robust than earlier peaks in contralateral recordings, as illustrated in **Fig. 15–3,** and show a clearer separation of waves IV and V than ipsilateral recordings.

The maturation of the auditory system begins at the periphery, where it is relatively adult-like at birth. The cortical regions are not fully mature until late adolescence (Ponton et al, 1996). During the first year of life the ABR matures rapidly; morphology of the response and latencies reach adult values at around 24 months. In premature infants the reliability of click-evoked ABR improves between 24 and 32 weeks gestational age; replicable waves I, III, and V are evident in the waveform at about 28 weeks gestational age (Eggermont and Salamy, 1988). Decreased latencies of waves III and V in the first 2 years of life are believed to be caused by decreased neural conduction time caused by completion of myelination in the proximal to distal direction in the central nervous system (Moore et al, 1996).

Pearl

- Because there are such pronounced changes in ABR latencies during the first 2 years, it is recommended that age-specific normative latency data be applied on a weekly basis during the preterm period, a biweekly basis during the 3-month period from term, and at monthly intervals thereafter until 18 to 24 months (Jacobson and Hall, 1994).

Choice of Stimulus for Auditory Brainstem Response Recordings

The first published reports of ABR recordings, using short duration clicks as the stimulus, appeared in the literature in the late 1960s and early 1970s. For many years clicks have been the favored stimulus for ABR recordings for neurological investigations of auditory pathways and estimating hearing sensitivity. This situation persists today, despite well-established evidence about the limitations of click ABR for frequency-specific hearing threshold estimation. A common misunderstanding is that the click ABR reflects hearing only in the high frequencies because it is mainly generated

by high-frequency cochlear regions in listeners with normal hearing (Coats and Martin, 1977; Hyde, 1985). Because of their rapid onset and short duration, clicks have a very broad frequency spectrum and hence the click ABR can be generated from any cochlear region with good hearing sensitivity. Consequently, click ABR thresholds can indicate normal hearing or underestimate hearing thresholds when there is a significant hearing loss, if the loss is restricted to part of the audiometric frequency range (Stapells and Oates, 1997; van der Drift, Brocaar, and van Zanten, 1987).

Because of the limitations of click ABR, tone burst ABR techniques have been developed that reliably estimate pure tone audiometric thresholds (Sininger, 2003; Stapells, 2002). There is considerable evidence that tone burst ABR more accurately estimates pure tone thresholds than click ABR (Stapells, 2002). The click ABR continues to have an important role in screening ABR and in the diagnosis of AD/AN, but should not be used for estimation of pure tone thresholds.

Clicks produce well-defined ABR waveforms because their rapid onset ensures optimal in-phase stimulation of high-frequency nerve fibers in the base of the cochlea (Kiang and Moxon, 1974). Recently an alternative to the click stimulus, known as a "chirp," has been suggested. The chirp contains a wide range of frequencies, but the frequency content is swept from a low to a high frequency at a rate that simulates cochlear traveling wave speed, to achieve simultaneous activation across the cochlear partition and maximize evoked response amplitude (Bell, Allen, and Lutman, 2002; Wegner and Dau, 2002). Because there are few published data on the use of chirp-ABR for diagnostic purposes, its use is still limited clinically.

Choice of Stimulus Polarity

Table 15–2 summarizes recommended stimulus parameters for the two main applications of ABR recordings in children, namely, threshold estimation and otoneurologic investigations. More detailed information on specific tone burst ABR stimulus and recording parameters can be found in Stapells (2002). Stimulus polarity refers to the onset phase of the stimulus. For rarefaction onset polarity, there is an inward movement of the transducer diaphragm, negative onset pressure in the ear canal, and an initial upward movement of the basilar membrane (Brugge et al, 1969). Traditionally, clinicians have used rarefaction clicks based on evidence for enhanced ABR amplitudes, including wave I and clearer wave IV and V separation. Alternating stimulus polarity is commonly used for tone bursts to cancel stimulus artifact,

Table 15–2 Stimulus Parameters Commonly Used for Different ABR Applications

Purpose of ABR Testing	Stimulus Type	Cycles	Rise, Plateau, and Fall Times	Polarity	Durations for Commonly Used Frequencies	Rate /s
Threshold estimation	Tone burst	5	2–1–2 cycles	Alternating	500 Hz = 10 milliseconds 1000 Hz = 5 milliseconds 2000 Hz = 2.5 milliseconds 4000 Hz = 1.25 milliseconds	39.1
Neurological investigation / auditory neuropathy	Click		Produced by delivering a "square" wave to transducer	Rarefaction and condensation	100 μs	17.1

because the relatively long duration of the stimuli means that the artifact may make it difficult to identify ABR peaks in the first part of the waveform (Foxe and Stapells, 1993). More recently, with increasing knowledge about the prevalence of AN/AD among children with hearing impairment (Rance et al, 1999; Sininger, 2002), there has been a move toward using both rarefaction and condensation polarities routinely for click ABR recording, to determine the presence of an abnormally large cochlear microphonic.

Tone Burst Auditory Brainstem Response

Optimizing Test Efficiency

Most commonly, infants will be in a state of natural sleep for ABR testing, although sometimes testing is done under general anesthesia. The ABR is unaffected by sedation and can be recorded in comatose patients (Hall and Harris, 1994). Sedation or general anesthesia may be necessary to complete testing in a timely fashion in an infant with suspected hearing loss or if a child is difficult to test, despite the associated risks (vomiting and asphyxia) and the need for resuscitation equipment and appropriately qualified medical staff. Universal newborn hearing screening and early confirmation of hearing thresholds using evoked potential audiometry when infants are more likely to sleep naturally will reduce the need for general anesthesia and sedation; however, this will still be required for some children. The American Speech-Language-Hearing Association (ASHA) has developed helpful guidelines on the use of sedation for ABR testing (ASHA, 1992).

Regardless of whether the child is sleeping naturally or sedated, test efficiency is critical and many authors have suggested a range of test protocols for ABR audiometry that maximize the information obtained per time invested, since it may be necessary at any stage to abandon testing (Elliott et al, 2000; Stapells, 2004). **Fig. 15–4** outlines a suggested test sequence that aims to obtain key information as quickly as possible so that, if the child wakes too soon, a decision can still be made about habilitation needs (hearing aids, cochlear implants, etc.).

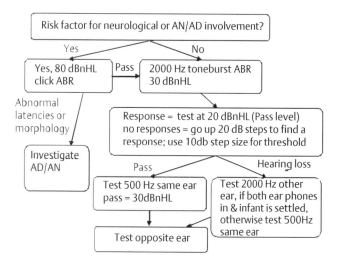

Figure 15–4 Recommended ABR test sequence.

The infant should be settled at the start of testing, ideally with insert earphones securely placed in each ear. It is best not to move the infant once testing begins, but may be necessary to place a bone vibrator or reposition transducers. Advantages of insert earphones for pediatric ABR testing include reduced stimulus artifact caused by the greater distance between the transducer and the electrodes (assuming electrodes and transducers are carefully placed at a distance from each other), greater comfort, avoidance of ear canal collapse, and increased interaural attenuation. Consequently, there is less need for contralateral masking, more reliable transducer placement, reduced interference from ambient noise if testing is not done in a sound booth, and improved infection control through use of disposable tips (Hall, 2007).

> **Special Consideration**
>
> • Supraaural earphones should be used only when inserts are not possible (e.g., ear canal atresia).

Examples of tone burst ABR recordings from an infant with normal hearing are shown in **Fig. 15–5**. Because the waveforms were very robust, it was possible to establish normal ABR thresholds at 500 and 2000 Hz very quickly in this infant. Repeat recordings are overlaid at the threshold levels. There is little noise in the recordings and the waveforms are very robust, so a baseline recording was not performed. A baseline recording with an inaudible stimulus level (such as -20 dB nHL) is recommended if there is any doubt about response reproducibility or it is difficult to determine threshold level.

B. Estimating Hearing Thresholds from Tone Burst Auditory Brainstem Response

Tone burst ABR and pure tone thresholds show close agreement but are not exactly the same, which is not surprising given that the ABR is a "farfield" evoked potential, recorded on the surface of the scalp far away from the neural generators. Stapells and colleagues determined how many infants with normal hearing had tone burst ABR at near-threshold levels and found that, at 20 dB nHL or lower, 52% and 96% of infants had a tone burst ABR at 500 Hz and 2000 Hz, respectively (Stapells, Gravel, and Martin, 1995). Ninety-two percent of infants with normal hearing had a 500-Hz toneburst ABR at 30 dB nHL or lower. Thus, recommended pass levels for tone burst ABR are 30–40 dB and 20–30 dB nHL at 500 and 2000 Hz, respectively (ASHA, 2004).

Various authors have demonstrated excellent correlations between tone burst ABR and pure tone thresholds (Stapells et al, 1995; 1990). The relationship between ABR and pure tone thresholds is not exactly one-for-one, however, as there is closer agreement when hearing thresholds are more severe than for milder hearing loss (Stapells et al, 1995). The relationship between ABR and pure tone thresholds also varies across stimuli (Stapells, 2002). Thus, it is difficult to have a simple, single correction factor when estimating the

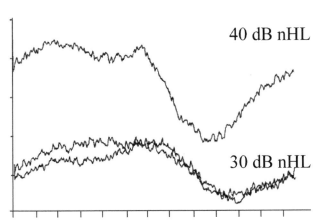

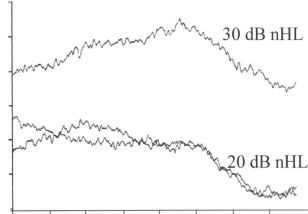

Figure 15–5 Air conduction ABR recorded to 500 Hz (left) and 2000 Hz (right) tonebursts from a four-month-old infant with normal hearing. The time window differs between stimuli (25 milliseconds at 500 Hz versus 15 milliseconds at 2000 Hz). For tonebursts at 30 dB nHL, wave V occurs at ~12 milliseconds at 500 Hz and 9 milliseconds at 2000 Hz. This latency difference is expected based on cochlear travel times (Don, Eggermont, and Brackmann, 1979)

audiogram from the tone burst ABR. One solution to this problem is to use a "look-up" table to estimate the audiogram, such as that shown in **Table 15–3**, based on the regression equations reported by Stapells and colleagues (1995).

Neurological Applications of Auditory Brainstem Response

The ABR is a sensitive indicator of brainstem status and has been used successfully to predict developmental outcomes in neonates who are at high risk for neurodevelopmental sequelae (Majnemer, Rosenblatt, and Riley, 1988). Abnormal findings associated with brainstem pathology or neuromaturational delay include absent or delayed waves, prolonged

Table 15–3 Estimated Pure Tone Thresholds (plus/minus 10 dB) for Three Tone Burst ABR Frequencies

ABR Threshold	Estimated Pure Tone Thresholds (dB HL)		
(dB nHL)	500 Hz	2000 Hz	4000 Hz
30	23	29	31
35	27	34	36
40	32	38	40
45	36	43	45
50	40	47	49
55	45	52	54
60	49	56	58
65	53	61	63
70	58	66	67
75	62	70	72
80	66	75	76
85	71	79	81
90	75	84	85
95	79	88	90
100	84	93	94

Abbreviations: HL, hearing level; nHL, normal hearing level.
Source: Stapells, D. R., Gravel, J. S., and Martin, B. A. (1995).

interwave intervals, and reduced wave V/I amplitude ratio (wave V small relative to wave I). Prolonged wave I-V intervals have been associated with brainstem pathology relating to perinatal asphyxia (Jiang and Tierney, 1996), prematurity and prenatal complications (Murray, 1988; Weber, 1982), and autistic spectrum disorder (Wong and Wong, 1991).

Using Auditory Brainstem Response to Diagnose Auditory Neuropathy/Auditory Dys-synchrony

A subset of children with sensorineural hearing loss have AN/AD, which is associated with unusual ABR findings. AN/AD is characterized by abnormal hearing thresholds, absent acoustic reflexes, otoacoustic emissions (OAEs), enlarged CM, and absent or abnormal ABR (Berlin et al, 2003; Starr et al, 1996). Speech recognition scores may be consistent with the audiogram, or may be much poorer than the audiogram would predict (Rance et al., 1999). OAEs may or may not be present (Rance et al, 2002). If OAEs are absent, the ABR findings will be key to the diagnosis of AN/AD. In children with AN/AD the ABR will be absent or abnormal and should contain evidence of cochlear activity (CM or abnormal positive potentials). **Fig. 15–6** shows an abnormal ABR recorded from the left ear of a 4-year-old with bilateral AN/AD. This child developed encephalopathy and required resuscitation at age 4 and was subsequently referred to audiology because his language had regressed. The ipsilateral ABR waveforms show a large CM and a late repeatable positive peak at about 8 milliseconds, which might be an abnormally delayed wave V.

Electrocochleography

ECoG is also used by some clinics for diagnosis of AN/AD. ECoG is a technique used for "near-field" recording of cochlear and eighth nerve potentials. This technique enhances the amplitude of the cochlear potentials (CM and summating potential) and the whole nerve action potential

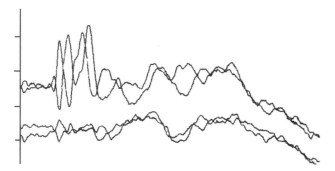

Figure 15–6 Ipsilateral (top) and contralateral (bottom) ABR waveforms recorded in the left ear of a 4-year-old child with bilateral AN/AD. Stimuli were 80 dB nHL clicks presented at 17.1/s to an insert earphone. Responses to rarefaction and condensation clicks are overlaid. There is a large CM at ~1–3 milliseconds in the early part of the ABR

(wave I of the ABR) because the recording electrodes are placed close to the generators of these responses. ECoG is performed either with a transtympanic electrode placed through the eardrum onto the promontory or in the round window niche or with extratympanic electrode placed in the ear canal. ECoG recorded with tonal stimuli allow accurate estimation of pure tone thresholds (Fjermedal, Laukli, and Mair, 1988; Wong, Gibson, and Sanli, 1997). General anesthesia is required for transtympanic ECoG in children and hence ABR is usually the preferred technique for diagnosis of AN/AD and threshold estimation.

Bone Conduction Auditory Brainstem Response

When a hearing loss is detected using air conduction ABR, the next step is to determine whether there is a conductive component, as this may determine treatment. Tympanometry and acoustic reflexes are helpful, but not entirely reliable. Reflexes will be absent when the hearing loss is more severe (Jerger et al, 1974). Tympanometry is not always reliable, especially in young infants, even when high-frequency probe tone tympanometry is used (Marchant et al, 1986). If tympanometry indicates the presence of middle ear disease, and ABR thresholds show a moderate or greater hearing loss, the size of the air-bone gap cannot be determined unless bone conduction (BC)-ABR testing is performed.

Ears with conductive hearing loss show consistently delayed latencies across stimulus levels. However, this "typical" pattern may not occur when there is an unusually shaped hearing loss. For example, Gorga and colleagues reported a case of steep high-frequency sensorineural hearing loss that resulted in a latency-intensity function that looked like the classical pattern for conductive hearing loss (Gorga, Reiland, and Beauchaine, 1985). Current guidelines (ASHA, 2004) recommend BC-ABR testing to more reliably determine whether there is a conductive component to the hearing loss.

Transducer placement and stimulus artifact cancellation are critical for successful BC-ABR recording (Foxe and Stapells, 1993). Another important consideration is the contribution of the opposite cochlea and whether masking is required. Stuart and colleagues (1990) and Yang et al (1987) investigated various bone vibrator placement options and

determined that the best placement for BC-ABR is "superoposterior," high on the mastoid, above and behind the pinna. This position optimizes ABR amplitude and minimizes stimulus artifact, if the reference electrode is placed low on the mastoid. It is not possible to attach the bone vibrator comfortably using the usual head band; hence, various attachment options have been explored, including handheld placement or a velcro/elastic headband. Handheld placement using a single finger in the center of the bone vibrator can provide the same signal quality as bone vibrator attachment with a conventional headband (Bachmann and Hall, 1998). Provided that sufficient care is taken to ensure consistent and appropriate placement, hand holding is an acceptable option if the decision to do BC-ABR is made after ABR testing is underway and it is awkward to attach the vibrator using a Velcro/elastic headband because of the position of the electrodes and sleeping infant.

Yang and colleagues noted that in young infants the bones of the skull are not fused, and there is greater interaural attenuation than in older children and adults (Yang et al, 1987). Thus, it is not always necessary to use masking, which can create masking dilemmas in children with bilateral atresia. The recommended approach when performing BC-ABR is to use two recording channels, with reference electrodes on the ipsilateral and contralateral ears. If, as is illustrated in **Fig. 15–7,** the response is larger and earlier in the ipsilateral recording channel, it must have been generated in the ipsilateral cochlea (Foxe and Stapells, 1993; Stapells and Ruben, 1989). **Fig. 15–7** shows an example of a BC-ABR recorded from a 3-month-old infant with unilateral atresia. The infant was in natural sleep and was tested with a handheld bone vibrator on the atretic side. Air conduction ABR thresholds in the atretic ear were 60 and 70 dB nHL at 500 and 2000 Hz, respectively. Wave V was earlier and larger in the ipsilateral recordings, indicating that the response was coming from the cochlea on the atretic side.

◆ Auditory Steady State Response

The focus of this chapter is on ABR, but ASSR is increasingly used for threshold estimation in infants (Han et al, 2006; Stapells et al, 2005). ASSR systems deliver either a single frequency, modulated pure tone signal, or multiple frequencies, to one or both ears simultaneously. When multiple frequencies and two ears are tested, different modulation rates are used so that the ASSR to each frequency in each ear can be separately detected. The recorded response consists of neural activity that corresponds to the modulation rate. A carrier tone at a particular test frequency activates the appropriate place in the cochlea, leading to modulated neural activity in the auditory pathways corresponding to that place of activation. The response to the modulated signal is detected as a "spike" or peak in the recorded neural activity at the same frequency as the modulation rate. **Fig. 15–8** provides an example of ASSR stimuli and responses. In this example, four tonal frequencies were tested simultaneously (500, 1000, 2000, and 4000 Hz), with each of these "carrier"

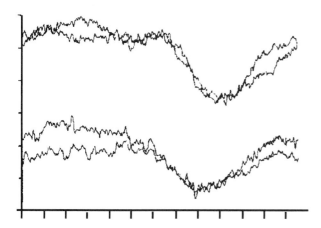

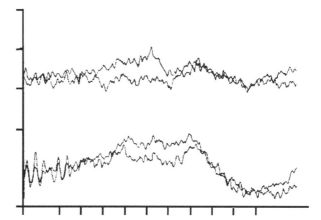

Figure 15–7 Two-channel BC-ABR recordings to 500 Hz (left) recorded at 10 dBnHL and 2000 Hz (right) recorded at 20 dBnHL from the atretic ear of a 3-month-old infant with unilateral atresia. Wave V is earlier and larger in the ipsilateral (below) compared with the contralateral (above) recordings, confirming that the response was generated by the ipsilateral cochlea on the atretic side.

tones amplitude modulated (100%) at a different rate (77, 85, 93, and 101 Hz, respectively).

Both amplitude (AM) and frequency (FM) modulation have been used for ASSR. Although FM increases the bandwidth of the signal, and therefore reduces frequency specificity of the response, it has been explored as an option for improving ASSR quality. For example, a combination of 100% AM and 20% FM improves ASSR amplitude and detectability in infants compared with AM alone (John et al, 2004). For both AM and FM, the modulation is sinusoidal, typically at a rate of 70 to 110 Hz. Steady-state responses can also be recorded at lower modulation rates, but background noise is more problematic at lower frequencies (Picton et al, 2003). At higher rates the ASSR is primarily generated in the auditory brainstem (Picton et al, 2003) and is not affected by sleep, so the high rate ASSR is suitable for estimating hearing sensitivity in infants.

As for tone burst ABR, there is good agreement between ASSR and pure tone thresholds (Lins et al, 1996; Rance, 2006), although ASSR thresholds show greater variability across normal hearing infants than tone burst ABR thresholds. Overall, the literature suggests that pure tone thresholds are more accurately predicted by tone burst ABR (Johnson and Brown, 2005; Rance, Tomlin, and Rickards, 2006). Another difficulty with ASSR relates to BC testing. Small and colleagues have shown that objective BC testing can be undertaken using ASSR in infants but artifactual BC-ASSR responses are possible at levels higher than 40 dB HL. Artifactual responses are also

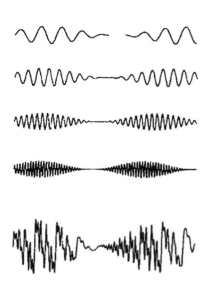

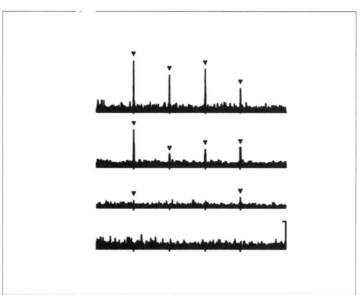

Figure 15–8 Left-hand panel shows four frequencies (500, 1000, 2000, 4000 Hz) amplitude modulated (100%) at rates of 77, 85, 93, and 101 Hz, respectively. The recorded response, shown in the right-hand panel, has peaks of energy at the frequencies corresponding to the four modulation rates. These peaks reduce in amplitude as stimulus level is reduced, and cannot be distinguished from the background noise at the softest stimulus levels tested, shown at the bottom of **Fig. 15–8.**

possible at high levels for air conduction ASSR testing (Small, Hatton, and Stapells, 2007; Small and Stapells, 2006).

Despite these limitations, ASSR does offer the advantages of objective threshold identification and efficient testing of multiple frequencies and ears simultaneously. ASSR systems use a variety of statistical approaches to automatically determine the lowest level at which a response is detectable. Unlike ABR, ASSR analysis occurs in the frequency domain rather than the time domain, and objective response detection algorithms use amplitude and phase characteristics of the recorded electrical activity. Different systems examine either phase coherence (degree of nonrandom phase behavior in the phase component of the ASSR), or amplitude and phase components (Picton et al, 2003). ASSR accuracy can be improved by extending test duration (Luts and Wouters, 2004), but this may not always be practical clinically.

♦ Middle Latency Response

The MLR occurs within about 100 milliseconds after stimulus onset and primarily represents responses from the thalamocortical pathways and primary auditory cortex (Kraus and McGee, 1993). The MLR can be used to assess hearing sensitivity, but is more affected by subject state and is more variable across and within subjects than ABR (Kraus and McGee, 1993), and therefore is not normally used for threshold estimation in children or adults. The MLR can be reliably recorded in infants at suprathreshold levels if recording and stimulus parameters are optimized (Tucker and Ruth, 1996). A recent study of children 7 to 16 years of age found no significant MLR latency and amplitude changes in school-aged children (Schochat and Musiek, 2006), but the authors concluded that this was probably due to the high degree of MLR intersubject variability.

Pearl

- The main usefulness of the MLR as a clinical tool for children relates to its sensitivity to central auditory pathology in children with auditory processing deficits (Arehole, Augustine, and Simhadri, 1995; Purdy, Kelly, and Davies, 2002). The MLR may also be useful for estimating thresholds when the ABR is absent because of central auditory pathology.

♦ Cortical Auditory Evoked Potentials

The "obligatory" cortical auditory evoked potentials (P1-N1-P2) occur within about 300 milliseconds after stimulus onset in adults, and within about 500 milliseconds after stimulus onset in children (Sharma and Dorman, 2006). CAEPs are referred to as obligatory because they are primarily de-

termined by the physical properties of the stimulus. Early attempts to objectively estimate hearing thresholds focused on cortical potentials and showed good agreement between CAEP and pure tone thresholds (Davis, 1965). CAEPs are not ideal for objective threshold estimation, however, because response detectability and amplitudes reduce during sleep (Cody et al, 1964; Purdy et al, 2005). Hence, infants need to be awake for testing.

The developmental time course of CAEPs has been extensively investigated (Kurtzberg et al, 1984; Sharma and Dorman, 2006). At birth and up to about seven years of age, the P2 peak is typically not evident in CAEPs recorded with a vertex-mastoid electrode configuration and the response is dominated by a large, late P1 response (Ponton et al, 1996). An example of a speech evoked CAEP recorded in an awake infant with normal hearing is provided in **Fig. 15–9**.

When appropriate test protocols are used, CAEPs are reliably present in young infants (Kurtzberg et al, 1984; Purdy et al, 2005). CAEP latencies and morphology are related to the amount of auditory deprivation in children with cochlear implants (Ponton et al, 1996; Sharma and Dorman, 2006). Because CAEPs can be evoked by longer duration stimuli, including speech sounds, they are useful for evaluating aided hearing in infants, to verify that cortical responses can be recorded to speech sounds at conversational speech levels. This is not a new idea, as some years ago researchers advocated the use of CAEPs to objectively evaluate unaided versus aided hearing in children (Gravel, 1989; Rapin and Graziani, 1967). With the advent of universal newborn hearing screening, however, there is now much greater need for reliable, objective, measures of hearing aid and cochlear implant success that can be used in infants. The ability to record aided CAEPs to a range of speech sounds is correlated with parental perceptions of aided hearing ability in infants with hearing loss (Golding et al, 2007).

Another potential application of CAEPs in children is in the area of AN/AD. Children with AN/AD who have poor speech perception outcomes have poor CAEPs for speech and tonal

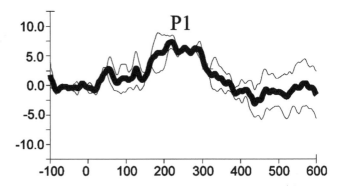

Figure 15–9 CAEPs recorded to the speech sound /m/ in a 7-month-old infant with normal hearing. The stimulus (80 milliseconds duration, 1125 milliseconds interstimulus interval) was presented via a loudspeaker at 50 dB SPL to the infant who was listening binaurally seated on his mother's lap and distracted by toys during testing. In young infants the CAEP waveform typically consists of a "P1" peak at ~200 milliseconds, with an amplitude of ~5–10 microvolts, as illustrated here.

stimuli compared with those with relatively good speech perception (Rance et al, 2002). The relationship between CAEPs recorded early in infancy and later speech perception outcomes in children with AN/AD is not yet known, however.

♦ Transducers and Stimulus Calibration

Insert earphones offer many advantages over supraaural earphones for evoked potential testing in children. Comfort and reliable placement are key considerations when testing sleeping infants for prolonged periods. Output impedance values for evoked potential systems can be higher (e.g., 300 ohms) than values for pure tone audiometric equipment, so it is important to check that transducers are appropriately selected and calibrated. Insert earphones used repeatedly with sleeping infants in awkward positions may be dropped more often than those used to test conscious adults, and frequent listening checks and regular calibration are important. The B-71 bone vibrator (Radioear Corp, New Eagle, PA, USA) is most commonly used and complies with audiometric standards and has a range of impedance options to suit different evoked potential systems. For soundfield delivery of stimuli (for example, for CAEP testing of aided hearing in infants) most clinical systems will require an external amplifier and loudspeaker. If this is not purchased with the ABR system, care needs to be taken to ensure impedances are matched and there is no distortion of the signal.

Sound levels for evoked potential stimuli are specified in dB HL for longer duration stimuli such as those used for ASSR and CAEP testing. For these stimuli the usual audiometric standards are relevant, although these do not specify reference levels for short speech sounds such as those used for aided CAEP testing in infants. For brief stimuli such as clicks and tone bursts, stimulus levels are specified in dB nHL ("normal hearing level"); this refers to the level of the stimulus relative to the normative threshold for otologically normal young adults. Calibration methods for clicks and tone bursts are described in the international standard IEC 60645–3 (Audiometers–Part 3: Auditory test signals of short duration for audiometric and neuro-otological purposes). This standard describes dB nHL levels and peak to peak equivalent sound pressure levels (dB ppeSPL) measurement techniques, but does not specify reference threshold levels.

Several publications contain reference values for tone burst ABR (Sharma, Purdy and Bonnici, 2003; Stapells, 2002, 2004). Reference threshold levels (0 dB nHL) for clicks and tone bursts vary with stimulus frequency and repetition rate but are typically 20 to 35 dB ppeSPL for air conduction stimuli. Interim reference threshold values have been published by the National Measurement Laboratory (NPL, 2005) and a draft international standard specifies reference levels for ABR stimuli (ISO 389–6 "Acoustics–Reference zero for the calibration of audiometric equipment–Part 6: Reference hearing threshold levels for test signals of short duration"). Helpful ABR calibration guidelines have been developed in the United Kingdom for Newborn Hearing Screening Program (NBSP, 2007).

- **Tips and Tricks for Successful Evoked Potential Recordings in Children**

1. Add waveforms to improve waveform quality. One or more repeat runs should be done at the level believed to be the ABR threshold to check for reliability of the response. Adding the two waveforms will normally improve the signal-to-noise ratio by enhancing wave V and reducing background noise, improving accuracy of peak identification.

2. Use disposable electrodes or keep reusable electrodes in very good condition. The use of disposable electrodes ensures a consistent high-quality electrode surface. Occasionally these may need to be secured to the head with tape, particularly if the infant is hot and sweating. If reusable electrodes are used it is possible to wear off the plating and expose the base metal, which will increase noise levels in evoked potential recordings. The same issues arise if reusable electrodes are tarnished or dirty.

3. Braid electrode cables. The electrode cables act as an antenna and can pick up electromagnetic artifact that will degrade the quality of the evoked potential waveforms. Braiding the cables together will reduce the amount of electromagnetic artifact pickup. The most common source of this electromagnetic artifact is from the transducer (bone vibrator, insert earphone, supraaural earphone), so cables should be placed as far as possible from the transducer. Potential sources of electrical artifact in the test environment should be kept away from the electrode cables (this includes mobile phones and other personal electronic devices).

4. Place electrodes low on the mastoid so that the bone vibrator can fit if needed. In adults the back of the earlobe and the mastoid are used interchangeably for ABR electrode placement. The mastoid is an easier location for electrode attachment in small infants but is also the place where the bone vibrator will be attached if BC-ABR is required. The negative electrode (also referred to as the noninverting or reference electrode) should be placed low on the mastoid so that, if BC-ABR is needed, the electrode is as far as possible from the electrode to minimize the chance of picking up electromagnetic artifact from the bone vibrator.

5. Use a vertex electrode. ABR amplitudes are enhanced by having the positive electrode (also referred to as the noninverting or active electrode) on the vertex rather than the forehead (Beattie et al, 1986; Stuart, Yang, and Botea, 1996).The vertex site is generally behind the fontanelle on most infants, so the fontanelle does not pose any problems for electrode attachment. Use of an abrasive paste such as NuPrep™ (wearer and Company, Aurora, co) on a Q-Tip® (cotton bud) should ensure skin impedances are sufficiently low (ideally lower than 5000 ohms). If an infant has thick hair, additional conductive paste may be needed to hold the electrode against the scalp and secure the electrode with tape.

6. Use four electrodes routinely. Four electrodes should be attached routinely (positive on the vertex; negative electrodes on the two mastoids; common on the forehead). If air conduction ABR testing indicates hearing loss and BC-ABR is required, it will then be easy to perform a two-channel (ipsilateral and contralateral) BC-ABR recording. Wave V amplitude and latency differences between channels, with ipsilateral earlier and larger than contralateral, provide confirmation that the BC-ABR is not a cross-heard response from the opposite cochlea (which would signal the need for masking).

7. Use masking when testing at high stimulus levels for air conduction ABR. At high stimulus levels the recorded ABR may be a cross-heard response from the opposite cochlea (Hall, 2007). Interaural attenuation values for insert earphones are 55 dB or better (Etymotic Research, 2007). A delayed waveform recorded at high levels may be difficult to interpret and a hearing loss asymmetry may not be evident if the clinician tested the poorer ear first, by chance, and then the infant woke up. To avoid this problem, contralateral broadband (white noise) masking should *always* be used when testing at stimulus levels of 70 dB nHL and higher.

8. Use an external amplifier to get stimuli louder for more severe hearing losses. Commercial evoked potential systems typically have maximum stimulus levels for air conduction testing of 80 to 100 dB nHL, depending on the stimulus type and toneburst frequency and transducer type. Louder levels are needed for more accurate threshold estimation in children with severe or profound hearing loss. Tone burst levels up to about 110 dB nHL can be readily achieved without distortion if an additional external amplifier is used. If an external amplifier is used, care should be taken to ensure stimulus and masking levels are appropriately calibrated.

the tone bursts. If there is a large discrepancy between low and high frequency tone burst ABR thresholds, and there is a severe-profound hearing loss at one frequency, it may be necessary to use ipsilateral masking to ensure that the response is coming from the frequency region of interest. At higher stimulus levels the response may be mediated by frequency regions more than an octave away from the nominal stimulus frequency.

3. It is possible to incorrectly interpret a repeatable artifact as a "true" response, leading to a false-negative result (missing a hearing loss). The "cross-check" principle is one of the cornerstones of pediatric audiology, and this applies to evoked potential testing as well as to behavioral audiometry. Other audiologic measures (OAEs, tympanograms, acoustic reflexes, case history, CT and MRI results) should be considered when viewing evoked potential results. When high stimulus levels are used artifactual responses may arise for both AC and BC ASSR. When high levels are used for tone burst ABR and care is not taken with transducer placement, a "ringing" stimulus artifact may contaminate a large portion of the waveform. It is also possible for large amplitude electrical noise in the environment to contaminate responses, and this may appear to be a repeatable evoked potential waveform. Strategies for avoiding such errors include good electrode maintenance and low skin impedances, watching out for electrodes that lift off during recordings, careful placement of transducers away from electrode cables, replication of responses at near threshold levels, "baseline" recordings with the stimulus level set below threshold, paying attention to sources of electrical contamination in the environment such as fluorescent lights, ensuring the latencies and amplitudes are and routinely checking threshold decisions with an independent observer.

Pitfalls

1. Unusual configuration hearing losses if only 500- and 2000-Hz ABR thresholds are available, the estimated audiogram may be inaccurate if there is an unusual hearing loss configuration, such as better or worse thresholds at 4000 or 1000 Hz. If possible, additional tone burst ABR frequencies should be tested (first 4000 Hz, then 1000 Hz) to "fill in" the audiogram.

2. Ipsilateral masking (e.g., notched noise) may be needed at high stimulus levels when thresholds differ substantially across frequencies. When the tone burst ABR technique was first investigated there was concern that the ABR would not be frequency specific due to "spectral splatter" resulting from the relatively short duration of

Discussion Questions

1. What is the relationship between tone burst ABR and behavioral thresholds?

2. At what age can objective hearing assessment be performed using ABR or ASSR?

3. What are the key features of the ABR that contribute to a diagnosis of AN/AD?

4. What is the role of MLR in pediatric audiology?

5. What are the merits of ABR versus ASSR for objective hearing assessment in infants?

References

Arehole, S., Augustine, L. E., and Simhadri, R. (1995). Middle latency response in children with learning disabilities: preliminary findings. Journal of Communication Disorders, 28, 21–38.

ASHA Ad Hoc Committee on Advances in Clinical Practice. (1992). Sedation and topical anesthetics in audiology and speech-language pathology. American Speech language-Hearing Association Supplement, 41–42.

ASHA. (2004). Guidelines for the Audiologic Assessment of Children from Birth to 5 Years of Age. American Speech-Language-Hearing Association.

Bachmann, K. R., and Hall, J. W. (1998). Pediatric auditory brainstem response assessment: the crosscheck principle twenty years later. Seminars in Hearing, 19, 41–60.

Beattie, R. C., Beguwala, F. E., Mills, D. M., and Boyd, R. L. (1986). Latency and amplitude effects of electrode placement on the early auditory evoked response. Journal of Speech & Hearing Disorders, 51, 63–70.

Bell, S. L., Allen, R., and Lutman, M. E. (2002). An investigation of the use of band-limited chirp stimuli to obtain the auditory brainstem response. International Journal of Audiology, 41, 271–278.

Berlin, C. I., Bordelon, J., St John, P., et al. (1998). Reversing click polarity may uncover auditory neuropathy in infants. Ear and Hearing, 19, 37–47.

Berlin, C. I., Hood, L., Morlet, T., Rose, K., and Brashears, S. (2003). Auditory neuropathy/dys-synchrony: diagnosis and management. Mental Retardation & Developmental Disabilities Research Reviews, 9, 225–231.

Brugge, J. F., Anderson, D. J., Hind, J. E., and Rose, J. E. (1969). Time structure of discharges in single auditory nerve fibers of the squirrel monkey in response to complex periodic sounds. Journal of Neurophysiology, 32, 386–401.

Coats, A. C., and Martin, J. L. (1977). Human auditory nerve action potentials and brain stem evoked responses: effects of audiogram shape and lesion location. Archives of Otolaryngology, 103, 605–622.

Cody, D. T., Jacobson, J. L., Walker, J. C., and Bickford, R. G. (1964). Averaged evoked myogenic and cortical potentials to sound in man. Transactions – American Otological Society, 52, 159–176.

Dallos, P. (1973). The auditory periphery: biophysics and physiology. New York: Academic Press.

Davis, H. (1965). Slow cortical responses evoked by acoustic stimuli. Acta Oto-Laryngologica, 206, 128–134.

Don, M., Eggermont, J. J., and Brackmann, D. E. (1979). Reconstruction of the audiogram using brain stem responses and high-pass noise masking. Annals of Otology, Rhinology, & Laryngology, 57, 1–20.

Eggermont, J. J., and Salamy, A. (1988). Development of ABR parameters in a preterm and a term born population. Ear and Hearing, 9, 283–289.

Elliott, C., Lightfoot, G., Parker, D., et al. (2000). Auditory brainstem response testing in babies using tone pip stimulation: a recommended test protocol.

Etymotic Research, I. (2007). ER-3A ABR Insert earphone. www.etymotic.com/pdf/er3a-abr-datasheet.pdf.

Fjermedal, O., Laukli, E., and Mair, I. W. (1988). Auditory brainstem responses and extratympanic electrocochleography: a threshold comparison in children. Scandinavian Audiology, 17, 231–235.

Foxe, J. J., and Stapells, D. R. (1993). Normal infant and adult auditory brainstem responses to bone-conducted tones. Audiology, 32, 95–109.

Golding, M., Pearce, W., Seymour, J., Cooper, A., Ching, T., and Dillon, H. (2007). The relationship between obligatory cortical auditory evoked potentials (CAEPs) and functional measures in young infants. Journal of the American Academy of Audiology, 18, 117–125.

Gorga, M. P., Reiland, J. K., and Beauchaine, K. A. (1985). Auditory brainstem responses in a case of high-frequency conductive hearing loss. Journal of Speech & Hearing Disorders, 50, 346–350.

Hall, J. W. (2007). Introduction to auditory evoked response measurement. In New handbook of auditory evoked responses (pp. 58–108). Boston: Allyn and Bacon.

Hall, J. W., and Harris, D. (1994). Auditory evoked respones in acute brain injury and rehabilitation. In J. T. Jacobson (Ed.), Principles and application in auditory evoked potentials (pp. 477–515). Boston: Allyn and Bacon.

Han, D., Mo, L., Liu, H., Chen, J., and Huang, L. (2006). Threshold estimation in children using auditory steady-state responses to multiple simultaneous stimuli. Journal of Oto-Rhino-Laryngology & Its Related Specialties, 68, 64–68.

Hyde, M. L. (1985). The effect of cochlear lesions on the ABR. In Jacobson, J. T. (Ed.), The auditory brainstem response (pp. 133–146). San Diego: College Hill Press.

Jacobson, J. J., and Hall, J. W. (1994). Newborn and infant brainstem response applications. In J. Jacobson (Ed.), Principles and applications in auditory evoked potentials. Boston: Allyn and Bacon.

Jerger, J., Harford, E., Clemis, J., and Alford, B. (1974). The acoustic reflex in eighth nerve disorders. Archives of Otolaryngology, 99, 409–413.

Jewett, D. L., and Williston, J. S. (1971). Auditory-evoked far fields averaged from the scalp of humans. Brain, 94, 681–696.

Jiang, Z. D., and Tierney, T. S. (1996). Binaural interaction in human neonatal auditory brainstem. Pediatric Research, 39, 708–714.

John, M. S., Brown, D. K., Muir, P. J., and Picton, T. W. (2004). Recording auditory steady-state responses in young infants. Ear and Hearing, 25, 539–553.

Johnson, T. A., and Brown, C. J. (2005). Threshold prediction using the auditory steady-state response and the tone burst auditory brain stem response: a within-subject comparison. Ear and Hearing, 26, 559–576.

Kiang, N. Y., and Moxon, E. C. (1974). Tails of tuning curves of auditory-nerve fibers. Journal of the Acoustical Society of America, 55, 620–630.

Kraus, N., and McGee, T. (1993). Clinical implications of primary and non-primary pathway contributions to the middle latency response generating system. Ear & Hearing, 14(1), 36–48.

Kurtzberg, D., Hilpert, P. L., Kreuzer, J. A., and Vaughan, H. G., Jr. (1984). Differential maturation of cortical auditory evoked potentials to speech sounds in normal fullterm and very low-birthweight infants. Developmental Medicine & Child Neurology, 26, 466–475.

Lins, O. G., Picton, T. W., Boucher, B. L. et al. (1996). Frequency-specific audiometry using steady-state responses. Ear and Hearing, 17, 81–96.

Luts, H., and Wouters, J. (2004). Hearing assessment by recording multiple auditory steady-state responses: the influence of test duration. International Journal of Audiology, 43, 471–478.

Majnemer, A., Rosenblatt, B., and Riley, P. (1988). Prognostic significance of the auditory brainstem evoked response in high-risk neonates. Developmental Medicine & Child Neurology, 30, 43–52.

Marchant, C. D., McMillan, P. M., Shurin, P. A. et al. (1986). Objective diagnosis of otitis media in early infancy by tympanometry and ipsilateral acoustic reflex thresholds. Journal of Pediatrics, 109, 590–595.

Moller, A. R. (2007). Neural generators for auditory brainstem evoked potentials. In R. F. Burkard, M. Don, and J. J. Eggermont (Eds.), Auditory evoked potentials: basic principles and clinical application (1st ed.). Baltimore: Lippincott Williams & Wilkins.

Moore, J. K., Ponton, C. W., Eggermont, J. J., Wu, B. J., and Huang, J. Q. (1996). Perinatal maturation of the auditory brain stem response: changes in path length and conduction velocity. Ear and Hearing, 17, 411–418.

Murray, A. D. (1988). Newborn auditory brainstem evoked responses (ABRs): prenatal and contemporary correlates. Child Development, 59, 571–588.

NPL. (2005). Newborn hearing screening programme (NHSP) ABR Reference levels for stimulus calibration. www.npl.co.uk/acoustics/research/theme1/reportret.pdf.

Picton, T. W., John, M. S., Dimitrijevic, A., and Purcell, D. (2003). Human auditory steady-state responses. International Journal of Audiology, 42, 177–219.

Ponton, C. W., Don, M., Eggermont, J. J., Waring, M. D., and Masuda, A. (1996). Maturation of human cortical auditory function: differences between normal-hearing children and children with cochlear implants. Ear & Hearing, 17, 430–437.

Purdy, S. C., Katsch, R., Dillon, H., Storey, L., Sharma, M., and Agung, K. (2005). Aided Cortical Auditory Evoked Potentials for Hearing Instrument Evaluation in Infants. Paper presented at the A Sound Foundation through Early Amplification, Basel, Switzerland.

Purdy, S. C., Kelly, A. S., and Davies, M. G. (2002). Auditory brainstem response, middle latency response, and late cortical evoked potentials in children with learning disabilities. Journal of the American Academy of Audiology, 13, 367–382.

Rance, G., Beer, D. E., Cone-Wesson, B. et al. (1999). Clinical findings for a group of infants and young children with auditory neuropathy. Ear and Hearing, 20, 238–252.

Rance, G., Cone-Wesson, B., Wunderlich, J., and Dowell, R. (2002). Speech perception and cortical event related potentials in children with auditory neuropathy. Ear and Hearing, 23, 239–253.

Rance, G., Tomlin, D., and Rickards, F. W. (2006). Comparison of auditory steady-state responses and tone-burst auditory brainstem responses in normal babies. Ear and Hearing, 27, 751–762.

Rapin, I., and Graziani, L. J. (1967). Auditory-evoked responses in normal, brain-damaged, and deaf infants. Neurology, 17, 881–894.

Schochat, E., and Musiek, F. E. (2006). Maturation of outcomes of behavioral and electrophysiologic tests of central auditory function. Journal of Communication Disorders, 39, 78–92.

Sharma, A., and Dorman, M. F. (2006). Central auditory development in children with cochlear implants: clinical implications. Advances in Oto-Rhino-Laryngology, 64, 66–88.

Sharma, M., Purdy, S. C., and Bonnici, L. (2003). Behavioural and electroacoustic calibration of air-conducted click and toneburst auditory brainstem response stimuli. Australian & New Zealand Journal of Audiology, 25, 54–60.

Sininger, Y. S. (2002). Identification of auditory neuropathy in infants and children. Seminars in Hearing, 23, 193–200.

Sininger, Y. S. (2003). Audiologic assessment in infants. Current Opinion in Otolaryngology & Head & Neck Surgery, 11, 378–382.

Small, S. A., Hatton, J. L., and Stapells, D. R. (2007). Effects of bone oscillator coupling method, placement location, and occlusion on bone-conduction auditory steady-state responses in infants. Ear and Hearing, 28, 83–98.

Small, S. A., and Stapells, D. R. (2006). Multiple auditory steady-state response thresholds to bone-conduction stimuli in young infants with normal hearing. Ear and Hearing, 27, 219–228.

Stapells, D. R. (2002). Threshold estimation by the tone-evoked auditory brainstem response: a literature meta-analysis. Journal of Speech-Language Pathology and Audiology, 24, 74–83.

Stapells, D. R. (2002). The tone-evoked ABR: why it's the measure of choice for young infants. Hearing Journal, 55, 14–18.

Stapells, D. R. (2004). Recommended recording parameters and stimulus parameters for clinical tone-evoked ABR in infants. From http://www.audiospeech.ubc.ca/haplab/TONE-ABR_PARAMETERS.html.

Stapells, D. R., Gravel, J. S., and Martin, B. A. (1995). Thresholds for auditory brain stem responses to tones in notched noise from infants and young children with normal hearing or sensorineural hearing loss. Ear & Hearing, 16, 361–371.

Stapells, D. R., Herdman, A., Small, S. A., Dimitrijevic, A., and Hatton, J. (2005). Current status of the auditory steady-state responses for estimating an infant's audiogram. In R. C. Seewald and J. M. Bamford (Eds.), A sound foundation through early amplification (pp. 43–59). Basel: Phonak, AG.

Stapells, D. R., and Oates, P. (1997). Estimation of the pure-tone audiogram by the auditory brainstem response: a review. Audiology & Neuro-Otology, 2, 257–280.

Stapells, D. R., Picton, T. W., Durieux-Smith, A., Edwards, C. G., and Moran, L. M. (1990). Thresholds for short-latency auditory-evoked potentials to tones in notched noise in normal-hearing and hearing-impaired subjects. Audiology, 29, 262–274.

Stapells, D. R., and Ruben, R. J. (1989). Auditory brain stem responses to bone-conducted tones in infants. Annals of Otology, Rhinology & Laryngology, 98, 941–949.

Starr, A., Picton, T. W., Sininger, Y., Hood, L. J., and Berlin, C. I. (1996). Auditory neuropathy. Brain, 119, 741–753.

Starr, A., Sininger, Y., Nguyen, T., Michalewski, H. J., Oba, S., and Abdala, C. (2001). Cochlear receptor (microphonic and summating potentials, otoacoustic emissions) and auditory pathway (auditory brain stem potentials) activity in auditory neuropathy. Ear and Hearing, 22, 91–99.

Stuart, A., Yang, E. Y., and Botea, M. (1996). Neonatal auditory brainstem responses recorded from four electrode montages. Journal of Communication Disorders, 29, 125–139.

Stuart, A., Yang, E. Y., and Stenstrom, R. (1990). Effect of temporal area bone vibrator placement on auditory brain stem response in newborn infants. Ear and Hearing, 11, 363–369.

Tucker, D. A., and Ruth, R. A. (1996). Effects of age, signal level, and signal rate on the auditory middle latency response. Journal of the American Academy of Audiology, 7, 83–91.

van der Drift, J. F., Brocaar, M. P., and van Zanten, G. A. (1987). The relation between the pure-tone audiogram and the click auditory brainstem response threshold in cochlear hearing loss. Audiology, 26, 1–10.

Weber, B. A. (1982). Comparison of auditory brain stem response latency norms for premature infants. Ear and Hearing, 3, 257–262.

Wegner, O., and Dau, T. (2002). Frequency specificity of chirp-evoked auditory brainstem responses. Journal of the Acoustical Society of America, 111, 1318–1329.

Wong, S. H., Gibson, W. P., and Sanli, H. (1997). Use of transtympanic round window electrocochleography for threshold estimations in children. American Journal of Otology, 18, 632–636.

Wong, V., and Wong, S. N. (1991). Brainstem auditory evoked potential study in children with autistic disorder. Journal of Autism & Developmental Disorders, 21, 329–340.

Yang, E. Y., Rupert, A. L., and Moushegian, G. (1987). A developmental study of bone conduction auditory brain stem response in infants. Ear and Hearing, 8, 244–251.

Chapter 16

Assessment and Management of Auditory Processing Disorders in Children

Gail M. Whitelaw

♦ **A Conceptual Framework for Auditory Processing**

♦ **Assessment of Auditory Processing Skills in Children**

Practical Considerations in Test Battery Development

Behavioral Assessments

♦ **Management and Treatment of Central Auditory Processing Disorders**

The Educational Environment

Compensatory Strategies

Compensatory Strategies

Direct Therapy and Auditory Training Programs to Address Central Auditory Processing Disorder

♦ **Summary**

Key Points

- Auditory processing disorders should be considered on the same continuum of auditory disorders as peripheral hearing loss.

- Assessment of auditory processing disorders is the scope of practice of the audiologist, although interdisciplinary input is necessary for accurate diagnosis.

- Peripheral hearing loss must be ruled out in any situation in which listening problems are suspected.

- A test battery approach must be used to accurately assess central auditory processing disorders—the test battery should include behavioral tests that use varying linguistic load and electrophysiologic tests.

- Electrophysiologic assessment of auditory processing disorders can provide a unique insight into the auditory system and can provide the ability to track changes in the auditory system.

- Management of auditory processing disorders is considered to incorporate three areas: environmental modifications, compensatory skills, and direct treatment by auditory training.

- Auditory training programs are available that take advantage of the current knowledge of auditory development and neural plasticity.

As noted in other chapters in this text, the practice of audiology in a pediatric population is both challenging and exciting. Assessment and management of auditory processing disorders (APDs) in the pediatric population is arguably one of the most exciting, challenging, and controversial areas in audiology. Understanding the clinical diagnosis of auditory processing disorders requires that the audiologist consider information beyond that obtained on the audiogram, use a breadth of professional knowledge that spans many areas, including auditory development, anatomy and physiology, and classroom acoustics, and participate as a member of an interdisciplinary team, often in the role of team leader.

Myklebust (1954) first described APDs in children, although he referred to it as *auditory imperception*. Since that time, the constellation of deficits that may contribute to auditory processing difficulties has received many labels; the current are CAPDs, also referred to as central auditory processing disorders (CAPDs). APD is not a new area in the profession of audiology. The popularity of attributing certain behaviors to the auditory system seems to peak every few years, as other professions claim to diagnose and treat these disorders with little understanding of the auditory system or its development. Clearly, the diagnosis and treatment of auditory processing disorders are in the scope of practice of the audiologist (ASHA, 2005b). However, APD is not identified and managed in isolation and may require input from a range of disciplines, including speech-language pathology, occupational and physical therapies, neuropsychology, pediatrics, and optometry, to name a few. In addition, input from parents and teachers is critical to effectively understand the strengths and limitations that the child demonstrates. Knowledge of the auditory system, the ability to control stimulus presentation, the environment in which assessment is performed, and education and skill in audiologic habilitation and rehabilitation make the audiologist uniquely qualified to address APDs in children.

The purpose of this chapter is to provide an introduction to broad concepts related to APD and to whet the reader's appetite to learn more about this area. Current issues related to APD are discussed, along with an overview of contemporary approaches to the diagnosis and treatment/management of APD in the pediatric population. The reader is challenged to view APD on a continuum of auditory disorders that can affect communication. The types of difficulties experienced by a child with APD share the similarity with hearing loss in that they present as an "invisible" disorder that may affect the development of speech and language skills, academic achievement, and listening abilities. However, APD often presents itself in a manner more subtle than peripheral hearing loss, requiring deeper investigation on the part of the audiologist. In addition, the audiologist faced with assessing APD is often part of a team providing a differential diagnosis, because behaviors consistent with APD may often be observed in other types of disorders, such as pervasive developmental disorder (PDD) or an attention deficit disorder (ADD).

◆ A Conceptual Framework for Auditory Processing

> **Pitfall**
>
> • Despite the fact that interest in auditory processing disorders is not new, providing a clear and concise framework for defining these disorders remains a challenge in the profession of audiology.

For many years, definitions of APD were criticized for being too lax, not modality specific, and not distinguishable from definitions of deficits in other areas such as peripheral hearing loss, cognitive, language-based, and supramodal attentional issues (Cacace and McFarland, 2005). In addition, the term *auditory processing* is used by other professions such as psychology or occupational therapy but is applied to a more global set of behaviors, further confusing the definition. Conversely, some audiologists doubt the existence of deficits that arise from the auditory system as explanations for certain behaviors, attributing these behaviors instead to disorders of nonauditory modalities such as attentional issues or language disorders.

Although there is no generally accepted comprehensive definition of auditory processing disorders, the challenges

of the past have led the profession to current definitions that address, at least in part, these criticisms. The American Speech-Language-Hearing Association (ASHA, 2005) defines APD as "the perceptual processing of auditory information in the CNS and the neurobiologic activity that underlies that processing and gives rise to electrophysiologic auditory potentials." Similarly, APD was defined in the recommendations of the Bruton conference as "a deficit in the processing of information in the auditory modality." (Jerger and Musiek, 2000). A critical issue not raised in either of these definitions that must be stated implicitly is that APD reflects deficits "in the formation and processing of audible signals not attributed to impaired hearing sensitivity or intellectual impairment" (Deconde-Johnson, Benson, and Seaton, 1997).

Auditory processes may be described as the auditory system mechanisms responsible for the following behaviors: sound localization and lateralization, auditory discrimination, temporal aspects of audition, auditory performance decrements when competing acoustic information is present, and auditory performance decrements when the auditory signal is degraded (ASHA, 1996). According to the ASHA statement, deficits in one or more of these areas would constitute an APD. Auditory processing difficulties may be present for speech and nonspeech stimuli (Rosen, 2005). These types of deficits result in the auditory system being less flexible than required for effective listening in the wide variety of environments faced by most children each day. This is particularly true in the classroom environment, in which unfamiliar linguistic information is being introduced in an often less than optimal acoustic environment. This taxes an auditory system that cannot effectively rise to the challenge.

A strict definition of APD also has clinical relevance. In some ways, APD is a field of dreams for families looking for answers, when applied in its broadest definition. Parents or educators who are shopping for explanations for academic underachievement may cling to APD as a holy grail, since they may find this to be a more palatable diagnosis than other possible options, such as cognitive impairment or autism spectrum disorder (ASD). The ready availability of information and misinformation regarding auditory processing on the Internet also fuels referrals for testing. The audiologist is encouraged to base decision making about auditory processing assessment on a strict definition of APD to minimize inappropriate referrals and to use time and resources most effectively.

In addition, APD is considered to be a low incidence disorder, as a relatively small number of children are thought to have this type of exclusive condition. Chermak and Musiek (1997) estimate that as many as 2 to 5% of school-aged children who are identified as having a learning disorder have APD. However, there is limited epidemiological information about APD, mainly because there is no general agreement on diagnostic markers. This is exacerbated by the potential overlap between the behavioral characteristics of APD and other types of neurobiologic disorders (Hind, 2006). As generally accepted definitions emerge and test batteries evolve, more accurate data about the prevalence of APD should become available.

Since the disorder represents individual differences in the brain, APD is idiosyncratic because individual subtle organizational abnormalities may have diverse presentations; therefore, APD can be as idiosyncratic as the individuals who experience it (Phillips, 2002). For most cases of APD in children, the actual etiology is unknown, but is attributed to poor underlying neurophysiologic representation of the auditory signal, a critical role of the central auditory nervous system (CANS) (Phillips, 1995). In some cases, the underlying etiology can be identified and may result from a head injury or neurologic disease. Delays in auditory development, related to factors such as chronic otitis media, may also be considered; however, some of the research in this area is contradictory and the causal relationship may not always be clear (Hall, Grose, and Pillsbury, 1995).

◆ Assessment of Auditory Processing Skills in Children

The challenge in assessing APDs is to develop a comprehensive test battery that provides adequate information to describe the functional parameters of the child's skills across a variety of auditory behaviors, provides a differential diagnosis, and guides appropriate treatment and management. Several tenets frame the development of the auditory processing battery. Historically, interest in assessing auditory processing skills arose from observations of adults who presented with complaints of difficulties listening in less than optimal environments, despite having no loss in hearing threshold sensitivity on an audiogram. Sensitized speech tests, which reduced the external redundancy of the speech signal by distorting it and reducing the intelligibility of the speech, were used to tax or challenge the auditory system as part of a site-of-lesion assessment in adults with pathologies of the CANS (Bocca, Calearo, and Cassarini, 1954). Several tests, using various methods of distorting the signal and challenging the auditory system, were developed during this period, including the Staggered Spondaic Word test (Katz, 1962) and dichotic consonant-vowels (CVs) (Berlin et al, 1973), which are still used today. These tests are sensitive to detecting retrocochlear and central pathologies in adults.

During the 1970s, interest in addressing auditory processing skills in children developed as observations were made of children with normal peripheral hearing acuity that presented difficulties similar to those demonstrated by adults with known CANS lesions. This interest coincided with the introduction of the term *learning disabilities* into the realm

of public education and the subsequent explosion in programs targeted at remediating learning disabilities, with a particular focus on processing and perceptual training (Hallahan and Mercer, 2002). The discussion of if and where APD fits into the learning disability continuum continues today, as the impact of APD on children in the classroom environment continues to be of interest. The first tests designed specifically to assess APD in school-aged children were introduced by Willeford (1977). Since that time, knowledge of auditory development and methods for assessing auditory skills in children have continued to evolve, and materials available for assessing auditory processing skills in children have expanded significantly.

All tests designed to assess auditory processing skills in children are based on several factors. Assessment of auditory processing is based on the assumption that the internal or intrinsic redundancy of the CANS is somehow compromised as a function of disease, delayed development, or some type of neurologic differences that may be thought of as miswiring. This intrinsic redundancy is responsible for the flexibility that the auditory system demonstrates, in being able to fill in missing information or focus on a primary message in the presence of background noise, for example. Tests included in the test battery, whether behavioral or electrophysiologic, tax the auditory system in some unique way by manipulating an aspect of stimulus presentation.

An understanding of the role in auditory development of auditory processing assessment is critical. All of the auditory processes highlighted earlier in this chapter have a specific developmental time course, some of which occur as late as adolescence. It is well established that children demonstrate poorer abilities compared with adults in terms of a variety of auditory behaviors and require a more favorable listening environment for performing auditory tasks in relation to adults (Olsho et al 1988; Hnath-Chisolm, Laipply, and Boothroyd, 1998; Hall et al, 2002). These differences are greater than those that could be explained by attention and motivation of the listener alone and have been attributed to the ongoing maturation of the CANS. It is critical that these differences are taken into consideration in developing a APD test battery for children that is based on the current knowledge of auditory development, and that has normative data collected across the age group for which the test is targeted.

Practical Considerations in Test Battery Development

An audiologist new to the area of APD will often seek a standard approach to testing, a cookbook approach, so to speak. Unfortunately, a standardized test battery has not been established at this time. Lack of a standardized test battery makes it difficult to compare studies and make comparisons across audiology practices or in the development of auditory skills, even in an individual child. A complicating issue is the diversity of philosophical approaches to APDs, despite advances in adopting a more uniform definition. Phillips (2002) indicates, "in practice however, this is often the state of a young science and any standardization of test materials that is appropriate will emerge as the scientific issues sort themselves out over time." Until a standardized test battery is developed and agreed on, audiologists assessing children for APD must rely on their knowledge and experience with this population and select a test battery based on several factors, including the population to be tested, the audience for whom the testing is performed (e.g., who is the referral source), and the purpose for which the information is requested. An assessment on a child to address concerns based on a referral from a neurologist may differ from a referral from a school-based speech-language pathologist. One test battery may require a greater reliance on electrophysiologic measures; another may be more heavily weighted toward behavioral testing. Tests that use a standard scoring method provide the benefit of being able to compare with results of other standardized educational testing, so that the results of an auditory processing assessment can be contrasted to those obtained in a speech-language or cognitive test battery.

As audiologists who perform APD assessments as part of their practice can attest, a prescreening procedure is beneficial to ensure that assessment of auditory processing skills is truly appropriate for the patient being referred.

> **Pearl**
>
> - A guiding tenet must be that if there is a concern regarding hearing or listening skills, a comprehensive audiologic evaluation must be scheduled regardless of age or other presenting issues to ensure that the child does not have peripheral hearing loss. A hearing screening alone is not sufficient.

Too often, parents or educators rely on hearing screenings performed in the schools to address these concerns; however, experience suggests that, because of the variability in personnel conducting the screenings, the environments in which they are performed, and the limited scope of the protocol, any concern related to hearing warrants a comprehensive diagnostic evaluation performed by an audiologist.

Many practices establish their own criteria for scheduling an auditory processing assessment. For example, an age criteria of 7 years typically is established in many practices. By age 7, the amount of variability in auditory skills noted in young children has decreased, the child has experience in the school environment, and normative data are available for a wide range of tasks. An additional criterion is the elimination from referral of children who have a history of

permanent hearing loss or cognitive impairment or who have been identified as having ASD. To explain, auditory processing difficulties may be inherent in each of these diagnoses; however, these difficulties are not specifically related to CANS dysfunction.

The population of children identified with ASD continues to grow. Audiologists are certainly involved in the team that contributes to this diagnosis by providing a comprehensive audiologic evaluation with what may be classified as a difficult-to-test population.

> **Special Consideration**
>
> - At this time, compared with general populations of children, there is no evidence that children with ASD have a higher incidence of comorbidity of APD or the behaviors that are attributed to auditory perception, not related to a more global sensory deficit (Eglehoff, Whitelaw, and Rabidoux, 2005; Downs, Schmidt, and Stevens, 2005; Gravel et al, 2001).

In addition to an audiologic assessment, a comprehensive case history should be considered one of the first tests in the APD test battery. Information should be obtained that addresses birth and developmental history, family history of learning or communication difficulties, medical history, academic history, information about general behavior, and social and emotional development. Records from previous assessments, including speech-language, medical, and cognitive are of significant value in understanding the child's skills and in providing a better understanding of presenting concerns. The results of a multifactored evaluation (MFE) and individualized education plan (IEP) from the child's school can provide significant insight into academic strengths and concerns, and provide input into the evaluation process from the school's perspective. Additional information about educator, parent, and child perceptions of hearing and listening skills can be obtained via an authentic assessment protocol. Authentic assessment is designed to evaluate a child's ability in the real world environment. Several questionnaires are available for the purpose of authentic assessments that are relatively quick to administer and are normed on children with APD and listening difficulties. These tools include the Children's Auditory Processing Scale (CHAPS) (Smoski, Brunt, and Tannahill, 1998), the Screening Inventory for Targeting Educational Risk (SIFTER) (Anderson, 1995), and the Fisher's Auditory Problems Checklist (Fisher, 1978).

Behavioral Assessments

A range of auditory skills must be assessed in the auditory processing test battery. This chapter will focus on general categories of skills that can be assessed; specific test materials are included in **Appendix 16–1**. The characteristics of each category are briefly highlighted here.

Monaural Low-Redundancy Tests

These test materials are presented to each ear separately. In each of these tests, the stimuli have been degraded in some way, which might include the frequency or temporal characteristics of the stimulus. Some examples of tests in this category would include low-pass filtered speech and auditory figure-ground tasks.

Temporal Processes   In recent years, the importance of temporal aspects of audition has become evident. Phillips (2002) notes that a vast number of auditory processes rely on temporal analysis of an incoming signal. Tallal, Miller, and Fitch (1993) report that deficits in temporal processing contribute to deficits in normal phonological development. These result in disorders in reading and speaking for at least a subpopulation of children. Tests in this category may include stimuli that measure the listener's ability in temporal ordering, discrimination, resolution, and integration, as suggested by ASHA (1996). Examples of tests that fall into this category include the Frequency Pattern Sequence test (Pinheiro and Ptacek, 1971; Ptacek and Pinheiro, 1971). Gaps-In-Noise test (Musiek et al, 2005), and Random Gap Detection Test (Keith, 2000b).

Binaural Interaction Tests   Tests in this category require that the listener integrate different auditory information presented between two ears to synthesize the information. The term *eye teaming* could be coined from what our optometry colleagues describe as the importance of two eyes working together; clearly, based on the binaural design of the auditory system, the ears are designed so that each ear does not function in isolation, but rather both ears work together as a unit. An example of this type of test is masking level difference (MLD).

Dichotic Listening Tests   In these tests, different acoustic stimuli are presented to each ear simultaneously. The listener's task is to separate each message; thus, these tasks may also be referred to as binaural separation tasks. These tasks can vary in linguistic load from CV stimuli to sentence materials. Dichotic listening tests provide insight into aspects of hemispheric dominance. In addition, this type of test stimuli has been studied for many years as a method for addressing neuromaturation of the auditory system. The right ear advantage (REA), superior performance for stimuli presented to the right ear compared with the left ear for dichotic stimulus presentation, is thought to be related to asymmetries in the pathways leading from the peripheral auditory system to the central auditory cortices. Traditionally, information presented to the right ear is believed to be transferred directly to the left auditory cortex; the left cortex is considered to be dominant for language. The REA is thought to be related to normal development: the difference becomes minimal between the two ears in adolescents and reaches adult-like values at that time. Examples of dichotic listening tasks include the Staggered Spondaic Word test (Katz, 1962), the Competing Sentences subtest of the SCAN-C/A (Keith, 1996, 2000a), and Dichotic CVs (Berlin et al, 1973).

As has been suggested, the APD test battery should include materials that vary the linguistic loading of the stimulus, use varying response modes, and tax the auditory system in a variety of ways. Another critical feature in behavioral testing is observing the behaviors that the child demonstrates during testing. The audiologist should make comments on several features of behavioral testing, including the speed of the child's response in relation to stimulus presentation, the types of strategies that the child may use to respond (e.g., verbal rehearsal in which the child may verbally "practice" their response before stating it for the examiner), and the level of the child's physical activity during the assessment (e.g., the child is pacing in the booth). These are all subjective observations, but with experience, the audiologist may be able to use these behavioral interpretations to support the differential diagnosis.

Pearl

- Administering APD tests to children and adults with typical auditory processing skills is a recommended exercise that allows the audiologist to gain experience observing normal auditory behaviors, and thus become proficient at APD assessment interpretation.

Electroacoustic Assessment

226-Hz tympanometry should always be performed as part of the APD test battery; to ensure that middle ear functioning is typical for a child of this age. In addition, ipsilateral and contralateral acoustic reflexes should be performed to assess the integrity of the brainstem pathways. This may add to a differential diagnosis related to APD assessment. Otoacoustic emissions (OAEs) should be used to confirm normal peripheral auditory function and may contribute to assessing the auditory system in a unique way. The contralateral suppression of the OAE procedure allows for the ability to isolate efferent auditory system function and address the "gating" function of the auditory system (Lauter, 2004). Abnormal function in these efferent auditory skills is thought to be associated with deficits in listening in speech-in-noise (Clarke et al, 2006). Preliminary studies suggest that children with APD may demonstrate less suppression of transient evoked otoacoustic emission (TEOAE) activity than in an age-matched control group (Munchnik et al, 2004). However, they present results that contradict this finding. Clearly, contralateral suppression procedures require additional attention because of the hypothesized relationship between efferent auditory activity and the ability to listen in the presence of background noise, since the inability to listen effectively in background noise is one of the most commonly reported behavioral observations in children with suspected APD. OAEs may provide a distinctive ability to isolate auditory system function related to other available tests that may be influenced by attention or motivation of the listener.

Electrophysiologic Assessment

As noted in the ASHA definition, eletrophysiologic assessment is considered to be a critical component of auditory processing assessment, a sentiment echoed by Jerger and Musiek (2002). The benefits of electophysiologic testing include the ability to use nonspeech stimuli or minimize linguistic load. This avoids concerns that the language processing skills are actually taxed in the assessment, the ability to minimize the impact of attention and motivation on the task, and provide a unique measure of auditory system improvement related to treatment or management programs (Jirsa, 2002). Limitations of electrophysiologic assessment may include the same lack of sensitivity and specificity of measures to identify an APD as with behavioral testing, the need to speculate between the results of the electrophysiologic measure, and the functional impact in the classroom, the assumptions inherent in a site-of-lesion approach that supports a disease model that may not apply in a developmental model, and the cost:benefit ratio.

Several electrophysiologic measures that provide a unique contribution to understanding auditory processing skills can be incorporated into the APD test battery. Although standard auditory brainstem evoked response (ABR) assessment may be of limited value in the test battery because it lacks sensitivity and specificity, incorporating complex stimuli (e.g., speech) into the ABR procedure provides a unique tool for assessing APD skills. An example of this procedure is the Biological Marker of Auditory Processing (BioMAP), developed based on research by Kraus and her colleagues (Johnson, Nicol, and Kraus, 2005). The BioMAP characterizes neural activity in response to the presentation of the CV /da/ and is described as an electrophysiologic response from the brainstem that "mimics characteristics of speech with remarkable fidelity." This test can currently be performed only on the Bio-Logic Navigator PRO (Natus Medical Inc., San Carlos, CA) equipment. This test may provide unique insight into auditory processing skills and identify children who would be strong candidates for an auditory training–based type of program and as a measure of treatment effectiveness.

Cortical evoked potentials have also been identified as having a significant role in the APD test battery. Electrophysiologic assessment provides for assessment of auditory processing skills independent of language skills. The later evoked potentials, such as auditory late response (ALR), mismatched negativity (MMN), and the auditory P300 response, can provide documentation of ADPs, either in conjunction with behavioral testing or independent of behavioral results. Increased latency of ALR responses have been noted in children with APD and have been correlated to slower processing speeds than in typically developing age-matched peers (Tremblay et al, 2001). MMN responses and the P300 response have been a focus in the assessment of auditory processing skills in children. Significant differences in response parameters (e.g., amplitude, latency) between children with APDs and children with typically developing auditory systems have been noted (Jirsa and Clontz, 1990); however, further investigation is needed to address the clinical relevance of these tests in the general pediatric clinical setting.

◆ Management and Treatment of Central Auditory Processing Disorders

Developing a comprehensive plan for the management and treatment of APDs is as complex as the process of assessment and should be linked to the assessment results. One of the fallacies of APD is that nothing can be done to treat it, so assessment of auditory processing skills is futile. This is based on the assumption that the only type of treatment or management results in a cure for the disorder, which is not consistent with how other types of pediatric auditory disorders are addressed. Clearly, fitting a hearing aid does not cure peripheral hearing loss; however, it this does not minimize the positive impact of the hearing aid on the management of hearing loss.

In the past, an audiologist would perform a assessment then provide a preprinted list of recommendations to address general aspects of APD. This approach often resulted in the observation from educators that if the list were provided, the evaluation would likely be unnecessary. This approach did not support the evidence-based approach to assessment discussed in this chapter and did not address a deficit-specific approach to treatment. Several approaches have been developed to profile results of auditory processing testing to customize a treatment plan to address the individual child's listening and learning needs. These are classified as predictable patterns of functional deficits and include the Buffalo model (Katz, Stecker, and Henderson, 1992) and the Bellis and Ferre model (1999). With a greater sophistication in assessment and profiling of results and a clearer understanding of neural plasticity, developing this deficit-specific approach to treatment/management is both necessary and possible. The ASHA (2005a) statement supports this premise

> [T]he quality and quantity of scientific evidence is sufficient to support the existence of APD as a diagnostic entity to guide the diagnosis and assessment of the disorder and to inform the development of more customized, deficit focused treatment and management plans.

A triad approach to management and treatment has been adopted to address the needs of the individual child with APD. This triad includes developing environmental modifications, helping the child to develop compensatory skills, and providing direct therapy. Another perspective is to address both context-centered management, such as the accommodations in the classroom, and person-centered management, such as direct therapy. An overview of approaches will be provided in this chapter; however, the reader is encouraged to explore management and treatment options in greater detail, both from exploring available research and from clinical application of options to individual patients.

As noted earlier in the chapter, a consistent focus of all aspects of management is to increase both the predictability and redundancy in the listening environment. Regardless of the approach, the audiologist is uniquely qualified to develop, implement, and oversee the treatment plan, based on knowledge of aural rehabilitation, accommodations for hearing and listening disorders, and the ability to coordinate an interdisciplinary team to meet the child's needs effectively.

The Educational Environment

Children spend most of their day in the classroom with a focus on listening as the means for learning. This can be fatiguing for a young child with normal peripheral hearing acuity and typically developing auditory processing skills, far more so for a child with hearing loss or APD. In the past, a common recommendation was preferential seating, placing the child close to the source of verbal instruction. Although this approach is inexpensive and has good face validity, it does not effectively address the listening and learning impact of poor acoustics on a child who would be classified as a high-risk listener (Johnson, 2000). Adults with normal hearing acuity and typically developing auditory processing skills require a +6 dB signal-to-noise ratio to maximize auditory learning, and typically developing children requiring a +10 dB signal-to-noise ratio in the classroom (Crandell and Smaldino, 2000). Speech-in-noise ratios have been consistently reported across classroom as +5 dB to -7 dB, much poorer than would be required for effective auditory comprehension for learning (Knecht et al, 2002). Leavitt and Flexer (1991), using the Rapid Speech Transmission Index (RASTI) approach, found that there was a significant loss of speech intelligibility unless the position of the speaker was very close (about 6 inches) to the source of the sound, dispelling the myth that preferential seating is an effective accommodation for a child with an APD. Most classrooms are no longer set up to establish a true preferential seat, and the distance of the student from the teacher is impractical for making a positive acoustic impact. However, some children may benefit from seating in the classroom that allows for unobstructed view of the teacher or for the teacher to be able to make comprehension checks.

Improving classroom acoustics can include addressing options for improving overall noise, reducing reverberation, and improving signal-to-noise ratio, all of which can have a significant impact on speech intelligibility in the classroom for all children. All efforts should be made to target the American National Standard Institute (ANSI) standard for classroom acoustics as the goal for every classroom (ANSI, 2002). In addition, the child with an APD may benefit from an assistive listening device, such as a frequency modulation (FM) system or infrared listening device, targeted at improving signal-to-noise ratio (Stein, 1998). However, use of an assistive listening device to address speech understanding issues in children with APDs is not a panacea, nor is it appropriate for all children. An overview of FM and infrared technologies can be found in Chapter 20. Children with CAPD obtain the same benefit from an improved acoustic environment as all other children and the benefits of soundfield amplification in the classroom are obvious.

The option of a personal FM system may also be worth considering. However, a critical issue is the fitting of personal FM technologies to a child with APD. By definition, these devices are being fit to children with normal peripheral hearing acuity, and care should be taken to ensure a transparent fit in which signal-to-noise ratio is enhanced without amplification that could damage normal hearing acuity. An FM receiver such as the Phonak EduLink or MicroEar, which is designed specifically for children with normal peripheral hearing acuity, should be considered on a trial basis to document benefits and limitations of the device and its impact on the child's listening in the classroom. The ASHA (1999) Guideline for Fitting and Monitoring FM systems provides a foundation for this type of fitting and authentic assessment, using the Listening Inventory for Education (LIFE) (Anderson and Smaldino, 1998) will assist in documenting performance with the system.

Compensatory Strategies

Children with APD often have poor ability to compensate for their listening limitations. Unlike learning to read, write, and spell, children are not directly taught the skills of listening. When a teacher tells their class to listen, a child with CAPD may have little understanding of what is required to be successful in the educational environment. Children may benefit from specific instruction in the steps that it takes to become an active and effective listener and in organizing incoming auditory information. Several programs have been described over the years that focus on developing specific listening skills in the classroom environment, such as that by Prelock (1993) and the Classroom Language and Auditory Strategies for Success (CLASS) (Taber, Foulkes, and Whitelaw, 1999).

It is critical to recall that auditory-oral communication is dually the responsibility of the teacher and the student in a classroom environment. If failure of communication occurs on the part of the listener, the speaker (or in this case, the teacher) should also be provided with strategies that can improve comprehension. An example of such an intervention program targeted at the speaker is the concept of clear speech, a set of intervention techniques designed to address parameters of the speech signal that can enhance speech intelligibility for the listener (Krause and Braida, 2002; Tye-Murray and Schum, 1994).

The child may benefit from developing additional metacognitive abilities that empower him to implement small but significant accommodations in the classroom, which gives him control over his own listening and learning environment. Several techniques and skills, including use of a pocket calendar/organizer and guided notes provided by the teacher, provide accommodation under the metacognitive approach. Metacognitive skills are often implemented in an interdisciplinary manner by a psychologist or speech-language pathologist.

Direct Therapy and Auditory Training Programs to Address Central Auditory Processing Disorder

Auditory training programs have long been implemented by speech-language pathologists working with children with APD in the school setting. Often these programs are implemented as part of language therapy program and target a top-down approach to listening. Some of these programs have also focused on addressing auditory aspects to build reading and literacy skills, such as the Orton-Gillingham or the Lindamood Phonemic Synthesis (LiPS) programs. These programs may include a multisensory approach to enhance auditory skills and often target global listening skills rather than addressing specific types of auditory processing skills that may be taught.

Recent interest in direct therapy and auditory training for APD capitalizes on the concept of neural plasticity and that the application of a challenging program can alter the CANS through alternating the CANS. Although auditory training programs have historically been applied to intervention for children with APD, current programs attempt to capitalize on intensive adaptive training methods applied using a specific type of stimuli via a computer game format, such as that developed for Fast ForWord, an auditory training program designed to address temporal processing (Tallal et al, 1998). Although the efficacy of using FastForWord as a treatment program for children with APD has been questioned, the options for computer-assisted auditory training have grown because of an improved understanding of the neuroscience principles that improve the efficacy and effectiveness with these types of programs and the ability to objectively and behaviorally measure this efficacy.

These techniques have been applied to specific areas of auditory training for APD. One example is the dichotic interaural intensity difference (DIID) training for binaural integration deficits (Musiek, 2004). This training technique presents a stimulus to the dominant ear at a less intense level than a stimulus presented to the poorer ear. Improvement in left ear deficits has been reported (Musiek, 2004). Temporal processing deficits have been addressed using training on temporal ordering tasks using the game SIMON™ as the vehicle for auditory training (Musiek, 2005).

These types of computerized auditory training programs will continue to grow as additional data are obtained about these programs and the ability to develop a deficit-specific program evolves. In addition, these programs are likely to have significant impact on developing auditory training as a means to build auditory processing skills in all younger children.

◆ Summary

Assessment and management of auditory processing skills in children is a time- and labor-intensive process, but a worthwhile investment on the part of the audiologist. Jerger (1998) states "the reality of APD can no longer be doubted. It is a distinct entity across the entire age range." This chapter focuses on the pediatric patient; however, assessment and management in APD across the lifespan are certainly within the scope of practice of audiology, which recognizes the role of the brain in hearing and listening and acknowledges that hearing and listening do not stop at the level of the inner ear. The auditory system's ability to learn and change supports why audiologists enter the profession—the ability to effectively identify an underlying disorder and intervene to improve the quality of the person's life and communication are germane to the area of APDs.

Discussion Questions

1. How does the audiologist develop an interdisciplinary team to assess auditory processing skills in children?

2. What issues might an audiologist consider in developing a AP test battery? What specific test materials might be included in the test battery, based on the issues and the audiologist's philosophical approach?

3. What is the role of the audiologist in the management and treatment of APDs?

4. What impact is a CAPD likely to have on a child in the classroom and why? What types of interventions can address these types of deficits in the classroom environment?

5. What does the current model of auditory development and knowledge of neural plasticity suggest about the efficacy of treatment related to APDs?

Appendix 16–1

Distributors for Auditory Processing Assessment Materials

Auditec of St. Louis

2515 South Big Bend Blvd

St. Louis MO 63143

800-669-9065

auditecinfo@auditec.com (e-mail)

www.auditec.com (website)

APD test materials include:

Auditory Fusion Test-Revised

Competing Sentences

   Dichotic Digits

   Dichotic Sentence Identification (DSI) Test

Masking Level Difference

Multiple Auditory Processing Assessment (MAPA)

Pitch Pattern Sequence (PPS) Test

Random Gap Detection Test (RGDT)

Time Compressed Sentences Test (TCST)

Time Compressed Sentences Test—Spanish version

Selective Auditory Attention Test (SAAT)

Staggered Spondaic Word Test—Spanish version

Educational Audiology Association

11166 Huron Street, Suite 27

Denver, CO 80234

800-460-7322

EAA@imigroup.org (e-mail)

www.edaud.org (website)

APD materials include:

Children's Auditory Performance Scale (CHAPs)

Fisher's Auditory Checklist

Listening Inventories for Education (LIFE)

Screening Identification for Targeting Educational Risk Listening Inventories for Education (SIFTER)

Harcourt Assessment, Inc.

19500 Bulverde Road

San Antonio, TX 78259

800-211-8378

http://harcourtassessment.com (website)

APD test materials include:

A Test for Auditory Processing Disorders in Children (SCAN-C)

A Test for Auditory Processing Disorders in Adults (SCAN-A)

Natus Medical Incorporated (Bio-Logic Hearing Diagnostics)

1501 Industrial Road

San Carlos, CA 94070

800-255-3901

www.blsc.com (website)

APD test materials include:

Biological Marker of Auditory Processing (BioMAP) software for Biologic Navigator Pro equipment

Precision Acoustics

505 NE 87th Ave Ste 150, Vancouver, WA

(360) 892-9367

APD test materials include:

Staggered Spondaic Word Test

Phonemic Synthesis Test

Competing Environmental Sounds (CES) Test

References

American National Standards Institute. (2002). ANSI S12.60-2002 American National Standard Acoustical Performance Criteria, Design Requirements, and Guidelines for Schools. Melville, NY.

American Speech-Language-Hearing Association. (1999). Guidelines for fitting and monitoring FM systems. ASHA desk reference. Rockville, MD.

American Speech-Language-Hearing Association (1996). Central auditory processing: current status of research and implications for clinical practice. American Journal of Audiology, 5, 41–54.

American Speech-Language-Hearing Association (2005a). (Central) Auditory Processing Disorders. www.asha.org/members/deskref-journals/deskref/default. Last accessed April 21, 2007.

American Speech-Language-Hearing Association (2005b). (Central) Auditory Processing Disorders-The Role of the Audiologist [Position statement]. www.asha.org/members/deskref-journals/deskref/default. Last accessed April 21, 2007.

Anderson, K. (1995). Screening Instrument for Targeting Educational Risk (SIFTER). Tampa: Educational Audiology Association.

Anderson, K., and Smaldino, J. J. (1998). The listening inventory for education (LIFE). Tampa: Educational Audiology Association.

Bellis, T. J., and Ferre, J. M. (1999). Multidimensional approach to the differential diagnosis of central auditory processing disorders in children. Journal of the American Academy of Audiology, 10, 319–328.

Berlin, C. I., Lowe-Bell, S., Cullen, J., and Thompson, C. (1973). Dichotic speech perception: an interpretation of right-ear advantage and temporal offset effects. Journal of the Acoustical Society of America, 53, 699–709.

Cacace, A. T., and McFarland, D. J. (2005). The importance of modality specificity in diagnosing central auditory processing disorder. American Journal of Audiology, 14, 112–123.

Cameron, S., Dillon, H., and Newall, P. (2006). The Listening in Spatialized Noise Test: an auditory processing disorder study. Journal of the American Academy of Audiology, 17, 306–320.

Chermak, G. D., and Musiek, F. E. (1997). Central auditory processing disorders: new perspectives. San Diego: Singular Publishing.

Clarke, E. M., Ahmmed, A., Parker, D., and Adams, C, (2006). Contralateral suppression of otoacoustic emissions in children with specific language impairment. Ear and Hearing, 27, 153–160.

Crandell, C. C., and Smaldino, J. J. (2000). Classroom acoustics for children with normal hearing and with hearing impairment. language, speech, and hearing services in schools. Language, Speech, and Hearing services in schools, 31, 362–370.

DeConde-Johnson, C., Benson, P. V., and Seaton, J. B. (1997). Educational audiology handbook. San Diego: Singular.

Downs, D., Schmidt, B., and Stephens, T. J. (2005). Auditory behaviors of children and adolescents with pervasive developmental disorders. Seminars in Hearing, 26, 226–240.

Egelhoff, K., Whitelaw, G., and Rabidoux, P. (2005). What audiologists need to know about autism spectrum disorders. Seminars in Hearing, 26, 202–209.

Fisher, L. I. (1978). Fisher's Auditory Checklist. Tampa: Educational Audiology Association.

Gravel, J. W., Dunn, M., Lei, W. W., Ellis, M. A. and Hood, L. (2001). Indices of basic auditory processes in children with autism. Proceedings of the American Auditory Society Meeting.

Hall, J. W. 3rd, Grose, J. H., and Pillsbury, H. C. (1995). Long-term effects of chronic otitis media on binaural hearing in children. Archives of Otolaryngology–Head and Neck Surgery, 121, 81–88.

Hallahan, D. P., and Mercer, C. D. (2002). Learning disabilities: historical perspective. Learning Disabilities Summit: Building a Foundation for the Future White Papers. National Research Center on Learning Disabilities.

Hind, S. (2006). Survey of care pathway of auditory processing disorder. Audiological Medicine, 4, 12–24.

Hnath-Chisolm, T. E., Laipply, E., and Boothroyd, A. (1998). Age-related changes on a children's test of sensory-level speech perception capacity. Journal of Speech, Language, and Hearing Research, 41, 94–106.

Jerger, J., and Musiek, F. E. (2000). Report of consensus conference on the diagnosis of auditory processing disorders in school-aged children. Journal of the American Academy of Audiology, 11, 467–474.

Jerger, J., and Musiek, F. E. (2002). On the diagnosis of auditory processing disorder: a reply to Clinical and research concerns regarding the 2000 APD consensus report and recommendations. Audiology Today, 14, 19–21.

Jirsa, R. E. (2002). Clinical efficacy of electrophysiologic measures in APD management programs. Seminars in Hearing, 23, 349–355.

Jirsa, R. E., and Clontz, K. B. (1990). Long latency auditory event-related potentials from children with auditory processing disorders. Ear and Hearing, 11, 222–232.

Johnson, C. E. (2000). Children's phoneme identification in reverberation and noise. Journal of Speech, Language, and Hearing Research, 43, 144–157.

Johnson K. L., Nicol, T., and Kraus N. (2005). The brainstem response to speech: a biological marker. Ear and Hearing 26, 424–443.

Katz, J. (1962). The use of staggered spondaic words for assessing the integrity of the central auditory nervous system. Journal of Auditory Research, 2, 327–337.

Katz, J., Stecker, N. A., and Henderson, D. (1992). Central auditory processing: a transdisciplinary view. St. Louis: Mosby Year Book.

Keith, R. W. (1996). Re: "Development of SCAN-A: test of auditory processing disorders in adolescents and adults." Journal of the American Academy of Audiology, 6, 286–292.

Keith, R. W. (2000a). Development and standardization of SCAN-C: test for auditory processing disorders in children—revised. Journal of the American Academy of Audiology, 11, 438–445.

Keith, R. W. (2000b). Random Gap Detection Test. St. Louis: Auditec.

Knecht, H. A. Nelson, P. B., Whitelaw, G. M., and Feth, L. L. (2002). Background noise levels and reverberation times in unoccupied classrooms: predictions and measurements. American Journal of Audiology, 11, 65–71.

Krause, J. C., and Braida L. D. (2002). Investigating alternative forms of clear speech: the effects of speaking rate and speaking mode on intelligibility. Journal of the Acoustical Society of America, 112, 2165–2172

Lauter, J. L. (2004). New approaches to understanding the human brain: three theoretical models and a test battery. Seminars in Hearing, 25, 269–280.

Leavitt, R., and Flexer, C. A. (1991). Speech degradation as measured by the Rapid Speech Transmission Index (RASTI). Ear and Hearing, 12, 115–118.

Munchnik, C., Ari-Even Roth, D., Othman-Jebara, R., Putter-Katz, H., Shabati, E. G., and Hildensheimer, M. (2004). Reduced medical oliviocochlear bundle system dysfunction in children with auditory processing disorders. Audiology Neuro-Otology, 9, 107–114.

Musiek, F. E. (2005). Temporal (auditory) training for CAPD. Hearing Journal, 58, 46.

Musiek, F. E. (2004). The DIID: A new treatment for APD. Hearing Journal, 57, 50.

Musiek, F. E., Shinn, J., Jirsa, R., Bamiou, D., Baran, J., and Zaiden, E. (2005). The GIN (Gaps-in Noise Test performance in subjects with confirmed central auditory nervous system involvement. Ear and Hearing, 26, 608–618.

Myklebust, H. R. (1954) Auditory disorders in children: a manual for differential diagnosis. New York: Grune and Stratton.

Olsho, L. W., Koch, E. G., Carter, E. A., Halpin, C. F., and Spetner, N. B. (1988). Pure-tone sensitivity of human infants. Journal of the Acoustical Society of America, 84, 1316–1324.

Phillips, D. P. (2002). Central auditory system and central auditory processing disorders: some conceptual issues. Seminars in Hearing, 23, 251–262.

Phillips, D. P. (1995). Central auditory processing and its disorders: a view from auditory neuroscience. American Journal of Otology, 16, 338–352.

Pinheiro, M. L., and Ptacek, P. H. (1971). Reversals in the perception of noise and tone patterns. Journal of the Acoustical Society of America, 49, 1778–1782.

Prelock, P. A. (1993). Managing the language and learning needs of the communication-impaired preschool child: a proactive approach. Clinics in Communication Disorders, 3, 1–14.

Ptacek, P. H., and Pinheiro, M. L. (1971). Pattern reversal in auditory perception. Journal of the Acoustical Society of America, 49, 493–498.

Rosen, S. (2005). "A riddle wrapped in a mystery inside an enigma": Defining central auditory processing disorder. American Journal of Audiology, 14, 139–142.

Smoski, W., Brunt, M., and Tannahill, J. (1998). Children's Auditory Performance Scale (CHAPS). Tampa: Educational Audiology Association.

Stein, R. (1998). Application of FM technology to the management of central auditory processing disorders. In Masters, M., Stecker, N, and Katz, J. (Eds.), Central auditory processing disorders: mostly management. Needham Heights: Allyn and Bacon. 89–102.

Taber, M. V., Foulkes, E., and Whitelaw, G. M. (1999). Classroom Language and Auditory Strategies for Success. Unpublished program. Columbus: The Ohio State University.

Tallal, P., Merzenich, M., Miller, S., and Jenkins, W. (1998). Language learning impairments: integrating basic science, technology, and remediation. Experimental Brain Research, 123, 210–219.

Tallal, P., Miller, S., and Fitch, R. (1993). Neurological basis of speech: a case for the preeminence of temporal processing. Annual NY Academy of Science, 682, 27–47.

Tremblay, K., Kraus, N., McGee T. J., Ponton, C. W., and Otis B. (2001). Central auditory plasticity: changes in the N1-P2 complex after speech-sound training. Ear and Hearing, 22, 79– 90.

Tye-Murray, N., and Schum, L. (1994) Conversation training for frequent communication partners. Journal of the Academy of Rehabilitative Audiology Supplement, 27, 209–222.

Willeford, J. A. (1977). Assessing central auditory behavior in children: a test battery approach. In Keith, R. (Ed), Central auditory dysfunction. New York: Grune and Stratton.

Part III

Hearing Access Technology for Infants and Children

Chapter 17

The Acoustic Speech Signal

Arthur Boothroyd

Key Points

- An essential first step in auditory-oral intervention is the provision and adjustment of hearing aids or cochlear implants to give audibility of the sound patterns of speech.

- Conversational speech, when it reaches the listener's ear, has an overall level around 60 dB sound pressure level (SPL).

- When examined in one third octave bands, the speech signal covers a range from around 100 Hz to higher than 8000 Hz; most of the energy is in the frequencies below 1000 Hz.

- Within each one third octave band, amplitude fluctuates from moment to moment over a range from around 15 dB above the average to 15 dB below it.

- This 30-dB range is responsible for the configuration of the normal performance versus intensity function, which rises from 0 to 100% over a range of 30 dB as the speech signal emerges from below threshold.

- Transferring the amplitude and frequency distribution of speech to the audiogram form produces the well-known speech banana.

- The utility of the speech banana is enhanced by an indication of the distribution of speech information within it—quantitatively, phonetically, and phonemically.

- The greatest concentration of useful information is found between 1000 and 3000 Hz. This is the region of the second vocal tract formant, which conveys information about place of articulation.

- Comparing the speech banana with a child's audiogram gives an impression of the audibility of speech and the potential benefits of hearing aids or cochlear implants.

- Difficulties of discrimination and noise susceptibility may remain even after the sound patterns of speech have been made audible.

♦ The Acoustic Speech Signal

Hearing and Spoken Language

Among the many requirements for acquisition of a first language, three are basic:

♦ Interaction with fluent users of language

♦ Full sensory access to the symbols of that language

♦ Feedback to the child, via the same sense, of his own efforts to reproduce those symbols

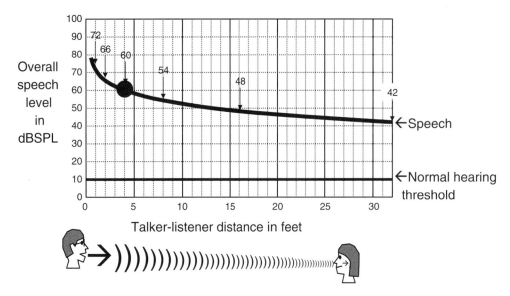

Figure 17–1 Effect of distance on the overall level of the acoustic speech signal (disregarding the effects of room acoustics). The black circle continues in Fig. 17–2.

For the hearing child of hearing parents, these three needs are met in relation to spoken language. For the deaf child of signing deaf parents, they are met in relation to signed language. But, for the deaf child of hearing parents, the second and third needs are not met. Without professional intervention, the developmental consequences of the resulting language deficits can be serious and far-reaching. However, these consequences begin with a simple fact—the child cannot hear (or cannot hear well) the sound patterns of speech—both her own and others. It follows that, once spoken language has been adopted as a goal of intervention, a first step is to give the child sensory access to the sounds of speech—in other words to optimize hearing. At the time of writing, the principal tools are hearing aids and cochlear implants. Their effective use, however, requires an awareness of the possibilities and limitations of the child's assisted hearing. Part of that understanding calls for some knowledge of the acoustic properties and informational content of the speech signal. In short, if our goal is for the child to develop spoken language, it behooves us to understand something about the acoustic speech signal.

Overall Amplitude and the Effect of Distance

Overall amplitude, measured in decibels, is one of the basic properties of the speech signal. A typical talker, speaking with conversational effort, at a distance of around 4 feet, generates speech with an overall level of around 60 dB SPL (roughly 50 dB above the normal threshold of hearing). This level, however, falls by 6 dB for every doubling of distance

(and increases by 6 dB for every halving of distance)[1] as shown in **Fig. 17–1**.

The Long-Term-Average Spectrum of Speech

The overall level of speech represents a summing of energy across frequency. If we examine the average level within narrow frequency bands, each one third of an octave wide,[2] we find that

- most of the energy is contained in the lower frequencies, below about 1000 Hz
- the level falls at the rate of about 5 or 6 dB per octave for frequencies above 500 Hz

A plot of speech level as a function of frequency is known as the long-term-average spectrum of speech (LTASS) and is used as a basis for the prescriptive fitting of hearing aids.[3]

Fig. 17–2 shows an example of a LTASS derived from a 20-second sample of speech from a woman talker. Also shown, for reference, is the normal soundfield hearing threshold (Robinson and Dadson, 1956; Sivian and White, 1933).

Variation of Amplitude with Time

The LTASS in **Fig. 17–2** is averaged over time and does not, therefore, reflect the short-term variations of speech amplitude. **Fig. 17–3** shows both the long-term average level and the maximum level as functions of frequency. The maximum

---

[1] Indoors, the 6 dB rule only applies up to a certain distance. Beyond this distance, the useful energy reaching the listener is determined by reflections from the room's boundaries. Unfortunately, these useful early reflections are accompanied by later reflections, or reverberation, which can have a negative effect on perception of the received signal (Boothroyd, 2004). The effects of room acoustics on the effectiveness of hearing aids and cochlear implants is an important and complex topic and beyond the scope of the present chapter.

[2] An octave band is a range of frequencies in which the highest frequency is twice the lowest. In a one third-octave band, the highest frequency is 1.26 times the lowest. The ear integrates energy over roughly one third of an octave.

[3] This spectrum is different for men, women, and children; it varies with talker within each of these groups; it changes with vocal effort; it changes with orientation of the talker with respect to the listener; and it changes somewhat with distance when close to the talker's mouth (Pittman et al, 2003).

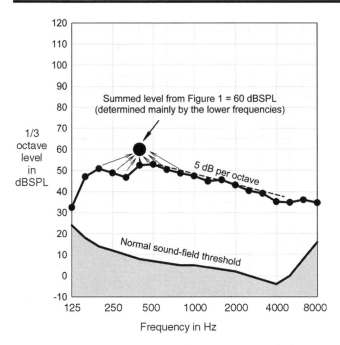

Figure 17–2 Long-term average speech spectrum, in one third octave bands, derived from a 20-second sample of a woman's speech. Talker distance is assumed to be 4 feet (see **Fig. 17–1**). The line continues in **Fig. 17–3**.

levels are measured over short periods lasting around .5 of a second. Also shown are the minimum levels below which there is unlikely to be any useful information. These levels are placed 30 dB below the maximum levels.[4] The result is an area on the amplitude-versus-frequency graph representing the boundaries of the distribution of useful information in the acoustic speech signal. This area is shown in **Fig. 17–3** along with the normal threshold of hearing.

The Performance versus Intensity Function

The 30 dB intensity range of speech is responsible for the 30 dB range of the normal performance versus intensity (P/I) function. This function records the percentage of speech units recognized as the average speech level rises from below threshold. The speech units can be phonemes (vowels and consonants), monosyllables in isolation, spondees in isolation, words in sentences, etc. **Fig. 17–4** shows the P/I function for phonemes in consonant-vowel-consonant (CVC) words. Phoneme recognition begins to rise above zero as the speech area first peeps above threshold and approaches 100% when the whole area is above threshold. Note that the speech area has been restricted to the region between 300 and 6000 Hz in **Fig. 17–4,** this being the region that contains most of the acoustic cues responsible for phoneme recognition. Note, also, that when roughly 50% of the speech area is above threshold, phoneme recognition is already around 80%—reflecting the ability of normally hearing users of

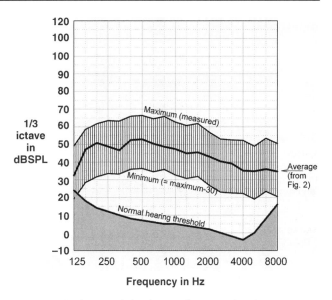

Figure 17–3 The speech level in any frequency band varies over a range of around 30 dB, from 15 dB above the average to 15 dB below it. The resulting speech area is shown here with vertical shading, in relation to the threshold of normal hearing. The shaded area continues in **Fig. 17–4**.

spoken language to take advantage of phonemic and lexical redundancy to compensate for an incomplete signal.[5]

Representing Speech on the Audiogram Form

So far, all representations of amplitude have been in SPL with sound level increasing as we move upward on the amplitude-versus-frequency graphs. This approach is widely used when dealing with hearing aid testing and fitting. In the intervention world, however, clinicians and educators are more familiar with the audiogram form. On this form, amplitude is measured in relation to the normal hearing threshold, and sound level increases as we move downward. The transformation is illustrated in **Fig. 17–5**. In this context, the speech area is commonly referred to as the speech banana. In the current example, the banana looks a little crumpled. These data, however, were derived from a 20-second sample of the speech of a specific talker. The more familiar representation shows the average of many talkers and is somewhat smoother, as shown in subsequent figures.

Information and Frequency

The information in speech is distributed unevenly across frequencies.

Pearl

- The highest concentration of information is found between about 1000 and 3000 Hz with progressively less at higher and lower frequencies.
---

[4] It is difficult to specify a meaningful minimum level because speech can contain breaks and pauses. It is generally accepted, however, that the useful information at any frequency is uniformly distributed over a range of around 30 dB. This assumption is incorporated into the computation of Speech Intelligibility Index (ANSI, 1997).

[5] Young children with hearing loss cannot be assumed to have the skills or knowledge needed to compensate for an incomplete signal. They need full access if they are to acquire them.

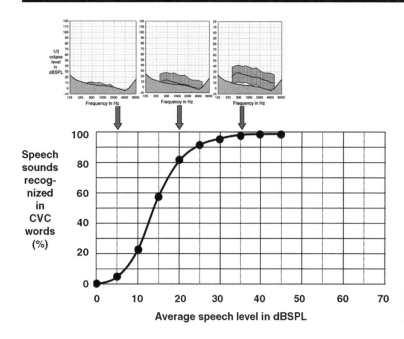

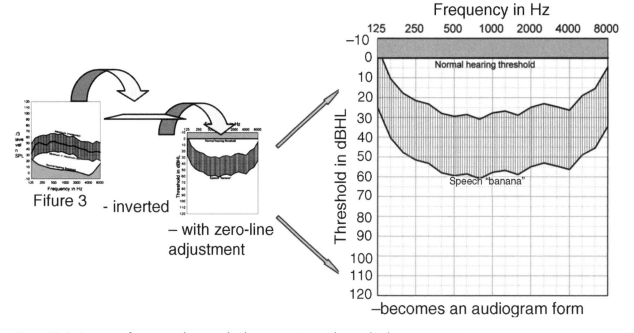

Figure 17–4 The decibel range of the performance versus intensity function reflects the short term amplitude range of the speech signal. CVC, consonant–vowel–consonant.

Figure 17–5 Conversion from a sound pressure level representation to a hearing level representation.

This point is illustrated by the concentration of dots in **Fig. 17–6**. There are 100 dots, so a little counting serves to identify the percentage of useful information in different frequency regions.[6] Also shown in **Fig. 17–6** are the frequency ranges of certain acoustic and phonetic features, discussed below.

[6] This way of representing the relative importance of different frequencies is based on the "count the dots" approach of Mueller and Killion (1990)

Acoustic Properties and Frequency

The concentration of information in the 1000 to 3000 Hz region is by no means coincidental. This is the region covered by the second vocal-tract formant. A formant is a peak in the short-term spectrum of speech caused by resonance in the oral cavities (Pickett, 1999). There are many formants, and they are numbered in order of increasing frequency. The second formant is produced by resonance of the cavity at the front of the mouth—from tongue to lips. For an adult male talker, its frequency varies over a 3:1 range from around 900 to 2700 Hz. (In women and

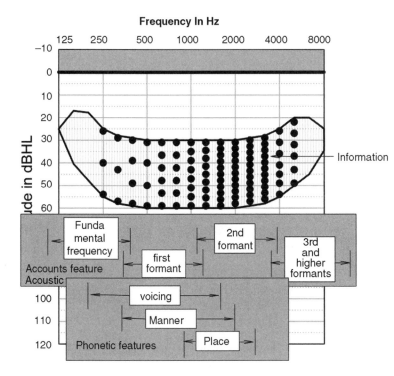

Figure 17–6 The relative importance of different parts of the speech banana is shown here by the distribution of dots. Also shown are the frequency ranges covered by some acoustic and phonetic features of the speech signal

children the values are somewhat higher.) The frequency at any moment is determined by a combination of the size of the lip opening and the location of the narrowest portion of the oral cavity, which depends mainly on the position and shape of the tongue. The frequency of the second formant (and the way it changes over time) provides the listener with information about the positions, shapes, and movements of tongue and lips. These articulators are responsible for many of the distinctions among the sound patterns of spoken language—hence the major importance of the frequency region covered by the second formant.

Of somewhat less importance, but also useful, is the first formant. This is produced by resonance of the whole oral cavity—from larynx to lips. For an adult male talker, its frequency varies over a 3:1 range from around 300 to 900 Hz. (Once again, in women and children the values are somewhat higher.) The frequency at any moment is determined by the vertical size of the oral cavity. The frequency of the first formant and the way it changes over time provide the listener with information about the raising and lowering of the jaw and tongue as well as the opening and closing of the lips.

The higher formants carry information about fricative sounds such as "sh" and "s" as well as bursts such as "ch" and "t." They also help the listener identify the talker.

The melodic pattern of speech is determined by voice fundamental frequency. This is the frequency at which the vocal folds vibrate. It covers a range of about 3:1 with an average around 100 Hz for men, 200 Hz for women, and higher for children. The value of fundamental frequency and its variation over time provide the listener with information, not just about talker age and gender, but also about

such things as syllable and word stress, phrase and sentence boundaries, and the talker's emotional state.

Pearl

- Interestingly, the listener does not need to hear the fundamental frequency but can acquire information about it from higher frequencies, especially from the region of the first formant.

Information about the frequency ranges covered by these acoustic cues is included in **Fig. 17–6**.

♦ Phonetic Features and Frequency

The acoustic properties mentioned above carry information about articulatory features that are responsible for defining the sound system of the language. Three features of consonant articulation are of special interest to clinicians and educators. These are voicing, manner of articulation, and place of articulation. Miller and Nicely (1955) published the results of a series of experiments on the effects of filtering on consonant confusions. From their data, Boothroyd (1978), determined, for each consonant feature, the frequency ranges containing the bulk of the useful information. This information is included in **Fig. 17–6**. The most striking feature of these data is that the range for identification of place of consonant articulation is very close to the range containing

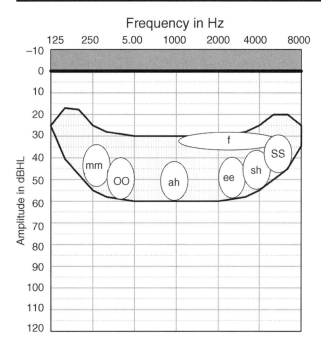

Figure 17–7 The locations of the key acoustic cues needed for recognition of selected speech sounds.

the highest concentration of information. This is not a coincidence. Consonants contribute considerably to intelligibility, and place of articulation carries more information about consonant identity than does either of the other two features. Moreover, the second vocal-tract formant is the primary cue for place of articulation.

Phonemes, Amplitude, and Frequency

Spoken vowels and consonants are identified by acoustic patterns. These patterns involve components that cover a wide range of frequencies, they change over time, and they are influenced by the sounds that precede and follow them. It is, therefore, difficult to allocate specific phonemes to specific locations within the speech banana. There are a few sounds, however, whose key acoustic cues are restricted to a relatively small frequency region, and we can be reasonably certain that they will not be recognized if those regions are inaudible. A sample of such sounds is shown in **Fig. 17–7,** which is based on experimental data (Boothroyd, Erickson, and Medwetsky, 1994).[7] Some of these sounds are

used in the Ling 5- or 6-sound test to confirm that a child can hear and identify speech patterns over an appropriate range of frequencies (Ling, 1989).

The Audiogram and the Speech Banana

When pure-tone thresholds are recorded on an audiogram form, the result is an audiogram. The line joining the Os or Xs divides the form into two regions. Above the line are inaudible sounds—the lost hearing. Below the line are audible sounds—the remaining or residual hearing. By examining the audiogram in relation to the speech banana, we can obtain a sense of the acoustic cues, the percent information, the consonant features, and even the types of speech sound that are available to the child through the sense of hearing. Consider, for example, the audiogram represented in **Fig. 17–8**. If we assume that this is the child's better ear, we can see that she should be able to recognize those sounds whose identity depends on low-frequency patterns, but she will be unable even to hear high-frequency sounds such as "sh" and "s" (also "ch" and "t"), let alone recognize them. And even though she will hear the "ee" sound, it will be indistinguishable from an "oo." If we were also to overlay this audiogram on **Fig. 17–6**, we would see that only about 30% of the useful acoustic information in the acoustic speech is available to this child—basically, that contained in the first formant and the variations of amplitude and fundamental frequency over time. We would also conclude that she will have great difficulty identifying (and, therefore, reproducing) place of consonant articulation.

Special Consideration

- Without appropriate intervention, this child (with what is commonly referred to as moderate hearing loss) will experience serious delays of language acquisition and will develop serious errors in her own speech.

The Aided Audiogram and the Speech Banana

Now contrast **Fig. 17–8** with **Fig. 17–9,** in which we compare the speech banana with the aided audiogram.[8] Most of the phonemes shown here have been rendered audible. There is, however, a restriction on the audibility of the highest frequencies, particularly, of the sound "s." This restriction occurs because current hearing aids are incapable of

---

[7] Illustrations such as this must be interpreted with caution. For example, the frequency range of the key resonance in the sound "s" tends to be much higher for women than for men; it varies within each gender group; and it is highly dependent on the preceding or following vowels (Boothroyd & Medwetsky, 1992). Recognition of the sound "ee" depends on audibility of the second formant (around 2500 Hz), but detection depends mainly on the first formant, which is almost identical to that of the sound "oo." If the second formant of "ee" is inaudible, "ee" and "oo" tend to be confused. More importantly, simple audibility of a given speech sound is no guarantee that it will be recognized or distinguished from similar sounds.

[8] The difference between the aided and unaided thresholds reflects the gain of the hearing aid, at least for very low inputs. With the introduction of wide-dynamic-range-compression hearing aids, the aided audiogram has become inappropriate as a way of estimating effective hearing aid gain. Because gain falls with increasing input, illustrations such as **Fig. 17** tend to overestimate gain for realistic speech inputs. Nevertheless, this remains a valid technique for deciding whether a given sound is audible via aided hearing – providing one keeps a clear distinction between audibility and recognition.

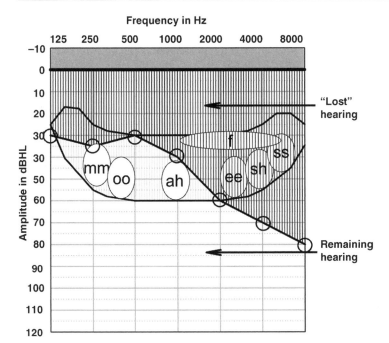

Figure 17–8 Examining a child's audiogram in relation to the speech banana provides insights into the child's access to acoustic speech information.

providing substantial gain at the higher frequencies (Stelmachowicz et al, 2001, 2002). One must also be very cautious when interpreting an illustration such as this. The damage to the hearing mechanism that produces the threshold shift also causes a loss of spectral and temporal resolution. As a result, the child may still have difficulty identifying and differentiating sounds, even when they have been made audible. In addition, reduced spectral and temporal resolution renders the listener highly susceptible to the interfering effects of background noise—a complaint of all hearing aid users. To emphasize these limitations, the higher frequency sounds in **Fig. 17–9** are shown with reduced font size.

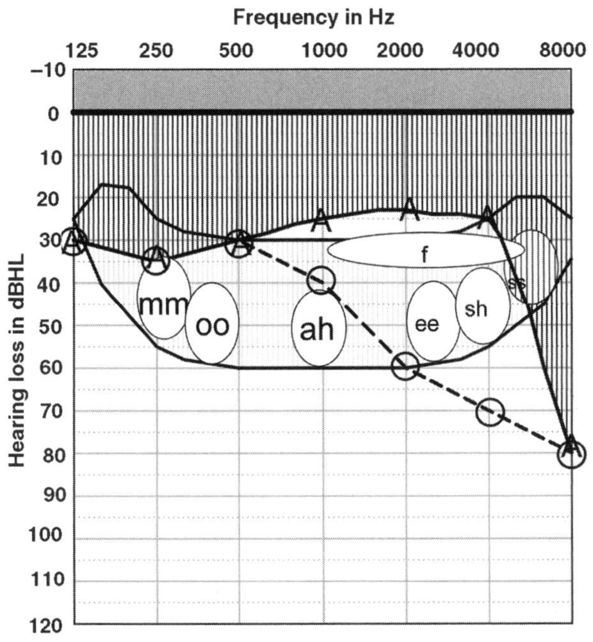

The Speech Banana and Cochlear Implants

Pearl

- A hearing aid amplifies speech and presents it in acoustic form to the ear. In contrast, a cochlear implant extracts information from the acoustic signal and recodes it in electrical form for direct presentation to the nerves of hearing, and in a manner that is matched (or mapped) to the individual's characteristics.

Instead, it depends on such things as the number of electrodes and their location in relation to independently stimulable auditory nerve cells. With modern implants, there is every reason to expect that temporal resolution will be preserved. The small number of independent channels of stimulation, however, are unable to provide normal spectral resolution. Appropriate mapping can usually provide audibility over a wide frequency range, including the high frequencies typically unavailable to the hearing aid user, as shown in **Fig. 17–10**. Because of reduced spectral resolution, however, the resulting hearing will exhibit problems of discrimination and noise susceptibility similar to those experienced by children with moderately severe hearing loss who use hearing aids. Again, this effect is emphasized in **Fig. 17–10** by a reduction of font size.

Figure 17–9 The effect of amplification on audibility of the speech signal is illustrated by showing the speech banana in relation to the aided soundfield threshold.

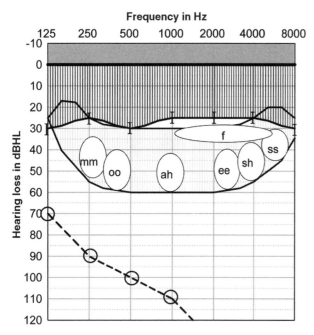

Figure 17–10 Modern multichannel cochlear implants can provide profoundly and totally deaf children with audibility of the speech spectrum over a wide range of frequencies. Unlike hearing aids, the implant is not constrained in terms of an upper frequency limit and it is not susceptible to acoustic feedback. The limited number of independent channels of stimulation, however, still leads to reduced spectral resolution when compared with normal hearing.

tration of useful information is between around 1000 and 3000 Hz. This is the range covered by the second vocal-tract formant, which conveys considerable information about place of articulation. At any frequency, the short-term amplitude varies between 15 dB above and below the average. The resulting range of 30 dB is reflected in the normal P/I function, in which recognition of speech elements rises from 0 to 100% over a range of about 30 dB as speech emerges from inaudibility to full audibility. Expressing levels in relation to normal hearing threshold, and transferring them to an audiogram form, results in the speech banana. Examination of this area in relation to a child's audiogram can provide insights into the acoustic cues, phonetic cues, and phonemes that are likely to be accessible to the child through the unaided sense of hearing. The same technique can be used to show the potential benefits of assistance with hearing aids or cochlear implants, providing one recognizes that the resulting hearing is not perfect and that difficulties of discrimination and noise susceptibility are likely to remain. Providing access to the information contained in the acoustic patterns of speech is an essential first step in auditory-oral intervention, but it is only the first step.

Acknowledgments   Preparation of this chapter was supported, in part, by NIH grant # DC006238 to the House Ear Institute.

♦ Summary

A first step in auditory-oral intervention is to optimize hearing so that the child has access to as much of the information as possible in the acoustic speech signal. This signal, which has an overall level of around 60 dB SPL when measured at a conversational distance, contains components that are distributed across a wide frequency range, from around 100 Hz to higher than 8000 Hz. Most of the energy is in frequency regions below 1000 Hz but the maximum concen-

Discussion Questions

1. Discuss the configuration of the normal P/I function.

2. Describe the utility of the speech banana.

3. Detail the difficulties that a child with a mild hearing loss will have discriminating speech in the presence of noise.

4. Why is a cochlear implant not an amplifier?

References

ANSI. (1997). American national standard methods for calculation of the speech intelligibility index. New York: American National Standards Institute.

Boothroyd, A. (1978). Speech perception and sensorineural hearing loss. In M. Ross and G. Giolas (Eds.), Auditory management of the hearing impaired child. Baltimore: University Park Press.

Boothroyd, A. (2004). Room acoustics and speech perception. Seminars in Hearing, 25, 155–166.

Boothroyd, A., Erickson, F., and Medwetsky, L. (1994). The hearing aid input: a phonemic approach to assessing the spectral distribution of speech. Ear & Hearing, 15, 432–442.

Boothroyd, A., and Medwetsky, L. (1992). Spectral distribution of /s/ and the frequency response of hearing aids. Ear and Hearing, 13, 150–157.

Ling, D. (1989). The Foundations of spoken language for hearing-impaired children. Washington, DC: A.G. Bell Association for the Deaf.

Mueller, G. H., and Killion, M. C. (1990). An easy method for calculating the articulation index. Hearing Journal, 9, 14–17.

Pickett, J. M. (1999). The acoustics of speech communication. Needham Heights: Allyn and Bacon.

Pittman, A. L., Stelmachowicz, P. G., Lewis, D. E., and Hoover, B. M. (2003). Spectral characteristics of speech at the ear: implications for amplification in children. Journal of Speech, Language, and Hearing Research, 46, 649-657.

Robinson, D. W., and Dadson, R. S. (1956). A re-determination of the equal loudness relations for pure tones. British Journal of Applied Physics, 7, 166–181.

Sivian, L. J., and White, S. D. (1933). On minimal audible sound fields. Journal of the Acoustical Society of America, 4, 288–321.

Stelmachowicz, P. G., Pittman, A. L., Hoover, B. M., and Lewis, D. E. (2001). Effect of stimulus bandwidth on the perception of /s/ in normal- and hearing-impaired children and adults. Journal of the Acoustical Society of America, 110, 2183–2190.

Stelmachowicz, P. G., Pittman, A. L., Hoover, B. M., and Lewis, D. E. (2002). Aided perception of /s/ and /z/ by hearing-impaired children. Ear & Hearing, 23, 316–324.

Chapter 18

Hearing Aids for Infants and Children

Harvey Dillon, Teresa Ching, and Maryanne Golding

The implementation of universal hearing screening programs makes it possible to detect hearing impairment early in life. Clinicians face multiple challenges in providing effective amplification to infants and young children, because methods that have been established for adults are not always directly applicable to young children.

There are three major reasons why special considerations apply to fitting hearing aids to children. First, they have smaller ears than adults, and their ear canal acoustics change rapidly over the first few years of life. This variation in ear canal acoustics potentially affects the accuracy of hearing thresholds. The changing resonant characteristics of a child's unaided ear canal over time requires that prescriptive targets be specified in terms of real-ear aided gain (REAG) rather than real-ear insertion gain (REIG) if the amplified levels at a child's eardrum are to provide consistent stimulation to the auditory system as the child grows. Second, infants have limited ability to provide reliable behavioral and verbal responses to stimuli. This necessitates the use of electrophysiologic measures in estimating hearing thresholds before reliable behavioral audiograms can be established, the use of coupler gain measures to verify that

REAG targets are matched in hearing aids, and the use of parental observations and electrophysiological measures in evaluating the effectiveness of hearing aids. Third, children rely on amplification to develop speech and language and to acquire knowledge of the world around them. They need better signal-to-noise (SNR) ratios than adults for perceiving speech, and they need access to sounds in their environment for incidental learning. Hearing aid technologies should be selected to meet the special needs of children.

♦ Selection of Hearing Aids: New Technologies

Wireless Compatibility

The passage of sound across a room inevitably degrades its quality. A hearing aid microphone detects the original sound, the reverberation of that sound around the room, noise from any other sources inside the room and possibly outside the room, and reverberation of the noise. Only the first of these signals helps the child understand speech; the rest degrade understanding. (As an exception, the very early echoes can also enhance intelligibility by increasing the level of speech, but most reverberant energy is detrimental to intelligibility.) By contrast, the wireless transmission of sound in the form of electrical energy can pass over huge distances with little or no degradation of sound quality. Wireless systems may be based on frequency modulation (FM) radio frequency or infrared transmission, or on magnetic loop induction.

Consequently, children are likely to benefit from wireless transmission of speech whenever they have to listen to someone from a distance of, say, 1 meter or farther. The greater the hearing loss and the greater the difficulty in understanding speech, the greater will be the benefit that wireless transmission offers. The primary limitation is achieving the cooperation of the person or persons talking. When there is just one talker, the situation is clear: the talker wears a transmitter, including a microphone mounted as close as possible to the mouth, and the child wears a receiver coupled to, or integral with, his hearing aids. In many situations, however, there are several people to whom the child needs to listen, including the child himself. The hearing aid must therefore appropriately combine the signal detected by the wireless receiver with the signal detected by the hearing aid microphone. Here the difficulties start because mixing the two signals can adversely affect the intelligibility of each, whereas a wireless signal can easily offer as much as a 20 dB improvement in SNR over acoustic reception. This will be substantially degraded (but still be beneficial) if the wireless and microphone paths are adjusted to have similar sensitivity.

The best mixing solution is when the receiver and hearing aid combination automatically gives high priority to the wireless signal whenever it recognizes voice activity in the wireless channel, and turns off the wireless channel when no voice activity is detected. Sadly, although such speech-operated switching systems have been available for at least 20 years, most wireless systems on the market do not have this feature. Consequently, the clinician must ensure that the hearing aid and receiver are adjusted to achieve the desired relativity between the wireless and hearing aid microphone signals. This is a difficult choice: too little and the advantage of the wireless system is largely lost; too great and the child will have inadequate audibility when someone other than the user of the transmitter is talking. Reflecting the difficulty of this choice, the ratio of wireless to microphone level at the output of the hearing aid has been recommended by different people (for a summary see Dillon, 2001) to be from 5 to 15 dB.

Wireless transmission to hearing aids has been available for 3 decades. The major change in this technology is that the receivers available are now small enough to clip onto the hearing aid, or be entirely contained within the hearing aid, rather than as large external devices.

Compression

There is no doubt that compression (nonlinear amplification) should be prescribed for children, and it is particularly beneficial for children too young to use a volume control. The major advantages of compression are that, relative to a linear amplifier with a fixed gain-frequency response, gain is increased for lower level sounds (increasing intelligibility) and decreased for higher level sounds (increasing comfort and acoustic safety). Although an adult or older child can achieve a similar result by using a volume control, an infant or younger child cannot. Fortunately, the gains prescribed by both major generic prescription rules, National Acoustic Laboratories (NAL)-NL1 and DSL[i/o], and by all proprietary prescription rules, inherently contain compression. Consequently, the clinician does not explicitly have to choose compression if hearing aids are adjusted to match these prescriptions.

Some clinicians have chosen not to provide compression for people (of any age) with severe to profound hearing loss. This choice may be based on some early research indicating that compression was mostly detrimental for people with such losses (Boothroyd et al, 1988). More recent research, aimed at discovering the optimal degree of compression, indicates that it is appropriate to provide compression for even these greater degrees of loss (Keidser et al, 2007a). In extensive listening trials in real-life conditions, a low compression ratio, particularly for the low frequencies, was preferred to either linear amplification or to higher compression ratios. Compression in moderation for severe or profound loss therefore appears to be the key. It is not known whether children should be prescribed fast- or slow-acting compression. Gatehouse, Naylor, and Elberling, (2006) have shown that for adults, the more alert the person and the more dynamic the listening environment, the greater the advantage of fast-acting compression over slow-acting, on average. The application of this to children remains unknown.

Noise Reduction and Speech Enhancement

Noise reduction or speech enhancement systems in hearing aids work by reducing the gain in a frequency region when the SNR in that region is poorer than in other frequency regions, or poorer than some preset criterion amount. Some hearing aids are designed to be sufficiently fast acting that the gain changes in the gaps between the syllables of speech; others are designed to be sufficiently slow acting that the gain fluctuates over periods of seconds or tens of seconds. In both cases, the result is that those frequency regions where noise dominates are deemphasized relative to other regions where speech is more dominant. Many studies over the decades (for a summary see Dillon, 2001) have shown that adults prefer noise suppression on the grounds that listening comfort is greater, and that noise is less salient, even though noise reduction has little or no effect on intelligibility. Although there are no experimental data about whether children have the same preferences, there does not seem to be any strong reason why their preferences should be different. Some have argued that the spectrum presented to children should not be altered while children are still learning to understand speech. However, the audible spectrum alters every time a different person talks, or the talker and listener move to a different room, or a different masking noise occurs. The spectral changes caused by noise suppression are relatively small compared with these and are always in the direction of making speech more salient. We therefore tentatively recommend that noise reduction systems in hearing aids be routinely enabled for children of all ages, just as they are for adults.

One particular form of noise suppression now available in hearing aids is transient suppression. This processing strategy recognizes when the waveform is changing at a rate so high it cannot be the result of a speech signal, and it reduces the gain of the signal during this portion of rapid change. The result is that the loudness of impulsive sounds such as doors slamming or hammering is greatly reduced (Keidser et al, 2007b). The processing has no adverse effect on speech and can be left permanently activated.

Directional Microphones

It is clear from physical principles that if a child is looking at a sound source, if the distance from the child to the source is not too much greater than the critical distance of the room, and if there is noise or reverberation in the environment, directional microphones will offer an improved SNR. Notwithstanding the ample evidence on the benefits of directional amplification for adults, this technology is rarely used in the fitting of young children for two reasons. First, it is not known in what proportion of a child's life the circumstances would be such that directional amplification would significantly improve SNR and speech perception. Second, there are no empirical data about the fundamental limitations of directional amplification that are due to head movements of children and the acoustics of their real-life environments. Young children do not always turn their heads to maintain eye contact with the talker in real-life situations. As such, fitting directional amplification may not lead to any benefits and may sometimes even limit children's access to incidental learning that results from sounds arriving from nonfrontal directions.

In laboratory settings, the benefit of directional microphones for school-aged children has been demonstrated by presenting speech from 0° azimuth and noise from 180° azimuth (Gravel et al, 1999). The children tested, ranging in age from 4 to 11 years, obtained an improvement of 5 dB on average when they used directional microphones to listen to words and sentences presented in multitalker babble than when they used omnidirectional amplification. Consistent with findings in earlier studies, children younger than 7 years required better SNR than older children to achieve the same level of performance.

In everyday life, children are often in situations where they listen to speech of a primary talker in the presence of other competing talkers and noises. When the target speech is spatially separated from competing sounds rather than spatially coincident, it has been shown that normally hearing children obtain an advantage of about 3 dB on average (Litovsky, 2005; Ching et al, 2006a). This is because they can combine information from both ears to partially reduce the impact of noise and benefit from binaural release of masking. However, many children with hearing loss from birth have deficits in binaural processing and are unable to

take advantage of the spatial separation between speech and noise (Litovsky, Johnstone, and Godar, 2006; Ching et al, 2006a). If evaluation of aided performance reveals that a child has a lot of difficulty listening to speech in noisy situations [e.g., by administering the Parental Evaluation of Aural/Oral Performance Children (PEACH) questionnaire, see below] or exhibits deficits in binaural processing (as shown in the absence of benefit from spatial separation, see below), the need for binaural directional amplification is very strong indeed. Results to date in a current NAL experiment investigating the efficacy of directional microphones in real-life listening situations suggest that once a child is old enough to routinely look at the person talking to him, directional microphones will provide benefit in most listening situations.

> **Pearl**
>
> • Enable directional microphones when the child is old enough to routinely look at the person talking to him.

Feedback Management and Canceling

Whenever the REAG of a hearing aid exceeds the attenuation of the signal as it leaks from the ear canal, out past the earmold, to the hearing aid microphone, feedback oscillation (whistling) is likely. Once it occurs, feedback oscillation reduces the amplification that the hearing aid can provide to external sounds, may mask perception of other sounds, and may be annoying to the child and to those in the vicinity. Feedback oscillation must therefore be prevented. There are two broad ways to achieve this.

The oldest method is feedback management, in which the gain of the hearing aid is reduced sufficiently to avoid oscillation, using one of the following options:

♦ Decrease the overall gain of the hearing aid.

♦ Decrease the gain of the hearing aid in a restricted frequency region, such as in one channel.

♦ Decrease the overall maximum gain that a broad-band compression amplifier can provide (which will always be the gain that applies in quiet situations).

♦ Decrease the maximum gain that the compression amplifiers in each channel of a multichannel hearing aid can provide.

Those methods further down the list are preferable to those higher up the list, because the gain reduction is increasingly restricted to frequencies and input levels at which the high gain is a problem. That is, although all the methods can prevent oscillation, the methods lower down the list do not reduce audibility to the same extent that methods higher up the list do. The terminology for achieving feedback management varies from hearing aid to hearing aid.

The second broad mechanism is to use feedback cancellation. Most advanced hearing aids now include a feedback canceling algorithm that automatically detects feedback oscillation and attempts to suppress it. Cancellation is achieved by a feedback path within the (digital) amplification sound path. The characteristics of this feedback path are automatically varied by the hearing aid so that the path has the same amplitude but the opposite phase (sometimes called anti-sound), to the external leakage that is causing the problem. As a consequence, the external leakage is canceled by the internal leakage. Unfortunately, exact cancellation is impossible. Feedback cancellation thus enables an additional 10 to 15 dB of gain to be achieved before oscillation occurs, rather than solving the problem. There can be some minor quality degradation when cancellation is actually occurring, but this is preferable to allowing oscillation. The other disadvantage is that many feedback cancellers can mistake sustained musical tones as feedback oscillation, and attempt to cancel them. For older children for whom listening to music is important, the ability to disengage feedback cancellation and use feedback management (in a second program of the hearing aid) may be advantageous. Feedback cancelling should otherwise routinely be selected for hearing aids for children, unless the loss is so moderate that feedback oscillation is unlikely to be a problem.

Transposition

Transposition (also called frequency compression) produces output in one frequency region (usual low or mid-frequency) in response to input signal energy in another frequency region (usually high frequency). They are usually intended to enable people to recover information from the high-frequency parts of speech, despite having no ability to directly recover information from high-frequency sound, either because it is inaudible, even after amplification, or because the person has no residual frequency selectivity. Evaluations of the effect of transposition on speech intelligibility over several decades have produced very mixed results. This is not surprising, as there are many varieties of transposition. First, there are the questions of which frequency range of speech is to be moved downward, and which frequency range it is to be moved to. This immediately raises the question of what should be done with the speech energy already in this lower frequency range. Some systems move this down also, others just superimpose the two signals within the same frequency range. Both methods have the potential to disrupt the extraction of information from this lower frequency range. Other systems attempt to avoid this problem by allowing transposition to occur only when no significant low frequency energy is present. In addition, there are several technical methods by which high-frequency information can be turned into low-frequency modulation (frequency shifting, frequency warping, vocoding), each producing its own inherent distortions. Lastly, there is the difficult question of which hearing loss profiles are most likely to benefit from transposition.

Based on the published literature (for a summary see Dillon, 2001), it is possible to conclude that transposition can sometimes increase intelligibility, but that not all transposition schemes have positive results. There is not yet a sufficient body of knowledge to conclude which forms of transposition will be beneficial for which clients. Consequently, it does not seem appropriate to fit transposition hearing aids to children who are still learning the sounds and uses of speech, as it is not clear how readily any speech patterns based on shifted energy could be relearned later in life. It may be reasonable to try transposition hearing aids on older children to determine if increased perception of high frequency sounds can be achieved without excessively affecting the intelligibility of other sounds. Fortunately, those children for whom conventional amplification is inadequate to communicate well are now extremely likely to benefit from cochlear implantation, so the need for an effective transposition hearing aid has diminished.

Trainability

A new concept in hearing aids is to make them trainable. A trainable hearing aid is one in which the hearing aid memorizes settings selected by the user, and desirably also measures and memorizes the characteristics of the speech and noise at the time the user made the adjustment (Dillon et al, 2006a). Over time, and over multiple adjustments, the hearing aid builds up a relationship between the acoustic characteristics of the input signals and the preferences of the user. The hearing aid can then automatically select the preferred characteristics each time input signals with similar characteristics occur. Sophisticated trainable hearing aids will also be able to predict, and automatically select, preferred characteristics for situations not previously encountered, by generalizing from the range of situations in which the hearing aids have been trained. A prototype trainable aid has proved to be effective, but has so far been evaluated only on adults (Zakis, Dillon, and McDermott, submitted).

Should children be allowed access to the trainability feature? The task asked of the hearing aid wearer is to adjust a control until the sound is clearest. This is little different in complexity than performing a paired-comparison task either in the clinic or at home with a two-program hearing aid. Children (with hearing impairment but no other developmental delay) aged 8 years or older are able to do both of these tasks reliably. Children of this age are also able to take direct responsibility for selecting between wireless input and combined wireless/hearing aid input, another task of similar complexity. It therefore seems reasonable to use trainability for children aged 8 years or older. Although there is no reason to expect that children will train the hearing aid to produce output levels intense enough to damage their remaining hearing, it would be beneficial if manufacturers provided the ability to limit the degree to which the hearing aid gain could be increased above the prescribed settings at each frequency, particularly for the gain applied to higher level sounds.

Earmolds

Earmolds for older children are little or no different from those for adults, but earmolds for infants are small! The very small size has several implications. First, when an impression is taken, a very small cotton block is needed if a sufficient insertion depth is to be achieved. Best results can be achieved with blocks custom made (from cotton-wool and thread) to best suit each ear, rather than the often-too-large ready-made ones. Second, the small size usually makes it impossible to fit in a vent or acoustic horn. Infants whose hearing loss is detected at birth usually have a sufficiently large loss that vents are not needed. If one is required, an external vent can be created by grinding a slit down the outside of the earmold. Far more commonly, the clinician would like to be able to stop leakage around the mold (rather than create it with a vent). The third issue arising from small ear canal size is that small ear canals grow rapidly, causing the earmold to become loose and leak, in turn causing feedback oscillation, or causing the earmold to fall out. Earmolds are likely to have to be made monthly up to 6 months of age, bimonthly up to 12 months, and three to four times per year up to the age of 3 years.

Earmolds for infants and younger children are usually made of soft materials, either because the softer materials are thought to have less leakage, or because they are inherently safer if the child's activities are likely to result in an accidental blow to the ear. Unfortunately, soft materials degrade faster, but this is not such a problem when they have to be regularly replaced because of ear canal growth. For ears prone to discharge, hard materials, and a spare set of molds to enable cleaning and drying, are advantageous.

Retaining hearing aids in place on small ears can be a problem. Devices that assist with this problem include double-sided sticky tape, extra-small earhooks, extra-stiff (moisture resistant) tubing, and Huggies to hold the hearing aid to the pinna. Finally, hyperallergenic coatings are available, and brightly colored earmolds are extremely popular.

Prescription of Hearing Aids

Once the diagnosis of hearing loss is confirmed, tympanometry, or high-frequency tympanometry, should be performed (Purdy and Williams, 2000, Feeney and Sanford, Chapter 13, this volume) to obtain information about middle ear function. In addition, acoustic reflex testing should be used to rule out retrocochlear pathology, and otoacoustic emissions testing should be carried out to determine if

further review for auditory neuropathy (Purdy and Kelly, Chapter 15; Austin Duff and Franck, Chapter 32, this volume) is necessary. To proceed with aiding, it is necessary to determine an audiogram, to adopt an approach that caters to the special needs of children, and to fit bilateral amplification according to a prescriptive procedure.

Audiogram

An optimal hearing aid fitting starts with an accurate audiogram. An important consideration in determining an audiogram for fitting is that the small ear canal sizes of infants and young children influence the validity of conventional audiometric measures. Because audiometers are conventionally calibrated such that an average adult has normal hearing thresholds of 0 dB hearing level (HL), constant across transducers, the same will not be true for children whose ear canals are shorter and narrower than those of adults. If insert earphones are used in determining thresholds, the volume of the ear canal directly affects the sound pressure level generated at the eardrum. As a child grows, the canal volume increases, and the sound pressure level (SPL) generated at the eardrum decreases. This in turn causes apparent hearing thresholds to "deteriorate" with increase in age. If soundfield assessment is used, the length of the ear canal determines its resonance properties or the real-ear unaided gain (REUG), and hence affects the threshold expressed as level in the undisturbed field. If headphones are used, both the volume and the length of the ear canal will affect thresholds. These effects render the audiometer dial readings inaccurate when measuring thresholds of anyone, including a child, who does not have an average adult ear canal. A consequence is that hearing thresholds measured using different audiometric transducers (insert earphones, soundfield loudspeakers, supraaural headphones) are not equivalent. To resolve this anomaly, there are two possible solutions. First, children's thresholds can be expressed in terms of dB SPL at the eardrum (Seewald and Scollie, 2003). This method involves measuring a child's real-ear-to-coupler difference (RECD) (i.e., the difference between the level of a signal in the ear canal and the level of the same signal in a coupler). The RECD can be used to convert hearing thresholds in dB HL to ear canal SPL. The equations used in the transformations are given in Bagatto et al (2005), and the calculation is done automatically in the desired sensation level (DSL) fitting software (Seewald et al, 1997; Scollie et al, 2005). This representation allows easy comparison of threshold levels with aided speech levels in the real ear. Second, an equally effective solution is to express thresholds in terms of adult equivalent hearing level. This is the threshold level that an average adult would have if the adult has the same threshold in dB SPL at the eardrum as the child (Dillon, 2001). The same techniques (using RECD) are used to determine the threshold SPL in the ear canal, but these thresholds are then converted to average equivalent hearing level by subtracting the average adult RECD (Ching and Dillon, 2003). The calculation is done automatically in the NAL fitting software (Dillon, 1999). As hearing loss is represented in terms of the familiar dB HL, the magnitude of the hearing loss is more easily grasped.

A second consideration in determining an audiogram for fitting arises from the fact that behavioral thresholds are often not available for children diagnosed with hearing loss soon after birth. Instead, auditory evoked potentials that provide frequency-specific information for each ear are used to estimate hearing thresholds. (Chapter 6 describes a behavioral evaluation technique that can successfully be used with infants.) The available electrophysiologic measures include auditory brainstem responses (ABRs; Stapells et al, 1995), auditory steady state responses (ASSRs; Rance et al, 2005), and electrocochleography (ECoG; Wong, Gibson, and Sanli, 1997). Threshold estimations obtained from auditory evoked potentials are referenced in dB normalized HL (dB nHL). This normative reference is defined differently across systems, but the calibration of systems invariably is based on obtaining behavioral thresholds from adults for the stimuli used in evoking auditory potentials (Stapells et al, 1995; see Bagatto et al, 2005 for a discussion). Correction figures for estimating behavioral thresholds in dB HL from ABR-derived thresholds in dB nHL have been derived by relating measured behavioral thresholds to ABR-derived thresholds of adults and older children with stimuli presented under headphones (Stapells et al, 2000a; 2000b) or insert earphones (Sininger et al, 1997). It is assumed that the normative reference defined by adults' hearing sensitivity would apply similarly to infants, had it been possible to measure behavioral thresholds for establishing a normative reference for infants. However, this is not likely to be a good assumption because the adult and the infant ear canals differ in volume and length. The same stimulus level presented via a headphone will result in different sound pressure levels at the eardrum, of the order of 2 to 7 dB smaller in the infant's than in the adult's ear for high frequencies (Voss and Herrmann, 2005). If insert earphones are used, the volume of the ear canal directly affects the sound pressure level generated at the eardrum. Higher sound pressure levels will be generated in the infant's than in the adult's ear for the same input level. The error implicit in assuming that the infant's behavioral threshold is 0 dB HL needs to be modified by incorporating the difference in RECDs between an adult and an infant in the correction figures.

Once estimates of behavioral thresholds for at least one low (e.g., 500 Hz) and one high frequency (e.g., 2 kHz) are available, amplification should be provided immediately to support early language development (see Thompson et al, 2001 for a review). The estimated thresholds should be confirmed by ear-specific audiometry to establish air conduction thresholds when reliable behavioral responses can be obtained, usually from about 7 months of age. If a child has a chronic conductive hearing loss, bone conduction thresholds have equal priority with air conduction thresholds. The effectiveness of amplification for providing auditory information to the child should be evaluated and monitored over time.

RECD/REAG/CG Adjustment Method

To achieve a consistent SPL at the eardrum, prescriptive targets should be specified in terms of REAG. This is the increase in signal level when aided, relative to the level in the sound field (Dillon, 2001, provides a detailed discussion). For a REAG prescription, the corresponding coupler gain (CG) targets are affected only by the difference between the coupler-measured gain and the real-ear gain, that is, the RECD. Therefore, an effective method to allow for differences in ear canal size is to measure the RECD (Moodie et al, 1994) before prescribing hearing aids, and to use the RECDs to calculate the CGs that will result in the target REAG. As a child grows, changes in the ear canal acoustics result in decreases in RECD (Feigin et al, 1989), and higher coupler gains will be required to provide the same REAG targets. If measurement of individual RECD is not possible, age-appropriate values may be used (Feigin et al, 1989; Bagatto et al, 2002) to derive coupler gain targets. Hearing aids can be adjusted and verified in a 2-cc coupler to match the prescribed values. This RECD/REAG/CG method is an integral part of the DSL Method (Bagatto et al, 2005) and is recommended to implement the NAL prescription for children younger than 5 years. For older children, either this method, or the insertion gain method used for adults is suitable.

Pearl

- CG = REAG − RECD, so small ear canals with large RECD values do not need as much CG to achieve a REAG target as would a large (adult) ear canal.

Both the DSL and the NAL hearing aid prescription software prescribe REAG targets (in addition to insertion gain targets), and calculate the required CG that will result in the REAG targets for an individual child. If the child's RECD has been accurately measured, and if tubing and venting effects have been allowed for, the match between target and measured gains in a 2-cc coupler will accurately predict the match between target and hearing aid performance in the real ear. Practical guides for adjusting and verifying hearing aids according to the DSL targets (Bagatto et al, 2005) and the NAL-NL1 targets (Ching et al, 2002) are available.

If open fittings are used with the RECD/REAG/CG fitting method, an additional consideration is necessary. The open fitting, effectively a very large vent, will cause a large negative RECD in the low frequencies. While this might seem to indicate that a very large CG is needed for low frequencies, this part of the prescription must be ignored for any low or medium frequency at which the target gain is less than a few dB. A gain of 0 dB will instead be achieved in the low frequencies by sound directly entering the ear canal.

Prescription of Gain and Output

The NAL-NL1 and the DSL [i/o] (and its new version, DSLm[i/o]) procedures for prescribing nonlinear hearing aids are widely used for prescribing amplification for children around the world. The DSL procedure prescribes more overall gain than the NAL procedure for all audiometric configurations. For sloping high-frequency loss, the NAL procedure provides less high-frequency gain than the DSL procedure because the NAL formula allows for the reduced contribution of audibility to speech intelligibility as hearing loss becomes severe in the high frequencies (Ching et al, 2001a; Dillon, 1999). For flat loss, DSL prescribes more low-frequency gain than the NAL procedure. Despite these differences in gain-frequency response prescribed by the two procedures, recent research has shown that both are similarly effective for children. A double blind crossover comparison of the prescriptions for 48 school-aged children with mild to moderately severe hearing loss indicated that on average, children perceived speech equally well with both prescriptions. The children also rated speech from 55 to 80 dB SPL amplified with either prescription to range from too soft to too loud on a seven-point loudness scale. Nevertheless, the children preferred more gain than that prescribed by NAL-NL1 for low input levels (Seewald et al, 2002; Ching et al, 2006b). Further, a randomized controlled trial of the two prescriptions has been conducted by assigning young children to either the NAL or the DSL prescription for first fitting after diagnosis. The assessments at 12 months post-fitting indicate that both groups of children developed language similarly well as their normal-hearing peers as long as the children were provided with amplification by six months of age (Ching et al, 2006c).

Pearl

- The evidence to date supports early fitting with either the NAL or the DSL prescription to facilitate normal development of language by children with hearing loss.

Prescription for Use with Cochlear Implants

Cochlear implants are more effective than hearing aids for intervention of children with profound hearing loss and for some children with severe hearing loss. On average, children who are profoundly deaf with unilateral cochlear implants achieved language and speech development similar to those of children with severe hearing loss who wore hearing aids (Boothroyd and Eran, 1994; Blamey et al, 2001). A survey of children who are deaf or hard of hearing has revealed that children with hearing loss greater than 118 dB HL and who received cochlear implants achieved auditory performance and academic abilities that were equivalent to children with unaided hearing levels of 80 to 104 dB HL who wore hearing aids (Stacey et al, 2006). These reports relate to performance of children who received a cochlear implant in one ear.

Recent research indicates that when children with a cochlear implant in one ear wore a hearing aid in the contralateral ear, they perceived speech and localized sounds better than when they wore a cochlear implant alone (Ching et al, 2006d; see Ching et al, 2007, for a summary). On average, children with hearing loss greater than 110 dB HL who wore a cochlear implant and a hearing aid in opposite ears demonstrated functional performance in real life that was equivalent to children with hearing loss of about 70 dB HL who wore bilateral hearing aids (Ching and Hill, 2007).

Pearl

- There is now international consensus that the standard of care for children who receive a cochlear implant in one ear and who have residual hearing in the opposite ear is to provide either binaural/bimodal fitting (fit a hearing aid in the nonimplanted ear) or bilateral implants (Offeciers et al, 2005).

No research as yet compares the efficiency of these two approaches. Although a cochlear implant by itself provides performance superior to a hearing aid by itself, it is feasible that bimodal fittings will be as good as, or even better than, bilateral implants because each device type provides information complementary to the other.

If bimodal fitting is considered, current evidence suggests that systematic fine-tuning of a hearing aid to complement a cochlear implant and balancing the loudness between ears enables better binaural hearing to be achieved (Ching et al, 2001b; 2004). Empirical data about amplification requirements of 48 children who used bimodal fitting revealed that the preferred frequency response slope was within 3 dB/octave of the response prescribed by the NAL-RP prescription (Byrne and Dillon, 1986; Byrne, Newall, and Parkinson, 1991), and the required gain was within 2 dB of the prescribed gain on average (Ching et al, 2007). The NAL procedure for adjusting a hearing aid to complement a cochlear implant includes three steps: prescribing and verifying hearing aid characteristics based on the NAL prescription, fine-tuning according to individual preferences based on intelligibility judgments, and finally balancing the loudness of the hearing aid with the cochlear implant in a systematic way (see Ching et al, 2004b for a step-by-step guide). The DVD that accompanies this book contains a video demonstration of the procedure, and a course on bimodal fitting is available via Cochlear College (www.cochlearcollege.com).

Pitfall

- Excessive cautiousness, such as prescribing conservative (i.e., insufficient) gain, or excessively delaying the decision to implant, can deprive a child of auditory experience during the first year of life when so many neural pathways are being developed.

◆ Verification and Evaluation of Hearing Aids

As the goal of amplification is to ensure that sounds are audible across the widest possible frequency range at a comfortable level, aided audibility is often used clinically to verify that the goal has been achieved. However, calculated audibility or measures of aided thresholds do not ensure that the amplification is optimally effective for an individual (Byrne and Ching, 1997). When fitting hearing aids to adults, it is common to fine-tune hearing aids depending on their verbal feedback. Because prescriptive targets are designed to be correct on average (for people with that degree of loss), fine-tuning is necessary for individuals who may differ in preferred gain and in perceptions of aided speech intelligibility and sound quality (Byrne, 1986; Leijon et al, 1990). When fitting hearing aids to children, a range of evaluation tools can be used to check that the amplification provided meets the needs of individual children. Methods of evaluation include speech tests (see Bess et al, 1996, for a summary, Madell, Chapter 10, this volume), paired-comparisons judgments (Eisenberg and Levitt, 1991; Ching et al, 1994) and subjective reports by parents and teachers (see Ching and Hill, 2007, for a summary).

Visual Displays of Audibility

Visual displays of audibility are useful for viewing how much of an assumed speech spectrum at a certain input level is audible to a child. Aided speech audibility can be computed from information about the child's hearing sensitivity, the long-term average speech spectrum, and gains provided by a hearing aid (in terms of REAG or CG) for different input levels across frequencies. Displays can be generated within the NAL and the DSL fitting software, and also by some types of real-ear gain analyzers.

It is important to recognize that displays of audibility do not indicate how well a child can extract information from an audible signal for understanding speech. Greater audibility can be achieved by providing more gain in hearing aids, but the increased audibility may result in saturation occurring more often in hearing aids, or in an increase in loudness, without any increase in speech intelligibility. The contribution of audibility to speech intelligibility depends on the amount of speech information that can be extracted from an audible signal. This is likely to decrease as hearing loss increases, especially in the high frequencies (Ching et al, 1998; 2001a; Hogan and Turner, 1998), and as the population of functioning inner hair cells in the cochlea diminishes (Moore, 2001). For this reason, audibility displays may be used to suggest the amount of audible information available to a child with mild or moderate hearing loss, but they should not be relied upon for estimating the information available to a child with more severe loss. The effectiveness of amplification in providing auditory information to a child has to be established by evaluating aided performance.

Aided Thresholds

The measurement of soundfield aided thresholds has traditionally been used to demonstrate a child's ability to detect the presence of sound in an audiometric test booth when the child is aided. However, aided thresholds do not provide information about a child's hearing ability at suprathreshold levels, or about sensation levels of amplified speech. Nevertheless, aided thresholds are useful for establishing whether a child's unaided thresholds are vibrotactile when hearing loss is profound. In such cases, aided and unaided thresholds will be approximately the same. When aided thresholds are used to supplement the RECD/CG approach to verifying hearing aids, the thresholds obtained should be compared with those prescribed by the prescription procedure used. The NAL prescription for nonlinear hearing aids includes aided threshold targets that can be used for this purpose.

Speech Tests

A realistic method to demonstrate aided improvement of a child with hearing loss to the family is to establish the child's speech reception threshold (SRT), and to compare the child's performance in aided and unaided conditions. For older children, a range of speech tests are available for assessing performance (see Bess et al, 1996, for a review; see Dillon and Ching, 1995, and Madell, Chapter 10 in this book for a discussion of selection and use of speech tests).

For assessing the binaural processing ability of children who are deaf or hard of hearing, the SRT for speech and noise presented from the same loudspeaker positioned at 0° azimuth can be compared with the SRT for speech presented at 0° azimuth and noise at +/−90° azimuth (Ching et al, 2006a). Children with normal hearing will display a 3-dB advantage from spatial separation, whereas children with congenital hearing loss will most commonly display no advantage.

For evaluating alternative amplification schemes to see which one is most effective, speech testing is not the method of choice despite its face validity. Not only are speech tests very time-consuming to perform, they are also limited in sensitivity to differences in hearing aid characteristics (Studebaker, 1982). If speech tests are administered for evaluating the effectiveness of amplification, they should be supplemented by assessments of functional performance in everyday situations.

Paired Comparison Testing

The paired comparison technique allows several schemes to be compared in pairs so that a listener can select the most preferred scheme for amplifying speech. Previous research with adults has shown that this method is more sensitive than speech perception tests to differences in amplification characteristics (Studebaker, 1982; Byrne, 1986). It can be used with school-aged children to compare the relative intelligibility of speech amplified with alternative frequency responses (Eisenberg and Levitt, 1991; Ching et al, 1999), and more reliable judgments can be obtained with audiovisual than with auditory-alone presentation of speech stimuli (Ching et al, 1994). The optimal frequency response for speech intelligibility was found to be the same, irrespective of the mode of stimuli presentation. Paired-comparisons testing, like speech testing, can be used only with older children. For young children, the available options for evaluating the effectiveness of amplification include subjective reports and objective electrophysiologic assessments.

Subjective Reports

Infants and young children are limited in their ability to provide verbal comment on the relative effectiveness of amplification for speech intelligibility and sound quality. Although self reports are useful for adults and possibly some older children (see Stelmachowicz, 1999, for a review), they are not applicable to young children. A variety of subjective report tools that rely on the observations of parents and teachers have been developed to guide audiologic intervention for young children, but these are limited in the range of ages and degrees of hearing loss to which they can be applied (see Ching and Hill, 2007, for a review). To address the need to evaluate amplification for children of a wide range of age and hearing loss, PEACH has been developed (Ching and Hill, 2007). The PEACH questionnaire, which is shown in **Appendix 18–1** and may be copied for use, consists of items that relate to usage of device, loudness comfort, functional performance in quiet and in noise, and alertness to environmental sounds. Parents are requested to observe and record their child's auditory and oral behaviors in everyday life situations in a diary, and the examples are solicited in a structured interview for scoring. PEACH can be used with children as young as 1 month through to school age, and for all degrees of hearing loss. Test-retest reliability is high, and critical difference values are published. Details of administration, together with instructions, questionnaire forms, and score sheets, are available on the NAL Web site (www.nal.gov.au), and the DVD that accompanies this book contains a video demonstration of the administration of the PEACH. Normally hearing children achieve near-perfect scores by about 3 years of age, but children with hearing loss exhibit deficits compared with their normal-hearing peers. By using the PEACH, the relative effectiveness of amplification for a child can be quantified in terms of deviations of his score from the normative mean. In addition, the scale also provides a "quiet" and a "noise" subscale score based on groups of items. In clinical applications, the "noise" subscale score is particularly useful in indicating the need for fitting FMs to individual children.

Appendix 18–1   Parents' Evaluation of Aural/Oral Performance of Children

Child's Name:		D.O.B.		Sex:				
Respondent:		Interviewer:		Date:				
		Frequency of reported behavior						
Preinterview questions:			**Never** 0%	**Seldom** 25%	**Sometimes** 50%	**Often** 75%	**Always** > 75%	
	Child's use of hearing aids/cochlear implants		0	1	2	3	4	
	Is your child upset by loud sounds?		4	3	2	1	0	
PEACH items:								
No	Scale	Item						
1	Q	Respond to name in quiet		0	1	2	3	4
2	Q	Follow verbal instructions in quiet		0	1	2	3	4
3	N	Respond to name in noise		0	1	2	3	4
4	N	Follow verbal instructions in noise		0	1	2	3	4
5	Q	Follow story read aloud		0	1	2	3	4
6	Q	Participate in conversation in quiet		0	1	2	3	4
7	N	Participate in conversation in noise		0	1	2	3	4
8	N	Participate in conversation in transport		0	1	2	3	4
9	Q	Recognize voice of familiar persons		0	1	2	3	4
10	Q	Converse on the phone		0	1	2	3	4
11	N	Recognize sounds in the environment		0	1	2	3	4

Obligatory Cortical Auditory Evoked Potential

With the rise of early identification of hearing loss programs, the need to evaluate hearing aid fittings in very young infants has gained increasing importance. In infants or older children with significant developmental delay, estimates of behavioral thresholds that are based on electrophysiologic thresholds are often used to derive target gain, but the need to evaluate the appropriateness of the fit remains. The recording of cortical auditory evoked potentials (CAEPs) to speech stimuli has the potential to provide such verification in these cases.

Various objective methods for evaluating the appropriateness of the hearing aid fit have been proposed over the years (for discussions on the application of ABRs see (Beauchaine et al, 1986; Hecox, 1983; Kiessling, 1982); and for discussions on the application of ASSRs in the evaluation of hearing aid fittings see (Dimitrijevic and John, 2004; Picton et al., 1998; Picton, Dimitrijevic, and John, 2002). CAEP testing, however, offers a rather unusual opportunity to present speech stimuli and record an electrophysiological response from the cortical region. The advantages of CAEP testing for hearing aid evaluation include the following:

♦ Unlike ABR, the test stimuli can have the same length as occurs for phonemes in natural speech, enabling hearing aids to respond to the sounds in a more realistic manner.

♦ Unlike ASSR, the response is not dependent on a particular amplitude modulation of the stimulus, which is advantageous because room acoustics will always decrease amplitude modulation before it reaches the listener.

♦ Unlike ABR and perhaps ASSR, signals have to pass through the entire auditory system before a response is generated, rather than just reach the brainstem.

A difference, which is sometimes an advantage and sometimes a disadvantage, is that CAEP testing is best done while the client is awake.

Stimuli

Obligatory CAEPs (cortically generated responses to any audible stimulus of an appropriate length) can be reliably evoked by virtually any suprathreshold speech sound or tonal stimuli in infants and adults (Agung et al, 2006). For most clinical purposes it seems reasonable to limit the choice of stimuli, bearing in mind the practicalities of keeping test time to a minimum. As an example, the spectra for the stimuli /m/, /g/, /t/, are shown in **Fig. 18–1.**

They have a spectral emphasis in the low-, mid- and high-frequency regions, respectively, and therefore have the potential to give diagnostic information about the perception of speech sounds in different frequency regions.

Parameters for Recording Cortical Auditory Evoked Potential in Infants

Table 18–1 shows parameters suitable for eliciting CAEPs in infants. The free-field test environment should regularly be calibrated to ensure that the test-speakers and room acoustics give a flat frequency response and hence do not distort the test signals, and that the intensity of the stimuli at the test-position (a comfortable lounge chair for the parent, who then holds the infant, is ideal) is correct. The employment of a colleague as a distracter is highly desirable to ensure that the child is occupied but quiet enough for quality recording to occur.

Infant Responses and Maturation

CAEPs can be reliably recorded in infants and children in response to speech stimuli in aided and unaided conditions (Cone-Wesson and Wunderlich, 2003; Gravel et al, 1989; Pang and Taylor, 2000) and a relationship between CAEPs and receptive language skills has been demonstrated (Kurtzberg, 1989). She reported that infants with normal CAEPs (defined as age-appropriate morphology, latency, and amplitude) to suprathreshold stimuli, were more likely to show normal

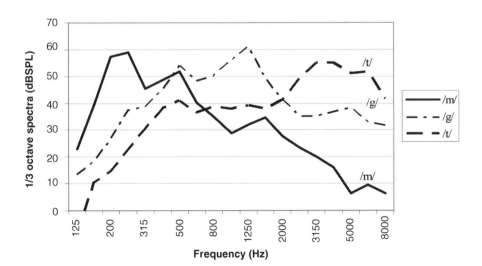

Figure 18–1   The one third octave spectra for the three speech stimuli /m/, /g/, /t/, are shown. They were extracted from continuous discourse that was spoken by a female with an average Australian accent and which had been filtered to match the International Long-Term Average Speech Spectrum.

Table 18–1   Parameters Suitable for Recording Cortical Auditory Evoked Potentials in Infants

Analysis Time: 100 milliseconds (or longer) prestimulus and 600 milliseconds (or longer) poststimulus onset
Filters: 0.1 to 30 Hz
Interstimulus interval: 1125 milliseconds
Electrode sites: vertex to mastoid
Artifact reject: $\pm$ 100 to 150 μ V
Number of accepted epochs: 50–100
Stimuli: speech segments presented in the freefield at suprathreshold levels
Infant state: awake but settled

receptive language function than those with abnormal responses at 1 year of age. There are, however, substantial differences in the average infant CAEP compared with adult CAEP waveforms. The newborn infant CAEP to speech stimuli is dominated by a prominent peak at 200 to 300 milliseconds when recorded at the midline (Kurtzberg, 1989; Sharma, Dorman, and Spahr, 2002; Stapells and Kurtsberg, 1991). Grand averaged CAEPs from 10 infants aged 3 to 7 months are shown in **Fig. 18–2.**

Pearl

- Obligatory CAEPs can be reliably recorded in young infants at suprathreshold levels, but intersubject variability of the response shape is high.

In this figure, the addition of a precortical response is also evident in response to /t/. This is consistent with a brain-stem-generated postauricular muscle response (PAMR), which is sensitive to abrupt onset stimuli (Agung et al, 2005). As infants with normal hearing mature, cortical responses change significantly with respect to the shape and

latency of the major components over the first 14 to 16 years of life (Hyde, 1997; Pasman et al, 1999; Rotteveel et al, 1986). These morphological changes with age likely reflect underlying developmental changes in the response generators such as improved synaptic efficiency arising from increased axon myelination and maturation of intra- and interhemispheric connections throughout the cortex (Cunningham et al, 2000; Eggermont and Ponton, 2003).

Response Detection

In common with most auditory evoked potentials, two or more averaged CAEP responses are often overlaid and inspected for repeatability before the examiner will conclude that a response has been detected. In addition, the latency of key response components may also be reviewed and compared with age-appropriate normative data before the response is considered to be normal. Age-appropriate normative data can, however, be misleading. First, substantial intersubject differences in wave morphology are not uncommon in CAEPs from infants with normal hearing CAEPs, even when tested in an ideal state (Wunderlich and Cone-Wesson, 2006). Second, latencies that are greater than normal have been observed in children who have had inadequate auditory stimulation for the early years of their lives (Sharma, Dorman, and Spahr, 2002). The rigid application of waveform templates to the individual CAEP response is therefore less reliable in defining abnormal and normal CAEP outcomes than is experienced in ABR testing. Given this intersubject variability, the clinical expertise required to identify a CAEP response in infants can be daunting, so the addition of a statistical test to aid in detection is highly desirable. The application of statistical measures in evoked potential detection is not new (for an excellent review of automated and machine scoring methods see Hall (1992)), but techniques that assume a certain waveshape are not likely to be successful in detecting CAEPs from infants or young children, particularly those who have previously been deprived of auditory stimulation. A new technique involving the application of the Hotelling's T2 statistic (Flury and Riedwyl, 1988) has been derived, and this technique requires minimal assumptions about the waveshape (Golding et al, 2007b). The result of this analysis is the probability that the observed average waveform arises just from random sources unrelated to the timing of the stimulus. The clinician can use this statistical outcome in combination with the displayed averaged response waveform to decide if a response to auditory stimulation has been detected.

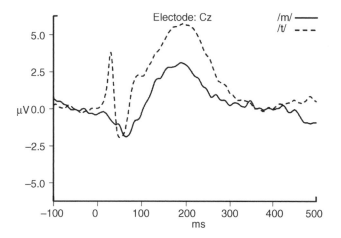

Figure 18–2   Grand average CAEP responses from 10 normal hearing infants are shown. The stimuli were /t/ and /m/ (durations of 31 milliseconds and 32 milliseconds, respectively) presented at 65 dB SPL in the soundfield.

Statistical detection of a response is of course not infallible, but is it more accurate than the human expert in detecting CAEPs? Certainly, the difficulties of subjective electrophysiologic response detection are well known (Hoppe et al, 2001; Hoth, 1993), particularly when the stimulus presentation level is just audible. In a recent experiment, the sensitivity and specificity in detecting CAEPs were compared for human experts and Hotelling's T^2. Adult responses were generated to stimuli presented at various sensation levels together with nonstimulus trials. Hotelling's T^2 was more accurate in discriminating a cortical response from no response, than the expert human observers (Dillon et al, 2006b). Although a similar (or even stronger) benefit from automated detection could be expected when CAEPs are generated from infants, this still needs to be confirmed.

The Relationship between Cortical Auditory Evoked Potential Detection and Behavioral Measures

In cooperative older children and adults, the CAEP threshold to tonal stimulation closely approximates the pure tone audiometric threshold. The difference between the two is, on average, 0 to 10 dB (Davis, 1965; Rickards, DeVidi, and McMahon, 1996). In infants, the difference may be similar if they can be kept quiet and unwanted physiologic noise can be kept to a minimum during recording (Cone-Wesson et al, 2003), but few data support this hypothesis. For speech stimuli presented at conversational level, aiding a child can often lead to a CAEP response where none existed when the child was unaided (Gravel et al, 1989).

Pearl

- Researchers reported in the 1960s that CAEPs, generated from a hearing-impaired infant, were better defined when hearing aids were fitted (Rapin and Graziani, 1967).

In a recent study of 28 aided infants and children aged 6 weeks to 3 years 5 months (mean age 8 months (SD 8.6) (Golding et al, 2007a), the presence or absence of CAEPs to three speech stimuli were compared with observed auditory behaviors that were recorded using the PEACH questionnaire (Ching and Hill, 2007). A positive correlation between the number of detected CAEPs to these speech stimuli (i.e., none to a maximum of three) and the age-corrected PEACH score was found. These results were significant using human expert and statistical detection methods.

Pearl

- Although the correlation between CAEP and questionnaire outcomes was not perfect, the results do suggest that detection of CAEPs to speech stimuli is a valid measure of aided functional performance in infants and young children.

Cortical Auditory Evoked Potential Detection and Aided Performance

Research to date suggests that the recording of CAEPs may assist in verifying hearing aid fitting in infants. Having prescribed the aid using electrophysiological estimates of threshold to determine gain across the frequency range, it seems appropriate to confirm that selected speech stimuli are detected, with hearing aids fitted, at the cortical level. If detection cannot be shown, one of several strategies may be required.

- As with any electrophysiological measure, the quality of testing should be reviewed. Apart from system checks (e.g., electrode integrity, stimulus intensity accuracy, functional performance of the hearing aids), the child may have been particularly restless during the assessment, leading to high response rejection rates that will undoubtedly obscure weak cortical responses, and a retest may be warranted.

- The original threshold estimates that were used in the prescription of the hearing aid should be checked in case the hearing aids were prescribed to have insufficient gain (Korczak, Kurtsberg, and Stapells, 2005).

- The CAEP test outcomes should be reviewed in the light of all other available information about the child, both behavioral and electrophysiological, before deciding on a course of action. The clinician may decide to adjust the hearing aid gain-frequency response, even if this means departing from the hearing aid prescription, or may choose to use the CAEP test outcomes to guide a behavioral test session if the child is nearing this stage of development. If the CAEPs were present to some but not all stimuli, for example, it may be appropriate to focus behavioral testing on stimulus presentations within frequency regions that did not elicit a CAEP response. An absence of CAEP responses, even when aided, is a particularly important piece of information when implantation is being considered, especially given the importance of implantation occurring within the first year of life (Ching et al, 2006c).

- In some cases of auditory neuropathy/dys-synchrony, CAEP responses may be detected when ABRs are absent (Hood, 1999; Rance et al, 2002). The case study of two infants who had been diagnosed with this condition was recently reported (Pearce, Golding, and Dillon, 2007). Both had otoacoustic emissions but lacked ABR responses to tonal stimuli at the time of diagnosis. One of these infants had repeatable CAEPs to speech stimuli presented at conversation levels. In this case, the severity of loss suggested by the ABR outcomes was inaccurate and could have led to overprescription of hearing aid gain. For children like this, a more conservative approach to the prescription of hearing aid gain that still enables detection of speech sounds, as evidenced by the CAEP responses, is appropriate. This will minimize the risk that the outer hair cells are damaged by amplified sound (Hood, 1998; Stredler-Brown, 2002). The child's progress should be monitored regularly.

Pearl

- Recording CAEPs to speech stimuli in the aided infant provides evidence that the stimuli are detected at the cortex and therefore strongly suggests that the stimuli are audible to the infant.

Special Consideration

- To ensure that an infant or young child is quiet but alert during testing, a variety of noiseless toys should be on hand. DVDs (without sound) can also be very useful forms of occupation.

Obligatory Cortical Auditory Evoked Potential and the Discrimination of Speech Stimuli

The presence of CAEPs to speech stimuli provides physiologic evidence that these stimuli have arrived at the cortex and are potentially audible to the infant with hearing aids fitted (Korczak, Kurtsberg, and Stapells, 2005). Detection is, however, the first step in the cognitive processes associated with discrimination of speech. Various studies have shown that the latency and amplitude of CAEP components may differ with changes in a feature of the stimulus (Hyde, 1997) such as voice onset time (Tremblay et al, 2006; 2003). Similarly, a cortical response to the change in spectrum during the transition from a fricative to a vowel in a consonant-vowel (CV) syllable (Ostroff, Martin, and Boothroyd, 1998) provides evidence that information sufficient to differentiate the two phonemes has made it to the auditory cortex. This suggests that examination of the latency and amplitude of the CAEP components and the detection of response differences by a statistical test may provide some evidence that differing perceptual processes are occurring for different speech sounds, and such differences may auger well for the development of speech discrimination ability. Much more work is needed in this area to fully understand how CAEPs might reflect these perceptual processes, particularly when the speech stimuli used to generate these responses are delivered through hearing aids with various signal processing characteristics (Tremblay et al, 2006).

Discussion Questions

1. Which features in hearing aids intended for adults should be disabled when fitted to children younger than 3 years?

2. What effects do small ear canals have on measured hearing thresholds?

3. What effects do small ear canals have on the REAG provided to infants?

4. How is the RECD measurement applied in pediatric audiology?

5. What are the options and advantages of different methods of evaluating the aided performance of children for (a) children younger than 12 months, (b) children aged 4 to 5 years, (c) children aged 6 years or older?

6. Should the recording of CAEPs be performed routinely in the assessment of all infants referred for hearing testing?

7. How might the detection of CAEPs form part of a routine evaluation of hearing aid fitting in infants?

8. If an infant is found to have CAEPs to speech stimuli but his ABRs to tonal stimuli are absent, what procedures should be followed?

Acknowledgments   We are grateful to Emma van Wanrooy and Leanne Skinner for their thoughts on some of the issues discussed in this chapter.

References

Agung, K., Purdy, S. C., McMahon, C., and Newall, P. (2006). The use of cortical auditory evoked potentials to evaluate encoding of speech sounds in adults. Journal of the American Academy of Audiology, 17, 559–572.

Agung, K., Purdy, S. C., Patuzzi, R. B., O'Beirne, G. A., and Newall, P. (2005). Rising-frequency chirps and earphones with an extende high frequency response enhance the post-auricular muscle response. International Journal of Audiology, 44, 631–636.

Bagatto, M., Moodie, S., Scollie, S., Seewald, R., Moodie, S., Pumford, J., and Liu, K. P. R. (2005). Clinical protocols for hearing instrument fitting in the desired sensation level method. Trends in Amplification, 9, 199–226.

Bagatto, M.P., Scollie, S. D., Seewald, R. C., et al. (2002). Real-ear-to-coupler difference predictions as a function of age for two coupling procedures. Journal of the American Academy of Audiology, 13, 407–415.

Beauchaine, K. A., Gorga, M. P., Reiland, J. K., and Larson, L. (1986). Application of ABRs to the hearing aid selection process: preliminary data. Journal of Speech and Hearing Research, 29, 120–128.

Bess, F. H., Chase, P. A., Gravel, J. S., Seewald, R. C., Stelmachowicz, P. G., Tharpe, A. M., and Hedley-Williams, A. (1996). Amplification for infants and children with hearing loss. American Journal of Audiology, 5, 53–68.

Blamey, P. J., Sarant, J. Z., Paatsch, L. E., Barry, J. G., Bow, C. P., Wales, R.J., Wright, M., Psarros, C., Rattigan, K., and Tooher, R. (2001). Relationships among speech perception, production, language, hearing loss, and age in children with impaired hearing. Journal of Speech Language and Hearing Research, 44, 264–285.

Boothroyd, A., Springer, N., Smith, L., and Schulman, J. (1988). Amplitude compression and profound hearing loss. Journal of Speech Language and Hearing Research, 31, 362–376.

Boothroyd, A., and Eran, O. (1994). Auditory speech perception capacity of child implant users expressed as equivalent hearing loss. Volta Review, 96, 151–168.

Byrne, D. (1986). Effects of frequency response characteristics on speech discrimination and perceived intelligibility and pleasantness of speech for hearing-impaired listeners. Journal of the Acoustical Society of America, 80, 494–504.

Byrne, D., and Ching, T. Y. C. (1997). Optimising amplification for hearing impaired children, I: Issues and procedures. Australian Journal of Education of the Deaf, 3, 21–28.

Byrne, D., and Dillon, H. (1986). The National Acoustic Laboratories' (NAL) new procedures for selecting the gain and frequency response of a hearing aid. Ear and Hearing, 7, 257–265.

Byrne, D., Newall, P., and Parkinson, A. (1991). Modified hearing aid selection procedures for severe/profound hearing losses. In Studebaker, G., Bess, F., and Beck, L. (Eds.), The Vanderbilt Hearing Aid Report II. Parkton, Maryland: York Press.

Ching, T. Y. C., Britton, L., Dillon, H., and Agung, K. (2002). RECD, REAG, NAL-NL1: accurate and practical methods for fitting non-linear hearing aids to infants and children. Hearing Review, 9, 12–20, 52.

Ching, T. Y. C., and Dillon, H. (2003). Prescribing amplification for children: adult-equivalent hearing loss, real-ear aided gain, and NAL-NL1. Trends in Amplification, 7, 1–9.

Ching, T. Y. C., Dillon, H., and Byrne, D. (1998). Speech recognition of hearing impaired listeners: predictions from audibility and the limited role of high frequency audibility. Journal of the Acoustical Society of America, 103, 1128–1140.

Ching, T. Y. C., Dillon, H., Katsch, R., and Byrne, D. (2001a). Maximising effective audibility in hearing aid fitting. Ear and Hearing, 22, 212–224.

Ching, T. Y. C., Dillon, H., Seewald, R., Britton, L., Joyce, J., and Scollie, S. (2006b). Hearing aid prescription for children: NAL-NL1 and DSL[i/o]. Paper presented at the 4th Widex Congress of Paediatric Audiology, Ottawa, May 19–21, 2006.

Ching, T. Y. C., Dillon, H., Day, J., et al. (2006c). Outcomes of children with hearing impairment: early vs later-identified. Paper presented at the British Academy of Audiology Conference, Telford UK, November 22–24, 2006.

Ching, T. Y. C., and Hill, M. (2007). The Parents' Evaluation of Aural/Oral Performance of Children (PEACH) scale: normative data. Journal of the American Academy of Audiology, 18, 221–237.

Ching, T. Y. C., Hill, M., Dillon, H., and van Wanrooy, E. (2004). Fitting and evaluating a hearing aid for recipients of unilateral cochlear implants: the NAL approach. Part 1. Hearing Review, 11, 14–22, 58.

Ching, T. Y. C., Hill, M., Birtles, G., and Beecham, L. (1999). Clinical use of paired comparisons to evaluate hearing aid fitting of severely/profoundly hearing impaired children. Australian & New Zealand Journal of Audiology, 21, 51–63.

Ching, T. Y. C., van Wanrooy, E., Hill, M., and Incerti, P. (2006). Performance in children with hearing aids or cochlear implants: Bilateral stimulation and binaural hearing. International Journal of Audiology, 45, S108–S112.

Ching, T. Y. C., Incerti, P., Hill, M., and van Wanrooy, E. (2006d). An overview of binaural advantages for children and adults who use binaural/bimodal hearing devices. Audiology & Neuro-otology, 11, 6–11.

Ching, T. Y. C., Newall, P., and Wigney, D. (1994). Audio-visual and auditory paired comparison judgments by severely and profoundly hearing impaired children: reliability and frequency response preferences. Australian Journal of Audiology, 16, 99–106.

Ching, T. Y. C., Psarros, C., Hill, M., Dillon, H., and Incerti, P. (2001b). Should children who use cochlear implants wear hearing aids in the opposite ear? Ear and Hearing, 22, 365–380.

Ching, T.Y.C., van Wanrooy, E., Hill, M., and Incerti, P. (2006a). Performance in children with hearing aids or cochlear implants: bilateral stimulation and binaural hearing. International Journal of Audiology, 45, S108–S112.

Ching, T. Y. C., van Wanrooy, E, and Dillon, H. (2007). Binaural-bimodal fitting or bilateral implantation for managing severe or profound hearing loss: a review. Trends in Amplification, 11, 161–192.

Cone-Wesson, B., and Wunderlich, J. (2003). Auditory evoked potentials from the cortex: audiology applications. Current Opinion in Otolaryngology and Head and Neck Surgery, 11, 372–377.

Cunningham, J., Nicol, T., Zecker, S., and Kraus, N. (2000). Speech-evoked neurophysiological responses in children with learning problems: Development and behavioural correlates of perception. Ear and Hearing, 21, 554–568.

Davis, H. (1965). Slow cortical responses evoked by acoustic stimuli. Acta Otolaryngologica, 59, 179–185.

Dillon, H. (1999). NAL-NL1: a new prescriptive fitting procedure for non-linear hearing aids. Hearing Journal, 52, 10–16.

Dillon, H. (2001). Hearing aids. Sydney, Australia: Boomerang Press.

Dillon, H., and Ching, T. (1995). What makes a good speech test? In G. Plant and K-E Spens (Eds), Profound deafness and speech communication. London: Whurr Publishers Ltd.

Dillon, H., Golding, M., Purdy, S. C., and Katsch, R. (2006b). Automated detection of cortical auditory evoked potentials. [Abstract] The Australian and New Zealand Journal of Audiology, 28, 20.

Dillon H., Zakis J., McDermott, H., Keidser, G., Dreschler, W., and Convery, E. (2006a). The trainable hearing aid: what will it do for clients and clinicians? Hearing Journal, 59, 30–36.

Dimitrijevic, A., and John, M. S. (2004). Auditory steady-state responses and word recognition scores in normal-hearing and hearing-impaired adults. Ear and Hearing, 25, 68–84.

Eggermont, J. J., and Ponton, C. W. (2003). Auditory-evoked potential studies of cortical maturation in normal hearing and implanted children: correlations with changes in structure and speech perception. Acta Otolaryngologica, 123, 249–252.

Eisenberg. L. S., and Levitt, H. (1991). Paired comparison judgments for hearing aid selection in children. Ear and Hearing, 12, 417–430.

Feigin, J. A., Kopun, J. G., Stelmachowicz, P. G., et al. (1989). Probe-tube microphone measures of ear-canal sound pressure levels in infants and children. Ear and Hearing, 10, 254–258.

Flury, B., and Riedwyl, H. (1988). Multivariate statistics: a practical approach. London: Chapman and Hall.

Gatehouse, S., Naylor, G., and Elberling, C. (2006). Linear and nonlinear hearing aid fittings, II: Patterns of candidature. International Journal of Audiology, 45, 153–171.

Golding, M., Pearce, W., Seymour, J., Cooper, A., Ching, T. Y. C., and Dillon, H. (2007a). The relationship between obligatory cortical auditory evoked potentials (CAEPs) and functional measures in young infants. Journal of the American Academy of Audiology, 18, 117–125.

Golding, M. Dillon, H., Seymour, J., Purdy, S., and Katsch, R. (2007b). Obligatory CAEP testing in infants: a five year review. Annual Report of the National Acoustic Laboratories, 2005–2006, 14–17. www.NAL.gov.au. Last accessed January 2007.

Gravel, J. S., Fausel, N., Liskow, C., and Chobot, J. (1999). Children's speech recognition in noise using omni-directional and dual-microphone hearing aid technology. Ear and Hearing, 20, 1–11.

Gravel, J. S., Kurtzberg, D., Stapells, D. R., Vaughan, H. G., and Wallace, I. F. (1989). Case studies. Seminars in Hearing, 10, 272–287.

Hall, J. W. (1992). Handbook of auditory evoked responses. Needham Heights: Allyn and Bacon.

Hecox, K. E. (1983). Role of auditory brainstem response in the selection of hearing aids. Ear and Hearing, 4, 51–55.

Hogan, C. A., and Turner, C. W. (1998). High-frequency audibility: benefits for hearing-impaired listeners. Journal of the Acoustical Society of America, 104, 432–441.

Hood, L. J. (1998). Auditory neuropathy: What is it and what can we do about it? Hearing Journal, 51, 10–18.

Hood, L. J. (1999). A review of objective methods of evaluating auditory 'neural pathways. The Laryngoscope, 109, 1745–1748.

Hoppe, U., Weiss, S., Stewart, R. W., and Eysholdt, U. (2001). An automated sequential recognition method for cortical auditory evoked potentials. IEEE Transactions on Biomedical Engineering, 48, 154–164.

Hoth, S. (1993). Computer-aided hearing threshold determination from cortical auditory evoked potentials. Scandinavian Audiology, 22, 165–177.

Hyde, M. (1997). The N1 Response and Its Applications. Audiology and Neuro-otology, 2, 281–307.

Keidser, G., Dillon, H., Dyrlund, O., Carter, L., and Hartley, D. (2007a). Preferred low- and high-frequency compression ratios among hearing aid users with moderately severe to profound hearing loss. Journal of the American Academy of Audiology, 18, 17–33.

Keidser, G., O'Brien, A., Latzel, M., and Convery, E. (2007b). Evaluation of a transient noise reduction algorithm. Hearing Journal, 60, 29, 32, 34, 38–39.

Kiessling, J. (1982). Hearing aid selection by brainstem audiometry. Scandinavian Audiology, 11, 269–275.

Korczak, P. A., Kurtsberg, D., and Stapells, D. R. (2005). Effects of sensorineural hearing loss and personal hearing aids on cortical event-related potential and behavioural measures of speech-sound processing. Ear and Hearing, 26, 165–185.

Kurtzberg, D. (1989). Cortical event-related potential assessment of auditory system function. Seminars in Hearing, 10, 252–261.

Leijon, A., Lindkvist, A., Ringdahl, A., and Israelsson, B. (1990). Preferred hearing aid gain in everyday use after prescriptive fitting. Ear and Hearing 11, 299–303.

Litovsky, R. Y. (2005). Speech intelligibility and spatial release from masking in young children. Journal of the Acoustical Society of America, 117, 3091–3099.

Litovsky, R. Y., Johnstone, P. M., and Godar, S. P. (2006). Benefits of bilateral cochlear implants and/or hearing aids in children. International Journal of Audiology, 45, S78–S91.

Moodie, K. S., Seewald, R. C., and Sinclair, S. T. (1994). Procedure for predicting real-ear hearing aid performance in young children. American Journal of Audiology, 8, 23–31.

Moore, B. C. J. (2001). Dead regions in the cochlea: diagnosis, perceptual consequences, and implications for the fitting of hearing aids. Trends in Amplification, 3, 1–34.

Offeciers, E., Morera, C., Miller, J., Huarte, A., Shallop, J., and Cavallé, L. (2005). International consensus on bilateral cochlear implants and bimodal stimulation. Acta Oto-Laryngologica, 125, 918–919.

Ostroff, J. M., Martin, B. A., and Boothroyd, A. (1998). Cortical evoked responses to acoustic change within a syllable. Ear and Hearing, 19, 290–297.

Pang, E. W., and Taylor, M. J. (2000). Tracking the development of the N1 from age 3 to adulthood: an examination of speech and non-speech stimuli. Clinical Neurophysiology, 111, 388–397.

Pasman, J. W., Rotteveel, J. J., Maassen, B., and Visco, Y. M. (1999). The maturation of auditory cortical evoked responses between (preterm) birth and 14 years of age. European Journal of Paediatric Neurology, 3, 79–82.

Pearce, W., Golding, M., and Dillon, H. (2007). Cortical auditory evoked potentials in the assessment of auditory neuropathy. Journal of the American Academy of Audiology, 18, 380–389.

Picton, T.W., Dimitrijevic, A., and John, M. S. (2002). Multiple auditory steady-state responses. Annals of Otology, Rhinology and Laryngology, 111, 16–21.

Picton, T. W., Durieux-Smith, A., Champagne, S. C., Whittingham, J., Morgan, L. M., Giguere, C., et al. (1998). Objective evaluation of aided thresholds using auditory steady-state responses. Journal of the American Academy of Audiology, 9, 315–331.

Purdy, S. C., and Williams, M. (2000). High frequency tympanometry: a valid and reliable immittance test protocol for young infants. New Zealand Audiological Society Bulletin, 10, 9–24.

Rance, G., Cone-Wesson, B., Wunderlich, J., and Dowell, R. (2002). Speech perception and cortical event related potentials in children with auditory neuropathy. Ear and Hearing, 23, 239–253.

Rance, G., Roper, R., Symons, L., et al. (2005). Hearing threshold estimation in infants using auditory steady-state responses. Journal of the American Academy of Audiology, 16, 291–300.

Rapin, I., and Graziani, L. J. (1967). Auditory evoked responses in normal, brain-damaged and deaf infants. Neurology, 17, 881–894.

Rickards, F. W., DeVidi, S., and McMahon, D. S. (1996). Cortical evoked response audiometry in noise induced hearing loss claims. Australian Journal Otolaryngology, 2, 237–241.

Rotteveel, J. J., Colon, E. J., Notermans, L. H., Stoelinga, G. B. A., de Graaf, R., and Visco, Y. M. (1986). The central auditory conduction at term date

and three months after birth, IV: Auditory cortical responses. Scandinavian Audiology, 15, 85–95.

Scollie, S., Seewald, R., Cornelisse, L. et al. (2005). The Desired Sensation Level multistage input/output algorithm. Trends in Amplification, 9, 159–197.

Seewald, R., Ching, T., Dillon, H., Joyce, J., Britton, L., and Scollie, S. (2002). Hearing aid selection procedures for children: Report of a collaborative study. Paper presented at the International Hearing Aid Research Conference, Aug 21–25, Lake Tahoe, NV.

Seewald, R. C., Cornelisse, L. E., Ramji, K. V., et al. (1997). DSL v4.1 for Windows: a software implementation of the desired sensation level (DSL[i/o]) method for fitting linear gain and wide-dynamic-range compression hearing instruments. Users' manual. London, ON: Hearing Health Care Research Unit.

Seewald, R. C., and Scollie. S. D. (2003). An approach for ensuring accuracy in pediatric hearing instrument fitting. Trends in Amplification, 7, 29–40.

Sharma, A., Dorman, M. F., and Spahr, A. J. (2002). A sensitive period for the development of the central auditory system in children with cochlear implants: implications for age of implantation. Ear and Hearing, 23, 532–539.

Sininger, Y. S., Abdala, C., and Cone-Wesson, B. (1997). Auditory threshold sensitivity of the human neonate as measured by auditory brainstem response. Hearing Research, 104, 27–38.

Stacey, P. C., Fortnum, H. M., Barton, G. R., and Summerfield, Q. (2006). Hearing-impaired children in the United Kingdom, I: Auditory performance, communication skills, educational achievements, quality of life, and cochlear implantation. Ear and Hearing, 27, 161–186.

Stapells, D. R. (2000a). Frequency-specific evoked potential audiometry in infants. In Seewald, R. C. (Ed.), A sound foundation through early amplification: proceedings of an international conference. Stäfa, Switzerland: Phonak AG, 13–32.

Stapells, D. R. (2000b). Threshold estimation by the tone-evoked auditory brainstem response: a literature meta-analysis. Journal of Speech-Language Pathology and Audiology, 24, 74–83.

Stapells, D. R., Gravel, J. S., and Martin, B. E. (1995). Thresholds for auditory brain stem responses to tones in notched noise from infants and young children with normal hearing or sensorineural hearing loss. Ear and Hearing, 16, 361–371.

Stapells, D. R., and Kurtsberg, D. (1991). Evoked potential assessment of auditory system integrity in infants. Clinics in Perinatology, 18, 497–518.

Stelmachowicz, P. G. (1999). Hearing aid outcome measures for children. Journal of the American Academy of Audiology, 10, 14–25.

Stredler-Brown, A. (2002). Developing a treatment program for auditory neuropathy. Seminars in Hearing, 23, 239–249.

Studebaker, G. A. (1982). Hearing aid selection: an overview. In G. A. Studebaker and F. H. Bess (Eds.), The Vanderbilt Hearing Aid Report: State of the art—research needs. Upper Darby, PA: Instrumentation Associates.

Thompson, D. C., McPhillips, H., Davis, R. L., Lieu, T. A., Homer, C. J., and Helfand, M. (2001). Universal newborn hearing screening: summary of evidence. Journal of the American Medical Association, 286, 2000–2010.

Tremblay, K. L., Billings, C. J., Friesen, L. M., and Souza, P. E. (2006). Neural representation of amplified speech sounds. Ear and Hearing, 27, 93–103.

Tremblay, K. L., Friesen, B. A., Martin, B. A., and Wright, R. (2003). Test-retest reliability of cortical evoked potentials using naturally produced speech sounds. Ear and Hearing, 24, 225–232.

Voss, S. E., and Herrmann, B. S. (2005). How does the sound pressure generated by circumaural, supra-aural, and insert earphones differ for adult and infant ears? Ear and Hearing, 26, 636–650.

Wong, S. H., Gibson, W. P. R., and Sanli, H. (1997). Use of transtympanic round window electrocochleography for threshold estimations in children. American Journal of Otolaryngology, 18, 632–636.

Wunderlich, J. L., and Cone-Wesson, B. (2006). Maturation of CAEP in infants and children: a review. Hearing Research, 212, 212–223.

Zakis, J. A., Dillon, H., and McDermott, H. J. The design and evaluation of a hearing aid with trainable amplification parameters. Ear and Hearing.

Chapter 19

Cochlear Implants for Infants and Children

George Alexiades, Myriam De La Asuncion, Ronald A. Hoffman, Rebecca Kooper, Jane R. Madell, Lori B. Markoff, Simon C. Parisier, and Nicole Sislian

---

Key Points

- Cochlear implants can provide auditory access for children with severe to profound hearing loss who do not receive sufficient benefit from hearing aids.

- Surgery is routine, except in cases of abnormal facial nerve anatomy, inner ear malformation, or ossification caused by meningitis.

- Complications of cochlear implantation are unusual, and usually minor.

- Candidacy criteria are expanding to include younger children, and children and adults with severe hearing loss.

♦ What Is a Cochlear Implant?

A cochlear implant is a small electronic medical device surgically implanted in the cochlea that provides access to auditory input for children and adults with severe to profound hearing loss. A cochlear implant does not provide normal hearing, but rather a representation of sound, which, through aural rehabilitation, can be interpreted by the user as speech. A cochlear implant comprises internal and external parts **(see Fig. 19–1)**. The external components include the microphone, a speech processor, and an external antenna with a magnet in the center. The internal parts include an antenna with a magnet in the center, a receiver/stimulator, and an electrode array. The external and internal portions communicate via radio frequency waves [frequency modulation (FM) signals] from the external to the internal antenna, which are kept in alignment by the magnets.

♦ How Does an Implant Work?

The microphone **(see Fig. 19–1)** of the cochlear implant is located at ear level, either on or behind the ear, and picks up sounds in the environment. It works in a similar fashion to the microphone of a hearing aid. Sound waves travel

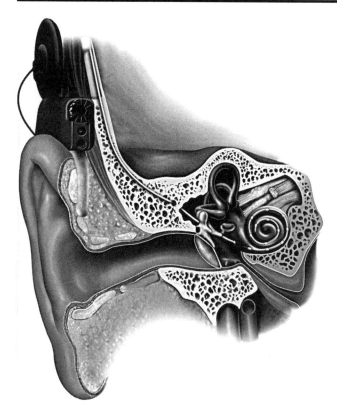

Figure 19–1 External and internal portions of a cochlear implant. (From Med El Corporation.)

through the air, and the acoustic energy is picked up. The microphone then transmits the signal to the speech processor, which is typically worn either behind the ear, in a pocket, or on the belt. The speech processor modifies the auditory signal and divides it into frequencies and intensities appropriate for the individual.

The electrode array is surgically placed within the cochlea and takes advantage of the tonotopic distribution of eighth nerve fibers along the cochlear partition. Higher frequency sounds are perceived at the basal end of the cochlea, and progressively lower frequencies are perceived as stimulation occurs up the basilar membrane toward the apex of the cochlea. This tonotopic distribution allows for pitch matching with specific electrodes. There is general agreement that the cochlear implant electrodes do not stimulate hair cells or nerve endings directly, but rather "ganglion cells," which are the collection of eighth nerve cells located in the bony modiolus of the cochlea. The frequencies that are stimulated are typically divided into 12 to 22 bands, depending on the type of implant used, and the speech-coding strategy chosen.

Once the speech processor has modified the information, the signal is sent from the external antenna to the internal antenna and then to the internal receiver. The signal is then extracted and decoded and sent to the electrode array. This sound, which is now in the form of electrical energy, is then transmitted to different regions of the cochlea, to the auditory (hearing) nerve, and subsequently to the brain where it is interpreted as sound.

◆ Electrode Arrays and the Cochlea

The electrode array is implanted inside the scala tympani, the portion of the cochlea that connects to the tympanic cavity of the ear (Goravalingappa, 2002). Once the cochlea has received the signal, it is sent to the eighth cranial nerve and up to the brain for processing.

Single versus Multichannel Electrode Arrays

The cochlear implant electrode array is separated into different bands, or channels. The first cochlear implants were single-channel devices, meaning that only one usable electrode was available. Single-channel devices distributed the sound to the auditory nerve as a whole, rather than to specific regions of the cochlea. With a single-channel device, the implant was useful for sound awareness, facilitated an increased ability to speech-read, and for some users, provided some basic speech discrimination cues. Today, electrode arrays are broken into many bands (typically 12 to 22, depending on the manufacturer). With multichannel devices, it is very common for a cochlear implant user to not only discriminate and recognize speech, but also to be able to speak on the telephone and enjoy music (Anderson et al, 2006).

Special Electrode Arrays

Split Array

The split electrode array is designed for patients who have ossified cochleas, usually as the result of meningitis. One part of the electrode is inserted into the basal end of the cochlea and the other into the apical end. In this way, some low and some high frequency stimulation can be obtained.

Short Electrode Array for Electrical and Acoustic Stimulation

A new type of cochlear implant is currently in clinical trials in the United States. This device is being developed to meet the needs of patients who have sloping hearing loss with good low-frequency hearing, but with severe to profound hearing loss in the high frequencies. These patients have not received good benefit from hearing aids because their high frequency hearing loss is so severe. Until recently, they would not have been considered candidates for cochlear implantation, since implantation would have damaged their good low-frequency hearing. Two manufacturers (Cochlear Corporation, Sydney, Australia, and Med-El Corporation, Innsbruck, Austria), have systems in clinical trial now that consist of a short electrode that provides high-frequency electrical information and, ideally, does not destroy the good low-frequency hearing. These devices can be used with a hearing aid, if needed, to amplify low frequencies.

Cochlear Implant Manufacturers

Specific information about current cochlear implants can be found on the manufacturers' Web sites:

♦ Advanced Bionics Corporation www.bionics.com

♦ Cochlear Americas www.cochlear.com

♦ Med El Corporation www.medel.com

♦ Cochlear Implant Candidacy

Older Children, Teens with Acquired Hearing Loss, and Adults

Cochlear implantation is considered when the person with hearing loss is not receiving sufficient benefit from hearing aids. Initially, only patients with profound hearing loss were eligible for implantation. The usual cochlear implant candidate had limited speech recognition, minimal telephone use, and did not benefit from standard hearing aids.

As implant technology has improved, and the benefits from implantation have become more evident, patients with less severe hearing loss have been receiving implants. Cochlear implants are now considered appropriate for teens and adults with a bilateral severe-to-profound sensorineural hearing loss (SNHL) [pure tone average (PTA) at least 70 dB hearing level (HL)], and speech perception of 40% or less. Typically, older children, teens, and adults who lose hearing postlingually (after the onset of language, or after about 5 years of age), and who wear hearing aids, will do well with a cochlear implant because their brains have been listening to sound and they have auditory memory. Older teens and adults with prelingual deafness or with postlingual hearing loss who have not been using hearing aids for many years may receive more limited benefit.

Age does not play a role in determining outcome. Studies have indicated a favorable association between shorter duration of deafness and good outcomes with a cochlear implant (Leung, Wang, and Yeagle, 2005). There is no age limit for a cochlear implant, and adults older than 90 years have been successfully implanted.

> **Pitfall**
>
> • Older teens with congenital deafness who do not have realistic expectations about cochlear implant benefit may be disappointed with results. It is important that the audiologist counsel the patient and family to be certain they have realistic expectations.

Infants and Children

U.S. Food and Drug Administration guidelines approve cochlear implantation for infants 12 to 24 months of age who have profound hearing loss (PTA 90 dB HL or poorer), and children 24 months of age and older with severe or profound hearing loss (PTA 70 dB HL or poorer). Many implant centers will implant children below the age of 1 year as long as the degree of hearing loss is confirmed and the child has had a hearing aid trial indicating insufficient benefit.

Determining candidacy for children is a team effort (see Chapter 22 about Team Management). A core evaluation for candidacy includes examination by an audiologist, a speech-language pathologist, and an otolaryngologist. In many cochlear implant centers, children will also meet with an educator and a psychologist, and in some centers, the family may meet with a social worker as well.

The audiologist is responsible for confirming degree of hearing loss, arranging for a trial of appropriate amplification, and determining if the child is receiving sufficient hearing aid benefit. The speech-language pathologist evaluates the child's speech, language, and auditory skills. The information obtained will establish baseline skills and assist in evaluating auditory potential. The otolaryngologist determines surgical candidacy (see Surgery section). The educator or teacher of the deaf works with the family in reviewing the child's educational options to ensure an optimal environment for learning with the cochlear implant. Auditory emphasis or, at the very least, a program that encourages the use of audition, is critically important for developing auditory skills and, in turn, developing speech and language. These skills do not develop automatically on activation of a cochlear implant, but require training. To optimize cochlear implant performance, the family needs to learn how to provide a good listening environment at home.

Social work services are helpful in assessing home and family issues. Access to a social worker who is knowledgeable about issues of childhood hearing loss can be critical to establishing realistic expectations and promoting success.

Although audiologic criteria, the degree of hearing loss, and performance with hearing aids are critical in determining candidacy, decisions about candidacy are not based solely on audiologic test results. For example, a child with profound hearing loss may have multiple disabilities, be enrolled in a therapy program that uses sign language exclusively, and have a home environment in which the parents work full time away from home. Such a child might be cared for by a babysitter who does not speak to the child and is inattentive to proper use of hearing aids. None of these problems individually would contraindicate implantation, but the combination makes success unlikely. Having the child evaluated by multiple clinicians as part of a team will increase the probability that all critical issues are identified and addressed. Success, although not guaranteed, will be more probable.

Children in general do well with cochlear implants because of their remarkable central nervous system plasticity. This plasticity is greatest from birth through about the age of 4 years. Typically, the younger the child is implanted, the better the speech and language outcome. Research suggests that children implanted at younger ages can be successfully integrated into the mainstream (Geers and Brenner, 2003; Chute and Nevins, 2006; Niparko et al, 2001). Children implanted before the age of 2 who are enrolled in an auditory-oral or auditory-verbal therapy program have the potential to develop speech and language skills at the same rate as their normal hearing peers (McConkey-Robbins et al, 2004). Those who have used hearing aids since early identification have good listening skills and, even when receiving an implant at a later date, can develop good use of audition. Older children, who are not experienced hearing aid users before implantation, will likely receive more limited benefit from implantation. Many such children, however, still receive enough benefit to make implantation worthwhile because they experience improved lipreading skills and better ability to identify environmental sounds.

The decision to implant is more difficult when children have severe hearing loss and receive some obvious benefit from their hearing aids. In these cases it is imperative to evaluate their speech perception ability at average and at soft conversational levels, which, if poor, may make them better candidates. (Refer to Chapter 10 for more information about evaluating speech perception.) Many children with severe hearing loss perform well for normal conversation in quiet but depend inordinately on hearing aid/FM systems. They manage to get through the school day but come home exhausted from the effort to listen. They are FM dependent (they rely on the FM system to understand conversation because their hearing aids allow only limited distance hearing.) Many of these children do very well with implants—much better than they did with their hearing aids. They find listening much less stressful and, although they use and benefit from FM systems, they are not dependent on them for listening in all situations because the cochlear implant allows better access to sound by extending distance hearing (Schafer and Thibodeau, 2006).

Another challenging group is children with auditory neuropathy/dysynchrony (see chapter 32). The current trend is to implant auditory neuropathy/dys-synchrony children early, if they do poorly with hearing aids.

Pearl

- Early implantation in infants and young children with severe and profound hearing loss provides the best opportunity for auditory access. Good brain access to the complete speech spectrum, in turn, typically results in superior benefit from implantation as evidenced by the child's ability to use hearing to learn language.

♦ Surgery

Presurgery Considerations

Cochlear implant surgery is a relatively straightforward otologic procedure. In the majority of cases, the temporal bone is normally developed, well pneumatized, and free of any disease.

Cochlear implantation is routinely performed on children 1 year of age and older. The main limiting factors in children younger than 1 year are anesthesia related. Children younger than 1 year of age who weigh less than 20 pounds may be at increased anesthesia risk (Young, 2002). Accordingly, children younger than one year are evaluated on a case by case basis. One factor that promotes early implantation is deafness secondary to meningitis. Deafness caused by meningitis

is often associated with ossification (obstruction by new bone formation) within the cochlea. Ossification can be rapidly progressive, limits full electrode insertion, and may lead to suboptimal postoperative performance. When a child younger than 1 year has had meningitis, early implantation is preferred.

A proper preoperative evaluation is the key to ensuring success in the operating room. A thorough history and physical exam should be performed to elucidate the etiology of hearing loss, identify past or present ear infections, and detect medical conditions that might interfere with general anesthesia. High-resolution computed tomography (CT) or magnetic resonance imaging (MRI) of the temporal bones should be performed preoperatively. A CT scan of the temporal bones details the bony anatomy of the ear, identifies the location of the facial nerve, delineates any congenital cochlear anomalies, and helps to identify bony ossification of the cochlea that can occur after meningitis. An MRI does not show bone well but excels at defining soft tissue. Accordingly, an MRI is the study of choice if there is concern about a cochlear nerve or central brain abnormality (Parry, Booth, and Roland, 2005). In addition, an MRI scan can help in identifying the degree of cochlear ossification because the MRI shows normal cochlear fluids when they are present. In certain situations, both imaging modalities are required.

Pearl

- Meningitis requires rapid evaluation and cochlear implantation because of the risk of postmeningitic bony obstruction of the cochlea when a severe to profound SNHL is encountered.

Surgical Considerations

The most important pieces of information from the surgeon's viewpoint include the patient's temporal bone anatomy, particularly facial nerve anatomy, cochlear anatomy, and cochlear patency (i.e., ossification), which is evaluated with a CT scan. Patients with abnormal cochlear anatomy or ossification must be counseled regarding the possibility of an incomplete electrode insertion and subsequent decreased postoperative performance with the implant. From a technical perspective, modified electrodes are available for implanting patients with cochlear malformations or an ossified cochlea.

Surgical Procedure

A brief overview of the surgical procedure helps one to better understand the challenges and risks involved. The skin incision is a routine postauricular incision **(see Fig. 19–2)** in the crease behind the ear.

The mastoid bone is identified and a "well" is created to house the body of the receiver/stimulator portion of the implant. The well is a circular area, several millimeters deep, drilled in the bone of the skull. To anchor the device to the skull so it will not move, small tunnels are created in the

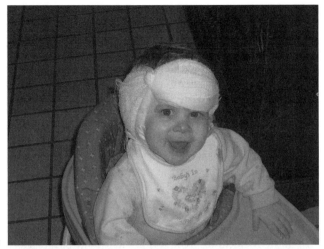

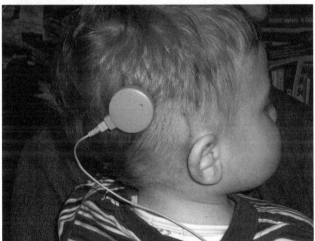

Figure 19–2   **(A)** Postoperative dressing. **(B)** Cochlear implant scar.

bone above and below the well. These tunnels secure sutures that are used to fix the device to the skull so that it will not move. A simple mastoidectomy, which involves removing the mastoid bone (air cells) with a drill, is then performed. A canal is then created in the bone between the well and mastoid to allow the electrode lead wire to rest in this channel and be protected from external trauma. Once the mastoidectomy is completed, a facial recess opening is performed. The facial recess connects the mastoid bone with the middle ear. To open the facial recess, the facial nerve must be surgically identified. A cochleostomy is then performed anterior and inferior to the round window, through the cochlear promontory. This creates an opening into the scala tympani, the largest and most inferior chamber of the cochlea. The receiver and stimulator are slid under the skin, in a subperiosteal pocket behind the well. The device is seated into the well and secured by a nonabsorbable suture. The electrode array is then inserted through the facial recess into the cochleostomy. The cochleostomy is packed with soft tissue around the electrode array to prevent leakage of perilymph. The wound is closed and a mastoid dressing is then applied. (The DVD accompanying this book has a short video showing cochlear implant surgery.)

Surgical Complications

Surgical complications are, happily, quite unusual with cochlear implantation. Facial nerve paralysis is a rare but serious complication of any ear surgery. The overall incidence of facial nerve injury in cochlear implantation is less than 1% in experienced hands (Fayad et al, 2003). Generally in such cases, there is a partial facial weakness that is delayed in onset with complete recovery anticipated in 2 to 6 weeks. Facial nerve injury is avoided by the surgeon having a thorough familiarity with normal facial nerve anatomy, the particular patient's anatomy as delineated on preoperative CT scans, and the use of real time intraoperative facial nerve monitoring. The incidence of facial nerve injury may be higher in patients where the facial nerve does not follow its usual anatomic course, as often happens with cochlear malformations.

Wound problems and infections occur in 3 to 4% of patients. These can be mild, with just some redness (erythema) of the wound, or can be a severe bacterial infection with resulting wound breakdown and extrusion of the device (Cunningham et al, 2004). Since the cochlear implant is a foreign body, all wound problems must be treated quickly and aggressively.

Dizziness for a few days after cochlear implantation is not unusual. Occasionally, the dizziness is of delayed onset, beginning 1 to 2 days after surgery. Dizziness rarely persists beyond a few weeks in children (Buchman et al, 2004).

The cochlea contains perilymph, which routinely leaks out during cochlear implant surgery. After the electrode array is implanted, the opening into the cochlea is sealed with fascia or periosteal tissue taken from within the surgical field. If perilymph leaks after surgery, it can lead to ongoing dizziness and, rarely, meningitis. Perilymph leakage and meningitis usually occur in association with a severely malformed cochlea. In the presence of a severely malformed cochlea, it is not unusual for there to be an abnormal communication between the cochlea and the cerebrospinal fluid space surrounding the brain. If a perilymph fistula occurs, it may need to be surgically repaired. Meningitis can be life threatening and must be treated with strong intravenous antibiotics. Because of the risk of meningitis, it is recommended that all children receive pneumococcal and *Haemophilus influenza* vaccines before cochlear implant surgery (CDC, 2003).

Delayed complications, weeks or months after surgery, are rare. Of particular concern in this regard, however, is excessive pressure between the external and internal magnets. Extreme pressure can block the blood supply to the skin and cause it to become devitalized and subsequently break down with infection or extrusion of the implant. Often, the first sign of impending skin breakdown is pain over this area. It is imperative that parents and audiologists routinely check to be sure that there is no redness or swelling over the internal magnet. Electrode and device migrations have been reported in the literature, but these are rare events (Hoffman et al, 1991; Roland et al, 1998).

Bilateral Cochlear Implant Surgery

Bilateral cochlear implantation has been gaining in popularity in recent years. Bilateral cochlear implantation can be performed simultaneously or sequentially. Simultaneous implantation occurs when both implants are placed as part of the same surgical procedure, with one anesthesia. Sequential implantation involves two separate surgeries, usually several weeks, months, or even years apart. Simultaneous implantation has the advantage of just one preoperative evaluation, one general anesthetic, and one period of recovery. However, postoperative discomfort is significantly higher in the simultaneous implant group. Should there be a postoperative fever, it can be difficult to determine which implant has the potential infection. Blood loss, which is usually not significant in a unilateral implant, does become an issue in younger children, whose overall blood volume is quite small. As a result, at our institution, we generally do not perform simultaneous cochlear implants in children younger than 2 years, unless there are other overriding factors such as ossification secondary to meningitis.

The overall complication rate with bilateral cochlear implantation is not significantly higher than for the unilateral group. Dizziness, which was an initial concern in bilateral implantation, has not been significantly higher in children. The risk of facial nerve paralysis remains quite small in experienced hands.

♦ Management following Implantation in Children

A few weeks after surgery, with healing complete, the habilitative process begins. For all cochlear implant devices, the speech processor program or MAP needs to be created in order for the child to have accessibility to sound. A MAP consists of a "setting" that includes threshold levels (the lowest amount of electrical stimulation needed to induce an auditory sensation) and maximum or comfortable levels (the amount of electrical stimulation that is comfortable or loud, depending on the manufacturer.) The difference between the threshold and maximum levels is known as the dynamic range (DR) (Clark, 2003). The DR essentially provides the patient with a range of hearing that is usable through the implant. Threshold levels are obtained using standard audiologic procedures [visual reinforcement (VRA) and conditioned play audiometry (CPA)]. The threshold and maximum levels change significantly from the initial stimulation over the first few months, and may continue to change over time. "Fine tuning" is necessary to verify that measurements continue to be optimal. Within each speech processor program, parameters can be changed or modified, affecting the habilitative outcomes. Most speech processors can store several programs, which may be set for different needs. For example, programs may be set with increasing loudness or for use with an FM system, music, or noisy situations. As children become older, their programming needs change. A teenager, for example, may require a phone program, or a "party" program, and these special programs can be set and changed accordingly.

In addition to cochlear implant mapping, every child should be evaluated in the test booth at a minimum of 3-, 6-, 9-, and 12-month intervals after initial stimulation, and twice yearly after the first year to be certain that the child is receiving the expected implant benefit. Evaluations will demonstrate at what levels the child is responding to sound and help determine if the device is programmed optimally. The child should be responding to sound at audible levels throughout the speech range (at the top of the speech banana) to permit her to have access to soft spoken language at distances. As soon as possible, audiologic evaluation should include speech perception testing (see Chapter 10). Information about specific speech perception errors can be used to modify the cochlear implant MAP to improve the child's speech perception capabilities.

Children are mapped using whichever behavioral technique (VRA or CPA) is age appropriate. Objective measures can also be used to establish MAPs. Using a program imbedded in the cochlear implant, it is possible to measure neural response telemetry or neural response imaging. These measurements determine the approximate threshold for stimulation of the auditory nerve without the need for a behavioral response. However, behavioral responses and objective measures do not always provide the same results and, in some cases, may differ significantly. Whenever possible, the audiologist should use behavioral responses to begin to create the MAP. The more reliable the behavioral responses, the more precise the MAPs will be for that specific child. An appropriate MAP facilitates speech detection and eventually speech perception, maximizing the potential of using audition to learn and develop speech and language.

♦ Using Two Ears: Bimodal Hearing and Bilateral Cochlear Implants

Traditionally, cochlear implantation has been performed monaurally; the nonimplant ear is preserved for future technologies. As the benefit of binaural hearing has become more evident, clinics have begun offering bilateral cochlear implantation more routinely. Current research is establishing the efficacy of implanting two ears.

The benefits of hearing with two ears is well documented for normal hearing listeners and for hearing aid users (Bronkhurst and Plomp, 1988; Byrne, Noble, and LePage, 1992; Simon, 2005) and includes increased speech intelligibility in quiet and in noise, improved sound quality, and better sound localization.

Binaural hearing listeners use interaural time differences and interaural level/intensity differences (ILDs) between the two ears for speech understanding in noise and for sound localization (Bronkhurst and Plomp, 1988; van Hoesel, Ramsden, and O'Driscoll, 2002). Unilteral implant users perform poorly in noise mainly because ILD cues are lost. (Bronkhurst and Plomp, 1989; Simon, 2005). Performance is also limited by the head shadow effect, squelch effect, and lack of binaural summation.

Head shadow refers to the benefit obtained as the noise source moves from the ipsilateral side to the contralateral side, so that the ear in use is shielded from the noise by the head. The term refers to the head acting as an acoustic barrier which causes attenuation in the high frequencies of the ear farthest from the sound. Hearing in the ear contralateral to the noise improves the signal-to-noise ratio in that ear. Improving the signal-to-noise ratio results in improved speech understanding in noise.

Binaural summation and squelch require binaural brain processing. Binaural squelch refers to the benefit resulting from the spatial separation between the signal source and the noise source (Schleich, Nopp, and D'Haese, 2004), due to signal processing by the brain of input from two ears. With two ears, the brain may have a better representation of the noise and speech and be better able to separate them. Binaural summation refers to the advantage of hearing with two ears when the signal arrives at both ears simultaneously (Schleich, Hopp, and D'Haese, 2004; Schon, Fuller, and Helms, 2002). Listening with two ears results in an improvement in hearing threshold of 3 dB (Schon, Fuller, and Helms, 2002).

Children who use only one cochlear implant may still benefit from using a hearing aid in the unimplanted ear. This is especially true as children with more residual hearing are being implanted. Even when a hearing aid does not provide good benefit on its own, a hearing aid with a cochlear implant can provide improved benefit. Several studies have demonstrated the improvement in performance with bimodal hearing (cochlear implant in one ear and hearing aid in the other ear) (Litovsky et al, 2004; Madell et al, 2005).

◆ Habilitation and Rehabilitation

Because children hear so much better with cochlear implants than they did with their hearing aids, families sometimes forget that implants alone are not enough. Every child *must* be involved in a therapy program that encourages the use of hearing. When children are implanted very young, cochlear implants can provide almost every child with sufficient hearing to develop speech and language using audition. Optimally, the child will receive therapy two or three times weekly, and the therapist will teach the family how to maximize auditory language stimulation within daily routines at home and at school. (See Chapters 21 and 25 for a discussion of therapy methods for working with children with cochlear implants.) As soon as possible, implanted children should begin to spend time with normal hearing children to enable them to develop the communication and social skills that will enable them to be mainstreamed. Older children are also better able to maximize their auditory skills with auditory therapy. Although in general, the expected benefit from implantation will vary depending on preimplant skills, with therapy and parental support listening skills can be maximized.

Children who receive one cochlear implant may benefit from using a hearing aid on their unimplanted ear to provide binaural hearing. Young children may not use a hearing aid at all initially. Older children, who are in school and who need to hear as well as possible during the day, may wear their hearing aids in school but are encouraged to use their implants alone at least 3 hours per day during the adjustment period to improve their ability to understand speech with this very different stimulus. Once the child is consistently hearing and understanding speech with the implant, a hearing aid can be used on the unimplanted ear full time.

◆ Cochlear Implants and Frequency Modulation Systems

Increasing numbers of children with cochlear implants are attending schools in mainstream settings. Although this affords them many educational advantages, poor classroom acoustics is an obstacle to success. Noise sources that contribute to poor acoustics include heating and air-conditioning systems, noise from computers and other projectors, and noise from hallways and outside traffic. In these noisy environments, children with cochlear implants demonstrate decreased speech recognition scores. Schafer and Thibodeau (2003) found that sentence recognition in noise decreased by 35% compared with scores obtained in quiet. FM systems can improve the signal-to-noise ratio (SNR) in the classroom. (See Chapter 20 for a discussion of FM systems and classroom acoustics.) Many FM options are now available for the student with a cochlear implant.

Personal FM systems include a transmitter worn by the talker, and a receiver that is coupled directly to the implant speech processor, either body worn or behind the ear. Personal FM systems provide the best SNR. Unlike hearing aids, however, where a normal hearing listener can monitor the FM signal by listening through the hearing aid, it is difficult to examine FM function with cochlear implants. As a result, a personal FM system may not be a good choice for a young child with poor language skills who cannot report equipment problems. Once a child is able to answer questions and repeat back what is said, it is easier to verify that the FM system is working appropriately.

A special consideration when fitting children using cochlear implants with personal FM systems is setting the mixing ratio. For children with cochlear implants, the mixing ratio is set by the implant audiologist during speech processor programming. At the time of the programming, the audiologist must decide the mixing ratio that will allow a good balance between the input from the microphone on the speech processor, and the input from the microphone on the FM transmitter. With the correct ratio, the child will be able to hear herself as well as the other students when the FM transmitter is on.

A desktop FM system consists of a small bag or case that houses an FM receiver that can be placed on the student's desk. The unit is light enough to be carried around from desk to desk or from classroom to classroom. These units are easy to monitor but do not have the portability of personal, wearable systems. Desktop systems work well only when the child is nearby. As the child moves away from the system, benefit diminishes. Nevertheless, a desktop FM device is the preferred system for children who cannot use a personal FM system. There are portable and wall-mounted soundfield systems that provide amplification for an entire classroom; however, these are less effective than a personal-worn FM or a desktop FM for a child with a cochlear implant (Anderson, 2005).

For most children, it can be expected that distance hearing will be best with a personal FM system. However, problems with interference can develop with any FM system, and it is important to be certain that the system selected works for the child using it. Ideally, the child should be tested in an audiology test booth with the cochlear implant alone, and then with the implant and FM together, to be certain that the signal the child is receiving is at least as good as that with the cochlear implant alone, and preferably, better (especially for perception of soft speech and speech in noise). The FM system should also be checked in the child's classroom to be certain that there is no interference in that environment.

◆ Conclusion

Cochlear implants provide excellent benefit for children with severe and profound hearing loss who do not receive sufficient benefit from their hearing aids. When candidates are suitably selected, when speech processors are correctly programmed, and when appropriate habilitation is provided, children can be expected to use their listening skills to develop good language and to have intelligible speech. These are youngsters who typically experience successful mainstreaming in their home schools.

Discussion Questions

1. What are the main components of a cochlear implant?

2. Briefly describe some potential complications of cochlear implant surgery.

3. Describe the advantages and disadvantages of bilateral cochlear implantation.

4. How does a cochlear implant differ from a hearing aid?

5. What is the difference between objective and behavioral measures used for programming cochlear implants?

References

Anderson, I., Baumgartner, W. D., Böheim, C., Nahler, A., Arnolder, C., and D'Haese, P. (2006). Telephone use: what benefit do cochlear implant users receive? International Journal of Audiology, 45, 446–453.

Anderson, K., Goldstein, H., Colodzin, L., and Iglehart, F. (2005). Benefit of S/N enhancing devices to speech perception of children listening in a typical classroom with hearing aids or a cochlear implant. Journal of Educational Audiology, 12, 14–28.

Bronkhorst, A. W., and Plomp, R. (1988). The effect of head-induced interaural time and level differences on speech intelligibility in noise. Journal of the Acoustical Society of America, 83, 1508–1516.

Bronkhorst, A. W., and Plomp, R. (1989). Binaural speech intelligibility in noise for hearing-impaired listeners. Journal of the Acoustical Society of America, 86, 1374–1383.

Byrne, D., Noble, W., and LePage, B. (1992). Effects of long-term bilateral and unilateral fitting of different hearing aid types on the ability to locate sounds. Journal of the American Academy of Audiology, 3, 369–382.

Centers for Disease Control and Prevention (CDC). Advisory Committee on Immunization Practices. (2003). Pneumococcal vaccination for cochlear implant candidates and recipients: updated recommendations of the Advisory Committee on Immunization Practices. Morbidity and Mortality Weekly Report, 52, 739–740.

Chute, P. M., and Nevins, M. E. (2006). School Professionals Working with Children with Cochlear Implants. San Diego: Plural Publications.

Clark, G. (2003). Cochlear implants: fundamentals and applications. New York: Springer-Verlag.

Cunningham, C. D. 3rd, Slattery, W. H. 3rd, and Luxford, W. M. (2004). Postoperative infection in cochlear implant patients. Otolaryngology–Head and Neck Surgery, 131, 109–114.

Fayad, J. N., Wanna, G. B., Micheletto, J. N., and Parisier, S. C. (2003). Facial nerve paralysis following cochlear implant surgery. Laryngoscope, 113, 1344–1346.

Geers, A. E., and Brenner, C. (2003). Background and educational characteristics of prelingually deaf children implanted before five years of age. Ear and Hearing, 24, 2S–14S.

Goravalingappa, R. (2002). Cochlear implant electrode insertion: Jacobson's nerve, a useful anatomical landmark. Indian Journal of Otology & Head & Neck Surgery, 54, 70–73.

Hoffman, R. A., Cohen, N., Waltzman, S., Shapiro, W., and Goldofsky, E. (1991). Delayed extrusion of the nucleus multichannel cochlear implant. Otolaryngology–Head and Neck Surgery, 105,117–119.

Leung, J., Wang, N. Y., and Yeagle, J., et al. (2005). Predictive models for cochlear implantation in elderly candidates. Archives of Otolaryngology Head & Neck Surgery, 131, 1049–1054.

Litovsky, R. Y., Parkinson, A., Arcaroli, J., et al. (2004). Bilateral cochlear implants in adults and children. Archives of Otolaryngology–Head and Neck Surgery, 130, 648–655.

Madell, J. R., Sislian, N. S., and Markoff, L. (2005). Bimodal Hearing: Hearing Aid on the Unimplanted Ear. Poster presented at Implantable Auditory Prosthesis Conference, August 1–5, Asilomar, C4.

McConkey-Robbins, A. D., Burton-Koch, M., Osberger, M. J., Zimmerman-Phillips, S., and Kishon-Rabin, L. (2004). Effect of age at cochlear implantation on auditory skill development in infants and toddlers. Archives of Otolaryngology Head and Neck Surgery, 130, 570–574.

Niparko, J., Kirk, K., Mellon, N., Robbins, A., Tucci, D., and Wilson, B. (2001). Cochlear implants: principles and practices. Philadelphia: Lippincott Williams and Wilkins.

Parry, D. A., Booth, T., and Roland, P. S. (2005). Advantages of magnetic resonance imaging over computed tomography in preoperative evaluation of pediatric cochlear implant candidates. Otology and Neurotology, 26, 976–982.

Roland, J. T. Jr. (2005) A model for cochlear implant electrode insertion and force evaluation: results with a new electrode design and insertion technique. Laryngoscope, 115, 1325–1339.

Roland, J. T., Fishman, A. J., Waltzman, S. B., Alexiades, G., Hoffman, R. A., and Cohen, N. L. (1998). Stability of the cochlear implant array in children. Laryngoscope, 108, 1119–1123.

Schafer, E., and Thibodeau, L. (2006). Speech recognition in noise in children with cochlear implants while listening in bilateral, bimodal, and FM-system arrangements. American Journal of Audiology, 15, 114–126.

Schafer, E., and Thibodeau, L. (2003). Speech-recognition performance of children using cochlear implants and FM systems. Journal of Educational Audiology, 11, 15–26.

Schleich, P., Nopp, P., and D'Haese, P. (2004). Head shadow, squelch, and summation effects in bilateral users of the med-e; combi 40/40+ cochlear implant. Ear and Hearing, 197–204.

Schon, F., Fuller, J., and Helms J. (2002). Speech reception thresholds obtained in a symmetrical four-loudspeaker arrangement from bilateral users of Med-El cochlear implants. Otology and Neurotology, 23, 710–714.

Simon, H. J. (2005). Bilateral amplification and sound localization: then and now. Journal of Rehabilitation Research and Development, 42, 117–132.

van Hoesel, R., Ransden, R., and O'Driscoll, M. (2002). Sound-direction identification, interaural time delay discrimination, and speech intelligibility advantages in noise for a bilateral cochlear implant user. Ear and Hearing, 23, 137–149.

Chapter 20

Classroom Acoustics: Personal and Soundfield FM and IR Systems

Joseph Smaldino and Carol Flexer

♦ **Classroom Acoustics: An Overview**

Effects of Signal-to-Noise Ratio (SNR)

Effects of Reverberation Time (RT)

Effects of Signal-to-Noise Ratio and Reverberation Time Together

♦ **Classroom Acoustic Guidelines and Standards**

Noise Effects on Student and Teacher Performance

Effects of Reverberation

Status of the ANSI S12.6 Acoustical Standard

♦ **Assistive Listening Devices: Personal FM, and Soundfield FM, and IR (Classroom Amplification) Systems**

Personal FM Unit

Use of a Personal FM at Home

Soundfield FM and IR Systems (Classroom Amplification Systems)

Who Might Benefit from Soundfield Distribution Systems?

Practical Issues for Assistive Listening Device Selection

Should an Audiologist Recommend a Personal FM System, a Soundfield System, or Both for a Given Child?

Measuring Efficacy of Fitting and Use of Technology

Functional Assessments as a Measure of Efficacy of FM and IR Technology

Equipment Efficacy for the School System

♦ **Conclusion**

Key Points

- The classroom is an auditory verbal environment in which accurate transmission and reception of speech between the teacher and students, or students and students is critical for effective learning to occur.

- Speech intelligibility is based on the science of signal-to-noise ratio (SNR), the relationship of the desired signal to all background and competing noise; children need the desired signal to be 10 times, or 15 to 20 dB louder than background noise to clearly discriminate words.

- Soundfield amplification technology is an exciting educational tool that allows control of the acoustic environment in a classroom, thereby facilitating acoustic accessibility of teacher instruction for all children in the room.

- Efficacy of technology use may be measured through educational performance, behavioral speech perception tests, direct measures of changes in brain development, or functional assessments.

The purpose of all environmental and technological management strategies is to enhance the reception of clear and intact acoustic signals to access, develop, and organize the auditory centers of the brain. Accordingly, this chapter will discuss classroom acoustics and the frequency modulation (FM) and infrared (IR) technologies that are necessary to improve access to the learning environment for all children.

◆ Classroom Acoustics: An Overview

The classroom is an auditory verbal environment in which accurate transmission and reception of speech between the teacher and students, or students and students is critical for effective learning to occur. Since information is exchanged in a classroom, it can be modeled using an information theory approach. The genesis of modern day information theory arose from Claude Shannon's 1948 paper titled, "A Mathematical Theory of Communication." By simplifying this theory, an understanding of the classroom acoustic environment and ways to maximize communication can occur. **Fig. 20–1** is an example of such an information transfer model.

In this model the speaker and listener bring important variables to the communication process. The speaker must speak loud enough for speech to be audible. This audibility variable is influenced by the vocal effort of the speaker and the distance between the speaker and listener. The speaker must also present a clear undistorted speech signal. Finally, the speaker can use speech that is either simple or complex, and the speech can be familiar or unfamiliar to the listener. The listener must have enough speech and language competency to use the efficiencies and redundancy resident in speech and language syntax, semantics, and phonology. In addition, the listener must have certain cognitive and processing competencies to retain and form auditory-linguistic linkages in the speech and language centers of the brain.

Separating the speaker and listener is the acoustic transmission path of the speech signal and encoding capacity of the listener. The transmission pathway can be quiet or it can be noisy. If noisy, the noise can derive from loss of information caused by inaudibility, background noise that masks information, or reverberation that distorts and ultimately masks information. The encoding capacity of the listener is a measure of the intactness of the peripheral, brainstem and central auditory mechanism. Loss of hair cells or auditory neurons also can reduce the child's encoding capacity—his ability to perceive the message.

Any of these variables can influence the adequacy of the communication between speaker and listener, and can occur in a multitude of combinations. For example, the best case scenario would be a speaker, whose speech was audible and clear using simple and familiar speech, standing close to a normal hearing listener with fully developed and normal speech, language and cognitive processes, in a room with little noise. The worst case would be a speaker whose speech is inaudible or distorted using complex and unfamiliar speech, some distance from an individual who is severely hearing impaired with incomplete speech, language, or cognitive processes in a room with a lot of noise. Classroom communication environments are somewhere between these two extremes.

Although there has been much research on the effects of room acoustics on speech perception of individuals with hearing loss, **Fig. 20–1** shows that hearing impairment is one of several variables that can be managed to improve information transfer. The other variables can and should also be managed if inadequacy in a variable produces loss of information transfer. Management could include auditory processing therapy, speech therapy, cognitive therapy, hearing assistive devices, and management of the noise in the transmission path. Also, **Fig. 20–1** shows that breakdowns in information transfers are not solely dependent on hearing status. In other words, students with normal hearing but with weaknesses in any other of the highlighted variables will also have an information transfer problem. In addition, some of the variables like speech and language competency or cognitive competency are developmental, so the younger the student the more impact these variables will have on information transfer, simply because they are not in final form. Each variable shown in **Fig. 20–1** is worthy of in-depth consideration, but this discussion will focus on the noise components.

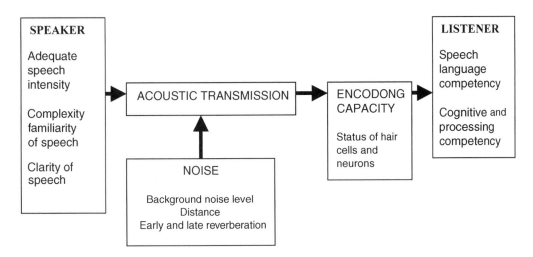

Figure 20–1   A simplified modification of Shannon's Mathematical Theory of Communication.

The acoustic characteristics of the classroom mainly determine the adequacy of the speech signal received by the students. Of importance is the Signal-to-Noise Ratio (SNR) of the teacher's speech received by the student and the reverberation time (RT) of the room. The SNR refers to the relative intensity of the teacher's speech compared with the level of any background noise present in the classroom as measured at the location of the student. RT refers to the length of time a signal persists in a room after the original signal has ended. Sometimes this persistence of sound is referred to as sound reflection or echoes in the classroom. Research has demonstrated that inappropriate levels of classroom noise or reverberation can compromise not only speech perception, but also reading scores, spelling ability, behavior, attention, and concentration in children with normal hearing and are even more deleterious to children with hearing loss or children who are at risk for listening and learning (see Crandell, Smaldino, and Flexer, 2005 for a review of these studies).

Effects of Signal-to-Noise Ratio (SNR)

Background noise in a room reduces speech recognition by covering up or masking important acoustic/linguistic cues in the message. This is especially true of the consonants that carry most of the intelligibility of speech necessary for accurate perception. (See Chapter 17 for a discussion of speech acoustics.) Background noise in a room tends to mask the weaker consonant phonemes significantly more than the more intense vowel phonemes. The most important factor for accurate speech recognition, in this regard, is the ratio of the intensity of the desired signal compared with the intensity of the undesired signal or noise. This ratio is reported as the decibel difference between the two intensities. For example, if the speech was 15 dB louder than the background noise, the SNR would be +15 dB. Speech perception is generally better when speech is considerably louder than the noise and decreases as the SNR of the environment is reduced (Finitzo-Hieber and Tillman, 1978). Speech-recognition ability in adults with normal hearing is not significantly reduced until the SNR is below 0 dB (Bradley, 1986). Ample evidence indicates that children require a much better SNR than adults (Boothroyd, 2004). The rationale for the better SNR is derived from the fact that children do not have fully developed auditory-linguistic and cognitive systems. Their immature systems limit the use of language redundancy and cognitive mechanisms, such as short-term memory, that can be used to overcome the masking effects on speech of too much background noise. To obtain speech recognition scores equal to those of normal hearers, listeners with sensorineural hearing loss

(SNHL) require the SNR to be improved by 4 to 12 dB (Killion, 1997). An additional 3 to 6 dB is needed in rooms with moderate levels of reverberation (Hawkins and Yacullo, 1984). Based on these data, acoustical guidelines for populations who experience hearing loss suggest that SNRs should exceed +15 dB for accurate speech recognition.

Effects of Reverberation Time (RT)

RT refers to the amount of time it takes for a steady state sound to decrease 60 dB from its peak amplitude. In a reverberant room, speech is reflected from various hard room surfaces, so that some of the speech elements are delayed in reaching the ear of the listener. The reflected speech overlaps with the direct speech signal (the signal not reflected before reaching the listener's ear) and covers up or masks certain acoustic speech components. Because vowels are more intense than consonants, a long RT tends to produce a prolongation of the spectral energy of vowels, which then covers up less intense consonant components. A reduction of consonant information can have a significant effect on speech recognition, as most acoustic information that is important for speech recognition is provided by consonants (French and Steinberg, 1947). Speech recognition, therefore, tends to decrease with increases in RT. Speech recognition in adults with normal hearing is not significantly degraded until the RT exceeds approximately 1 second. Listeners with SNHL, however, need considerably shorter RT (0.4 to 0.5 seconds) for optimal communication (Crandell, Smaldino and Flexer, 2005). Because of this increased difficulty, acoustical guidelines for populations who experience hearing loss suggest that RT should not exceed 0.4 to 0.5 seconds in communication environments frequented by these individuals (ASHA, 1995; 2005).

Effects of Signal-to-Noise Ratio and Reverberation Time Together

The effects of RT and SNR interact. That is, when the factors are combined (which is the case in virtually all real-world listening environments), the combination affects speech recognition more than either of the factors alone. Finitzo-Hieber and Tillman eloquently demonstrated this combination effect in 1978. A summary of their findings is shown in **Table 20–1**.

Table 20–1 shows the mean speech recognition scores of children with normal hearing and children with SNHL for monosyllabic words across various SNRs and RTs. At an SNR of +12 dB and RT of 0.4 seconds, children with normal hearing do not recognize speech perfectly (83%) and children with hearing impairment perform even more poorly (60%). As the SNR becomes poorer or as the RT lengthens, speech recognition decreases to the worst case studied (SNR = 0 dB; RT = 1.2 seconds), where children with normal hearing achieve a 30% score and children with hearing loss recognize virtually none of the speech (11%). Both of these listening conditions have been reported in classroom environments. Imagine trying to succeed in school perceiving only 11% of what is presented orally by the teacher!

Another dramatic example of the interplay between classroom acoustics and speech was reported by Leavitt and

Table 20–1 Mean Speech Recognition Scores (% correct) by Children with Normal Hearing and Children with Sensorineural Hearing Loss for Monosyllabic Words Across Various Signal-to-Noise Ratios (SNR) and Reverberation Times (RT)

Condition	Normal Hearing	Hearing Impaired
RT 0.0 seconds		
Quiet	94.5	83.0
+12 dB	89.2	70.0
+6 dB	79.7	59.5
0 dB	60.2	39.0
RT 0.4 seconds		
Quiet	92.5	74.0
+12 dB	82.8	60.2
+6 dB	71.3	52.2
0 dB	47.7	27.8
RT 1.2 seconds		
Quiet	76.5	45.0
+12 dB	68.8	41.2
+6 dB	54.2	27.0
0 dB	29.7	11.2

Abbreviation: RT, reverberation time

Source: Table adapted from Finitzo-Hieber and Tillman (1978).

Flexer in 1991. Using the Rapid Speech Transmission Index (RASTI), they demonstrated that 83% of the speech energy, delivered in the front of a classroom, was available to a listener in the front row of a typical classroom-sized environment. However, in the back row of the same classroom, only about 50% of the speech energy was available. RASTI is a measure of speech energy as it traverses a room and is an index of the amount of energy available to be perceived when influenced by SNR and RT, not the amount perceived. Even less of the signal would be available if the listener has hearing loss or reduced auditory and language processing. These factors would hamper the student's actual perception of the available speech energy. That is, add the impact of the classroom acoustical environment to the distortion imposed by a damaged auditory or linguistic system, and it becomes apparent why simply using a hearing aid is not likely to result in satisfactory communication in the classroom.

◆ Classroom Acoustic Guidelines and Standards

In 2002, the American National Standards Institute (ANSI, 2002) issued standard S12.60 entitled, Acoustical Performance Criteria, Design requirements and Guidelines for Classrooms, which stipulated a background noise level of no more than 35 dB(A). As noted previously, speech recognition in adults with normal hearing is not severely compromised until the SNR of the listening environment is about 0 dB. However, normal hearing children who are learning speech and language and those with listening deficits caused by hearing loss or other listening and learning risk factors require a much better SNR. For listeners with SNHL,

investigators have suggested that SNRs in learning environments should exceed +15 dB (see Crandell, Smaldino, and Flexer, 2005 for a review of these studies). This recommendation is based on the finding that the speech recognition of listeners with hearing impairment tends to remain relatively constant at SNRs in excess of +15 dB but deteriorates at poorer SNRs. In addition, when the SNR decreases below +15, persons with hearing loss have to spend so much attentional effort listening to the message that they often prefer to communicate through other modalities (e.g., sign language or written materials).

To accomplish a +15 SNR, in most settings, it appears that unoccupied room noise levels cannot exceed 30 to 35 dB(A) or approximately an NC 25 curve (ANSI, 2002; Crandell, Smaldino and Flexer, 2005). Studies have reported that these acoustic criteria are infrequently achieved in the academic setting (Crandell and Smaldino, 1995; Knecht, et al, 2002). Crandell and Smaldino (1995) reported that none of 32 classrooms studied met recommended criteria for background noise. Similarly, applying the ANSI (2002) classroom acoustics standard, Knecht, et al (2002) found that most of the 32 elementary grade classrooms they studied did not meet the recommended background noise level of 35 dB(A).

Noise Effects on Student and Teacher Performance

In addition to affecting speech recognition directly, background noise can also compromise academic achievement, literacy, and attendant listening and learning behaviors in the classroom (Anderson, 2001). Rosenberg (2005) completed a comprehensive review of studies that have explored the effects of undesirable levels of background noise. What is striking from reading these studies is that no matter what the variable under study, a better performance was obtained as the SNR improved in virtually every case.

The widespread nature of excessive noise in the classroom was underscored in a 1998 survey of school administrators. The General Accounting Office found that inappropriate classroom acoustics was the most commonly cited problem that affected the learning environment (Access Board Web site, 1998). In addition, the negative effects of undesirable levels of background noise on teachers have been reported. Sapienza, Crandell, and Curtis (1999) showed that teachers exhibit a significantly higher incidence of vocal problems than the general population. It is reasonable to assume that these vocal difficulties are caused, at least in part, by teachers having to increase vocal output to overcome the effects of classroom noise during the school day (Blair, 2006).

Effects of Reverberation

As previously discussed, speech recognition in adults with normal hearing is not significantly affected until the RT exceeds about 1.0 second. For listeners with SNHL, most investigators have recommended that listening environments should not exceed about 0.4 second (through the speech frequency range: 500, 1,000, and 2,000 Hz) to provide optimum communicative efficiency. In 2002, the American National Standards Institute (ANSI, 2002) issued S12.60

Acoustical Performance Criteria, Design Requirements and Guidelines for Classrooms that recommended a RT of 0.6 seconds for moderately sized learning environments. A review of the literature suggests that appropriate RTs for persons with hearing loss are rarely achieved. Crandell and Smaldino (1995) reported that only nine of 32 classrooms (27%) displayed RTs of 0.4 second or less. Knecht et al (2002) applying the ANSI (2002) criteria for reverberation found that most of the 32 elementary grade classrooms they studied did not meet the 0.6-second maximum RT recommended in the standard.

Status of the ANSI S12.6 Acoustical Standard

Compliance with the ANSI classroom performance criteria is, at this writing, completely voluntary. It is hoped that in the future adequate acoustics will be thought of as a necessary requirement in a learning environment, not a luxury. In the future, universal building codes might be modified to include good acoustics, making the classroom listening environment no less important than items already in the codes such as adequate lighting and ventilation. Every effort should be made to meet the background noise and reverberation stipulations of the standard as a first step in improving listening and learning environments for all children. Because of expense, meeting the ANSI (2002) stipulations is often not possible by physical room modification alone.

Pearl

• Meeting the ANSI acoustic performance stipulations does not guarantee adequate acoustic accessibility for children with special listening and learning needs. Other enhancing technologies must also be considered.

◆ Assistive Listening Devices: Personal FM, and Soundfield FM, and IR (Classroom Amplification) Systems

Even though hearing aids are the initial form of amplification for infants and children with hearing loss, hearing aids are not designed to deal with all listening needs. Their biggest limitation is their inability to make the details of spoken communication available under the following conditions: when there is competing noise, when the listener cannot be physically close to the speaker, or when both conditions exist together. Because a clear and complete speech signal greatly facilitates the development of oral expressive language and reading skills, some means of improving the SNR must be provided in all of a child's learning domains (Anderson, 2004; Estabrooks, 2006; Ling, 2002).

Assistive listening device (ALD) is a term used to describe a range of products designed to solve the problems of noise, distance from the speaker, and room reverberation or echo

that cannot be solved with a hearing aid alone (Boothroyd, 2002). ALDs enhance the SNR to improve the intelligibility of speech, expand the baby's or child's distance hearing, and enable incidental learning.

There are many categories of ALDs, ranging from listening devices (which will be discussed in this section) to telephone devices and alert/alarm devices. The types of ALDs most relevant to children might be referred to as SNR-enhancing devices, which include personal FM systems and soundfield IR and FM (classroom) amplification systems. By enhancing the SNR, these devices augment the audibility and intelligibility of the speaker's voice.

Special Consideration

• A pediatric or educational audiologist must be involved in the recommendation and fitting of all hearing aids and assistive listening devices.

Personal FM Unit

A personal FM unit is a wireless personal listening device that includes a remote wireless microphone placed near the desired sound source (usually the speaker's mouth, but it could also be a tape recorder or TV) and a receiver for the listener who can be situated anywhere within about 50 feet of the talker. No wires are required to connect the talker and listener because the unit is really a small Frequency Modulation radio that transmits and receives on a single frequency (**see Fig. 20–2**).

Because the talker wears the remote microphone within 6 inches of his mouth, the personal FM unit creates a

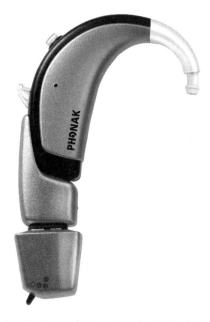

Figure 20–2 Personal FM receiver boot attached to a hearing aid. (Photo from Phonak, with permission).

listening situation that is comparable to a parent or teacher being within 6 inches of the child's ear at all times, thereby allowing a positive and constant SNR (Sexton, 2003). The close proximity to the microphone also eliminates the effects of reverberation, because only direct (not reflected) sound reaches the microphone for transmission. Personal FM systems, therefore, offer a direct communication connection between the talker and listener in any communication situation (ASHA, 2000; Launer, 2003). Personal FM units are essential for a child with any type and degree of hearing loss, from minimal to profound, who is in any classroom or group learning situation (Anderson et al, 2005; ASHA, 2000; Flynn, Flynn, and Gregory, 2005). Several models of personal FM equipment are available, costing approximately $2500 per unit. The most common styles include ones where the FM receiver is built into the ear-level hearing aid case or another where a small FM receiver boot is attached directly to the bottom of the ear-level hearing aid, or to a cochlear implant speech processor. Most recently, wearable personal FM systems designed for children with normal hearing, but who are challenged by poor SNRs, such as children with auditory processing disorders, have become available.

A sampling of manufacturer Web sites is offered at the end of the chapter for product information about wireless personal FM systems and soundfield amplification systems. In addition, refer to ASHA (2002) for "Guidelines for Fitting and Monitoring FM Systems."

Use of a Personal FM at Home

Traditionally, personal FM systems coupled to hearing aids have been used for school-aged children in the classroom setting, but growing evidence suggests that children of all ages also can benefit from personal FM systems used at home. Moeller, et al (1996) compared two groups of children; one group was encouraged to use an FM system at home, and another group used hearing aids alone. The families who wore the FM systems at home were provided with training about how to operate the units. Subjective reports from parents suggested that appropriate use of the FM at home facilitated effective communication in a variety of listening situations. Some parents of young children report that having the FM transmitter around their neck is a reminder to "talk, talk, talk" to their children, increasing the auditory input the child receives. Another reported advantage was that two of the children felt an increased sense of security when they could hear their parents from a distance.

In another study about home FM use, Gabbard (2003) reported preliminary information that was gathered from the Colorado Loaner FM Project. The Project used the FM Listening Evaluation for Children as a way to gain an understanding of the use and benefit of hearing aids and FM systems with children. Parents were asked to complete the evaluation form at least 3 to 6 months following FM fitting and then again at quarterly intervals. Some of the parents' comments regarding perceived benefit of the FM included "being mobile while continuing to hear," "consistent sound whether noisy or not," "provides the best amplification to help auditory skills," and "keeps him focused on the speaker." Flynn, Flynn, and Gregory (2005) agreed that FM use at home improved speech understanding as measured by functional auditory assessment tools.

Soundfield FM and IR Systems (Classroom Amplification Systems)

Soundfield technology is an exciting educational tool that allows control of the acoustic environment in a classroom, thereby facilitating acoustic accessibility of teacher instruction for all children in the room (Crandell, Smaldino, and Flexer, 2005). A soundfield system looks like a wireless public address system, but it is designed specifically to ensure that the entire speech signal, including the weak high-frequency consonants, reaches every child in the room. **(See Figs. 20–3A and 20–3B.)**

By using this technology, an entire classroom can be amplified through the use of one, two, three, or four wall- or ceiling-mounted loudspeakers.

The teacher wears a wireless microphone transmitter and his voice is sent via radio waves (FM) or light waves (IR) to an amplifier that is connected to the loudspeakers. There are no wires connecting the teacher with the equipment. The radio or light wave link allows the teacher to move about freely, unrestricted by wires. The loudspeakers are designed and positioned to uniformly improve the SNR throughout the areas where instruction occurs in the room.

Who Might Benefit from Soundfield Distribution Systems?

It could be argued that virtually all children benefit from soundfield amplification systems because the improved SNR creates a more favorable learning environment. Studies continue to show that soundfield amplification systems facilitate opportunities for improved academic performance

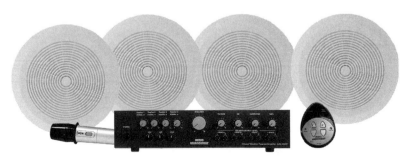

A

Figure 20–3 (A) A classroom soundfield system has a wireless teacher-worn microphone, a pass-around microphone for students, an amplifier, and evenly dispersed ceiling-mounted loudspeakers.

(Continued)

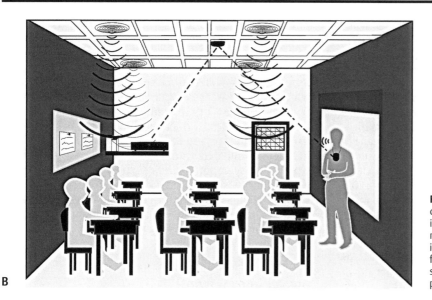

B

Figure 20–3 *(Continued)*   **(B)** Infrared is the most commonly used mode of transmission where the infrared signal is sent (emitted) from the teacher microphone to the diode in the center of the ceiling, to the amplifier on the wall, and then to the four loudspeakers in the ceiling. (Photo and schematic from Audio Enhancement; used with permission)

(Crandell, Smaldino, and Flexer, 2005; Flexer and Long, 2003; Mendel, Roberts, and Walton, 2003).

If children could hear better, more clearly, and more consistently, they would have an opportunity to learn more efficiently (Edwards and Feun, 2005; Rosenberg et, al, 1999). No one disputes the necessity of creating a favorable visual field in a classroom. A school building would never be constructed without lights in every classroom. Recognizing the positive impact of better SNR in classrooms, some school systems have as a goal the amplification of every classroom in their districts (Knittel, Myott, and McClain, 2002).

Pitfall

- Because "adequate acoustics" is an invisible and ambiguous concept, the necessity of creating a favorable acoustic environment may be questioned by school personnel.

The populations that seem to be especially in need of SNR-enhancing technology include children with fluctuating conductive hearing loss (ear infections), unilateral hearing loss, "minimal" permanent hearing loss, auditory processing problems, cochlear implants, cognitive disorders, learning disabilities, attention problems, articulation (speech) disorders, and behavior problems.

Teachers who use soundfield technology report that they also benefit. Many state that they need to use less energy projecting their voices; they have less vocal abuse and are less tired by the end of the school day (Blair, 2006). Teachers also report that the unit increases their efficiency as teachers, requiring fewer repetitions, thus allowing for more actual teaching time.

With more and more school systems incorporating principles of inclusion, children who previously would have been educated in self-contained classrooms are in the mainstream classroom. Soundfield amplification systems offer a way of enhancing the classroom learning environment for the benefit of all children. Soundfield technology is a win-win situation.

Pearl

- About 90% of today's population of children who are identified with hearing loss at birth likely will go directly into general education classrooms by 5 or 6 years of age. Those classrooms must be acoustically ready for them.

To summarize, classroom amplification facilitates the reception of consistently more intact signals than those received in an unamplified classroom, but signals are less complete than those provided by using a personal FM unit (Crandall, Smaldino, and Flexer, 2005). In addition, the equipment, especially the loudspeakers, must be installed appropriately, and teachers must be trained about the rationale and effective use of the technology.

Pearl

- A primary value of soundfield amplification is that the better SNR can focus the pupils and facilitate attention to relevant information. To that end, the clever use of the sound system's microphone can be a powerful teaching tool. Teachers need to be trained about how to use the microphones and their voices to create a listening attitude in the room; the purpose of the improved SNR is to quiet and focus the room, not to excite or distract the children.

Practical Issues for Assistive Listening Device Selection

Many issues need to be evaluated when selecting classroom amplification systems or when an audiologist recommends a soundfield rather than a personal FM system for a particular child, and few data are available to guide these decisions (Crandell, Smaldino, and Flexer, 2005; Flexer, 2004a). Following is a list of questions that an audiologist should consider in making decisions about classroom amplification.

♦ What steps can be taken to improve the classroom's acoustics by reducing noise and reverberation?

♦ Have teachers been given thorough in-service training about the auditory basis of classroom instruction and subsequent rationale for the use of soundfield technology?

♦ What type of microphone should be used: lapel microphone, boom (head worn) microphone, or collar microphone?

♦ Who will be the contact person in the district or building to troubleshoot and maintain equipment?

♦ Will loaner equipment and spare parts be available?

♦ Is there administrative support for project coordination?

♦ How many loudspeakers should be installed in a given room?

♦ Where should the loudspeakers be installed?

♦ What is the best SNR made possible by the equipment?

♦ Is the equipment durable, high quality, and flexible?

♦ What is the carrier frequency for the radio signal of the unit and the potential for interference (from cellular phones, pagers, etc.)?

♦ What is the fidelity of the unit?

Should an Audiologist Recommend a Personal FM System, a Soundfield System, or Both for a Given Child?

Once it is determined that a child has a listening problem that interferes with acoustic accessibility, the first step is to try to modify the physical characteristics of the classroom to approximate the ANSI classroom acoustics standards. The next step involves recommending, fitting, and using some type of SNR-enhancing technology.

> **Pitfall**
>
> • Preferential seating can improve visual accessibility to speech in some situations but does not control the background noise and reverberation in the classroom, stabilize teacher and pupil position, or provide for an even and consistent SNR.

In many instances the best listening and learning environment can be created by using both a soundfield FM or IR and a personal FM system at the same time. The soundfield FM or IR unit, appropriately installed in a mainstreamed

classroom, improves acoustic access for all students in the classroom. For children especially challenged by the effects of poor SNR and reverberation, such as hearing loss or auditory processing problems, a personal FM system might be more effective. The teacher need wear only a single transmitter if the child's personal FM transmitter is coupled to the audio-out port of the soundfield system, using an appropriate patch cord. The child with hearing loss (or who is otherwise listening challenged) greatly benefits from having access to the two microphones of the soundfield system. He also benefits from having a quiet environment in the classroom and a specific auditory focus. Because of the added complexity of using two technologies, teachers do require training about both technologies, including how to trouble-shoot and use them.

Whatever type of SNR-enhancing technology is selected, the following common-sense tips could facilitate use and function of the technology:

♦ **Try the equipment** People must experience SNR-enhancing equipment for themselves; they cannot speculate about function.

♦ **Be mindful of appropriate microphone placement** Microphone placement dramatically affects the output speech spectrum. Specifically, high frequencies are weaker in off-axis positions. A head-worn microphone provides the best, most complete, and most consistent signal. A collar microphone, worn around the teacher's neck, also allows some level of control of microphone distance. If a lapel microphone is worn, it should be placed midline on the chest about 6 inches from the mouth.

♦ **Check the batteries first if any malfunction occurs** Weak battery charge can cause interference, static, and intermittent signals.

♦ **Audiologists should write clear recommendations** for FM or IR equipment, specifying the rationale, type of SNR-enhancing technology needed, equipment characteristics, coupling arrangement chosen, parent and teacher training, and follow-up visits.

A 36-minute videotape, Enhancing Classrooms for Listening, Language, and Literacy, can be useful in conveying the above concepts to parents, teachers, and therapists (Flexer, 2004b).

Measuring Efficacy of Fitting and Use of Technology

Efficacy can be defined as the extrinsic and intrinsic value of a treatment (Crandell, Smaldino, and Flexer, 2005). The recent focus on evidence-based practice underscores the importance of demonstrating that interventions work. Even though the literature shows that the uses of FM and IR technologies clearly have value (Rosenberg, 2005), some efficacy measurements need to be made to show that the individual baby or child in question is obtaining benefit. Benefit can be measured through educational performance, behavioral speech perception tests, direct measures of changes in brain development, or through functional assessments (Tharpe, 2004).

Functional Assessments as a Measure of Efficacy of FM and IR Technology

Functional assessments as a measure of efficacy are typically conducted by having the teacher, student, or parent complete a questionnaire before and after use of the personal FM or soundfield system. The SIFTER, LIFE, CHILD, and CHAPPS are functional assessment tools that are readily available and widely used as efficacy measures for classroom interventions.

SIFTER— Screening Instrument for Targeting Educational Risk

The SIFTER is a one-page form that is easily filled out by the teacher or teachers at multiple intervals during a school year (Anderson, 1989). The form allows the teacher to observe and rate the student's performance compared with typical students in the class according to the five content areas are: academic, attention, communication, class participation, and school behavior. The total score in each area is recorded as pass, marginal, or fail. Even though the SIFTER was originally developed to identify students at risk for listening problems, it has proven to be useful in establishing efficacy of intervention in the classroom. When used in a pre-test, post-test paradigm, any change in the child's classroom performance as a result of the FM intervention can be noted and documented.

LIFE— Listening Inventories for Education

The LIFE is an extension of the SIFTER (Anderson and Smaldino, 1998). The LIFE also uses a teacher self-report questionnaire, but it adds a self-report questionnaire that is filled out by the student. The addition of student input about his personal classroom listening difficulties improves the overall validity of this subjective approach to efficacy.

CHILD—Children's Home Inventory of Listening Difficulties

The CHILD (Anderson and Smaldino, 2001) is a further extension of the LIFE, wherein teachers in the classroom environment, and parents and children in the home environment can assess the adequacy of the environment for listening, and observe changes as a result of intervention both at school and in the home.

CHAPPS—Children's Auditory Performance Scale

This questionnaire, appropriate for children aged 7 and older, consists of six subsections that were selected to represent the most often reported auditory difficulties experienced by children diagnosed as having APD (Smoski, 1990). The 36-item scale concerns six listening conditions: quiet, ideal, multiple inputs, noise, auditory memory/sequencing, and auditory attention span. Parents or teachers are asked to judge the amount of listening difficulty experienced by the child in question compared with that of a typical child of similar background and age.

Equipment Efficacy for the School System

The key to securing technology from the school system is to obtain data documenting need (Ackerhalt and Wright, 2003). A multifactored comprehensive evaluation, which is a thorough evaluation by a multidisciplinary team, is necessary to document the need for a child to receive special services (see Chapter 23 for more information about laws). The last category on most multifactored comprehensive evaluation forms is Assistive Technology Needs. In order for assistive technology to be recommended within any legislative framework, some type of evaluation must be conducted. It must be documented that the child in question cannot obtain an appropriate education unless a personal FM system or an FM or IR soundfield system is used. Can the child's access to and performance in the general education environment be linked to hearing difficulties in the classroom? What tests can be administered to document acoustic access and listening difficulties in the classroom?

◆ Conclusion

Improving listening and learning environments is a primary focus of pediatric and educational audiologists. This focus should include home, daycare, and classroom environments.

The ANSI classroom acoustic stipulations are an important goal for every classroom. Acoustical modifications in the form of personal FM or soundfield FM or IR SNR-enhancing technologies are viable and cost-effective means for assuring signal saliency and auditory focus for children, whether or not they have diagnosed hearing problems. Numerous studies suggest that every classroom ought to have a well-installed and used soundfield system as a necessary learning condition for all children.

Discussion Questions

1. Why do efficacy measures need to be conducted after acoustic interventions such as personal FM or soundfield amplification are implemented?

2. What common sense questions should the audiologist consider when deciding on the use of SNR-enhancement technology?

3. Compliance with ANSI classroom acoustics standard is currently voluntary. Why should the standard be compulsory for all classrooms?

4. What are the possible advantages of using SNR-enhancing technology in the home environment?

5. Why are certain populations, who do not exhibit hearing loss per se, candidates for SNR-enhancing technologies?

Sampling of Manufacturer Websites   www.audioenhance-ment.com (personal FM, FM and IR classroom amplification)

www.avrsono.com (FM boots, Logicom Personal FM)

www.comtek.com (personal FM and classroom amplification)

www.lexisfm.net (Oticon Amigo Personnel FM)

www.lifelineamp.com (personal FM, FM and IR classroom amplification)

www.lightspeed-tek.com (personal FM, FM and IR classroom amplification)

www. phonak.com (Smartlink, Microlink, EduLink, MyLink Personal FM Systems)

www.sennheiserusa.com (personal FM, FM and IR classroom amplification)

www.widex.com (SCOLA personal FM)

Dedication   We lost our very good friend and colleague Carl Crandell a little more than a year ago. Although he did not physically contribute to this chapter, his thoughts and spirit run through every word. Carl was a passionate proponent of the use of SNR-enhancing technologies to improve listening and learning for all children. His wish was for others to become advocates for children, and we hope that by reading this chapter you will understand that that is our wish too.

References

Access Board Web site (1998). www.access-board.gov. Last accessed January 14, 2008.

Ackerhalt, A. H., and Wright, E. R. (2003). Do you know your child's special education rights? Volta Voices, 10, 4–6.

American National Standards Institute. (S12.60-2002). Acoustical Performance Criteria, Design Requirements, and Guidelines for Schools. New York: American National Standards Institute (ANSI S12.60).

American Speech-Language-Hearing Association. (2002). Guidelines for Fitting and Monitoring FM Systems. www.asha.org/members/deskref-. Last accessed January 14, 2008.

American Speech-Language-Hearing Association. (1995). Guidelines for acoustics in educational environments. ASHA, 37, 15–19.

American Speech-Language-Hearing Association. (2005). Guidelines for Addressing Acoustics in Educational Settings. www.asha.org/members/deskref-journals/deskref/default. Last accessed January 14, 2008.

Anderson, K. L. (1989). Screening instrument for targeting educational risk (SIFTER). Tampa: Educational Audiology Association. www.hear2learn.com. Last accessed January 14, 2008.

Anderson, K. L. (2001). Voicing concern about noisy classrooms. Educational Leadership, 58, 77–79.

Anderson, K. (2004). The problem of classroom acoustics: the typical classroom soundscape is a barrier to learning. Seminars in Hearing, 25, 117–129.

Anderson, K. L., Goldstein, H., Colodzin, L., and Inglehart, F. (2005). Benefit of S/N enhancing devices to speech perception of children listening in a typical classroom with hearing aids or a cochlear implant. Journal of Educational Audiology, 12, 14–28.

Anderson, K., and Smaldino, J. (1998). The listening inventory for education: an efficacy tool. (LIFE). Available for free download. www.hear2learn.com. Last accessed January 14, 2008.

Anderson, K., and Smaldino, J. (2001). Children's home inventory for listening difficulties (CHILD). Available for free download. www.hear2learn.com and Phonak.com. Last accessed January 14, 2008.

Blair, J. C. (2006). Teachers' impressions of classroom amplification. Educational Audiology Review, 23, 12–13.

Boothroyd, A. (2002). Optimizing FM and sound-field amplification in the classroom. Paper presented at the American Academy of Audiology National Convention, Philadelphia.

Boothroyd, A. (2004). Room acoustics and speech perception. Seminars in Hearing, 2, 155–166.

Bradley, J. S. (1986). Speech intelligibility studies in classrooms. Journal of the Acoustical Society of America, 80, 846–854.

Crandell, C. C., Kreisman, B. M., Smaldino, J. J., and Kreisman, N. V. (2004). Room acoustics intervention efficacy measures. Seminars in Hearing, 25, 201–206.

Crandell, C., and Smaldino, J. (1995). An update of classroom acoustics for children with hearing impairment. Volta Review, 1, 4–12.

Crandell, C. C., Smaldino, J. J., and Flexer, C. (2005). Sound-field amplification: applications to speech perception and classroom acoustics (2nd ed.) New York: Thomson Delmar Learning.

Edwards, D., and Feun, L. (2005). A formative evaluation of sound-field amplification system across several grade levels in four schools. Journal of Educational Audiology, 12, 57–64.

Estabrooks, W. (Ed.) (2006). Auditory-verbal therapy and practice. Washington, DC: Alexander Graham Bell Association for the Deaf and Hard of Hearing.

Finitzo-Hieber T., and Tillman T. (1978). Room acoustics effects on monosyllabic word discrimination ability for normal and hearing-impaired children. Journal of Speech and Hearing Research, 21, 440–458.

Flexer, C. (2004a). The impact of classroom acoustics: listening, learning, and literacy. Seminars in Hearing, 25, 131–140.

Flexer, C. (2004b). Classroom amplification and the brain. (Videotape). Layton, UT: Info-Link Video Bulletin.

Flexer, C., and Long, S. (2003). Sound-field amplification: preliminary information regarding special education referrals. Communication Disorders Quarterly, 25, 29–34.

Flynn, T. S., Flynn, M. C., and Gregory, M. (2005). The FM advantage in the real classroom. Journal of Educational Audiology, 12, 35–42.

French, N., and Steinberg, J. (1947). Factors governing the intelligibility of speech sounds. Journal of the Acoustical Society of America, 19, 90–119.

Gabbard, S. A. (2003). The use of FM technology for infants and young children. Paper presented at ACCESS Conference, Chicago, IL.

Hawkins, D. B, and Yacullo, W. (1984). Signal-to-noise ratio advantage of binaural hearing aids and directional microphones under different levels of reverberation. Journal of Speech and Hearing Disorders, 49, 278–286.

Killion M. (1997). SNR loss: I can hear what people say, but I can't understand them. Hearing Review, 4, 8,10,12,14.

Knecht, H. A., Nelson, P., Whitelaw, G., and Feth, L. (2002). Background noise levels and reverberation times in unoccupied classrooms: predictions and measurements. American Journal of Audiology, 11, 65–71.

Knittel, M. A. L., Myott, B., and McClain, H. (2002). Update from Oakland schools sound field team: IR vs FM. Educational Audiology Review, 19, 10–11.

Launer, S. (2003). Wireless solutions: the state of the art and future of FM technology for the hearing impaired consumer. Paper presented at ACCESS Conference, Chicago, IL.

Leavitt, R., and Flexer, C. (1991). Speech degradation as measured by the rapid speech transmission index (RASTI). Ear and Hearing, 12, 115–118.

Ling, D. (2002). Speech and the hearing impaired child (2nd ed.). Washington, DC: Alexander Graham Bell Association of the Deaf and Hard of Hearing.

Mendel, L. L., Roberts, R. A., and Walton, J. H. (2003). Speech perception benefits from sound field FM amplification. American Journal of Audiology, 12, 114–124.

Moeller, M. P., Donaghy, K. F., Beauchaine, K. L., Lewis, D. E., and Stelmachowicz, P. G. (1996). Longitudinal study of FM system use in nonacademic settings: effects on language development. Ear and Hearing, 17, 28–41.

Rosenberg, G. G., Blake-Rahter, P., Heavner, J., Allen, L., Redmond, B. M., Phillips, J., and Stigers, K. (1999). Improving classroom acoustics (ICA): a three-year FM sound field classroom amplification study. Journal of Educational Audiology, 7, 8–28.

Rosenberg, G. (2005). Sound field amplification: a comprehensive literature review. In C. C. Crandell, J. J. Smaldino, and C. Flexer. (Eds.). Sound-field amplification: applications to speech perception and classroom acoustics (2nd ed.). New York: Thomson Delmar Learning, pp. 72–111.

Sapienza, C. M., Crandell, C., and Curtis, B. (1999). Effect of sound field FM amplification on vocal intensity in teachers. Journal of Voice, 13, 375–381.

Schafer, E. C., and Thibodeau, L. M. (2003). Speech-recognition performance in children using cochlear implants and FM systems. Journal of Educational Audiology, 11, 15–26.

Sexton, J. (2003). FM as a component of primary amplification. Educational Audiology Review, 20, 4–5, 43.

Shannon, C. (1948). A mathematical theory of communication. Bell System Technical Journal. 27, 379–423, 623–656.

Smaldino, J. (2004). Barriers to listening and learning in the classroom. Volta Voices, 11, 24–26.

Smaldino, J. J., and Crandell, C. C. (Eds.). (2004). Classroom acoustics. Seminars in Hearing, 25, 113–206.

Smoski, W. (1990). Use of CHAPPS in a children's audiology clinic. Audiology Society, 11, 53–56.

Tharpe, A. M. (2004). Who has time for functional auditory assessments? We all do! Volta Voices, 11, 10–12.

Part IV

Educational Management of Hearing Loss in Children

Chapter 21

Communication Approaches for Managing Hearing Loss in Infants and Children

Carol Flexer

Key Points

- The main communication approaches first discussed with families typically include the following: those that focus on listening and spoken language (LSL), the two branches are auditory-oral (A-O) – now called auditory-verbal education by some (AVEd), and auditory-verbal therapy (AVT); cued speech; sign language (BiBi); and total communication (TC).

- Families need to be provided with full information about each approach; one way to begin the communication options conversation is to ask families about their desired outcome for their baby or child.

- The professional must recognize that about 95% of children with hearing loss are born to hearing and speaking families; these families are very interested in having their child learn to listen and talk.

- Some communication approaches are primarily auditory in orientation, and some are primarily visual.

- Not every child will do well in every approach.

A variety of communication approaches are available for managing hearing loss in infants and children (Schwartz, 2007). The decision about selecting the best approach for a particular child and her family is usually overwhelming because parents are asked to make these important decisions at a time when they have just learned that they have a baby or child who is deaf or hard of hearing, and when they have had little or no experience with hearing loss, hearing aids, or cochlear implants.

The purpose of this chapter is to present a summary overview of the various communication approaches, and to provide a list of resources and Web sites that offer additional and detailed information about each approach.

♦ What Are the Communication Approaches?

Multiple approaches are available for teaching babies and children who are deaf or hard of hearing to communicate. Some approaches are primarily auditory, and some are primarily visual; these different orientations likely will lead to different outcomes.

Auditory Approaches

An auditory approach is based on the assumption that a baby or child with hearing loss can have primary access to auditory information through the use of hearing aids or cochlear implants (Estabrooks, 2006; Ling, 2002; Flexer, 1999; Nicholas and Geers, 2006). The goal of an auditory approach is to develop spoken language and communication through listening, leading to full and independent integration of the child into the general hearing community (Cole and Flexer, 2007; Pollack, Goldberg, and Caleffe-Schenck, 1997). The main auditory approaches historically have been A-O and AVT. Recently, a new certification program has been developed called the LSLS (Listening and Spoken Language Specialist) that recognizes the unity and similarities in both listening and spoken language approaches. There are two branches of the LSLS program: LSLS Cert. AVEd (Auditory-Verbal Educator), and LSLS Cert. AVT (Auditory-Verbal Therapist). For more information about the LSLS program, please refer to www.agbellacademy.org.

Pearl

- If spoken communication is the family's desired outcome for their baby, auditory brain access through the use of technology followed by extensive, parent-centered auditory language enrichment is essential.

Cued speech may be placed in the spoken language category, because even though it uses a visual system of hand shapes and signals that the family must learn, the goal of cued speech is to facilitate programming, mainstreaming and spoken communication, not to develop a sign language system.

Visual Approaches

Visual approaches, on the other hand, focus on looking, not on listening. They are based on the assumption that a baby or child who experiences hearing loss cannot access her auditory environment in a foremost way and cannot become proficient in spoken communication, even with amplification. The goal of a visual approach is to use sign language as the primary communication, and to be part of

the deaf community (Schwartz, 2007). Families must become proficient in sign language to communicate with their children beyond the preschool level. Examples of visual approaches are BiBi, American Sign Language (ASL), Manually Coded English (MCE), and Conceptually Accurate Signed English (CASE). **(See Table 21–1.)**

Some approaches attempt to teach both spoken and sign language communication (Watkins, Taylor, and Pittman, 2004). Examples are Simultaneous Communication, Sign-Supported Speech and Language, and Total Communication (TC). The terms *simultaneous communication* and *total communication* often are used interchangeably.

Approach Issues

There are advantages and disadvantages to each approach (Kretschmer and Kretschmer 2001) depending in part on

- the nature and needs of the child and family
- the ability of the family to do what it takes to implement a particular approach
- the presence of qualified providers to work with and support the family

In addition, reports vary about how successful or unsuccessful a particular approach might be (Moog and Geers, 2003).

Not every child will do well in every approach. It is not unusual for a family to select one approach or even to combine approaches, and then change their mind as they acquire more information and experience (Luterman and

---

Pearl

- Success can be defined as reaching the desired outcome expressed by the family through the implementation of the chosen communication approach.

Table 21–1 Visual Languages, Systems, and Strategies

Communication Approach	Characteristics of Communication
ASL	ASL is a visual-gestural language that is used by some deaf people in the United States and Canada. It has its own set of language rules that are separate from spoken or written English. It is not possible to speak English and sign ASL at the same time. Speech is not used, and the goal is to communicate using sign language, not spoken language. Different sign language systems are used in different countries.
CASE or PSE	Signs from ASL are used in English word order. The focus is on conceptual accuracy to augment understanding and no attempt is made to provide a one-to-one relationship with spoken English. Specific features of ASL, such as facial expression and use of space, may be used. These sign systems rely on context and mechanisms such as initialization to support meaning.
MCE: Signed English; Signing Exact English; Seeing Essential English	These systems were constructed by educators to teach English. The sign systems attempt to represent English by combining ASL signs, English word order, and some invented signs to represent grammatical markers (e.g., plurals, possessives, tenses) in English. Each word, including each morpheme, is signed. An example would be to sign the word "*working*" by signing the word "*work*" and then signing the ending "*ing*." All structure words, such as "*the*" and "*to*," are signed in this system.

Abbreviations: ASL, American Sign Language; CASE, Conceptually Accurate Signed English; MCE, Manually Coded English; PSE, Pidgin Signed English.

Note: Teachers or interpreters with special skills in each of these visual modes will be required to implement the communication approach. In addition, family members will need to become proficient in these visual approaches to communicate with their children beyond a preschool-level.

Maxon, 2002). The selection of a particular communication approach at any point in the habilitative process is influenced by many variables, including

♦ the child's age at the time of diagnosis of hearing loss

♦ other problems, disabilities, or challenges not related to hearing loss that the child may have or that may surface as the child ages

♦ the family's ability to help instruct the child over time

♦ the quality of intervention programs that are available for infants and school-aged children in the family's geographic area

Summary of Approaches

Many Web sites and books explain each approach in detail; some of these resources are included at the end of this chapter. **Tables 21–1 and 21–2** summarize these approaches.

Table 21–2 Summary of Communication Approaches and Philosophies

Communication Approaches and Philosophies	Definition
A-O Approach (now called AVEd by many professionals)	This approach has spoken language as a desired outcome. Active listening, enhanced by the use of hearing aids or cochlear implants, is accompanied by speech reading to receive instructional and conversational information (Clark, 2006). The use of natural gestures is acceptable; sign language is not used. Children with hearing loss may be grouped together in auditory-oral classrooms for specialized oral instruction, at least in preschool and kindergarten, with mainstreaming being a goal. Family members will need to learn how to manage auditory technology, and how to provide an enriched spoken language environment for their child.
AVT Approach (AVT has also been called "unisensory" and "acoupedic")	This is primarily an early intervention therapeutic approach in which technology (hearing aids or cochlear implants) is paired with specific techniques and strategies that teach children to listen and understand spoken language. The 10 Principals of Auditory-Verbal Practice focus on parent coaching to foster cognition, speaking, reading, and learning through the auditory modality. Visual cues (lip reading and sign language) are not used or taught during therapy so that the child can develop the auditory system through directed listening practice. The foremost goals of A-V therapy are to guide parents and caregivers as the primary facilitators for helping their children develop intelligible spoken language through listening, and to advocate for their children's inclusion in regular schools. AVT uses one-on-one teaching of parent or caregiver and child, focusing on strong family involvement; children are mainstreamed from the beginning (Estabrooks, 2006). However, some children will require additional auditory support after entering the mainstream. Parents are key partners in AVT.
BiBi	A person who achieves fluency in ASL and English (or another language) is bilingual. Using this approach, ASL is often taught as the first language and English is taught as a second language to develop literacy skills. English may be taught by using a sign system or through print – spoken English is not featured. The child will need to be in an ASL self-contained classroom, or require an ASL interpreter if placed in a general education classroom. Family members will also need to learn ASL and the English-based sign system to communicate with their child.
Cued Speech	A supplement to spoken English, Cued Speech is intended to make important features of spoken language fully visible, since about 60% of the phonemes are not visible through speech reading. This system enhances speech reading by employing phonemically based gestures to distinguish between similar visual speech patterns. The goal of Cued Speech is the reception and expression of spoken communication. Family members will need to learn Cued Speech to communicate with their child. Children are expected to be able to drop the use of cues once their oral language skills are firmly established.
Sign-Supported Speech and Language	Signs are used occasionally to support spoken language development. Signs function as a bridge to enhance the meaning of oral communication. The signs also can serve to enhance understanding in certain challenging situations such as noisy environments or when a hearing device is not in use. Family members will need to learn sign language in addition to oral communication techniques to communicate with their child.
Simultaneous Communication	This is the concurrent use of signs and speech. To provide language using two modalities simultaneously, a sign system, rather than a signed language, is used. This visual representation of the oral language is accomplished using manual symbols and signs. If not in a self-contained classroom that uses sign language, the child will require a sign language interpreter. Family members will need to learn both sign language and oral communication techniques to communicate with their child.
TC has also been called a multisensory approach.	Introduced in the 1960s, this philosophy aims to make use of several strategies or modes of communication including sign, speech, auditory, written, and other visual aids. First developed by Roy Holcomb, the choice of modalities depends on the particular needs and abilities of the child, and professes to provide whatever is needed to foster communicative success. Children will need to be placed in a TC classroom, or have an interpreter if in general education classrooms. Family members also will need to learn sign language and other prescribed techniques to communicate with their child.

Abbreviations: AVEd, Auditory–Verbal Education; A-O, Auditory-Oral; ASL, American Sign Language; AVT, Auditory Verbal Therapy; BiBi, Bilingual Bimodal; TC, Total Communication

(Developed with Arlene Stredler Brown – see Chapter 24 for more information about early intervention practices)

Families need to be provided with full information about each approach (Joint Committee on Infant Hearing, 2007). One way to begin the communication options conversation is to ask the famiy about their desired outcome for their baby or child. That is, how do they want their child to communicate in the family constellation, in school, and in the community? The professional must recognize that about 95% of children with hearing loss are born to hearing and speaking families (Mitchell and Karchmer, 2004); these families are very interested in having their child learn to listen and talk. The conversation then needs to focus on what is takes from both the family and a qualified interventionist to implement each approach, because every approach requires family involvement (Watkins, Taylor, and Pittman, 2004).

Factors to Consider

A family might consider many factors when choosing how to communicate with their child (Ling, 2002; Luterman, and Maxon, 2002; Watkins, Taylor, and Pittman, 2004):

◆ Is the communication approach in the best interest of the child and family?

◆ Does the communication approach allow the child to have control and influence over the environment, to converse about needs, and to take part in the world of abstract thought?

◆ Does the communication approach allow all family members to communicate deeply—not only on the surface— with the child?

◆ Does the communication approach permit the child to feel part of the family unit through pleasurable and significant interaction?

◆ How will the child communicate with peers, with extended family, and with the community as a whole?

◆ Is the family ready to take on the commitment that the communication approach requires?

◆ Will the child be equipped by school age with the necessary language, thinking, and learning skills?

Programming decisions are very difficult and can be made only after a great deal of thought. Before a family makes a communication approach decision, they are advised to do the following (Watkins, Taylor, and Pittman, 2004):

◆ Visit the various programs and individual therapists in the community

◆ Meet and speak with parents of other children with hearing loss who are enrolled in different programs

◆ Meet and speak with older teens and adults wiht hearing loss who have been taught using the various approaches, keeping in mind that they were born at a time that did not have newborn hearing screening, early intervention, cochlear implants, or digital hearing aids.

◆ Summary

Every communication approach decision should be reviewed regularly. Not every program is right for every child, and families may change approaches over time. As the child grows and learns, the family and therapists will discover more about what is best for the child.

> **Pearl**
>
> ◆ A key issue is expectations. In this time of early identification and multiple technologies, parents and family ought to have high expectations for outcomes, if all parties do what it takes.

During the beginning stages of therapy, the child's progress should be reviewed often, and diagnostics should be a part of therapy sessions. If the selected approach does not seem to be a match for the child or family, or if the child is not progressing as originally expected, an approach change should be investigated.

Discussion Questions

1. How might the pediatric audiologist initiate a communication approach conversation with a family?

2. What is the role of a pediatric audiologist relative to a family's choice and implementation of a communication approach?

3. Does the management of hearing loss play a role in every communication approach? Why or why not?

4. Does the recommendation of amplification technology play a role in visual approaches as well as in auditory approaches?

◆ Web-Based Resources

General Information

www.ncbegin.org

http://www.handsandvoices.org/

http://www.babyhearing.org/

Information about Listening and Spoken Language (LSL) Approaches: Auditory-Oral (A-O) – now called Auditory-Verbal Education (AVEd) by some; and Auditory-Verbal Therapy (AVT):

www.agbellacademy.org

www.oraldeafed.org

www.listen-up.org

www.johntracyclinic.org

Information about Cued Speech

www.cuedspeech.org

www.dailycues.com

www.tecunit.org

www.language-matters.com

Information about ASL and Visual Approaches

www.deafchildren.org

www.nad.org

http://deafness.about.com/cs/communication/a/total-comm.htm

http://clerccenter.gallaudet.edu/

http://www.seecenter.org/

References

Clark, M. (2006). A practical guide to quality interaction with children who have a hearing loss. San Diego, CA: Plural.

Cole E., and Flexer, C. (2007). Children with hearing loss: developing listening and talking, birth to six. San Diego, CA: Plural Publishing.

Estabrooks, W. (Ed.). (2006). Auditory-verbal therapy and practice. Washington, DC: Alexander Graham Bell Association for the Deaf and Hard of Hearing.

Flexer, C. (1999). Facilitating Hearing and Listening in Young Children, 2nd ed. San Diego: Plural Publishing.

Joint Committee on Infant Hearing (2007). Year 2007 position statement: principles and guidelines for early hearing detection and intervention programs. Pediatrics; 102(4): 893–921.

Kretschmer, L., and Kretschmer, R. (2001). Children with hearing impairment. In T. Layton, E. Crais, and L. Watson (Eds.), Handbook of early language impairment in children: nature (pp. 560–584). Albany, NY: Delmar Publishers.

Ling, D. (2002). Speech and the hearing impaired child (2nd ed.). Washington, DC: Alexander Graham Bell Association of the Deaf and Hard of Hearing.

Luterman, D.M., and Maxon, A. (2002). When your child is deaf: a guide for parents (2nd ed.). Austin: Pro-Ed.

Mitchell, R. E., and Karchmer, M. A. (2004). Chasing the mythical ten percent: parental hearing status of deaf and hard of hearing students in the United States. Sign Language Studies, 4, 138–163.

Moog, J. S., and Geers, A. E. (2003). Epilogue: major findings, conclusions and implications for deaf education. Ear and Hearing, 24, 121S–125S.

Nicholas, J. G., and Geers, A. E. (2006). Effects of early auditory experience on the spoken language of deaf children at 3 years of age. Ear and Hearing, 27, 286–298.

Pollack, D., Goldberg, D., and Caleffe-Schenck, N. (1997). Educational Audiology for the Limited-Hearing Infant and Preschooler: An Auditory-Verbal Program. Springfield, IL: Charles C. Thomas.

Schwartz, S. (2007). Choices in deafness: a parent's guide to communication options (3rd ed.). Bethesda: Woodbine House.

Watkins, S., Taylor, D. J., and Pittman, P. (Eds.). (2004). SKI-HI curriculum: family-Centered programming for infants and young children with hearing loss. Logan, UT: HOPE, Inc.

Chapter 22

Collaborative Team Management of Children with Hearing Loss

Jane R. Madell and Carol Flexer

Key Points

- The goal of team management is to have all involved professionals provide services in a coordinated way and with a unified philosophy to a child with hearing loss and his family.

- The child and family are always at the center of the team.

- A system of communication, shared among clinicians and the family, needs to be formulated that will provide information about how a child is performing; some families have found a communication notebook to be a useful tool for sharing information among team members in multiple settings.

- For team coordination to work well, someone must be assigned to be the case manager; as the child's needs change over time, the case manager may change.

- Disagreements among clinicians need to be handled in a way that does not involve families in interprofessional disputes.

♦ The Goal of Team Management

Multiple professionals are involved in providing services to children with hearing loss and their families. Even though the professionals may do their best individually, they do not always work together as a coordinated team or communicate with each other when planning and implementing services. As a result, the totality of services that the child actually receives can be far from optimal (Madell et al, 2003).

The goal of team management is to have all involved professionals provide services in a coordinated way to a child with hearing loss and his family. Sometimes all services are provided by a single program in one location. In other instances, services are provided by clinicians working out of different programs, including clinicians working in hospital-based audiology programs, in schools, and in private practices. Whether at one or at multiple centers, services should be delivered with a unified philosophy and by clinicians who communicate regularly with each other (Madell et al, 2003).

Teaming can be a very positive experience for professionals and families, in the following ways:

- Observations made by one clinician are helpful to other clinicians in understanding the child's overall performance and behaviors, and can help clinicians rethink and improve their individual recommendations.

- Collaborating with service providers from other specialties helps clinicians expand their knowledge-base, and helps them better understand all children they serve.

- Collaboration with a team provides each professional with a broader view of the effects of hearing loss on the child and the family.

This chapter will discuss the composition of a team and the roles of team members. The critical position of the team manager will be detailed. The chapter will end with four case studies that illustrate the value of a coordinated team, and the recognition that the role of team manager shifts as the child's primary needs change over time.

◆ Who Is on the Team?

The composition of the team will be different for every child and will depend on the child's individual needs (**see Fig. 22–1**). The child is always at the center of the team. All team efforts focus on the child, the family, and their needs. In some cases, the family refers only to the parents. In other cases, extended family members (grandparents, aunts, uncles, siblings, and other caregivers) also are included.

Audiologist

For every child with hearing loss or auditory processing disorders (APDs), a pediatric audiologist is a key member of the team. The audiologist is responsible for:

- identifying hearing loss

- monitoring hearing loss over time

- evaluating auditory behaviors

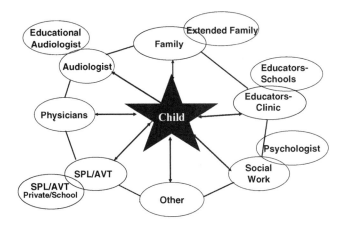

Figure 22–1 The team. AVT, auditory-verbal therapist; SPL, speech-language pathologist.

- evaluating speech perception capabilities

- selecting and fitting amplification technologies (hearing aids, cochlear implants, frequency modulation [FM] systems)

- monitoring use of technologies to be certain that they are providing the necessary benefit

- evaluating the need for and selection of assistive technologies including personal FM and classroom listening systems

- counseling parents and other team members about hearing loss and technology

- identifying other auditory problems such as APDs.

Because the audiologist sees the child less frequently than some of the other team members, he can and should observe the child's progress over time, including the child's speech, language, and auditory development. If the child is not making appropriate progress, the audiologist needs to discuss concerns with other team members and encourage them to reevaluate the child's developmental, listening, and linguistic status.

Once a child enters school, an educational audiologist frequently joins the team. The educational audiologist will be responsible for monitoring personal technology in school, selecting and monitoring assistive technology (including FM systems), and teaching school staff how to use the systems appropriately. In some schools, the educational audiologist is responsible for educating classroom teachers about hearing loss, and maximizing learning in the classroom for children with hearing loss. In other schools, training school personnel is the responsibility of the teacher of the deaf. In some cases, the educational audiologist may provide all the audiology services a child requires, and the child may not receive audiologic services from an outside clinic or hospital. In other cases, the school audiologist will not deal with personal technology and will deal only with school equipment. A few audiology centers employ an educational audiologist in-house who may provide both clinical and educational audiologic services.

Medical Professionals

Every child with hearing loss will receive medical services from at least two physicians: a pediatrician and an otolaryngologist. The pediatrician will manage routine medical issues, and the otolaryngologist will be responsible for ear issues.

Infants with hearing loss ought to have the benefit of a medical home (American Academy of Pediatrics, 2002), which the American Academy of Pediatrics defines as an approach to providing health care services where care is accessible, family-centered, continuous, comprehensive, coordinated, compassionate, and culturally competent. For most children, the medical home will reside with the pediatrician; however, this may not be the case for every child.

All children with hearing loss should see an otolaryngologist at least annually. Obviously, it is necessary for pediatricians and otolaryngologists to work well together so that medical issues can be treated in a timely fashion. These key physicians will be responsible for making referrals to other medical personnel as needed, including referrals for genetics evaluations, neurology, and ophthalmology consultation. (See Chapter 3 for a complete discussion of medical management of the child with hearing loss.)

Speech-Language-Auditory Therapist (SLP)

A speech-language pathologist with specific training in the provision of auditory therapy for children with hearing loss, or an auditory-verbal therapist needs to be involved in the evaluation and management of all children with hearing loss (see Chapter 25). As soon as the hearing loss is identified and at least annually thereafter, the child's speech-language skills and functional listening skills should be assessed. This evaluation will include assessing and monitoring the child's performance with his technology, and participating in determining the need to change technology (e.g., to new or more powerful hearing aids or to shift from hearing aids to cochlear implants). After speech-language and auditory assessments are conducted, recommendations are made for appropriate therapies and for providing training and coaching to parents to enable them to carry over therapy at home. When a child reaches school age, services may move from the clinic to the school. However, if the school speech-language pathologist does not have the skills to work with children with hearing loss, it may be necessary for the child to continue to receive services outside the school environment or to train school personnel to work with children with hearing loss.

Educational Personnel

A teacher of the deaf typically is involved in the management of all school-aged children with hearing loss. (The title of this teacher may vary, and may include teacher of the deaf, teacher of the hearing impaired, or teacher of the deaf or hard of hearing.) In some areas of the country, a teacher of the deaf will be involved with preschool children also (see Chapters 26 and 30). For children enrolled in self-contained classes for children with hearing loss, the teacher of the deaf will be the primary provider of educational services. For children who are mainstreamed, a general education teacher will be responsible for providing academic instruction. As a support, the teacher of the deaf may provide individual or resource room instruction on a daily basis or several times per week to preview material that will be covered in the mainstream class, and to review material previously covered. The teacher of the deaf, in some schools, will also be responsible for monitoring the FM equipment and for teaching the regular school staff about hearing aids, cochlear implants, and FM systems.

Social Worker

Social workers meet with newly diagnosed families to help them deal with their feelings about having a child with hearing loss, and to help them work through the paperwork involved in procuring services and technology for their children. Social workers can help families enroll in Early Intervention, obtain Medicaid funding as appropriate, and navigate insurance issues. In some centers, they work with families who are trying to decide the value of shifting from hearing aids to cochlear implants. They provide crisis intervention when a child has a decrease in hearing or a cochlear implant device failure, or for family issues that are not related to hearing loss. In some centers, the social worker may run support groups for teenagers and for parents. Support groups could be run by the social worker alone or collaboratively with other staff members.

Psychologist

School systems and other clinics may have an educational psychologist who evaluates children on a regular basis (usually every 3 years) to assess learning strengths and weaknesses, and to make recommendations for educational placement and special service needs. Psychologists also may offer the support services provided by social workers as described above, including counseling for newly diagnosed hearing loss, managing support groups, and providing assistance in crisis intervention.

Family

Families play a critical role in a child's success. The word *family* is used here in its broadest definition. *Family* certainly implies parents, but also can include grandparents, siblings, and other relatives or caregivers (nannies, etc.) who are involved in a child's day-to-day care. Even the most talented group of clinicians will not be successful in educating a child if the family is not involved. Language learning must take place all day long. Infants and young children are at home many hours each day. If the family is not working with the child for many hours every day, the child will not reach the outcomes desired by the family.

A family who has selected an auditory-oral or auditory-verbal program for their child needs to be responsible for making sure that the child's technology always is working optimally. In addition, they need to know how to talk, talk, talk to the child to build language and communication (Cole and Flexer, 2007). Families who have selected sign language as a communication mode for their child need to learn sign language way above the level of baby and preschool signs. They need to communicate with the child using sign language in the same way and at the same level of language complexity used to communicate with their hearing children in order for the child's language to develop to age-appropriate levels.

In addition to working with their child at home, a family needs to transport their children to and from therapy. Once the child is in school, the family must be sure that the child goes to sleep early enough so that he is bright and alert and ready to learn when at school. Further, the family needs to check and assist with homework. The family needs to know what is happening at school and in therapy to be sure the child is receiving the services he needs. In addition, the family needs to verify that professionals working with the child have high enough expectations, and that the child is doing the best that he can do.

Providing support for typically developing children is very often stressful for parents. Children with special needs, including children with hearing loss, require even more effort on the part of the family. Even though parents are primarily responsible, grandparents and others can be very helpful in providing the necessary assistance.

Occupational and Physical Therapists

Many children who are deaf or hard of hearing, especially in the preschool years, need the services of physical or occupational therapists. Services include strengthening fine and gross muscle development as well as vestibular development and sensory integration. These services may be provided in schools or may be obtained from clinicians outside of school.

Professionals in the Community

When children receive services from clinicians in more than one center or from individual providers, everyone on the team must make a commitment to open communication. A child may receive speech-language services from a provider at one center and audiology services from a provider at another. The audiologist can deliver the best possible audiology services only when he knows how the child is performing with hearing aids at home and at school. For example, the speech-language pathologist, auditory therapist, and classroom teacher should be able to tell the audiologist what specific phonemes the child is not hearing, or that the child is having difficulty hearing soft speech. With this information, the audiologist can adjust technology to improve functioning.

A system of communication, shared among clinicians, needs to be formulated that will provide ongoing information about how a child is performing. Certainly everyone working with a child should send diagnostic and evaluation reports to others on the team. However, evaluations usually do not occur frequently, so any problems that develop between evaluations may not be reported to team members in a timely fashion.

Some families have found a communication notebook to be a useful tool for sharing information among team members. The notebook travels with the child to every setting and team member. Then, everyone who works with the child writes down what is happening during each contact including concerns about performance, homework, and questions for others on the team. Some families have developed a Web site or blog where everyone involved with the child can share information. Paper or electronic notebooks are effective only if everyone, including parents, is committed to both writing a summary of contact with the child and reading other clinicians' entries.

Figure 22–2 is an example of another communication tool that can be useful. It is an information sheet that can be shared between the audiologist and speech-language

OBSERVATION OF AUDITORY PERCEPTION

Child's Name_____ Date: _____
Observed by: _____ Title: _____

Cochlear Implant: _____Advance Bionics____Cochlear Corp. _____Med-El
Speech Processor: _____
Program #_____   Volume #_____   Sensitivity #_____
Program #_____   Volume #_____   Sensitivity #_____
Program #_____   Volume #_____   Sensitivity #_____
Program #_____   Volume #_____   Sensitivity #_____

Hearing Aid Type: Right Ear_____ Left Ear _____
Volume: Right Ear_____   Left Ear_____
Program Information: _____

Changes in Perception since last MAP or Hearing Aid Adjustment
Date(s) of Observation:_____

Has the child demonstrated misperceptions since the last MAP/Hearing Aid adjustment?_____
_____
_____

Has the child demonstrated phonemic confusion since the last MAP/Hearing Aid adjustment?_____
_____
_____

Have there been changes in voice quality?_____
Have there been changes in resonance?_____
Has the child asked for more repetitions of information?_____
Has the child been clipping syllables or lengthening vowels?_____
_____

Has the child had difficulty adhering to word boundaries? _____
Have there been changes in FM usage? _____

Additional Comments or Observations:

Figure 22–2 Communication between the speech-language-auditory therapist and audiologist: Observation of auditory perception.

pathologist. Because the speech-language pathologist or auditory verbal therapist sees the child frequently, she is in a good position to specifically identify a child's auditory problems. Sharing this information with the audiologist in a clear and concise way, places the audiologist in a good position to make changes in equipment to improve listening skills.

◆ The Case Manager

For team coordination to work well, someone must be assigned to be the case manager. There must be a go-to person, or critical problems may remain unsolved. The case manager is responsible for

- collecting information from everyone working with the child
- being sure that the information is distributed to all team members
- determining the services that are needed
- addressing problems as they arise
- ensuring that the child actually is receiving all the necessary services
- being available to provide support to the family
- communicating with all clinicians either at case conferences or by phone, mail, or email

If a child is receiving services from many facilities, the parents will often be responsible for coordinating services. Although the parents are certainly ultimately responsible for their child, it can be difficult for them to negotiate differences of opinion between clinicians. Therefore, it is often useful if one of the clinicians involved in the case acts as the coordinator. As the child's needs change over time, the coordinator may change.

When audiologic issues are paramount, such as when a child is initially diagnosed or when hearing loss is fluctuating, the audiologist usually assumes the case manager role. On the other hand, when patients are receiving ongoing habilitation services, especially in preschool years, the speech-language pathologist or auditory therapist is usually the case manager. When a child requires integrated educational planning, a teacher of the deaf typically becomes the case manager. When there are complex otologic medical issues, the otologist will be the case manager.

Team Meetings

The optimal way for all players to communicate is to have periodic interdisciplinary team meetings. If many children are seen by the same group of clinicians in one location, or in different locations, it will be beneficial for the team members to meet monthly or bimonthly to discuss all children as needed. However, if clinicians from different facilities are involved in providing services, it can be difficult for

them to meet in one room at the same time. A conference call may be useful for discussing specific issues as they arise and in planning for joint recommendations. For children who are in school, the annual individual education plan (IEP) meeting is frequently a good time to have a team meeting. Clinicians from the community center can go to the school or can participate by phone. When there are multiple clinicians from one facility, they can meet to discuss the case and have one representative participate at the IEP meeting. (See Chapter 30 for discussion about facilitating services between schools and clinics.)

Dealing with Disagreements among Team Members

The child and family will benefit most from receiving a consistent message from all clinicians about goals for the child and ways of achieving the goals. If, for example, one clinician works with the child using American Sign Language and another uses auditory-based therapy, the child is not receiving consistent intervention. Moreover, the family is put under a great deal of stress as they attempt to determine what is best for their child while managing very divergent treatments that have different desired outcomes.

Even though clinicians may have legitimate disagreements about recommendations for the child, they should try to work out differences with each other before discussing recommendations with families. Disagreements among clinicians need to be handled in a way that does not involve families in interprofessional disputes. When there is a serious disagreement, such as whether a child should receive a cochlear implant, or whether one educational placement is better than another for a child, parents should be advised of the different opinions, presented with complete information, and given assistance in making their decision. Clinicians are experts in their own areas; however, the family is always the final arbiter about what is best for their child. Professionals must behave professionally and respectfully toward parents and other professionals, regardless of the decisions made by the family.

◆ Case Examples and Discussion of Case Management Issues

Case 1: "Vic" (not his real name) is a preschooler who is ready to transition to his local school district. Vic has hearing loss that was identified at 12 months of age; he was fitted with hearing aids and an FM system at that time. He received in-home early intervention that included services provided by a speech-language pathologist and a teacher of the deaf. The speech-language pathologist was the initial case manager.

Before Vic reached 2 years of age, the audiologist, speech-language pathologist, and teacher of the deaf met to discuss the case. It was determined that Vic was not receiving sufficient benefit from his hearing aids. When wearing his hearing aids, he was detecting sounds in the moderate hearing loss range; an insufficient loudness to provide access to the speech spectrum at average and soft conversational levels.

Everyone working with Vic recognized that he could function well only when it was quiet or when he was listening through the FM system. He was not able to hear well at a distance or when there was competing noise. A cochlear implant was recommended, and Vic received the implant at 2 years of age. Three months later, he started wearing a hearing aid on the unimplanted ear.

At age 3, Vic entered an auditory-oral preschool program at a school for the deaf. In addition, he attended a mainstream preschool two afternoons per week. The teacher of the deaf from the Hearing and Speech Center became the case manager and coordinated services between the center, the school for the deaf program, and the mainstream preschool. Even though Vic was doing very well with his cochlear implant, he continued to detect sound at only moderate hearing loss levels with the hearing aid. So, at 4 years of age, he received a second cochlear implant. Testing with two cochlear implants indicated that Vic could now detect sound at borderline normal hearing levels. Word recognition scores, obtained during an audiologic evaluation using the NuChips test (Elliot and Katz, 1980), were 84% at a normal conversational level of loudness (50 dB hearing level [HL]), and 60% at a soft conversational level (35 dB HL). In his speech-language-listening evaluation (Kirk et al, 1995), Vic obtained listening scores of 80 to 100% on the LNT and Common Phrases (Osberger et al, 1991) test. Language testing indicated an age equivalent of 5.5 years on the PPVT-III (Dunn and Dunn, 2007), and he was in the 75th percentile on the CELF-P (Wigg et al, 1992).

The team, comprised the audiologist and teacher of the deaf consultant from the Hearing and Speech Center, the speech-language-listening therapist, and the teachers from both the mainstream preschool, and preschool deaf infant program, met again and determined that Vic was ready to be transitioned back to his local school district. The teacher of the deaf attended the IEP team meeting at the school district, and discussed the services that Vic would require to be successfully mainstreamed.

When Vic started school, the teacher of the deaf visited the mainstream class and met with the staff to provide training about hearing loss and ways to maximize Vic's auditory performance. The teacher of the deaf from the Hearing and Speech Center remained in touch with both the school and clinic staffs to make sure that Vic was performing well in school.

Case 2: "Gail" (not her real name) is an example of auditory neuropathy/dys-synchrony   Gail passed otoacoustic emissions screening at birth; however, as time went on, she demonstrated delayed speech and language development. The parents reported their concern to the pediatrician on several occasions, and finally, at 18 months she was referred for an audiologic evaluation. At that time, she was identified with a moderate, bilateral sensorineural hearing loss. At 19 months, a click auditory brainstem response (ABR) confirmed moderate, bilateral hearing loss; however, ABR testing at that time did not include tonal air and bone thresholds and did not test reversed polarity to check for auditory neuropathy/dys-synchrony.

Although Gail wore her hearing aids consistently, participated in a good preschool therapy program, and had parents who worked consistently with her, she was not making good progress. Her speech and language skills were slow to develop and she was not able to use hearing to understand speech. The school suggested that the family consider moving Gail to a program using American Sign Language (ASL) because of her lack of progress developing auditory skills. At 2.5 years of age, the family sought a second opinion about her diagnosis. The audiologist at the second opinion center was concerned about Gail's performance and poor auditory skills; with her hearing aids, Gail was detecting sound at borderline normal levels and was involved in a good auditory therapy program, but was not making the expected progress. Consequently, the ABR was repeated including testing with reversed polarity. This time, testing suggested auditory neuropathy/dys-synchrony.

Gail's case was reviewed at a team meeting. The audiologist became the case manager. Bilateral cochlear implants were recommended. Gail received the implants at 38 months of age. She remained in the auditory-oral preschool and made excellent progress. At the 6 month cochlear implant evaluation, word recognition tests indicated NuChips test (Elliot and Katz, 1980) scores of 93% at 50 dB HL, 87% at 35 dB HL, and 80% at 50 dB HL +5 dB SNR. Speech and language evaluation at 4.5 years of age indicated delayed language (PPVT) with performance at a 3 year 7 month age level. Expressive language scores were at 3.7 years. Speech production was excellent at 5.5 years.

Gail's case management then shifted from the audiologist to the teacher of the deaf as education issues became paramount. The team met again and decided to return Gail to her local school district in an integrated kindergarten class because her language scores were not sufficient for her to be in a mainstream class. Services now included speech-language-auditory services and teacher of the deaf services, each delivered five times weekly. A personal FM system was recommended for school use. The teacher of the deaf from the Hearing and Speech Center met with the school to confirm that Gail was going to receive all necessary services. She visited the school, observed the class, and met with the staff to provide training about hearing loss and ways to maximize Gail's auditory performance. She continued to be in touch with the school and clinic staff to ensure that Gail was making good progress.

Case 3: "Suzy" (not her real name) is an example of shifting case management over time   Suzy is now a college student who had profound hearing loss identified as a toddler. As a toddler, Suzy was fitted with hearing aids and an FM system; however, her hearing aids allowed her to detect sound only at moderate hearing loss levels. Early psychological testing indicated normal intelligence, and Suzy was enrolled in an Auditory-Verbal therapy program. The speech-language pathologist was the first case manager.

Suzy did not make the progress that was expected. She was clearly intelligent but could not seem to learn auditorally, and her speech and language skills were delayed. Because Suzy was not making sufficient progress, when the team met they felt that they could not recommend a mainstream kindergarten placement. The team discussed Suzy's lack of progress with the family and recommended an alternate therapy program such as Cued Speech or ASL. Because the family was anxious to attempt mainstreaming

Suzy, they decided to try Cued Speech. Consequently, Suzy entered kindergarten with a Cued Speech interpreter. The Cued Speech interpreter then became the next case manager.

Suzy continued to receive speech-language-auditory therapy. With the use of the Cued Speech interpreter, Suzy was able to improve her speech and language skills, but her auditory skills remained poor.

At 7 years of age, the family decided to consider a cochlear implant. Following implantation, Suzy's auditory skills improved dramatically. Within a year, Suzy felt that she no longer required the Cued Speech interpreter. Her mother and the other clinicians involved in Suzy's management were skeptical about Suzy attending school without an interpreter. As a result, the interpreter remained in the class for another 6 months; however, she provided less and less assistance. Finally, everyone was comfortable having Suzy in the classroom without that support.

Responsibility for case management shifted again and returned to the speech-language-auditory therapist who continued to provide services. By fourth grade, Suzy began using a note-taker and when she entered high school, she stopped receiving speech-language services.

Suzy's mother now became the case manager. Suzy received Communication Access Real-time Translation (CART) services in high school for academic subjects. At the time she entered high school, she also decided to receive a cochlear implant for her second ear. Suzy then returned to auditory therapy for 1 year after receiving the second cochlear implant. She is now a freshman in college, majoring in psychology. She receives CART services in the classroom and extended time for tests. Her grades are good. She is now her own case manager.

Case 4: "Lenny" (not his real name) is an example of Down Syndrome   Lenny's auditory management began when he was 5 months old. Lenny experiences Down syndrome, and he failed his newborn hearing screening. Follow-up behavioral and ABR testing indicated moderate hearing loss by air conduction, but bone conduction thresholds were within normal limits. He had flat tympanograms, consistent with middle ear pathology. Lenny was referred to an ear, nose, and throat specialist. Otologic evaluations revealed very narrow external auditory canals and bilateral serous otitis media.

Management issues were discussed. Should Lenny receive myringotomy tubes? Should he receive hearing aids? In either case, he needed speech-language-auditory therapy. Management became the responsibility of the otologist because medical issues were paramount. The decision was made by the team to not use myringotomy tubes. The surgeon felt surgery might be too difficult because of the small size of the ear canals. In addition, since it was now spring, it was hoped that Lenny's health would improve and his ears would clear of fluid.

Subsequently, Lenny was fitted with amplification and was doing well, even though fluid was still present in his middle ears. He was closely monitored otologically and received several courses of antibiotics. Middle ear disease cleared up for short periods of time but returned with associated hearing loss that negatively affected his speech and language development.

Responsibility for case management moved to the audiologist to deal with amplification issues. Lenny received speech-language-auditory therapy and was enrolled in a special education preschool. At 3 years of age, hearing testing continued to indicate a primarily mild hearing loss with moderate thresholds in the low frequencies. Unaided word recognition testing indicated poor word recognition scores (48%) at a normal conversational level (50 dB HL), 0% at soft conversational levels (35 dB HL), and very poor word recognition (24%) at a normal conversational level with competing noise added. Fortunately, testing with hearing aids revealed excellent word recognition scores (86 to 94%) in all three conditions.

The case was discussed again with the team. The otologist felt that the situation in Lenny's ears had changed sufficiently so that myringotomy tubes could be inserted. Surgery was performed and hearing improved slightly, but hearing aids were still necessary.

Case management then moved to the speech-language-auditory therapist who was now the primary provider. When Lenny entered kindergarten in a special education class, management was shared between the classroom teacher and the speech-language-auditory therapist who continued to provide services to Lenny.

◆ Summary

Although providing collaborative services requires increased effort on the part of all involved, the extra work is more than worth the effort because collaboration is essential for the provision of quality services to infants and children. In some ways, teaming makes the jobs of all professionals easier, because collaboration enables each to work in designated areas of expertise and allows other team members to contribute their unique knowledge. Each team member values his place on the team and respects and appreciates the roles of the others. Furthermore, having multiple clinicians provides more support to families.

The case manager typically changes over time, and eventually, the family usually takes over that responsibility. When children reach college age, many are capable of taking over responsibility for their own services. Self-advocacy is, of course, the ultimate goal.

Discussion Questions

1. What factors should be considered when determining which professional should be the team manager for a child with hearing loss at any point in time?

2. How are members of the team selected?

3. What are some ways that team disagreements might be resolved?

4. What strategies and techniques will allow all team members to stay in communication with one another?

References

American Academy of Pediatrics. (2002). The medical home. Pediatrics 110, 184–186.

Cole, E., and Flexer, C. (2007). Children with hearing loss: developing listening and talking, birth to six. San Diego: Plural Publishing.

Dunn, L. M., and Dunn, L. M. (2007). Peabody Picture Vocabulary Test, 4th Edition, (PPVT-4 Scale). New York: Pearson Assessments.

Elliot, L., and Katz, D. (1980). Development of a new children's test of speech discrimination. St Louis: Auditec.

Kirk, K. I., Pisoni, D. B., and Osberger, M. J. (1995). Lexical effects on spoken word recognition by pediatric cochlear implant users. Ear and Hearing. 16, 470–481.

Madell, J. R., Hoffman, R. A., Kooper, R., Cheffo, S., Heymann, L., Rothschild, P., Seth, C. M., Sorkin, D., Rafter, K., Johnson, C. D., Houston, K. R. (2003).

Coordination of Cochlear Implant Services, Audiology Today October FT1–FT 20.

Madell, J. R, Hoffman, R. A., Cheffo, S., Heymann, L., and Ying, E. (2006). Team management of children with hearing loss. Workshop presented at the Alexander Graham Bell Association for the Deaf conference, Pittsburgh, PA, July.

Osberger, M. J., Miyamoto, R. T., Zimmerman-Phillips, S., Kemink, J. L., Stroer, B. S., Firszt, J. B., and Novak, M. A. (1991). Independent evaluation of the speech perception abilities of children with the Nucleus 11-Chanel cochlear implant system. Ear and Hearing, 12, 66S–80S.

Wigg, E., Secord, W., and Semel, E. (1992). Clinical Evaluation of Language Fundamentals–Preschool (CELF-P). New York: The Psychological Corporation.

Chapter 23

Education and Access Laws for Children with Hearing Loss

Donna L. Sorkin

Key Points

1. Underlying a child's or adult's eligibility for services under U.S. laws is the need to demonstrate a disability that limits one or more major life activities.

2. U.S. disability laws support the provision of services needed to allow children and adults to attend school, live and work in the mainstream with full access to telecommunications, communication access, and other services that support their needs as people with hearing loss.

3. Passage of laws does not guarantee access to needed services. Children with hearing loss should be involved in the individualized education plan (IEP) and all discussions of their needs from a young age, so that they can develop the knowledge and skills that they will need to be their own best advocates.

Many parents still experience periodic frustrations when seeking services and appropriate placement options, but overall families can expect that their children who are deaf or hard of hearing will attend a neighborhood school with her hearing peers and with needed services; go to college with full communication opportunities; enter the workforce supported by whatever accommodations she requires;

and enjoy meaningful access to a wide range of telecommunications products and services. In the past 30 years there has been a dramatic expansion in the application of federal laws to address the needs of people with disabilities. Children and young adults with hearing loss have benefited from such legislation in diverse and important ways.

We have now moved from an environment in which a child with a significant hearing loss could expect to work in a "deaf" trade (such as typesetting) and spend her life in the deaf community, to a largely open society in which a young person who is motivated and has received appropriate services and support can pursue whatever academic and professional career she chooses, regardless of her level of hearing loss or communication modality. Not long ago those of us who were deaf relied on telecommunications relay volunteers to call our family members or our business associates. I still vividly remember waiting my turn for a volunteer relay assistant to become available to help me make a telephone call so I could speak to a client. If I happened to find someone who could type quickly without too many errors, I proceeded to make all the calls I needed to make that day in nonstop fashion.

Our perspective now in the United States and in many parts of the world is that services and support should be available to provide full access for a child with hearing loss. The scope of our national disability laws has been broadened to require freedom from discrimination as a result of a disability; full use of available technologies like cell phones and broadcast and cable television; appropriate services and support for families during early intervention and for school-aged children at school; consideration of workplace needs; and communication access in public places such as theaters, museums, and transportation facilities. By and large, the laws are in place. Still, passage of laws is one thing; ensuring that a child or a young adult has what she is entitled to is another matter entirely.

This chapter is designed to provide the information needed to undertake three important tasks as an audiologist: (1) mentor and coach a family and child to become advocates for the hearing impaired child's needs; (2) become familiar enough with the laws to help families know what they are entitled to under our legal system; and (3) point them to additional resources—beyond what you can realistically offer—that they can tap into now and as the child ages and her needs progress. With regard to the last task—as with all children—just when we think we have the hang of parenting, our children enter a new phase of their lives and parents are forced to adjust to a whole new set of challenges. Children with hearing loss are no different in this regard. For that reason, it is important to provide families and patients with resources and skills that will aid them over the long term.

◆ The Concept of Disability

Patients today will grow up in a society that views disability very differently than was the case in our country 50 or even 25 years ago. Our new model for disability has been evolving for some time now, but the new thinking is that there is no pity or shame in having a disability. Rather, the stereotyping and fears about disability, and ultimately the discrimination that occurs because of a lack of access to services, are the real problems. We have moved away from trying to hide the fact that someone cannot hear or see. We encourage people to be open about their disabilities and instead focus on what they need to fully participate.

A public example of the way this new perspective has played out involves President Franklin Delano Roosevelt. Roosevelt contracted polio as a young man, before being elected governor of New York, and never walked again after his illness. Although it was widely known that he had difficulty moving about because of the paralysis, the fact that he used a wheelchair and could not walk was little known by the average American. He was never photographed in his wheelchair and on those occasions when he appeared in public, he wore painful leg braces and was assisted by others when he walked. None of this was publicly discussed until well after his death because of the stigma associated with being confined to a wheelchair and having a significant disability.

In 1997, a national memorial honoring FDR was completed in Washington, D.C. The initial design gave no hint that Franklin Roosevelt used a wheelchair. The larger than life statue of President Roosevelt at the memorial site

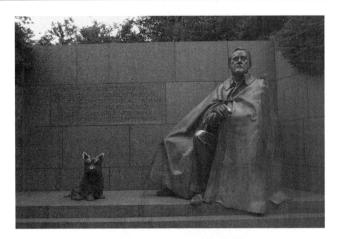

Figure 23–1 The initial statue of President Franklin Delano Roosevelt at the FDR Memorial in Washington, DC conceals the fact that he was seated in a wheelchair.
(Photo by Donna Sorkin.)

(Fig. 23–1) shows him seated, with a cape draped over his legs, in such a way that his wheelchair is entirely hidden. Disability advocates were furious that a memorial of this magnitude on the national mall in Washington, D.C. purposely concealed the fact that Roosevelt used a wheelchair. They felt it was a continuation of past practices in which society hid people with disabilities, or in this case, intentionally veiled the fact that a powerful and charismatic person was not able-bodied. Disability organizations successfully argued that an additional statue be added to the memorial, a statue that shows FDR in his wheelchair. Although his disability was never revealed to the public during his lifetime, advocates stated that if he were alive today, Roosevelt would have wanted the public to know that he served as president of the United States—the most powerful position in the world—with a significant disability (Sorkin, 2004). Another statue of FDR in his wheelchair **(Fig. 23–2)** was added in 2000 to coincide with the 10th anniversary celebration of the passage of the Americans with Disabilities Act and was formally dedicated by President Bill Clinton.

That viewpoint provides the basis for our federal laws that require nondiscrimination and access. Underlying an individual's eligibility for coverage under most U.S. laws that provide services or accessibility for a child or an adult with hearing loss is the need to demonstrate a known disability. For example, under the Americans with Disabilities Act (ADA), the definition of disability was construed broadly to include anyone who has a physical or mental impairment that substantially affects one or more major life activities. Hearing loss is considered to be one of these life activities.

But what if assistive technology so improves the individual's condition that he is no longer limited in life activities? There have been several Supreme Court cases in which the definition of an individual with a disability was narrowed. In one case, individuals were denied jobs as commercial airline pilots because they were nearsighted (*Sutton v. United Airlines*, 1999). With eyeglasses, their vision was corrected to

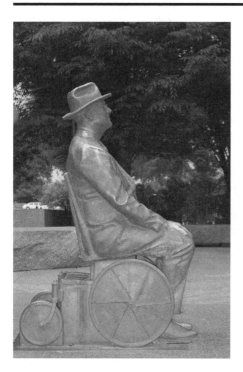

Figure 23–2 Several years after the FDR Memorial opened, a second statue was added that clearly shows President Roosevelt in his wheelchair. Although no such photographs were published of FDR during his lifetime, 50 years after his death public perspectives dictated a more open approach to his disability.
(Photo by Donna Sorkin.)

20/20. Those individuals felt that they should have been protected by the ADA because without glasses their vision was a significant limitation. The court ruled in favor of the airline stating that those individuals had too much sight with corrective glasses to fall within the definition of an individual with a disability to be protected under the ADA.

The *Sutton v. United Airlines* court decision suggests that an individual who receives substantial benefit from assistive technology like hearing aids or cochlear implants could also lose the protection (or possibly services) of disability laws if the correction provided by technology provides the equivalent of normal hearing. An audiologist may be asked by families to discuss their child's hearing loss and her need for services. This expertise can be invaluable in demonstrating functional or practical aspects of hearing loss as well as the specific services that a child needs to keep up with her peers. At present, no hearing technology provides the equivalent of normal hearing for a child with hearing loss, so it is important to demonstrate and discuss the impact of a child's hearing loss on listening and learning.

Pearl

• For example, using HINT (hearing in noise test) scores or single words in quiet or noise to demonstrate how much a child is missing may help demonstrate the impact of the hearing loss on her functional performance.

Still another aspect of the issue relates to a reticence by some families to think of their child with a hearing loss as having a disability. Some families so desperately want their child to be normal that they are reluctant to call attention to her hearing loss and consequently do not pursue services such as a frequency modulation (FM) system that could help her. Even parents of children with profound hearing loss who use cochlear implants have been known to minimize the impact of the child's deafness and boast that their child does not need services at school. Without delving into the psychological aspect of this kind of thinking and the impact that it could have on the child, it is important to acknowledge and understand that the concept of disability underlies the framework for laws that ensure educational services and accessibility features that allow children and adults to engage in various activities and be included in all of the same opportunities in life as anyone else.

Although the person's disability determines eligibility, our laws in America emphasize the individual's ability and our commitment as a society to provide what is needed to allow inclusion. Within this context, an agency or organization—public or private—is prohibited from discriminating on the basis of a person's disability. It is also expected that organizations will provide reasonable accommodations and services that will make their offerings accessible to children and adults with hearing loss.

Three categories of laws will be covered in this chapter:

♦ Education

♦ Telecommunications

♦ General access in public places and in the workplace

There is some overlap between these categories. For example, some laws that primarily concern general access can be applied to educational settings for children who do not qualify for coverage under the Individuals with Disabilities Education Act (IDEA), and there are general access laws (such as the ADA) that have telecommunications components.

♦ Education Laws

The Individuals with Disabilities Education Act

IDEA is the primary federal program that requires state and local aid to address the requirements of children with disabilities in educational settings. The legislation was originally passed in 1975 because America's educational system was not meeting the needs of children with disabilities. At the time that IDEA was first signed into law by President Gerald Ford, only one in five children with disabilities attended public school. After passage of IDEA, school attendance and matriculation rates for children with disabilities dramatically increased (U.S. Department of Education, Raising the Achievement of Students with Disabilities: New Ideas for IDEA, August 2006).

IDEA was most recently updated as the 2004 Reauthorization of the Individuals with Disabilities Education Improvement Act of 2004. The 2004 law maintains the basic structure and civic rights guarantees of the original IDEA law. As with all federal legislation, IDEA was passed by Congress and signed into law by the president. Regulations explaining how the IDEA law is to be implemented by states and local school districts were then developed by the U.S. Department of Education with input from diverse organizations. At this writing in 2007, the most recent regulations were published in the *Federal Register* on August 14, 2006 and include revised language relating specifically to children with hearing loss. Since IDEA is a funding statute, states and local school districts must follow these procedures to receive federal funds for public education.

An audiologist's expertise is vital to the families they serve in helping to demonstrate the importance of specific and appropriate services for a child who is deaf or hard of hearing. Like most federal programs, IDEA has its share of jargon, and even experienced audiologists can be intimidated by the alphabet soup of acronyms that comprise the regulations. Nonetheless, the audiologist's expertise is in understanding the audiologic needs of patients, and such information is invaluable in helping children receive the early intervention or school-based services they need to excel.

Part B of the Individuals with Disabilities Education Act

Part B of IDEA focuses on school-based services and covers children 3 to 21 years of age. The cornerstone of the law, since its initial passage, has been the concept of a free and appropriate public education (FAPE) that provides for special education and related services that are specifically designed to meet the needs of a child with a disability. The legal intent is to allow children with disabilities full access to an education while addressing their special learning or access needs. The following glossary of terms covering FAPE and other key concepts is intended to help best understand terms within the IDEA framework.

Free and Appropriate Public Education

A free and appropriate public education (FAPE) is to be provided to the child with a disability as described in the IEP (the document that describes how the child's needs will be met). The services to be provided are free. Families cannot be charged if the services are identified in the child's IEP. The word *appropriate* is important and emphasizes that the school district must consider the individual needs of the child.

Individualized Education Plan

The IEP is a written legal document that provides detail on the special education and related services that a child needs to receive an education. The IEP should be developed in a collaborative way between the family and school personnel. It should outline both the child's needs and how his school placement and services will address his unique needs. An IEP should include: (1) the child's current educational performance; (2) goals for the school year and how these goals will be met with specific educational or related services; (3) whether and how the child will participate in regular education programs; and (4) criteria for evaluating the child's progress against the goals. It is very important to have the IEP provisions in writing. Although we generally think of the IEP process as being an annual event, if there is significant change in the child's status (such as undergoing cochlear implant surgery over winter break or experiencing a decline in hearing or any occurrence that affects the child's ability to access her educational program), parents can ask for a review of the IEP and this can be done at any time.

Least Restrictive Environment

Least restrictive environment (LRE) emphasizes that the child will be educated, to the extent possible, with children who do not have disabilities. IDEA emphasizes that children should be removed from the regular classroom only to the extent needed to provide special services. LRE requirements, as described in the 2006 regulations, are "a strong preference, not a mandate, for educating children with disabilities alongside their peers without disabilities" (U.S. Department of Education, 2006).

The LRE concept can be a source of controversy when families and school personnel disagree on what placement is best for the child. There are many instances in which a school district's perspective on LRE for a child is driven by what programs or options are already in place, rather than by what placement would best serve the child. School districts are required by the law to offer a continuum of alternative placements to meet the needs of students but the reality is that a continuum of placements is not available in some areas of the country.

It is helpful to think of LRE and the continuum of placements as a line along which the student may move according to his needs, usually (though not always) from a more restrictive environment to a lesser one. See **Fig. 23–3** for an example of the continuum of public school placements. One

Continuum of Public School Placements

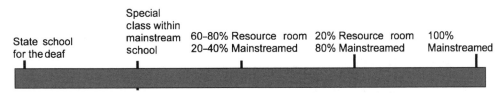

Figure 23–3   Continuum of public school placements.

child might best be served by an initial placement in a resource room (or self-contained classroom with other children who are hearing impaired) for most of the day. Over the course of his school career, he might spend less time in the resource room and eventually he might be better served in a mainstream classroom with accommodations for his hearing loss (such as an FM system). Another child might spend his entire public school time in a state school for the deaf. Still another child might be best served by a 100% mainstreamed placement from first grade onward. IDEA law requires that the child's needs drive the placement. As the child's hearing care expert, the audiologist has a key role in helping the child and her family work with the school district to ensure she has a placement (and services) that is determined by her unique needs and not a placement that is driven by the too frequently used adage, "This is what we offer."

Mainstreaming

Mainstreaming is sometimes equated with the LRE. It is not the same; rather, mainstreaming is one example of how the LRE concept can be applied. For many families, the goal is to eventually have their children who are deaf or hard of hearing attend school with their normally hearing peers in a mainstream classroom. Other families believe that their children are best served in a classroom with other children with hearing loss. When and if a child is ready for a mainstream placement should be a function of the child's readiness, both academically and socially. Some school districts discourage mainstream placement because they do not offer itinerant services, so it is difficult to serve children with hearing loss who are not clustered in one location.

Special Education

Schools must design and provide instruction that is specially designed to meet the unique needs of the individual child.

Related Services

These are services that help the child benefit from special education and may include speech and audiology services, physical or occupational therapy, and psychological services. The most recent version of the IDEA regulations specify that routine checking of hearing aids and cochlear implants are appropriately covered as a related service although replacement of the cochlear implant device and mapping is not the responsibility of the local school district (U.S. Department of Education, 2006).

Helping a Family with the Individualized Education Plan

A child's audiologist and the other hearing care professionals who serve her and her family (including the teacher for hearing-impaired children, the speech pathologist, and the auditory-verbal therapist) should provide guidance and documentation to support the development of the IEP. Such materials might include information on the child's communication skills; hearing status; cognitive abilities; assessment of the listening environment she will be placed in and whether acoustical improvements are needed; assistive technology needs (i.e., hearing aid, cochlear implant, FM system); social and emotional factors; related services required (speech, educational audiologist, listening therapy); communication access needs such as interpreters, note-taking, or captioning; in-service training for teachers and others including classmates; and provision for daily troubleshooting the child's technology (hearing aids, cochlear implant, FM). Keep in mind that the IEP is a binding document, but services will be provided only if they are written into the IEP. If the audiologist feels that the patient is ready and would benefit from the mainstream, she has a key role in helping the family demonstrate the child's readiness and to identify and justify those services she needs in the mainstream to learn and achieve.

Pearl

- As the expert on your patient's hearing needs, you have a key role in supporting the family to ensure everything the child needs is specified clearly in the written IEP document.

Recent Guidance on Individuals with Disabilities Education Act Regulations

The 2004 IDEA Regulations, published in August 2006, highlighted several topics of note to audiologists. Several legal decisions would have required school districts to provide mapping or programming services for children with cochlear implants as an audiology service. The 2004 Regulations make it clear that schools are not responsible for "post-surgical maintenance, programming, or replacement of the medical device" (U.S. Department of Education, 2006). The school responsibilities for hearing aids and cochlear implant processors are similar in that schools are required to ensure that hearing aids and external components of surgically implanted medical devices are functioning properly, which includes routine troubleshooting and assistive technology such as FM systems are provided when needed and maintained.

There has been some question as to whether a student may use school-purchased assistive technology such as an FM system at home or in other settings outside of school. The new regulations state that the child's team may approve such use if it is needed to receive FAPE. Children often do have learning opportunities outside of school, so parents could argue that the FM system is needed to access spoken language in those settings.

Interpreting services in the new regulations are identified as a related service. The definition of interpreting services has been expanded to include various forms of captioning and note-taking. Additionally, all of the various types of interpreting are covered, including Cued Speech, oral transliteration, and sign language interpreting.

Part C of the Individuals with Disabilities Education Act

Part C of IDEA addresses early intervention (EI) services for children up to 3 years. This part of IDEA provides grants to states to develop early intervention programs for infants and toddlers if they have developmental delays or have a diagnosed condition that could impact the child's development. Children with hearing loss often experience language delays and are usually eligible for services under Part C. Unlike Part B, early intervention services are coordinated by a designated state agency, which controls the implementation and provision of services at the local level. The state agency varies by state and may be the state school for the deaf, social services, health department, or a special early intervention agency.

Individualized Family Service Plan

Part C services are provided through the Individualized Family Service Plan (IFSP), which addresses the needs of the child and family members, rather than just the child, as is the case with Part B. IFSP services vary by state and might include

- speech language pathology and audiology services
- auditory therapy by a certified auditory-verbal therapist or by someone who is not certified
- home-based, deaf education services
- family training, counseling, and home visits
- occupational or physical therapy
- hearing aids or FM systems
- psychology or social work services
- sign language instruction for the child and family
- information about, and exposure to, Deaf Culture
- service coordination
- transportation

A key role of early intervention professionals in any of these functions is to train the family in how to encourage language development in their child who experiences hearing loss. Since many families are new to hearing loss, and because young children are likely to develop language as part of their family interactions, communication is an appropriate emphasis.

As part of the IFSP, a family will be assigned a service coordinator who will help the family obtain services as a function of the child's needs, the state's offerings, and the resources allocated by the state for early intervention. As the child's audiologist, you have a key role in helping the family and the service coordinator determine services and providers that will address the child's hearing loss, the family's preferences as to the child's language modality, family goals, and any other special needs that the child may have. About 40% of children with hearing loss have an additional disorder (Perigoe and Perigoe, 2005). Such other issues can affect a child's ability to develop language and should be considered alongside of hearing loss.

One final word about the early intervention process is in order. Given that most families will be new to hearing loss

and that they are starting on a long journey with their children, it is important that professionals recognize from the start the importance of helping parents develop the skills they will need to negotiate the early intervention (and later the school system) as well as the medical and psychosocial aspects of raising a child who is deaf or hard of hearing. IDEA recognizes that parents have the right to make key choices for their children. Some states have recognized the need to provide such encouragement by establishing parent mentoring programs such as Wisconsin's Guide- by-Your-Side, which is also offered by the parent organization Hands and Voices (Hands and Voices, 2006). If the state early intervention (EI) agency does not provide such mentors for parents, they should be encouraged to do so.

Pearl

- You might also assist parents by establishing your own informal mentoring network, linking parents of newly identified children with more experienced families.

No Child Left Behind Act of 2001

IDEA focuses on providing access to an educational program; No Child Left Behind (NCLB) spotlights academic achievement. The law holds schools accountable for ensuring that all students, including those with disabilities, meet specific standards. NCLB highlights the responsibility of states, school districts, and individual schools to target resources to improve the achievement of students with disabilities and to closely monitor the quality and impact of services provided under IDEA.

In the past, students with disabilities were often excluded from assessments and accountability systems. NCLB is a useful mechanism to further highlight and address the needs of pediatric patients in those instances in which the audiologist, other service providers, or the family feels that the child's IEP is not sufficiently providing quality services that allow her to meet the same high standards as her peers. The law authorized new federal monies to states and districts for activities designed to strengthen teacher quality in areas like reading, math, science, and English fluency. The extra support and attention that can be applied due to NCLB can translate into greater emphasis on gaining a high level of performance for students with hearing loss.

Section 504 of the Rehabilitation Act and the Americans with Disabilities Act

Section 504 mandates that all entities receiving federal funds must not discriminate and must offer services that provide access to their programs. Since all public schools and most colleges and universities receive federal funds, they are subject to the requirements of Section 504. Some children with hearing loss who are performing at grade level have been categorized by their school districts as not having an educationally significant hearing loss and thus are not eligible for an IEP. If this is the case, Section 504 can be used to provide related services such as FM systems, interpreters, and captioning.

Colleges and universities (receiving federal funds) are not required to substantially modify their academic programs for students with disabilities, but under Section 504 they are required to make adjustments that will allow equal opportunity. For example, an art course might be substituted for music or a student may need to be provided with more time to complete academic requirements than is customary. The college student will not have an IEP team to help her, so she must request and work out such adjustments that allow her access to her college program.

The ADA can be applied in similar fashion to Section 504 because the ADA requires that programs open to the public be communications accessible. The ADA's Title III (Public Facilities) applies to public schools (K-12) as well as to college and universities, regardless of whether or not they receive Federal funding.

A summary of IDEA provisions and the three other laws covered in this section is provided in **Table 23–1**.

Table 23–1

Education Laws	Coverage	Relevant Federal Agency	Web Resources
IDEA Public Law 108–446	Primary federal law addressing the educational needs of children with disabilities. Requires that states and local school districts provide free and appropriate early intervention and educational services that address the child's specific needs.	Department of Education	
Part B	Focuses on school-based services and covers children 3 to 21 years of age.	Department of Education	www.ed.gov/legislation/FedRegister/finrule/2006-3/081406a.pdf www.ed.gov/policy/speced/guid/idea/modelform-iep.pdf
Part C	Part C of IDEA addresses EI services for children up to 3 years. Provides grants to states to develop early intervention programs for young children who have a diagnosed condition that could impact on the child's development	Department of Education	www.nectac.org/idea/idea.asp
NCLB, 2001	By focusing on academic achievement, the law's intent is to hold schools accountable for ensuring that all students—including those with disabilities—meet specific standards. IDEA focuses on access to the child's educational program, whereas NCLB provides a mechanism for monitoring the quality and impact of services provided under IDEA.	Department of Education	www.ed.gov/policy/elsec/guid/edpicks.jhtml?src=fp www.whitehouse.gov/news/releases/2002/01/20020108.html
Section 504 of the Rehabilitation Act	For children who do not qualify for special education services under IDEA, Section 504 can be utilized to provide related services such as FM systems or captioning. See General Access below on other Sec 504 elements.	Relevant Federal Agency	www.usdoj.gov/crt/ada/cguide.htm#anchor65610 www.section508.gov/index.cfm?FuseAction=Content&ID=15
ADA, Title II (public schools) and Title III (private schools)	Can be applied in similar fashion to Section 504. Private schools and higher education institutions are required to make their programs communications accessible.	Access Board (guidelines) Department of Justice (enforcement)	See General Access

Abbreviations: ADA, Americans with Disabilities Act; EI, early intervention; FM, frequency modulation; IDEA, Individuals with Disabilities Education Act; NCLB, No Child Left Behind Act.

♦ Telecommunication Laws

Before the telecommunications revolution, a lack of telephone access was one of the most limiting aspects of having a hearing loss. I can clearly remember what it was like before the ready availability of all of the telecommunications options we now have, including landline and wireless telephones with volume control and telecoil compatibility, telecommunications relay services provided by state agencies (rather than volunteers), email and instant messaging, and captioned television and video programming. This set of services has made an extraordinary difference in the lives of young people who are deaf or hard of hearing, regardless of their level of hearing loss or mode of communication. A child with a hearing loss today will make heavy use of text messaging and email, putting him on a par with her hearing peers who are using the same technology.

A bit of history is in order as we review the framework for today's telecommunications laws. Ironically, the telephone was invented by Alexander Graham Bell, a teacher of the deaf, in part because of his abiding concern in augmenting communication opportunities for people who are deaf and his related interest in acoustics. Bell's mother and wife Mabel were both hard of hearing. He was interested in teletype machines as a mechanism of providing reliable messaging options for people with hearing loss, an interest that eventually led to his invention of the telephone. How ironic that his discovery actually produced extraordinary frustration and isolation for people with hearing loss for nearly a century, until relatively recent federal legislation mandated that telephone equipment and services provide access for people with hearing loss.

Hearing Aid Compatibility Act

Wireline Telephones

The Hearing Aid Compatibility (HAC) Act of 1988 required that all wireline and cordless (not wireless) telephones manufactured after 1989 incorporate the ability to connect internally with the telecoil in hearing aids. (Wireless telephones were originally exempt from the HAC rules; see below for 2003 rules, which later were expanded to include wireless.) A negotiated rulemaking completed in 1996 added the requirement that all wireline and cordless phones manufactured after 1998 also provide volume control with minimum gain of 12 dB and additional boost options up to 18 dB; there is also an option to provide even more gain if the phone has an automatic reset mechanism. The rulemaking also specified public locations where wireline phones were required to be HAC. These include

- the workplace
- hospitals and residential health care facilities
- coin-operated and credit-card–operated telephones
- emergency telephones (i.e., elevators, tunnels, highways)
- hotel rooms

Having this requirement in place has greatly expanded the likelihood that people using hearing technology will have the telephones they need when they are in various familiar or unfamiliar environments.

There are large variations in how well various telephones work for different individuals. In a setting like a hotel room or a phone at rest stop on the highway, where someone does not expect to be using a given telephone again, one does the best one can. But if the setting is one's regular workplace (where someone will be relying on a particular piece of equipment regularly) and the individual finds that the phone does not work well, she should take the initiative to request that her employer work with her to find equipment that provides acceptable access. Individuals of all ages should be encouraged to advocate for themselves and search for other telephones if one particular technology does not work well for them.

Wireless Telephones

The first wireless telephones were analog and did not create major accessibility problems for people using hearing technology, although few (if any) of these first wireless phones were HAC (i.e., included a method to internally connect with a telecoil). When Congress passed HAC 1989, it exempted wireless telephones, though it left the door open for inclusion of some phones in the future if specific criteria were met (i.e., if removing the exemption was in the public interest).

In 1995, a new type of digital wireless telephone technology began appearing in the United States, some years after its introduction in Europe and other parts of the world. The reported experiences of hearing aid wearers in those regions where digital wireless phones were being used were not promising. Before long, digital wireless technology took the country by storm. Advocates for people with hearing loss quickly realized this was a significant problem that needed to be addressed within the federal regulatory framework. As a result of ongoing advocacy by consumers and their organizations over a period of almost 10 years, the Federal Communications Commission (FCC) eventually did agree to lift the wireless exemption for hearing aids under HAC. The FCC established technical standards set forth in the American National Standards Institute (ANSI) Standard C63.19. The FCC further required that each manufacturer or mobile service provider offer at least two digital wireless handset models that meet a specific interference standard by September 16, 2005, and that at least 50% of their offerings comply with the standard by February 18, 2008. Additionally, each manufacturer or service provider was required to offer at least two models that met the standard for inductive coupling (with the telecoil of a hearing aid) by September 18, 2006 (Federal Communications Commission, Hearing Aid Compatibility Order, 2003).

In providing guidance to patients, it is helpful to explain and reference the ratings that telephone handset manufacturers are required to include with the written materials about their products in stores and on their Web sites. Handsets that receive a compatibility rating of M3 or M4 have met (M3) or surpassed (M4) the ANSI compatibility standard for hearing aids set in microphone mode, as adopted by FCC. The higher the M-rating, the higher the signal quality (and the lower the interference level) the handset will have. Handsets that receive a telecoil rating of T3 or T4 have met (T3) or surpassed (T4) the required standard as adopted by the FCC. The higher T-4 rating will generally provide a better result for the user.

Although this rating scheme was specifically developed for hearing aid users, because it is a measure of radio frequency interference, it is also appropriate as a guide for cochlear implant or Baha users. Patients should be advised to use these ratings to assist in their selection of telephone models, but to always test a telephone before buying because what works for one person may not work for another.

Telecommunications Act of 1996

Section 255

Section 255 of the Act required that telecommunications products and services be accessible to, and usable by, people with disabilities, if readily achievable to do so. The law covers wide-ranging products and services, including telephones (wireline, cordless, wireless); answering machines; pagers; and services such as call waiting, voice mail, and interactive voice response systems, that have implications for people with hearing loss. The legislation was important in that it brought attention to the importance of thinking about the diverse needs of people with disabilities as part of the design of new products, a concept known as universal design.

Pearl

- The universal design paradigm will be important to children of today as new products that have not been offered before are conceptualized and developed for our use.

There is some overlap between the Telecommunications Act and HAC. HAC is absolute, whereas the Telecommunications Act allows companies to fall back on the readily achievable language as grounds for not providing access. Section 255 has been important in requiring manufacturers to address the compatibility of their products with specialized equipment used by consumers who are deaf or hard of hearing. A good example of this is the compatibility of wireless telephones with TTYs and assistive listening devices.

Section 713 (Closed Captioning)

Closed captioning of television programming allows children and adults with hearing loss to view the audio portion of a TV program as text on the television screen. (**Fig. 23–4** demonstrates captioning of the children's TV program "Arthur.") All televisions sold in the United States with screens larger than 13 inches include the capability to display captions, a consequence of a 1990 federal law—The Television Decoder Circuitry Act. Section 713 of the

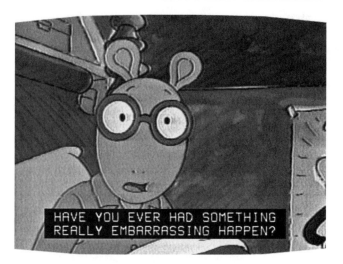

Figure 23–4   The children's television program Arthur with closed captions, as mandated by the Telecommunications Act.

(Image by Marc Brown and WGBH/Boston.)

Telecommunications Act made captioning a reality in America by mandating that all television programming, including broadcast, cable, and satellite, follow a specific schedule for implementing captioning. Although there are some exemptions (such as overnight programs that air between 2:00 a.m. and 6:00 a.m.), 100% of all new English language TV programming must now be closed-captioned and 75% of previously developed programming (first shown before 1/1/1998) must be captioned by 2008. Spanish language programming follows a different schedule. As a result of this important legislation, people with hearing loss of all ages have nearly full access to television programming.

Unless paid for by the federal government (see Section 508 below), videos (DVD or VHS format) developed by private companies are not required to be closed captioned, although most entertainment videos produced today are captioned.

Pearl

- Ironically, most educational videos developed for use in school settings are not captioned.

Section 508 of the Rehabilitation Act

Section 508 establishes requirements for electronic and information technology developed, maintained, procured, or used by the federal government. Section 508 requires federal electronic and information technology to be accessible to people with disabilities, including employees and members of the public. Federal agencies must comply with specific accessibility requirements when they procure or develop electronic and information technology. This requirement has important implications for employees or potential employees with hearing loss, as the standards effectively address key areas that often present barriers for people with hearing loss: telephones, TVs, videotapes, DVDs, multimedia websites, interactive voice response systems, and information kiosks. Although Section 508 applies only to those who are federal employees or those using federal programs, it also serves as a model that other employers can emulate in providing accessible workplaces.

Americans with Disabilities Act, Title IV

Title IV of the ADA requires that telephone companies provide interstate and intrastate telecommunications relay services 24 hours a day, 7 days a week at no cost to the caller. Telephone relay services enable a person with hearing loss, who cannot understand speech on the telephone, to communicate with others through a relay assistant who types (or signs) what the hearing person is saying. A variety of options are available to relay users, including captioned telephone, in which a computer, PDA, or wireless device can be used to make a call, without special telephone equipment. Captions provided on a computer screen can accommodate persons with low vision because they can take advantage of the large text, variable fonts, and colors that are available. Relay services continue to evolve and improve.

A summary of telecommunications laws reviewed in this section is provided in **Table 23–2**.

Table 23–2

Telecommunication Laws	Coverage	Relevant Federal Agencies	Web Resources
(HAC) Act of 1988 Final negotiated rulemaking 1996	Requires all new wireline and cordless (not wireless) phones provide both coupling with the telecoil in a hearing aid and volume control. Wireless phones initially exempted from HAC rules (see below).	FCC	www.fcc.gov/Bureaus/common_carrier/ FAQ/faq_hac.html www.access-board.gov/telecomm/ marketrep/guidelines/43i.htm
Hearing Aid Compatibility Rules for Wireless Telephones, 2003	The FCC later broadened HAC definition to include usability by people without telecoils via acoustic coupling. The rules directed digital wireless manufacturers to develop phones that are usable with hearing aids and to provide labeling and information about usability.	FCC	www.fcc/cgb/consumerfacts/hac.html www.aboutus.vzw.com/accessibility/ digitalPhones.htm www.ce-mag.com/archive/01/ Spring/Hollihan.html
Telecommunications Act of 1996 Section 255	Requires that companies make products and services accessible to, and usable by, people with disabilities, if readily achievable. Covers telephones (wireless, cordless, wireline), answering machines, pagers, and services such as call waiting, voice mail, and interactive voice response.	FCC	www.fcc.gov/cgbl/dro/section255.html www.fcc.gov/telecom.html
Telecommunications Act of 1996 Section 713	As of 2006, 100% of all new English television programming must be closed-captioned. 75% of programming first shown before 1/1/1998 must be captioned by 2008. Spanish language programming follows a different schedule. Some exceptions exist such as overnight programs (2:00 a.m.– 6:00 a.m.) and for those for whom captioning would constitute an undue burden.	FCC	www.fcc.gov/cgb/consumerfacts/ closedcaption.html

Table 23–2 *(Continued)*

Section 508 of the Rehabilitation Act of 1973	Federal agencies must comply with specific accessibility requirements when they procure or develop electronic and information technology. Impacts telephones, televisions, DVDs, videotapes, multimedia Web sites, interactive voice response systems, information kiosks, pagers.	Relevant federal agency	www.access-board.gov/508.htm www.section508.gov www.opm.gov/disability/
ADA, Title IV (Telephone Relay Services)	Requires telephone companies to provide interstate and intrastate telecommunications relay services 24 hours a day, 7 days a week at no cost to the caller.	FCC	www.fcc.gov/cgb/dro/title4.html

Abbreviations: ADA, Americans with Disabilities Act; FCC, Federal Communications Commission; HAC, Hearing Aid Compatibility Act.

◆ General Access

Section 504 of the Rehabilitation Act

Section 504 of the Rehabilitation Act forbids organizations and employers from excluding or denying individuals with disabilities an equal opportunity to receive program benefits and services. The act applies to any federal agency or entity or program receiving federal funds, and it broadly defines discrimination as not being accessible to someone with a disability. Any grant, loan, or contract to a public or private entity or program requires that entity to follow the regulations of the act. It applies to employers, hospitals, human service programs, public schools, colleges, and universities—that receive federal funds.

Section 504 can be used to ensure that a child (or a person of any age) receives the accommodations she needs to fully participate in a program. It can be used to access services like FM systems, interpreting, captioning, and note-taking. It may even be possible to use the act to obtain acoustical improvements in the built environment. Like most federal laws, Section 504 has a specific complaint process. What is a bit different is that this law allows each federal agency to have its own set of Section 504 regulations that apply to its own programs and the entities that receive aid from them.

Although we tend to think of applying Section 504 at school, the law may also be used to gain access to any educational or cultural program that a child might wish to participate in outside the usual school setting. As the child ages, Section 504 also applies to the workplace and to other institutions. The child's audiologist should encourage the child and his family to develop the skills and knowledge to seek whatever accommodations he needs to participate. This kind of thinking will serve the child now and throughout his life.

The Americans with Disabilities Act

The ADA was intended to provide people with protection from discrimination in all aspects of their lives. There are four parts of the ADA that address access to: (1) employment; (2) state and local government services (which include educational institutions) and transportation; (3) public accommodations, which means anywhere the public goes (stores, theaters, places of entertainment, hotels and motels, health care facilities); and (4) telecommunications relay services (see above in Telecommunications). The overriding goal of all these parts was to ensure that people with hearing loss could use, benefit from, and enjoy the same services and opportunities as everyone else.

Title I–Employment Provisions of the Americans with Disabilities Act

Title I, employment provisions of the ADA, requires any employer with 15 or more employees not to discriminate on the basis of a person's disability and further to remove barriers that prevent a qualified person from performing a job. The ADA does not say that an employer is required to hire someone who could not perform the essential functions of the job. For example, if a person cannot hear well enough to reliably respond to questions on the telephone, an employer would not be legally required to hire that person as a telephone receptionist. However, if an employee is qualified for a job and can do everything relating to her job except access spoken information during large group training activities, the employer would be required to provide communication access (such as a FM system, captioning or interpreter) as a reasonable accommodation to meet the employee's needs. An employer is required to provide such accommodations unless they are deemed burdensome. The courts have generally viewed accommodations like these access services as reasonable and not burdensome. As with all parts of the ADA, there is a specific process for lodging complaints should that be necessary.

Title II–State and Local Governments

Title II requires that state and local governments give people with disabilities equal access to the programs, services, and activities they sponsor. This part of the ADA is similar to Section 504; the main difference is that Section 504 applies to recipients of federal government monies, whereas Title II of the ADA pertains to all state and local governments regardless of size. For a child with hearing loss, this means that all offerings accessed by the child and her family—library, recreation, social services, etc.—must be made accessible unless doing so would result in an undue financial or administrative burden.

Title II also addresses public transportation such as city buses or rail transit. Both the service and the communication systems that support the service (i.e., information kiosks, telephone information lines) are to be made accessible. In theory, this means that voice announcements on transit systems should also be provided in a text format.

Title III–Public Accommodations

Title III, public accommodations, covers businesses and non-profit organizations that offer services to the general public. Any entity that normally conducts business with the public, including restaurants, hotels, stores, movies, theaters, convention centers, doctors' offices, sports stadiums, fitness clubs, and private schools, is subject to the ADA Title III provisions. One area where there has been considerable effort by advocates is captioning at the movies and at live theater offerings. Although movie theaters are required to provide assistive listening devices, including a means to link to the telecoil of a hearing aid, movies were exempt in the original ADA language from being required to show open captioned movies. Several court cases upheld advocates' position that although theaters are not required by the ADA to provide open captioning, closed captioning is a needed and appropriate method of providing communications access. Many live theaters now provide one or two sign interpreted or captioned showings per run for a particular show. (**Fig. 23–5** demonstrates one technology for providing closed captioning in movie theaters and other places of entertainment.)

The specifics of how the ADA is to be performed is described in detail in the Americans with Disabilities Act Accessibility Guidelines (ADAAG), which were last revised and updated in 2004. In early 2007, the new guidelines were published (U.S. Access Board, 2004) but had not been formally accepted by the Department of Justice; hence the 2004 ADAAG is not legally binding until Justice Department acceptance. The following changes in the regulations are of interest to children and adults with hearing loss:

- Technical standards for assistive listening systems (ALS) used in public places are required (for the first time) to ensure consistency in the quality and strength of the auditory signal.

- Neckloop attachments must be provided to allow inductive coupling between the ALS receiver and the telecoil in hearing aids or cochlear implants.

- Public telephones must have volume control with gain up to 20 dB.

- The number of required TTYs in public places was increased.

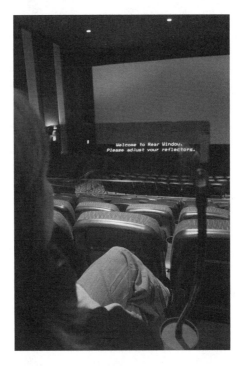

Figure 23–5   Rear Window is a closed captioning technology developed by WGBH National Center for Accessible Media in Boston used in movie theaters around the country and at select attractions at Walt Disney World and other theme parks. Rear Window displays reversed captions on a light-emitting diode text display, which is mounted in the rear of the theater. Transparent acrylic panels, which attach to the seat in a theater, reflect the captions for people with hearing loss.

(Photo by Jeffrey Dunn for WGBH.)

- Fire alarm alerts, audible and visual, shall be permanently installed in a specific percentage of hotel rooms.

A summary of Section 504 provisions as well general access provisions under the ADA appears in **Table 23–3**.

◆ Helping the Child Become Her Own Best Advocate

One of the most important lessons we can teach our children with hearing loss is that they must learn to be their own best advocates. We should help them understand that the laws are there to help them fully benefit from all life has to offer, and the accommodations that we reviewed here—at school, in the workplace, at the movies, when traveling, for telecommunications access—are basic rights in America. From an early age, we should involve children in the IEP process. The IEP should not be something that is done for the child; rather it should be a collaboration that allows the child to eventually become a full participant. The child's involvement can be something very simple to start. For example, the child might serve punch to the IEP team and discuss how his technology helps him. The next year, he would be expected to contribute a bit more. As time goes on, we want

Table 23–3

General Access	Coverage	Relevant Federal Agency	Web Resources
Section 504 of the Rehabilitation Act of 1973 (Non-Discrimination under Federal Grants and Programs)	Requires that any federal agency, organization or program receiving federal funds not discriminate based on disability. Nondiscrimination means that such organizations must be fully accessible to people with disabilities. Any grant, loan, or contract to an entity or program—public or private—requires that entity to follow the regulations of the act. Applies to employers, hospitals, human service programs, public schools, colleges, and universities—if they receive federal funds.	Relevant federal agency	www.section508.gov/index. cfm?FuseAction=Content&ID=15 www.usdoj.gov/crt/ada/cguide.htm
ADA, 1990	Title I: Employment Title II: State & Local Government & Transportation Title III: Public Facilities (private and nonprofit services open to the general public) Title IV: Telephone Relay (see above)	Title I: EEOC Title II: Transportation complaints to Federal Transit Administration Title II-IV Access Board (for guidelines and standards), Department of Justice (enforcement)	www.access-board.gov/ada-aba/index.htm www.jan.wvu.edu/links/ADAtam1.html www.usdoj.gov/crt/ada/cguide.htm www.access-board.gov/Adaag/about/index.htm www.ada.gov/pcatoolkit/chap1toolkit.htm

Abbreviation: ADA, Americans with Disabilities Act

our children to transition into being full partners in the IEP process, articulating their own needs and helping formulate their goals. In some cases, we are seeing teens who are running the meeting, which is highly desirable and will serve those adolescents well as they begin their college careers in a different setting without the support of their teams. This does not happen overnight, so we need to begin the process of teaching children to advocate for themselves while they are still young. In so doing, we are instilling in our children the understanding that laws are there to help address their needs. However, to enjoy the benefits of our federal laws, we must (1) know and understand our rights; (2) speak up about what we need; and (3) know how to politely but firmly negotiate the system. Whether we are talking about hiring the type of interpreter we want at school or ensuring that a facility is providing an assistive listening system, our children will only benefit from the wide-ranging laws reviewed here if they know how to advocate for themselves.

Many parents have difficulty resisting the temptation to do everything for their children. When the child has a disability, the urge to do it for her is even more likely to take over. As the child's audiologist, you can make a positive contribution to your patients' success beyond the hearing loss by coaching families in the importance of helping children develop their own advocacy skills. Many resources are available to help you accomplish that.

Discussion Questions

1. Children with hearing loss are now being identified at birth and fit early with technology that is considerably improved from what was available 10, or even 5, years ago. Regardless of their level of hearing loss, many children are learning language that is equivalent to their hearing peers. What kinds of issues does this create in terms of eligibility under various disability laws, and what is your role in advising parents and school professionals?

2. What are the differences between legal intent and practice as it applies to each of the three categories of laws reviewed in the chapter?

3. How should we teach a child to advocate for herself, and at what age should that process begin?

4. What if you do not agree with the school district's decision about placement and services for a patient? What is your role vis-à-vis the child, her family, and the school-based personnel?

5. Does your role as a hearing health professional include or exclude being an advocate for the child and her family? What are the boundaries?

References

Federal Communications Commission (2003). Hearing Aid Compatibility Order, 18 FCC Red at 16780 Paragraph 65; 47 C.F.R. Section 20.19(c).

Hands and Voices (2006). Guide-by-your-side program. www.handsandvoices.org/services/guide.htm. Last accessed January 5, 2008.

Perigoe, C., and Perigoe, R. (2005). Multiple challenges—multiple solutions: children with hearing loss and special needs. Volta Review, 104, 4, 211.

Sorkin, D. L. (2004). Disability law and people with hearing loss: we've come a long way (but we're not there yet). Hearing Loss, 25, 13–17.

Sutton v. United Airlines. (1999). 527 U.S. 471.

U.S. Access Board. (2004). Americans with Disabilities Act (ADA) Accessibility Guidelines for Buildings and Facilities. Architectural Barriers Act (ABA) Accessibility Guidelines. Preamble and Final Rule. http://www.access-board.gov/ada-aba/final.htm

U.S. Department of Education. (2006). Assistance to states for the education of children with disabilities and preschool grants for children with disabilities, final rule. Washington, DC: *Federal Register*, August 14, 2006.

Additional Readings

Breslin, M., and Silvia, Y. (Eds.). (2002). Disability rights law and policy: international and national perspectives. Ardsley, NY: Transnational Publishers.

Federal Communications Commission (2003). Section 68.4 of the commission's rules governing hearing aid-compatible telephones, report and order wt dkt. 01-309.

Georgia Tech Research Corporation. (2004) Information technology technical assistance and training center. Speak out! About inaccessible information and telecommunication technology. www.ittatc.org/technical/speakout/. Last accessed January 5, 2008.

Sorkin, D. L. (2004). FM technology: reimbursement and the law. Access: achieving clear communication, employing sound solutions. Proceedings of the first international FM conference. Warrenville, IL: Phonak.

Strauss, K P. (2006). A new civil right: telecommunications equality for deaf and hard of hearing Americans. Washington, DC: Gallaudet University Press.

Tucker, B. (1998). IDEA advocacy for children who are deaf or hard of hearing. San Diego: Singular Publishing Group, Inc.

U.S. Department of Justice. (2006). ADA tool kit. www.ada.gov/pca-toolkit/chap1toolkit.htm. Last accessed

Resources and Helpful Web Sites

1. Alexander Graham Bell Association for the Deaf and Hard of Hearing provides books and other resources on education and advocacy for people with hearing loss with a focus on children: www.agbell.org. Last accessed January 5, 2008.

2. Hands and Voices is a parent organization that emphasizes unbiased advisement on options, parent information and support: www.handsandvoices.org. Last accessed January 5, 2008.

3. Hearing Loss Association of America provides materials on advocacy, access laws, and telecommunications: www.hearingloss.org/advocacy/TC06.asp. Last accessed

4. NICHCY has technical assistance materials relating to the education of children with disabilities: www.nichcy.org. Last accessed January 5, 2008.

5. No Child Left Behind Web site: www.ed.gov/nclb/landing.jhtml. Last accessed January 5, 2008.

6. National Early Childhood TA Center: www.nectac.org. Last accessed January 5, 2008.

7. Technical Assistance Alliance for Parent Centers (PACER): www.taalliance.org. Last accessed January 5, 2008.

8. US Access Board has extensive online guidance materials on the ADA and Section 504: www.access-board.gov. Last accessed January 5, 2008.

9. U.S. Department of Education. Assistance to states for the education of children with disabilities and preschool grants for children with disabilities, final rule. Published in the Federal Register August 14, 2006. www.copag.net/pdf/reqsonly.pdf. Last accessed January 5, 2008.

10. US Department of Education. Raising the Achievement of Students with Disabilities: New Ideas for IDEA. August 2006. www.ed.gov/admins/lead/speced/ideafactsheet.html. Last accessed

11. Wrightslaw provides materials on education law for attorneys and advocates: www.wrightslaw. Last accessed January 5, 2008.

Chapter 24

The Importance of Early Intervention for Infants and Children with Hearing Loss

Arlene Stredler-Brown

♦ **Case One**

Part C of the Individuals with Disabilities Education Act (IDEA)

♦ **Case Two**

Early Intervention Providers and Their Qualifications

♦ **Case Three**

Consultants

♦ **Case Four**

Curriculums
Services to the Family
Strategies to Foster Child Development
Techniques That Affect the Quality of Parent–Child Interaction

♦ **Case Five**

Family-Centered Intervention

♦ **Case Six**

Evidence-Based Practice
Transition to Preschool

♦ **Summary**

Key Points

- Several federal initiatives support early intervention for infants and toddlers with hearing loss. The Individuals with Disabilities Education Act (IDEA), Part C, mandates services for children younger than 3 years. The Early Hearing Detection & Intervention (EHDI) initiative is supported by the Walsh Bill. This initiative provides funding to states to develop their screening, audiologic diagnostic, and intervention programs.

- Early intervention for children with hearing loss is a relatively new profession. Providers often rely on in-service training to meet quality standards.

- Consultants can support the early interventionists. They can provide hands-on training to teach an interventionist a new communication approach. Consultants offer guidance about motor skills, functional vision, cognitive development, and other domains that influence development.

- Family-centered intervention is a three-pronged approach that includes information and support for parents, outcomes for the child, and the dynamics of the parent–child interaction. There are specific curriculums for each of these domains.

- Very young children practice communication in their daily routines. Parents and other family members are the recipients of the early intervention. Families learn appropriate and effective communication techniques that are the essence of parent-centered intervention.

- In 2007, the goal for infants and toddlers with hearing loss is to achieve communication and language skills commensurate with their hearing peers. Evidence-based practice makes this outcome possible and measurable.

Case studies have been used to illustrate the six key points in this chapter. These vignettes are based on events in families' lives. Each anecdote encourages the reader to think about the way he delivers information to families.

◆ Case One

An 8-week-old child failed her newborn hearing screening test. The audiologist has just used state-of-the-art diagnostic tests to confirm hearing loss. The family has much to learn about the early intervention system in their community.

Part C of the Individuals with Disabilities Education Act (IDEA)

IDEA (2004) ensures that children with disabilities have access to services. Part C of IDEA addresses the needs of children from birth to 36 months of age. This federal law establishes minimum guidelines, and each state develops its own state plan. In most states, a child younger than 3 years with bilateral hearing loss is eligible for early intervention services. However, children with minimal hearing loss may not meet a state's eligibility criteria. A survey conducted by the National Center for Hearing Assessment and Management (2006) reviewed eligibility criteria in each state. Some states provide services to children with all degrees and types of hearing loss. Other states require a child to have a moderate to severe degree of hearing loss to qualify for services. Some states exclude children with mild, unilateral, or other minimal degrees of hearing loss. If a child is denied services, it is often possible to appeal the decision.

Pitfall
• A state's eligibility criteria can change over time, so it is important for the audiologist to verify criteria and stay current.

The law entitles infants and toddlers with disabilities, and their families, to receive several different services. First, each family has the right to have a service coordinator. The service coordinator is the point of entry into early intervention. For a child with hearing loss, the service coordinator is a conduit between the diagnosing audiologist and the early intervention provider. The service coordinator helps parents obtain the services they need, facilitates timely delivery of these services, and helps the family to coordinate the services that are provided by different professionals from various agencies.

The law states that it is appropriate for the service coordinator to be from the profession most immediately relevant to the infant's or toddler's or family's needs (IDEA, 2004). Indeed, families often ask about the experience of the service coordinator. Since most families embark on an unknown journey into audiology, early intervention, and therapy, they want to know if the service coordinator is familiar with the type and degree of hearing loss of their children. Families typically want to know the impact hearing loss can have on the development of speech and language. Most families want the different communication approaches that are used with children with hearing loss to be demonstrated. Hopefully, the service coordinator can answer these questions and provide this information. Each state is responsible to develop a system of service coordination to meet the needs of families (Marge and Marge, 2005).

Some states have a system of specialty service coordinators. These service coordinators are experts on hearing loss in young children. The positive impact of specialty service coordination has been demonstrated in the State of Colorado. Colorado has a group of 10 specially trained service coordinators who are experts on hearing loss who reside in different regions in the state. These specialty service coordinators are familiar with the early intervention services and programs in their regions. They provide information to families. They also provide emotional support to family members as they cope with their child's diagnosis. The average age of entry into early intervention in Colorado was 3.5 months in 2004 (Colorado Department of Public Health and Environment, 2005), and this network of specialty service coordinators is credited with this early start of services.

A second entitlement in the law ensures access to funding. Each state plan identifies specific eligibility criteria for Part C services. If a child with hearing loss meets eligibility criteria, the state system is responsible to fund early intervention services.

When a child is eligible for services, a meeting is conducted. One outcome of this meeting is the creation of an Individual Family Service Plan (IFSP) that must include specific information. The components of the IFSP are identified in **Table 24–1**.

The law is clear about the importance of this plan, because the IFSP guides intervention, identifies specific services, and identifies who will provide each service. The IFSP

Table 24–1 The Individual Family Service Plan

1. A statement of the child's present level of development
2. A statement of the family's resources
3. A statement of the family's priorities and concerns
4. A statement of the major outcomes expected
5. The criteria, procedures, and timelines used to measure outcomes
6. A statement of necessary early intervention services
7. A statement of the natural environments, to the maximum extent appropriate, in which services will be provided (or a justification when services should not be provided in a natural environment)
8. The projected dates for the start of services and the anticipated duration of services
9. Identification of the service coordinator
10. The steps to be taken to support the transition of the child to preschool services when the child is $2^1/_2$ years of age (IDEA, 2004)

also identifies the agency or individual who will pay for each service.

Implicit in the IFSP is the need to collect data to monitor progress. A measurement of the child's development is conducted and reported in the IFSP. The IFSP is reviewed at 6-month intervals and a new plan is created annually. Each time a new IFSP is created, a new measurement of the child's development is obtained and reported.

Pearl

- The collection of developmental information over time is crucial because this is how parents know that the early intervention program is effective for their child.

◆ Case Two

A family has just met with their service coordinator and knows that programs are available in their community. They need to select the program that provides what they want. The parents look to one another. How will they make a choice?

Early Intervention Providers and Their Qualifications

Before the start of newborn hearing screening programs, early interventionists were found in large metropolitan areas. Sometimes, if a family was fortunate, an early intervention provider lived in a rural area. However, this scenario is changing now that states have established EHDI programs. In the past 10 years, much more attention is being given to the "I," that is to say the "intervention," in EHDI programs. Each state continues to offer unique programs.

When considering early intervention programs, the family needs to consider the delivery model. Services can be family centered or child centered. Both are reasonable options. However, Part C strongly endorses family-centered practices for children younger than 3 years.

In family-centered intervention (Dunst et al, 2002) all family members are the clients. The interventionist delivers information about hearing loss to family members and provides emotional support. And, in short order, the interventionist starts to teach family members specific techniques to use with their child.

Pearl

- The goal is to develop the child's communication and language so that these skills remain on track with their hearing peers.

Communication and language exist in relationship. For a young child, family members and caregivers are the primary communicators in the child's life. Therefore, it is logical that the adults are the clients. They are the ones who need to learn to communicate effectively with the child. Adaptations and adjustments to communication and language are made to foster language learning, in spite of the condition of hearing loss.

Child-centered therapy is always a viable option. In this paradigm, the professional works directly with the child to investigate, identify, and implement specific communication strategies. Parents may observe these therapy sessions, but the intent is for the professional to provide direct one-on-one instruction to the child.

Another consideration is the environment in which intervention occurs. Part C of IDEA strongly endorses treatment in natural environments by stating that early intervention services, "to the maximum extent appropriate, are provided in natural environments, including the home and community settings, in which children without disabilities participate" (34 CFR 303.12[b]). Part C defines natural environments as "settings that are natural or normal for the child's age peers who have no disabilities" (34 CFR 303.18). A home is a natural environment. The grocery store, a community park, and a children's museum are all natural environments.

There is one more consideration for children with hearing loss. These children require a setting that supports a language-rich environment (DesGeorges, Johnson, and Stredler-Brown, 2006). A language-rich environment is one in which language is complete, expanded, and reinforced to provide appropriate repetition. When a child who is deaf or hard of hearing is immersed in a language-rich environment, there is potential to override the potential influences of hearing loss. Fortunately, federal law provides an opportunity to justify why a child's early intervention may be conducted in settings other than natural environments. In addressing this issue, the law states that "the provision of early intervention services for each eligible child occurs in a setting other than a natural environment only if the IFSP team determines that early intervention cannot be achieved satisfactorily for the child in a natural environment" (34 CFR 303.12[2]).

Next, consider the qualifications of the early interventionist. Historically, interventionists have been a hybrid group. They come from a variety of preservice training programs. A survey of 16 states (Arehart et al, 1998) reported that most professionals received preservice training in three types of programs: teacher education for the deaf and hard of hearing, speech-language pathology, and audiology. A small number of providers received preservice training in early childhood education or early childhood special education.

Unfortunately, a graduate degree in any one of these training programs does not guarantee that the professional has the requisite competencies to work with these children and their families. Therefore, families must determine that the early interventionists have the skills, competencies, knowledge, and experience to effectively teach young children with hearing loss. These competencies and skills are identified in **Table 24–2**.

Table 24–2 Competencies for an Early Interventionist Providing Parent-Centered Intervention

- Communicating with family members
- Forming collaborative partnerships
- Working with families
- Assessing, interpreting assessments, and monitoring progress
- Developing and implementing a therapy plan
- Managing sensory devices
- Maximizing auditory potential
- Facilitating communication development
- Facilitating cognitive development

Source: Colorado Infant Hearing Advisory Board and Membership of the Screening, Assessment, and Early Intervention Task Forces (2003). Guidelines for Infant Hearing Screening, Audiologic Assessment, and Early Intervention (Colorado Infant Hearing Advisory Committee). Denver, CO: Colorado Department of Public Health and Environment.

◆ Case Three

My 18-month-old child has just been diagnosed with a sensory-motor disability. Will my early interventionist have the skills to work with this disability too?

Consultants

A significant number of infants and toddlers with hearing loss have additional disabilities. Some studies show that 33 to 38% of children, birth to 3 years of age, have an additional developmental disability (Schildroth and Hotto, 1996; Moeller et al, 1990). One state's data tracking system identified 40% of their infants and toddlers with hearing loss with an additional disability (Clinical Health Information Records of Patients, 2004). This disability may be a visual acuity problem, a functional vision disability, a motor delay, a cognitive delay, sensory-integration dysfunction, attention deficit disorder, a learning disability, or some other disability.

When are additional disabilities identified? Who performs the diagnostic evaluation to make a diagnosis? Who treats the disability? Testing should be conducted at regular intervals. Part C of IDEA recommends assessing the baby or child at 6-month intervals. Most important, testing should be conducted by a multidisciplinary team of qualified professionals. A team approach, in and of itself, provides the opportunity to identify a child with additional challenges. Only an appropriately credentialed professional can confirm a diagnosis of additional disabilities. This professional could be an occupational therapist, a physical therapist, a vision specialist, a social worker, or a psychologist, among others.

Once a diagnosis is made, the diagnosing professional or therapist has two tasks: (1) Diagnose and treat the secondary disability; and (2) Teach the parents and the primary interventionist (this is the person with expertise working with hearing loss) to integrate appropriate strategies into therapy sessions and daily routines.

A child with multiple disabilities does not necessarily require multiple treatment programs. A transdisciplinary model of intervention integrates the expertise of different professionals as they serve children with complicated needs (Linder, 1993). For example, a speech-language pathologist may focus on the development of communication skills while a physical therapist identifies adaptive seating for optimal physical support. In a transdisciplinary approach, the speech-language pathologist will position the child in the adaptive seat while working on communication skills. Likewise, the physical therapist can practice communication skills while establishing the best seating positions. Both professionals learn to employ techniques from another discipline; one discipline complements the other. This approach is powerful for the parents. They also are learning to integrate multiple techniques into their daily routines.

Consultants serve another important role. To explain, most early interventionists learn one communication approach in their preservice training program. However, parents might select an approach that does not match the interventionist's experience and expertise. In this situation, a consultant with expertise in the family's chosen approach can provide training to the primary interventionist.

Pearl

- A mentor can effectively change a professional's clinical practices (Rall and Brunner, 2006).

One example of a mentor training paradigm is offered by Rall and Brunner (2006), who describe a five-step process. First, the interventionist needs to have a collegial relationship with his mentor. Once this rapport is established, the mentor observes an intervention session with the family. Next, the mentor models new techniques. The interventionist then practices these techniques while receiving guidance from the mentor. After guided practice, the interventionist practices the new techniques independently. Another meeting with the mentor provides an opportunity for the interventionist to evaluate their new skills. This cycle repeats itself while the interventionist learns the skills he needs to meet the expectations of the parents and the needs of the child.

◆ Case Four

At our IFSP, we scheduled sessions with an early interventionist six times each month. We identified many outcomes and procedures. What exactly can we expect our early interventionist to teach us?

Curriculums

Family-centered early intervention includes many content areas. These content areas fall into three categories: (1)

services to the family; (2) strategies to foster the child's development; and (3) techniques that influence the quality of parent–child interaction.

Services to the Family

In a parent-centered approach, the parents are the clients. Parents and other caregivers learn to understand hearing loss and its potential impact on development. Most parents, especially those who do not have experience with hearing loss, have an emotional reaction (Moses, 1985). The intervention process can support family members emotionally. Because hearing loss has a significant impact on communication and language, parents must implement specific techniques to foster communication and language. The early interventionist teaches these strategies to the parents and other caregivers.

Strategies to Foster Child Development

Many developmental domains need to be considered, and all affect the child's learning. The first consideration is cognitive development. For a young child, cognition is exhibited and measured through play. In addition, motor skills, personal-social skills, and self-help skills all contribute to development. A child's growth in each of these domains needs to be observed carefully over time because a disability in any of these developmental areas can have a negative impact on development. If problems occur, techniques to support the child's progress need to be taught. When development in these domains is age appropriate, the child's inherent skills can be harnessed to enhance communication and language.

Then, there is the primary focus of the early interventionist, which is to promote the development of communication. Communication includes any and all of the following domains: auditory skill development, speech, preverbal communication (e.g., vocalizations and gestures), and verbal communication (starting with first words). Verbal communication, or language, includes four specific domains. They are described in **Table 24–3**.

With guidance from the professionals, a family selects a communication approach. See Chapter 21 for an overview of communication approaches.

Techniques That Affect the Quality of Parent–Child Interaction

Communication is reciprocal; it is a dynamic process that happens between two or more people. Therefore, the interventionist must consider the attributes of the communicative dyad. Mahoney and Powell (1986) state that, "interventions impact child development to the extent that parents are supported and encouraged to engage in responsive interactions with the child." The venues that support responsive interactions include frequent play, matching a child's interests, having parent and child take an equal number of turns, and increasing responsive comments (Cole and Flexer, 2007). Daily practice of these strategies is recommended.

It is important to have an optimal interactive match (Bailey and Simeonsson, 1988). The premise here is to allow the child's mode of communication to influence the modality used by the parents. The parent is encouraged to recognize and imitate the mode used by the child. This reinforces the child's communicative intents. In addition, the parent can communicate by using a different mode to encourage more sophisticated communication.

Parents have a lot to learn. Many states create a resource guide specifically for parents of children who are deaf or hard of hearing. There are many topics in these resource guides, including a description of hearing loss; the potential effects of hearing loss; information about amplification, cochlear implants, and assistive listening technology; access to early intervention in one's community; intervention programs with expertise in hearing loss; communication approaches; support for evidence-based practices; funding for amplification and intervention; and lists of organizations in the state and country that focus on hearing loss.

◆ Case Five

Our early interventionist meets with our family regularly. She works with the adults for most of the session. Only some of her time is spent with our child. I am confused about the purpose of intervention. Who is the client? Is the intervention for the adults or is it for our child?

Family-Centered Intervention

Parents have many questions about hearing loss and its impact on communication. When intervention starts, information is provided to the family. There is an endless list of issues, and the interventionist needs to answer the parents' questions first.

Table 24–3

Components of Language Learning	Description
Semantics	The study of word meanings and word relations
Syntax	The aspect of language that governs the rules for how words are arranged in sentences
Morphology	The study of the minimal units of language that are meaningful, such as /–s/ for plural nouns or third-person verb tenses, /–ing/ for present progressive, and /–ed/ for past tense
Pragmatics	The functional use of language

Source: Schow and Nerbonne (2002).

Pearl

- Parents know what they want to learn. The interventionist must respect the rate at which different parents acquire information.

Next, communication and intervention techniques are taught to the adults. The characteristics of the parent–child interaction can be prescriptive. The techniques that are taught may focus on preverbal communication, receptive language, expressive language, listening skills, speech skills, play skills, and others. The goal is for each adult in the child's life to use these techniques and to use them daily. A rubric of a home visit is illustrated in **Fig. 24–1**.

At a home visit, the interventionist first reconnects with family members and reviews the events since the last visit. The early interventionist learns about the experiences of each family member. The interventionist often needs to set aside his agenda to address the current events in the family's life.

Next, family members identify their priorities. Of course, the interventionist has a well-developed plan for each session. However, the family's questions, concerns, and accomplishments are of paramount importance, because the specific strategies that will be taught during the session must be appropriate for the child and for the family.

The next step in the rubric is a familiar one for the interventionist. A brief explanation of a strategy or technique is offered. Then, the play begins. The interventionist shows the craft underlying communication. The family members are active and engaged in the communication and intervention process. The interventionist uses coaching strategies to explore, with the family, the techniques that work. Several strategies can be explored during one session. This process helps parents feel competent and confident.

Each session includes assessment and evaluation of the family and child's progress. The early interventionist and the parents discuss the child's skills before, during, and after each technique is taught. The purpose is to identify the effectiveness of the communication strategy. Did the child's

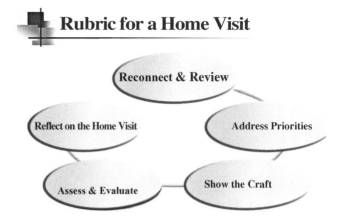

Figure 24–1   Rubric for a home visit (*Contributors*: A. Stredler-Brown, M.P. Moeller, R. Gallegos, P. Pittman, J. Corwin, M. Condon).
Source: Stredler-Brown et al (2004).

behavior change because of it? If so, how did it change? If not, why not?

In a family-centered program, evaluation also includes consideration of the family members. The interventionist helps each family member to comment on his comfort with the new strategies. Parents are expected to integrate these strategies into their daily routines, and to do so, they must be comfortable using the technique.

As the home visit time draws to an end, the family members reflect on the session. The interventionist is looking for input from the parents. Were particular strategies or techniques successful? Were the questions from family members answered? Were family members satisfied with the information they received? Are they ready to use the new information and novel strategies in their daily routines?

Experienced professionals working with infants and toddlers with hearing loss assert there is an art and a science to early intervention (Stredler-Brown, 2005; Stredler-Brown et al, 2004). These relationship-based techniques provide information and emotional support to parents. These techniques are called tools of the trade. The tools are described in **Table 24–4**.

Table 24–4   Tools of the Trade

Information resource: The early interventionist has an exhaustive amount of information about hearing loss. Specific information can be gathered in response to the questions from family members.

Coach and partner: The interventionist is an observer and provides reinforcement. The interventionist points out desirable behaviors. As the early intervention process unfolds, parents begin to recognize what is important. Family members learn to identify what is working for them and for their child.

Sounding board: The interventionist uses active listening (Rogers, 1961) and reflects what is heard back to the family. The interventionist can notice the content of the message. Of equal importance, the interventionist can listen for the emotions the family members reveal.

News commentator (Moeller and Condon, 1994): The early interventionist provides an on-the-spot commentary. This gives immediate feedback to the family. This technique is used as parents discover the effectiveness of a specific strategy.

◆ Case Six

Our early interventionist says our 24-month-old child is making progress. We're happy to hear this. But, our child's communication is not like her hearing peers. Is there a way to measure her progress?

Evidence-Based Practice

Children are identified with hearing loss, in increasing numbers, at a very young age. There is a call to action to measure the developmental outcomes of all of these children who are receiving early intervention (Dunst et al, 2002). How can outcomes be quantified? Do we have the appropriate tests to do this? Who would administer the tests? The answers are a resounding "yes" to each of these questions.

Now that systems support children entering early intervention by 6 months of age, it is appropriate to raise our expectations. No longer should one hear, "He is doing well for a deaf child." Rather, the expectation is for a child with hearing loss of any degree who has received early intervention by 6 months of age to be doing well. The communication and language skills of a child with hearing loss can be commensurate with their hearing peers. For children with cognitive disabilities, the standard will be their developmental age, rather than their chronological age. The key issue when providing evidence-based practice is to document the effectiveness of the intervention, a goal supported by research (Yoshinaga-Itano et al, 1998; Moeller, 2000) that documents the effectiveness of early identification and an early start of intervention.

Evidence is compelling. Each interventionist can collect evidence to document the progress made by each child. Informal assessment is an integral part of each session. Formal testing is completed at 6-month intervals and documented on the IFSP. Each program, subsequently, can take the individual child data and analyze it to identify program trends.

Assessment serves several purposes. First, the data provide an ongoing record of progress. Is the one for one rule being met (Johnson, 2005)? The one for one rule expects a child to make 1 year's growth in 1 year's time. For the infants and toddlers, progress is measured more frequently. The expectation for these very young children is 1 month of progress in 1 month's time or 3 months of progress in 3 month's time. Outcome data are used to acknowledge the efficacy of the individualized intervention program. If the requisite amount of progress is being made, the program must be a good fit. The number of sessions, the communication approach, and the skills of the interventionist and parents all contribute to the child's development. Conversely, if progress is not being made, there is due cause to review the strategies being used.

Assessment also benefits the administrative unit. Collecting data is a powerful way for a program to measure outcomes. By aggregating the data, a program can document its achievements, prioritize initiatives, and designate funding appropriately.

The areas of development that merit assessment are identified in **Table 24–5**.

Table 24–5 Developmental Domains for Assessment

✓ Communication and language
✓ Functional auditory skills
✓ Speech
✓ Play and cognition
✓ Parent–child interaction
✓ Social-emotional development
✓ Physical development
✓ Vision
✓ Family needs and environment

Source: Clark et al (2004).

Transition to Preschool

The transition from early intervention to preschool services starts when a child is 2¹/₂ years old. The early interventionist can support parents as they learn about preschool placements. There are several types of programs. The least restrictive option places the child with hearing loss in a preschool program with hearing children. This could be a publicly funded preschool program or a private preschool. Another option enrolls the child with hearing loss in a noncategorical preschool program which has children with different types of disabilities in the same classroom. A third option, often found in larger metropolitan areas, is a center-based program, which enrolls as many children with hearing loss as possible in one classroom. To have this critical mass of children, students may be transported to one school from different catchment areas. All these options, to varying degrees, can enroll peers who do not have disabilities. These peers serve as models for typical development.

Parents are encouraged to visit the preschool programs. A checklist to guide these observations was developed by Johnson, Beams, and Stredler-Brown (2005). The considerations are listed in **Table 24–6**.

Table 24–6 Criteria for Selecting a Preschool Program

• Total number of students in the classroom
• Number of students with hearing loss in the classroom
• Adult-to-child ratio
• Communication approach used by each child in the classroom
• Accommodations for amplification
• Related services (e.g., speech/language pathologist, educational audiologist, occupational therapist, physical therapist, psychologist)
• Parent support
• Physical environment
• Acoustic accommodations
• Curriculums
• Communication between school and home
• Family involvement in day-to-day preschool activities
• Role models who are deaf or hard of hearing
• Assessment

Source: Johnson, Beams, and Stredler-Brown (2005).

♦ Summary

Early intervention is complex. It must start early—within weeks of the diagnosis of hearing loss. It must be provided by well-trained providers. An individualized curriculum must be created. Progress must be monitored. More and more often, young children with hearing loss, birth to 3 years of age, exhibit communication and language skills at age level (Yoshinaga-Itano, 2004). In the not-too-distant future, this benchmark can become a standard for children with hearing loss.

There is an art and a science to early intervention. Technological advances contribute to the science, and the skills of the providers and the prescriptive nature of intervention represent the art.

Discussion Questions

1. How does a family learn about the early intervention programs in their community?

2. What are the criteria for selecting a program that meets the family's and the child's needs?

3. What are the qualifications for an early interventionist working with children with hearing loss?

4. What is included in a curriculum for an infant or toddler with hearing loss?

5. Why is family-centered programming valued?

6. How does evidence-based programming benefit a child and the child's family?

References

Arehart, K., Yoshinaga-Itano, C., Thomson, V., Gabbard, S., and Stredler-Brown, A. (1998). State of the states: the status of universal newborn hearing screening, assessment and intervention systems in 16 states. American Journal of Audiology, 7, 101–114.

Bailey, D., and Simeonsson, R. 1988. Family assessment in early intervention. Columbus: Merrill.

Clark, K., Abraham, H., Lambourne, M., Madsen, M., and Welch, P. (2004). Assessment. In S. Watson, D. J. Taylor, and P. Pittman (Eds.), SKI-HI curriculum: family-centered programming for infants and young children with hearing loss. Logan, UT: HOPE, Inc.

Clinical Health Information Records of Patients (CHIRP): 2004 [Electronic data]. Denver: Colorado Department of Public Health and Environment.

Clinical Health Information Records of Patients (CHIRP): 2005 [Electronic data]. Denver: Colorado Department of Public Health and Environment.

Cole, E., and Flexer, C. (2007). Children with hearing loss: developing listening and talking, birth to six. San Diego: Plural Publishing

Colorado Infant Hearing Advisory Board and Membership of the Screening, Assessment, and Early Intervention Task Forces (2003). Guidelines for Infant Hearing Screening, Audiologic Assessment, and Early Intervention (Colorado Infant Hearing Advisory Committee). Denver: Colorado Department of Public Health and Environment.

DesGeorges, J., Johnson, C. D., and Stredler-Brown, A. (2006). Natural environments: a call for policy guidance for infants and toddlers (0–3) who are deaf/hard and hearing. Unpublished manuscript.

Dunst, C. J., Boyd, K., Trivette, C. M., and Hamby, D. W. (2002). Family-oriented program models and professional helpgiving practices. Family Relations 51, 221–229.

Individuals with Disabilities Education Improvement Act of 2004, 20 U.S.C. § 1400 et seq. (2004).

Johnson, C. D. (2006). One year's growth in one year, expect no less. Hands & Voices Communicator, 9, 3.

Johnson, C. D., Beams, D., and Stredler-Brown, A. (2005). Preschool-Kindergarten Placement Checklist for Children who are Deaf and hard of Hearing. www.cde.state.co.us/cdesped/download/pdf/dhh-PS-KPlcmntCklst.pdf.

Linder, T. W. (1993). Transdisciplinary play-based intervention: guidelines for developing a meaningful curriculum for young children. Baltimore: Paul H. Brookes Publishing Company.

Mahoney, C., and Powell, A. (1986). Transactional Intervention Program. Farmington, CT: University of Connecticut School of Medicine.

Marge, D. K., and Marge, M. (2005). Beyond newborn hearing screening: meeting the educational and health care needs of infants and young children with hearing loss in America. Report of the National Consensus Conference on Effective Educational and Health Care Interventions for Infants and Young Children with Hearing Loss, September 10–12, 2004. Syracuse, NY: Department of Physical Medicine and Rehabilitation, SUNY Upstate Medical University.

Moeller, M. P. (2000). Early intervention and language development in children who are deaf and hard of hearing. Pediatrics, 106, E43.

Moeller, M. P., and Condon, M. C. (1994). D.E.I.P.: A collaborative problem-solving approach to early intervention. In J. Roush and N. D. Matkin (Eds.), Infants and toddlers with hearing loss (pp. 163–194). Baltimore: York Press.

Moeller, M. P., Coufal, K. L., and Hixson, P. K. (1990). The efficacy of speech-language pathology intervention: hearing-impaired children. Seminars in Speech and Language, 214, 227–247.

Moses, K. (1985). Infant deafness and parental grief: psychosocial early intervention. In F. Powell, T. Finitz-Hieber, S. Friel-Patti, and D. Henderson (Eds.), Education of the Hearing Impaired Child. San Diego: College-Hill Press.

National Center for Hearing Assessment and Management (NCHAM). (2006). Criteria for infants and toddlers with hearing loss to be eligible for early intervention services under IDEA. www.infanthearing.org/earlyintervention/eligibility.pdf. Last accessed December 15, 2006.

Rall, E., and Brunner, E. (2006). Mentoring in audiology. Seminars in Hearing, 27, 92–97.

Rogers, C. R. (1961). On becoming a person: a therapist's view of psychotherapy. Boston: Houghton Mifflin Company.

Schildroth, A. N., and Hotto, S. A. (1996). Changes in student and program characteristics, 1984–85 and 1994–95. American Annals of the Deaf, 141, 68–71.

Schow, R. L., and Nerbonne, M. A. (2002). Overview of audiologic rehabilitation. In R. L. Schow and M.A. Nerbonne (Eds.), Introduction to audiologic rehabilitation. Boston: Allyn and Bacon.

Stredler-Brown, A. (2005). The art and science of home visits. ASHA Leader, January 18, 6–7,15.

Stredler-Brown, A., Moeller, M. P., Gallegos, R., Corwin, J., and Pittman, P. (2004). The art and science of home visits (DVD). Omaha: Boys Town Press.

Yoshinaga-Itano, C. (2004). The impact of early access to language and communication for children with hearing loss. In D. Powers and G. R. Leigh (Eds.), Education of deaf children: global perspectives. Washington DC: Gallaudet University Press, pp. 69–84.

Yoshinaga-Itano, C., Sedey, A. L., Coulter, D. K., and Mehl, A. L. (1998). The language of early- and later-identified children with hearing loss. Pediatrics 102, 1161–1171.

Chapter 25

Speech/Language/Auditory Management of Infants and Children with Hearing Loss

Elizabeth Ying

Key Points

- The role of a speech-language pathologist (SLP) encompasses diagnostic and therapeutic responsibilities for a child who is deaf or hard of hearing.

- The need to assess functional listening distinguishes the communication evaluation of a child with hearing loss from the communication evaluation of a normal-hearing child.

- Audition is the most effective and efficient modality for acquiring and monitoring spoken language skills.

- The primary objective of aural habilitation and rehabilitation training is to develop functional listening skills for continued language learning and enhanced communicative interactions.

- Advances in amplification technology and early identification and intervention have facilitated more children with hearing loss to acquire functionally adequate listening and age-appropriate spoken language skills.

Since passage of the Walsh Act in 1997, most states now implement programs of universal newborn hearing screening. As a result, hearing loss is being identified at earlier ages compared with even a decade ago, and more families and their infants or toddlers are seeking assessment and treatment of the communication deficits accompanying hearing loss by the time the child is 1 to 3 months of age. Advances in technology options (including digital hearing aids and cochlear implants) as well as the increased availability of parent-child-focused early intervention programs that emphasize auditory skill development and the comprehension and use of spoken language, have significantly altered what are considered as functionally adequate progress and performance. Whereas in the recent past, it was considered exceptional for a child with significant hearing loss to achieve age-level communication skills by any age, it is now commonly expected that children whose hearing loss was identified early will function receptively and expressively on a par with their typically hearing peers by preschool or kindergarten. This evolution of the student with severe to profound hearing loss from a functionally deaf to a functionally hearing student places unique social and educational management challenges on professionals and school systems alike.

♦ Role of the Speech-Language Pathologist

It is widely accepted that an SLP is an integral member of the interdisciplinary diagnostic team that serves children with hearing loss. Traditionally, findings from an initial speech-language evaluation yield the following baseline information about a child who is deaf or hard of hearing: vocabulary and receptive-expressive language functioning; and speech production stimulability and capability. These important findings will determine initial training needs and serve as comparative data for the measurement of therapy benefit and progress.

The communication profiles of children with any degree of hearing loss are characterized by a wide variability in functional listening skills and linguistic competency. Therefore, for any child with hearing loss, the communication evaluation should encompass a functional listening assessment. This component is needed to obtain critical information about speech perception abilities (e.g., the nature and extent of a hearing aid or implant user's reliance on auditory input for continued language learning and enhanced communicative interactions). This functional listening assessment requirement distinguishes the speech-language assessment of a child with hearing loss from the communication assessment of his normal-hearing peers, because formulation and implementation of aural habilitation/rehabilitation training also fall within the professional domain of the SLP.

Pitfall

- Few graduate training programs offer the coursework or practical experiences that are necessary to prepare the average SLP with skills to work with children with hearing loss. The academic preparation of an SLP should prepare clinicians to conduct the evaluation and treatment programs for pediatric patients with hearing loss. Furthermore, SLPs must be prepared to assume additional responsibilities for the student with hearing loss who is enrolled in general education settings (e.g., monitoring amplification, serving as a resource to the classroom teacher, providing preteaching of classroom vocabulary and content, and facilitating social interactions).

♦ Diagnostic Evaluations

There are two major purposes for conducting speech-language evaluations and functional listening assessments: (1) to identify communicative strengths and weaknesses (during the initial assessment); and (2) to monitor progress over time (during progress assessments). Identifying the purpose of the assessment is essential to determining the scope of the assessment and in selecting the most appropriate assessment tools.

Upon receiving a referral for evaluation, it is first absolutely critical to review the audiologic findings and general case history. The SLP must understand the child's hearing loss, including aided and unaided hearing. In addition, the SLP must make sure that the child's technology is

working and that the child has auditory access to the information presented in the SLP assessments.

Initial Assessment

Findings from an initial speech-language evaluation/functional listening assessment identify areas of strength and weakness in several skill domains, including

- phonemic awareness (encompasses assessment of detection, discrimination, and identification of vowel elements and consonants as they occur in isolation or in different positions with words)

- vocabulary (encompasses the assessment of the understanding or expressive use of real words or sound associations representing real words, e.g., *woof-woof* for *dog*)

- language comprehension (encompasses the assessment of the understanding and contingent response to spoken language including acting upon directions and questions by performing actions, manipulating objects, pointing to pictures, or verbally responding)

- expressive language (encompasses the assessment of nonverbal and verbal behaviors produced to intentionally convey meaning)

- speech production (encompasses the assessment of the articulation of speech sounds in isolation, repeated and alternated syllables, words, and word combinations as well as overall voice quality, prosody, and intonational characteristics)

- pragmatic functioning (encompasses the assessment of how spoken language is used for various communicative purposes such as labeling, commenting, requesting, directing, and questioning)

Performance data yield critically needed information to determine future habilitation and rehabilitation management as well as educational placement and related services needs.

During the communication assessment, additional information is also gathered about factors (listed below) that account for much of the variability in the performance of pediatric hearing aid or cochlear implant users. Through formal and informal measures, the SLP obtains information about: (1) age of identification (Yoshinaga-Itano et al, 1998); (2) previous communication modality (Geers et al, 2003); (3) cognitive factors (such as attention span and memory) (Geers et al, 2003; Pisoni and Geers, 2000); (4) environmental considerations such as everyday communicative demands and expectations (Quittner, Leibach, and Marciel, 2004); and (5) parental input/language proficiency (Cole and Flexer, 2007; Stallings et al, 2004).

Testing may also reveal areas that should be addressed to ensure that there is sufficient and appropriate support for the child with hearing loss both at home and in school. Considerations such as consistency of present technology use, realistic understanding of the impact of hearing loss on language learning, and availability of aural habilitation and rehabilitation training should be identified during the initial diagnostic assessment. Most important, it should be possible to formulate aural habilitation training objectives and strategies based on the results of a comprehensive communication evaluation.

Progress Assessments

In contrast, subsequent assessments (routinely occurring at 6-month intervals or annually) provide all of the above, but also slightly different, information. Comparative analysis of performance on criterion-referenced or standardized measures affords an objective means of monitoring progress and benefit (of both therapy and technology) for the child who is deaf or hard of hearing. Subsequent assessments also present the necessary information for making changes in the child's aural habilitation/rehabilitation training.

◆ Determining the Focus of Therapy

Children entering the aural habilitation and rehabilitation process fall within four major age groupings: infants, preschool-aged, school-aged, and teenagers. Each of these developmental groups has distinctly differing diagnostic and training requirements. Recognizing the unique needs of each group is critical in both selecting the appropriate diagnostic tools as well as in interpreting the test findings and formulating appropriate training programs.

Infants

It is increasingly more common to be asked to conduct a speech-language evaluation and functional listening assessment on an infant who has only recently been diagnosed with hearing loss or who is just beginning a hearing aid trial process. Because of their young ages, infants exhibit few skills that can be formally assessed. Therefore, a large part of the evaluation process involves parent questionnaires of observed auditory and basic communication behaviors. Parental responses on such questionnaires provide important information about parental understanding of the impact of hearing loss on future language learning and social-communicative interactions and parental understanding of amplification use and aural habilitation training on the development of desired skills.

Frequently, the infant or toddler has already undergone some type of global early intervention (EI) eligibility assessment. Rarely, however, has there been any attempt during such assessments to observe or document the auditory responsiveness and stimulability of the infant-toddler with hearing loss. Generic early intervention providers may have limited experience with hearing loss (and even less experience in determining potential candidates for more advanced technologies such as FM devices or cochlear implants as the child's primary amplification at home.

Early intervention or speech–language pathologists often lack special training or experience that can support the necessary preimplant training or that can assist in the infant's or toddler's initial acclimation to either hearing aids or cochlear implants. Also, the concept of fast tracking an infant or toddler for cochlear implantation is often misinterpreted as affording minimal services to the child and family until an implant is fitted, when, in fact, the early interventionist should be an active participant in preparing the baby and parents for the implant procedure.

During the hearing aid trial, it is valuable to attempt to establish some prerequisite behaviors to the onset of speech and environmental sounds, such as developing visual attending skills, sustained attention to sound-making toys, and exposure to a variety of low-frequency listening and vibrotactile experiences.

Preschoolers

The primary component of the evaluation process for the preschool-aged child is to assess the present level of functioning in light of the child's amplification history and previously delivered aural habilitation training. If the preschooler with hearing loss has been fortunate enough to have had some auditory-verbal training but had achieved minimal gains, the evaluator might assume that the child has limited potential to use auditory input from hearing aids or implant programs (e.g., MAP) that are currently being used. In contrast, if previous early intervention programming has been more visually based or used sign support, one must question if there has been sufficient focus on auditory skill emergence to determine ultimate benefit from the hearing aid trial or implant program (e.g., perhaps the lack of auditory progress is an artifact of training as opposed to either a subject-specific or device-related issue). This communication modality issue becomes particularly important in borderline cases for cochlear implantation (e.g., for children whose audiograms suggest that they should be hearing better with hearing aids). At times, potential implant recipients might exhibit behaviors during formal testing that suggest they are more stimulable (e.g., have greater auditory potential) than reported by the parents or their ongoing speech-language clinicians. This finding would, in turn, suggest that changes are needed in the preschooler's aural habilitation objectives and strategies.

Depending on the child's age, exploration of present or future school-based aural habilitation services might also be a component of the evaluation process. When the child with hearing loss continues to exhibit limited functional listening or oral communication skills, the most appropriate evaluation measures may be largely parent-report inventories or criterion-referenced assessment tools; keeping in mind that it is critical to include some tool to assess the nature and consistency of the preschooler's auditory and communicative demands.

School-Aged Children

At this level, communication mode (total communication versus auditory-oral and auditory-verbal) and current communication skills impact on both the diagnostic and therapeutic management of a child with hearing loss. Potential first-time implant candidates in this age group are assumed to have missed the window of opportunity for optimal verbal language learning (unless the referral for implantation is being made because of a change in hearing). This may create a need to assess the child's level of linguistic competency in her first language (e.g., a manual communication system). In addition, when the school-aged child is being evaluated for implant candidacy, assessment measures should also be used to determine whether parents and professionals (who have often initiated the implant process) have realistic expectations of the ultimate benefit for the particular implant candidate.

It is expected that the school-aged hearing aid user or implant recipient can take formal standardized testing, preferably administered in the child's primary mode of communication. In addition, if the present or future educational placement for this aged child is a regular classroom setting, it is strongly recommended that tests standardized on children with normal hearing versus children with impaired hearing be used. This will provide a more representative sample of how the skills of the school-aged student with hearing loss compare with those of her classroom peers. The results of this evaluation are used to determine the child's areas of strengths and weaknesses, to serve as a baseline from which to measure future progress, and to identify specific modifications needed in his ongoing aural habilitation and rehabilitation management.

Teenagers

Teens and parents who enter the evaluation or rehabilitation process often do so in response to having experienced a change in hearing status or a failure in some aspect of their social-communicative interactions. If considering cochlear implantation, the device may be viewed as a potential cure for deafness. Other precipitating variables for pursuing a cochlear implant in this age group, however, include a progression in the severity of the teenager's hearing loss or simply the relaxing criteria for implant candidacy.

The requirements of the communication evaluation for a teenager are the same as those for the school-aged child. However, it is also critical to actively involve the teen in the decision-making process regarding future amplification devices (including trying a digital hearing aid, using an FM, or obtaining a cochlear implant). Similarly, it is unrealistic to expect that any progress will be made in the recommended therapy programming without the teen's motivation and commitment to such training. If the teen has restricted language skills, it is difficult to determine if her limited understanding of the issues will allow her to offer an informed consent.

Professionals who are actively involved in the diagnostic and therapy processes with teenagers recognize that teens who have adjusted to the compromised auditory input over many years may perceive increased or continuous sound from present technology as bothersome and aversive. The usen of social-communicative questionnaires such as the "L.I.F.E.," the Listening Inventory for Education (Anderson and Smaldino, 1998) has been found to be extremely useful in assessing if the teen and parents have realistic expectations of an amplification device, the listening environment, or present level of functioning. Similarly, sharing test results

and training strategies throughout the habilitation and rehabilitation process is motivating, but also ensures that the teen maintains realistic expectations about her course of management and develops a better understanding of what is needed for her own self-advocacy.

Special Consideration

- None of the hearing aid or implant manufacturers have developed commercially available products that captivate the interest of this digital generation and also impart critically needed information about devices, programming, and training issues. Partnering with mainstream print and video advertisements to include teens with hearing loss by using available products (e.g., batteries, iPods, phones) might initially attract the interest of a teen to further investigate manufacturers' informational materials (brochures and Web sites) that are been developed specifically to address the concerns of this age group.

In recent years, there has been a growing group of children from all developmental groups who reenter the evaluation and hearing habilitation process to receive a second cochlear implant. (Special note should be made that ideally a hearing aid trial has already been completed as part of the evaluation process for the second cochlear implant, involving the full-time use of a hearing aid in the unimplanted ear). Particularly for the teen who received an initial implant at a young age, the child likely has few memories of the time commitment or training required to achieve benefit from the first device. Determining whether the teen and family have realistic expectations for the second device (compared with the dramatic gains received from the first) is a critical component of the evaluation procedure for this group. The second CI can be expected to improve hearing in competing noise, extend distance hearing, and assist in localization. Little increased benefit may occur in quiet for some children. Therapeutically, the challenge lies in devising a motivating and effective protocol for integrating the likely different signals that the implant user initially receives from each implant.

♦ Selection of Test Protocols

The need to ensure accurate reception/perception of verbal test stimuli distinguishes the test administration for a child with hearing loss from that of her normal-hearing peers. Accordingly, all technology must be carefully checked to determine that it is functioning as intended before any speech-language-listening assessments are conducted. Furthermore, as previously cited in this chapter, assessing functional listening at the suprasegmental, phoneme, word, and sentence level is also a necessary component of a comprehensive speech-language assessment for this population. Depending on the child's age, selected diagnostic protocols may involve informal and formal measures. These measures, in turn, might involve criterion-referenced or norm-referenced tools. The advantage of norm-referenced diagnostic measures is that they permit comparison of the child's performance data to those of typically developing peers.

The components of a comprehensive communication evaluation should consist of three distinct skill domains: (1) auditory perception measures in contrasting listening environments; (2) receptive and expressive language functioning: and (3) speech production measures in contrasting listening environments. **Table 25–1** provides an organizational framework for conducting such an assessment. Given the wealth of available diagnostic tools, it is clearly evident that no single test can appropriately meet the requirements of all of the necessary skill domains. A suggested protocol of tests has been included in **Appendix 25–1A** of this chapter to offer a model for designing an appropriate diagnostic protocol.

Table 25–1 Functional Listening Assessment

Functional Listening Assessment						
Background Information						
Name:			Device: (RE) (LE)			
Date:			Settings: (RE) (LE)			
	Listen Alone (Quiet)			**Listen Alone (Noise)**		
Linguistic Level	RE	LE	Bin.	RE	LE	Bin.
Suprasegmental						
Phoneme						
Word						
Sentence						
Connected Speech						
	Look and Listen			**Look and Listen**		
	(Quiet)			**(Noise)**		
Linguistic Level	RE	LE	Bin.	RE	LE	Bin.
Suprasegmental						
Phoneme						
Word						
Sentence						
Connected Speech						
Speech Production						
Verbal Comprehension	**Expressive Language**					
Standard Score Percentile Rank Age Equivalent	Standard Score %ile Rank Age Equivalent					
Pragmatic functioning						

Abbreviations: LE, left ear; RE, right ear.

Pearl

- More information may be obtained by using an assortment of subtests from various tests to obtain a more representative sample of the child's level of functioning and management needs rather than using one prescribed test completely. Using tests normed on children with hearing loss often yields ceiling effect scores and an inflated view of child's present level of functioning.

◆ Service Delivery

The SLP provides direct instructional services to a child with hearing loss, either individually or within a group setting. The mandate for an early interventionist to provide services within the child's natural environment (United States Department of Education, 1991) has substantially altered the delivery of services to children under the age of 3 years. The focus of such services has been modified to address the social-communicative interactions of the child within family dynamics and daily home routines. Previously, it was not uncommon for an infant or toddler to be taken to a hospital or clinic setting where frequently the parents were either not present in the session or they passively observed the therapy session. The expectation of naturalistic early intervention programming is that the parent or caregivers are actively involved in the training sessions, taking conversational turns and using the clinician's modeled techniques for stimulating functional listening and speech-language skills (Cole and Flexer, 2007).

This commitment to active parental involvement is not unique to early intervention. Quite the contrary, one of the primary tenets of the auditory-verbal and auditory-oral approaches from their inception has been the importance of active parental involvement (see Chapter 21). Skilled clinicians within clinical settings have been able to effectively implement naturalistic training tasks to facilitate the child's acquisition of a target skill (in a less distracting environment), with active parent involvement. The expectation is that because the parents have been actively involved, they will be able to reinforce the skills within naturally occurring situations at home.

Similarly, the education initiatives of the 1980s and early 1990s, which require that the general education classroom must change to accommodate the individual learning needs of all students, has most influenced the delivery of support services to the student with hearing loss, from the preschool years throughout the college experience (National Council on Disability, 1989). Ideally, instructional flexibility should be written into the child's individualized educational plan (IEP), allowing for push-in and pull-out services as needed. In a push-in delivery model, the student's auditory and speech and language training objectives are provided within the classroom setting; a pull-out model affords training outside the classroom

During pull-out therapy sessions, the SLP can work in a less distracting environment on areas of weakness that are difficult to address in a classroom setting (e.g., resolving

specific phonemic confusions or addressing the child's pre-teaching needs). On the other hand, by going into the classroom environment, the SLP has the valuable opportunity: to observe the imposed communicative demands, teacher talk used by the classroom teacher to navigate the behavior of her students, and to engineer social-communicative interactions between peers and adults while concomitantly addressing the child's individual training objectives.

Pitfall

- In both service delivery models, care needs to be taken to avoid having the student become overly dependent upon the service provider, and therein fostering less independent functioning in the classroom than the student is capable of demonstrating.

◆ Components of Hearing Habilitation/Rehabilitation Training

In the absence of appropriately programmed hearing aids or speech processors (the external device of a cochlear implant), limited benefit can be gained from ongoing aural habilitation/rehabilitation. Therefore, periodic audiologic assessments are warranted to monitor the auditory status and to make changes in the device programming for a child with hearing loss. During the early stages of language learning, audiologic testing or device reprogramming is recommended every 3 months. (Auditory Verbal International Principles and Rules of Ethics Cite AVT International, 1993). However, to benefit optimally from this ongoing audiologic management, there should be an interactive exchange between the audiologist and the aural habilitation and rehabilitation provider.

Because the SLP or auditory therapist has many opportunities to closely monitor and document the nature of the child's phonemic confusions, the SLP could and should share this information with the audiologist, who can then optimize modifications to the hearing aid or speech processor. Current digital hearing aids and cochlear implant speech processors have numerous features to enhance specific listening environments. They can be programmed with distinctly differing programs to capitalize on specific acoustic or perceptual features to coincide with or facilitate particular training targets.

Perhaps the most valuable input needed by the audiologist for device programming is a descriptive analysis of any observed positive or negative changes in the child's auditory responsiveness reported by the SLP, including

- tolerance to specific sounds or device settings
- attention-getting responses
- distance listening
- phonemic confusions

Therapy Environment

The optimal listening and learning environment for any child acquiring language is a quiet, child-friendly setting that affords a variety of sensory experiences and permits independent exploration. The structured auditory training session can occur within a range of environments from natural home environments to quiet or noisy classroom settings or acoustically controlled clinic settings, depending on the purpose of the therapy session. It seems counterintuitive to attempt to facilitate critical listening in a distracting environment with competing background noise; however such may be the purpose of an advanced listening session.

Equally as critical is that auditory therapy should be a parent-child directive (e.g., actively involving the parent or caregiver in the ongoing training tasks). Regardless of the frequency of training sessions, it is indisputable that the parents will be the most consistent source of auditory and speech-language stimulation to the child. It is, therefore, essential to guide the parents in acquiring skills and strategies for eliciting their child's most optimal listening, comprehension and production responses within naturally occurring daily routines (Cole and Flexer, 2007).

Now that the fitting of bilateral devices (two hearing aids or cochlear implants, or one cochlear implant with an appropriate hearing aid on the unimplanted ear) is considered best clinical practice, the structural organization of individual training sessions has been forever altered. Particularly during the adjustment period of having amplification on both ears, some portion of each therapy session should be directed toward listening with each device separately and under bilateral conditions. Realizing that one of the expected benefits of bilateral device use is improved listening in noise, training tasks should be used where the hearing aid or implant user is expected to follow spoken language in the presence of competing background noise. Potential noise sources could be commercially available four talker [SW2] Babble audiotapes (Carver, 2000) or even talk radio. Over time, the signal-to-noise ratio between the speech and noise should be decreased to afford practice in listening environments that better simulate those encountered in everyday social interactions.

Pitfall

- The national mandate to conduct early intervention sessions within the home environment is sometimes erroneously viewed by clinicians and parents alike as an opportunity for parents to merely observe or opt-out of participating in the sessions (e.g., using therapy as a break or opportunity to complete household chores while the child is otherwise engaged).

Direct Intervention Services

The primary objectives of providing hearing habilitation and rehabilitation to pediatric hearing aid or implant users is to develop and expand functional listening skills for the purposes of continued language learning and enhanced communicative interactions. Young children fitted with either conventional amplification or cochlear implants require direct instruction to master the vocabulary and linguistic structure of the language being directed to and around them. Their active involvement in meaningful social-communicative interactions with their typically developing and normal hearing peers significantly enriches their language learning efforts.

However, the increased auditory access afforded by a cochlear implant has been observed to facilitate more incidental learning (e.g., learning from mere exposure) relative to their profoundly hearing-impaired peers fitted with conventional hearing aids. During the critical language learning period (between birth and 3 years of age), the process of attaching meaning to auditory cues occurs with an ease and naturalness that is not observed when listening and speech are initiated at later ages.

Ongoing parent-child–centered training should be provided to an infant or young child with hearing aids or a cochlear implant at least twice a week for 60-minute sessions. Regardless of how often direct therapy services can be delivered, auditory-verbal or auditory-oral intervention is recommended if the family's desired outcome for their child is spoken language. (See Chapter 21 for more information about different communication approaches.) In accordance with the child's age and exhibited skills upon entering the hearing habilitation process, she can be expected to achieve greater auditory performance from those baseline levels, if provided with appropriate technology and sufficient auditory-based speech and language training.

Systems like Signed English or Cued Speech (Yoshinaga-Itano, 2000) coupled with auditory training may be the appropriate intervention for some older children who were taught visually in earlier intervention and educational programs, or who do not have sufficient auditory access. Yoshinaga-Itano (2000) reported that it is indeed possible to map acoustic cues and speech production cues onto an existing or intact sign language system. Both Signed English (i.e., a manual communication system) and Cued Speech (i.e., a phonemic-based system that uses hand shapes and body positioning to correspond to speech) would afford an older child who is attempting to advance her auditory skills with the best match between the what he hears and sees. In contrast, American Sign Language (ASL) is a separate language with its own syntax and grammar; it is not designed to be used with spoken language. If paired with spoken language, a mismatch is created that may complicate the language-learning process.

Pitfall

- Some teachers and clinicians report that they use ASL with English word order. However, because these systems are incompatible, the child will have incomplete access to both spoken English and ASL as functional language systems

Training Strategies

Several published auditory curriculums offer parents and professionals hierarchical guidelines for auditory skill emergence and a variety of useful training activities (Moog, Biedenstein, and Davidson, 1995; Koch, 1999). Such programs are sometimes inappropriately viewed as cookbooks to address the individual training needs of a child fitted with hearing aids or cochlear implants. However, a thorough understanding of the underlying principles and training strategies of both the auditory-verbal and auditory-oral intervention models best compliments the current trend of providing evidenced-based intervention to this diverse population. These approaches emphasize the development and reliance upon auditory cues to receive, comprehend, and use spoken language in the context of meaningful, real-life experiences.

◆ Conclusions

Documenting auditory skill emergence and speech-language progress over time is the final component of the comprehensive, communication management of children who are deaf or hard of hearing. The professional literature is expanding with the results from a diverse body of research efforts, directed toward identifying critical prognostic indicators of success or benefit from current technology and training options. As a result, SLPs now have quantifiable evidence with which to determine the effectiveness of the hearing habilitation and rehabilitation programming they afford. However, documentation from ongoing diagnostic training, in combination with regularly scheduled comprehensive assessments, should direct future intervention for an individual child. Information from research and clinical domains, in turn, motivates the manufacturers to improve the programming schemas of digital aids and cochlear implant speech processors to meet the needs of an increasingly younger and more diverse population of oral communicators with significant hearing loss.

Discussion Questions

1. What variables most influence the acquisition of optimal functional listening skill emergence and age-appropriate speech and language skills?

2. What role do realistic expectations and consistent communicative demands play in the emergence of listening and spoken language skills?

3. How does an SLP identify the present level of functioning and training needs for a child that cannot respond on formal test measures?

4. Why should the teenager be actively involved in the decision-making process regarding her communication management?

References

Anderson, K., and Smaldino, J. (1998). Listening Inventory for Education (L.I.F.E.). Denver: Educational Audiology Association.

Auditory-Verbal International. (1993). Suggested protocol for audiological and hearing evaluation. Easton, PA: AVI Principles and Rules of Ethics.

Boothroyd, A., and Minnear, D. (2001). Evaluation of the computer-assisted speech perception test (CASPA). Journal of the American Academy of Audiology, 27, 134–144.

Carver, W. (2000). Four talker babble audiotape. St. Louis: Auditec of St. Louis.

Carrow-Woolfolk, E. (1995). Oral and written language scales. Circle Pines, MN: American Guidance Service, Inc.

Cole, E., and Flexer, C. (2007). Children with hearing loss: developing listening and talking birth to six. San Diego: Plural Publishing Company.

Dawson, J., Stout, C., and Eyer, J., (2003). Structured photographic expressive language test -3. DeKalb, IL: Janelle Publications.

Dunn, L., and Dunn, L. (1997). Peabody picture vocabulary test (3rd ed.). Circle Pines, MS: American Guidance Service, Inc.

Fenson, L., Marchman, V., Thal, D., Dale, P., Reznick, S., and Bates, E. (2006). MacArthur-Bates communicative development inventories (CDIs) (2nd ed.). Baltimore: Paul H. Brookes Publishing Co.

Geers, A. E., Nicholas, J. G., and Sedey, A. L. (2003). Language skills of children with early cochlear implantation. Ear and Hearing, 24, 46S–58S.

Goldman, R., and Fristoe M. (2000). Goldman Fristoe 2 test of articulation. Circle Pines, MN: American Guidance Service, Inc.

Kirk, K., Pisoni, D., and Osberger, M. (1995). Lexical neighborhood test (LNT). St. Louis: Auditec of St. Louis.

Koch, M. (1999). Bringing sounds to life, Parkton, MD: York Press.

Little ears auditory questionnaire. (2006). Innsbruck, Austria: Med-El Corporation.

Moeller, M.P. (2000). Early intervention and language development in children who are deaf and hard of hearing. Pediatrics, 106, E43.

Moog, J., and Geers, A.E. (1990). Early speech perception test. St. Louis: Central Institute for the Deaf and Hard of Hearing.

Moog, J., Biedenstein, J., and Davidson, L. (1995). Speech perception instructional curriculum and evaluation (SPICE), St. Louis, MO: Central Institute for the Deaf.

National Council on Disability. (1989). The education of students with disabilities: where do we stand? A report to the President and the Congress of the United States, National Council on Disability, American Psychological Association. Washington, DC.

Nilsson, M., Solli, S., and Sullivan, J. Hearing in noise test (HINT) sentences, St. Louis: Audiotec of St. Louis.

Pisoni, D.B., and Geers, A.E. (2000). Working memory of deaf children with cochlear implants: correlations between digit span and measures of spoken language processing. Annals of Otolaryngology, Rhinology, Laryngology, 109, 63–64.

Quittner, A.L., Leibach, P., and Marciel, K. (2004). The impact of cochlear implants on young children: new methods to assess cognitive and behavioral development. Archives of Otolaryngology—Head and Neck Surgery, 130, 547–554.

Reynell, J., and Gruber, C. (1997). London, The Reynell developmental language scales III (3rd ed.). nfer Nelson.

Robbins,A., Renshaw, J., and Osberger, L. (1995). The common phrases test. Indianapolis: Indiana University School of Medicine.

Semel, E., Wing, E., and Secord, W. (2003). Clinical evaluation of language fundamentals (4th ed.). San Antonio: Harcourt Assessment Inc.

Stallings, L.M., Kirk, K.I., Chin, S., and Gao, S. (2004). Parent word familiarity and the language development of pediatric cochlear implant users. Volta Review, 102, 237–257.

Tramell, J., Farrar, C.M., Francis, J., et al. (1981). Test of auditory comprehension. Portland, OR: Foreworks Publications.

U.S. Department of Education. (1975). Public Law 94-142, The education act.

U.S. Department of Education. (1991). Public Law 102-119, The disability education act, P (IDEA, Part H).

Wetherby, A., and Prizant, B. (1993). The communication and symbolic behavior scale. Baltimore: Paul H. Brookes Publishing Co.

Ying, E. (1990). Speech and language assessment: communication evaluation, in hearing impaired children in the mainstream. Parkton: MD, York Press.

Yoshinaga-Itano, C. (2000). Early intervention and language development in children who are deaf and hard of hearing. Pediatrics, 106, 594–602.

Yoshinaga-Itano, C., Sedey, A., Colter, D., and Mehl, A. (1998). Language of early and late identified hearing loss. Pediatrics, 102, 116–171.

Zimmerman-Phillips, S., Osberger, M. J., and Robbins, A. M. (1997). Infant-toddler meaningful auditory integration scale. Sylmar, CA: Advanced Bionics Corporation.

Zimmerman, I., Steiner, V., and Pond, R. (2002). Preschool language scale-4 (4th ed.). San Antonio: Psychological Corporation.

Appendix 25–A

The following diagnostic protocol affords a listing of commercially available tests and how they could be used to meet the requirements of a comprehensive functional listening assessment and speech-language evaluation. This listing is by no means exhaustive or suggestive that other test measures might not also be useful. Please see **Appendix 25–1B** for more descriptive information about the tests and where they can be obtained.

Auditory Perception

Tests	Infants	Preschool	School-Aged	Teenage	Bilateral
IT-MAIS	X	X			
Little Ears	X	X			
ESP	X	X	X	X	X
TAC		X	X	X	x
Potato Head		X	X		
Common Phrases		X	X	X	X
AB List (C.A.S.P.A.)		X	X	X	X
PBK			X	X	X
LNT			X	X	X
HINT			X	X	X

Language Functioning

Tests	Infants	Preschool	School-Aged	Teenage	Bilateral
CSBS	X	X			
MacArthur-Bates	X	X			
Reynell	X	X	X		
PLS-4		X	X		
PPVT-III		X	X	X	X
CELF-4			X	X	X
SPELT-3		X	X	X	X
OWLS			X	X	X

Speech Production

Tests	Infants	Preschool	School-Aged	Teenage	Bilateral
GFTA-2		X	X	X	X
Intelligibility Measure			X	X	X

Appendix 25–B

Test	Stimuli	Skill Domain	Availability
Infant Toddler-Meaningful Integration Scale (IT-MAIS)	Detection, discrimination, recognition environmental sound, speech (phonemes and word level)	Speech Perception	Advanced Bionics
Little Ears Auditory Questionaire (2006)	Detection, discrimination, recognition environmental sound, speech (phonemes, word, and sentence level)	Speech Perception	Med-EL Worldwide Headquarters Imsbruck, Austria
Early Speech Perception Test (ESP)	Suprasegmentals, Phonemes, Words	Speech Perception	CID St. Louis, MO
Potato Head Test	Words. Sentences	Speech Perception	IU School of Medicine DeVault Reseach Laboratory Web site
Common Phrases	Sentences	Speech Perception	IU School of Medicine DeVault Reseach Laboratory Web site
AB List (Computer Assessed Speech Perception Assessment)	Phonemes, Words	Speech Perception	J. American Academy of Audiology
Phonetically Balanced Kindergarten List	Phonemes, Words	Speech Perception	ASHA Washington, DC
Lexical Neighborhood Test	Phonemes, Words	Speech Perception	Audiotec of St. Louis St. Louis, MO
Hearing in Noise Test	Sentences	Speech Perception	Audiotec of St. Louis St. Louis, MO
Communication Skills Behavior Scales (CSBS)	Suprasegmentals, Phonemes, Words, Sentences	Receptive/Expressive	Paul H. Brookes Baltimore, MD
MacArthur-Bates Communication Development Inventories	Words, Phrases	Receptive/Expressive	Paul H. Brookes Baltimore, MD
Reynell Developmental Language Scales (Reynell 1997)	Words, Sentences	Receptive/Expressive	Super Duper Publications Greenville, SC
Preschool Language Scale - 4	Words, Sentences	Receptive/Expressive	The Psychological Corp. San Antonio, TX
Peabody Picture Vocabulary Test - 3	Words	Receptive Language	American Guidance Service Circle Pines, M]N
Clinical Evaluation of Language Fundamentals (CELF-4)	Words, Sentences, Paragraphs	Receptive/Expressive	Psych Corp San Antonio, TX
Oral & Written Language Scales	Words, Sentences, Paragraphs	Receptive/Expressive	American Guidance Service Circle Pines, M]
Goldman-Fristoe Test of Articulation-2	Phonemes, Words, Sentences	Articulation	AGS Circle Pines, MN

Chapter 26

Educational Placement Options for School-Aged Children with Hearing Loss

Susan Cheffo

♦ **Preschool Options**

Mainstream Preschool

Schools and Programs for the Deaf

♦ **Options for School-Aged Children (5 to 21 Years of Age)**

Mainstream Schools

General Education Class

Inclusion Class

Self-Contained Class

Collaborative Class

Schools and Programs for Children Who Are Deaf

♦ **Related Services**

Teacher of the Deaf

Speech-Language Pathology Services

Teacher Assistant/Aide/Shadow/Intervention Assistant

Interpreter

Educational Consultant

Classroom Modifications

♦ **Summary**

Key Points

- There are various educational placement options in the mainstream or in schools for the deaf.

- Related services are provided both in and out of class for students who need them.

- Schools are required to provide assistive technology as needed by students.

- Modifications and testing accommodations must be offered as needed.

- All educational services must be listed on a child's Individualized Education Plan (IEP) or 504 plan.

Numerous educational placement options are available for the school-aged child with hearing loss. With legislative changes and expansion of educational programs, the choices of educational placements for children 3 to 21 years of age have increased. Advances in technology, providing children with hearing loss greater access to sound, have led deaf education from segregated schools for the deaf to traditional school settings. Within these settings, quality support services and classroom modifications are required to help the child with hearing loss succeed. Knowledge of the laws augmented by a creative school staff experienced in working with children with hearing loss will enhance the educational opportunities for children in the mainstream. For families who opt to keep their children in schools for the deaf, there has been movement from sign language to auditory-oral communication. Whether a mainstream or self-contained placement is chosen, individualization within that setting must occur so that the child's hearing, educational, and social needs are met. This chapter will address the various school placement options for children 3 to 21 years of age. Along with placement options, appropriate services, modifications, and testing accommodations will be discussed. The IEP/504 plan (see Chapter 23) drives the educational services for the child. All services listed on the IEP/504 must be carried out by the school. Therefore, including all services, modifications, and accommodations on the IEP will ensure their implementation. A positive reciprocal relationship between school districts, professionals, and family will help create appropriate school services.

♦ Preschool Options

Preschool is usually the time young children with hearing loss first separate from their parents and attend a full- or part-time program. Youngsters develop their preacademic skills, build their listening and verbal skills, and start socializing in preschool; the foundations for education begin at this time.

When children who are deaf or hard of hearing transition from early intervention (EI) (see Chapter 24), to preschool, they need to be evaluated to select appropriate school placement. These evaluations, scheduled with parental consent, include audiology, speech-language, psychological, motor skills, educational readiness, determination of necessary classroom adaptation, and social history. The Individual Family Service Plan (IFSP) is developed by the team after the evaluations are complete and describes the child's abilities and areas of concern. Preschool educational placement will be decided at the IEP meeting. Parents, ultimately, make final decisions about placement. Finding a good match for preschool should not be difficult when information is available about the child's abilities and when the parents have information about various options. In spite of having good information, parents may feel insecure about their decisions. It is important to remember that if the placement is not successful, the committee can reconvene to determine whether a different type of placement or service is necessary. There needs to be flexibility in creating the appropriate environment for a young child beginning school.

Pearl

- If a preschool placement is not meeting a child's needs, the IEP team can reconvene, and a change in placement can be arranged.

Mainstream Preschool

The mainstream or traditional preschool is one option for youngsters who are deaf or hard of hearing, who have attained age-appropriate or near age-appropriate speech and language skills. Many parents and clinicians feel that the mainstream preschool experience provides better language role models offered by children with typical hearing. In addition, placement in the mainstream enhances their child's preparation for the larger world (Zwolan and Sorkin, 2006).

There are private and public preschool options. If a parent chooses a private preschool, payment is out-of-pocket. For a public, universal preschool program, funding is provided by the federal government. For parents seeking a private preschool, finding one close to home is preferable. There are a variety of philosophies for preschool education, all of which need to be carefully evaluated by educators and parents.

Whether public or private, preschools that have served children with hearing loss in the past may be most beneficial. Enthusiasm about having a child with hearing loss and a willingness to collaborate with a team of professionals and parents are positive characteristics. Parents may want to bring an educator from EI, their speech-language pathologist, or a clinician from the audiology center to accompany them when visiting different schools. Professional advice may help them make an informed decision as to which program is the best match for their child.

Schools and Programs for the Deaf

Private oral schools called OPTION schools are located in various cities in the United States for children with hearing loss. These schools provide education to children who are deaf or hard of hearing by training use of residual hearing. Sometimes children are enrolled in these programs for early, intensive development of spoken language in their preschool years. There may be an extension of these programs through elementary grades to establish reading skills (Chute and Nevins, 2002). A certified teacher of the deaf (TOD) is usually the class instructor, although an early childhood educator or speech-language pathologist may be in charge. Knowledge of early childhood education and how typically hearing children develop language is important.

During the last few years, schools or programs for the deaf that have traditionally used sign language are developing effective auditory-oral programs for their preschool students. Many State Schools for the Deaf (4201 schools) have begun auditory-oral infant/preschool programs. State mandated newborn hearing screenings has led to early identification of hearing loss, earlier hearing aid use, as well as earlier cochlear implantation. All of these advances have increased children's ability to perceive soft speech at a very early age, and develop speech and language similar to their peers with typical hearing (Geers, 2003). These programs have become another appropriate auditory-oral option for early identified children.

Some of these schools/programs for children with hearing loss provide an integrative model, where typical peers attend classes at the site (reverse mainstreaming), or children with hearing loss attend traditional preschool classes part-time. There is usually a liaison from the school for the deaf to work with the mainstream preschool staff, explaining technology, ramifications of hearing loss, teaching strategies, and providing resources. Having hearing children in class can improve language, communicative interaction, and social skills. The pace of instruction and teacher expectation in integrated classes has been observed to increase compared to programs in which all children are hearing impaired. For parents who decide to place their children in a self-contained program for children with hearing loss where there is no mainstreaming, it is recommended that their child attend after-school activities with typical peers. This will give children the opportunity to interact socially and enhance auditory and verbal skills. Some activities, such as dance, sports, arts and crafts, gymnastics, or library may be helpful. Not all activities are costly. Family gatherings and play dates should also be encouraged.

Although parents may be faced with various placement alternatives and some difficult decisions, it is important for them to remember they are not alone. Professionals can guide families in making choices and supporting parent decisions. A decision may not be 100% satisfactory, and placements may need changing. The school district supports families and will revisit the IEP to make program modifications as needed. Disagreements between parents and the school district may require resolution through alternative means, such as mediation or due process hearings; however, such proceedings are generally not necessary.

✦ Options for School-Aged Children (5 to 21 Years of Age)

Mainstream Schools

Many children who are deaf or hard of hearing are returning to local school districts to continue their education beyond preschool. The law states that children with disabilities are entitled to a free and appropriate education (FAPE) in the least restrictive environment (LRE) (ASHA, 2006) (see Chapter 23). Attending school in the child's local school district is a goal of many parents, and can be a positive and fulfilling experience. Children who are deaf or hard of hearing can attend school with neighborhood friends, while participating in school activities along side their typical peers. Elementary school is a time when children are generally more sensitive to special needs and accepting of differences. It is also a time when lifelong friendships can be developed. During middle and high school, academics are critical and social interactions can positively or negatively affect the school experience. The following options within school districts are similar for students 5 to 21 years old, although readily available options may vary from district to district.

General Education Class

A general education class usually consists of 20 to 25 children, sometimes more. One teacher is in charge of all the children and teaches all subjects. By fourth or fifth grade, departmentalization may be in effect. This is the first time more than one teacher is introduced, and students move from room to room throughout the day. The children in the class are independent learners and require little support. Children with hearing loss who attend general education classes usually have age-appropriate language and cognition. They are motivated, articulate youngsters with excellent communication skills.

Inclusion Class

There are approximately 20 to 25 children in class, but a percentage of the youngsters have an IEP that mandates special education support and accommodations. There is a full-time classroom teacher, and, in addition, a special education teacher who may be in the room part or all day. There is usually also a teacher assistant all day. Having the classroom teacher and assistant present in the classroom permits special education children to have individual support throughout the day. It is important to observe the inclusion class to ensure that the needs of the other classified children do not conflict with the needs of the child who is deaf or hard of hearing. Inclusion classes may be called by other names (blended or collaborative class), but the design of the class is similar.

Self-Contained Class

Children who are unable to participate in a general education or inclusion class may benefit from a self-contained, special education class within the local public school. The class size is small. The teacher is certified in special education and there is usually a full-time teacher assistant. The children reap the benefit of individualization and small group learning. This class is designed to help youngsters develop the necessary skills to eventually attend an inclusion or general education class. As skills improve, the child may be able to move into a regular education class for part of the day. Behavior may be an issue in this type of class, so observation is important to determine if the class is appropriate for the child in question.

Collaborative Class

Some schools have the ability to create a collaborative experience similar to inclusion, except all the IEP children have hearing loss. Instead of a special education teacher sharing the class, the special education teacher is a TOD. Having a general education teacher and TOD coteach can be an ideal teaching situation. The children gain the benefit of appropriate curriculum and expectation, with the specific guidance and support of a TOD. A collaborative class is not common in many areas, but this model has been successful.

Pearl

- Parents seeking a mainstream option for school-aged students have usually enrolled early-amplified infants and toddlers in auditory-oral or mainstream preschools. Family members are active participants during this process.

Schools and Programs for Children Who Are Deaf

Children who attend schools for the deaf from 5 to 21 years of age usually have more severe disabilities, or their parents have chosen these schools for cultural or communication reasons. Many of the children who attend these schools or programs require additional educational support and a more restrictive environment. These schools and programs are usually day classes, but residential placements are still available in some areas. There typically is a nurturing, protective environment and an affiliation with other students and adults who are deaf or hard of hearing. There is no cost to parents for state-sponsored schools or programs for the deaf.

Within these schools are various communication options that include

- auditory-oral, where children use amplification to listen, including frequency modulation (FM) systems, and speech reading is used to support communication

- total communication that incorporates any means to communicate with children who are deaf, including a sign language system that is based on English, finger spelling, gestures, and any other means of helping a child understand English

- American Sign Language, a manual language not based on English syntax, that is used within the deaf community, and English is taught as a second language (BEGINNINGS, 2005)

◆ Related Services

All students who are deaf or hard of hearing require some level of support service throughout their schooling. Whether a child attends a mainstream program or a school for the deaf, related services are part of his educational plan.

The types of related services offered on elementary, middle, and high school levels are similar to those provided in preschool. However, the delivery of service to an older child is different because there is greater emphasis on academics once a child turns 5. There is also a need for highly qualified providers to deliver these services; educators who are experienced, receive ongoing training, and achieve good results with their students. Although dedication and a nurturing sensibility are evident characteristics in those working with children who are deaf or hard of hearing, knowledge about how to implement these special services is key. There is a need for ongoing staff development training to keep up with changes in the field, as well as advances in technology. Related service providers must expand their knowledge base to understand new curriculums, state tests, revisions to the law and school curriculum, and today's deaf or hard of hearing child who may have more subtle hearing needs.

Related services are determined at the child's IEP/504 meeting. The committee decides on the appropriate services, the amount of time the service will be provided, as well as the location of service provision. There is no cost to parents for related services as long as the services appear on the child's IEP or 504 plan. School districts pay for this service, which is reimbursed in part by the state. There are various related services detailed below, the most important ones beingTOD, speech-language pathology, and FM assistive technology.

Pearl

- The most frequently used services in the mainstream for children with cochlear implants include speech-language pathology (75%), FM systems (65%), and deaf education services (54%) (Zwolan and Sorkin, 2006).

Teacher of the Deaf

The TOD is state certified and has specific training in working with children who are deaf or hard of hearing. In the mainstream setting, the TOD works individually with a student for a determined amount of time. This individual is the VIP to the child who is deaf or hard of hearing throughout his schooling. The major areas of need to consider when including students with special needs in regular classroom settings are modifying the physical environment, providing appropriate levels of support, and monitoring the child's progress (Dinnebeil and McInerney, 2000).

First, the TOD observes the acoustic environment and suggests modifications where necessary. He ensures that appropriate and consistent use of amplification is provided, performs listening checks to be certain equipment is working properly, and performs troubleshooting as needed. Second, the TOD analyzes the child's language, teaches vocabulary, and encourages verbal interactive communication skills. Behavior and social skills may also need to be addressed. Previewing and reviewing academic material, the crux of TOD sessions, can begin during preschool and continue through high school. Third, by assessing the child's progress through evaluations and reporting on IEP goals, the TOD knows where deficits or successes are, and if services need increasing or decreasing. In order to make sure all providers and parents collaborate, the TOD also oversees a communication notebook, a system of sharing information with all professionals and the child's family. TOD services are provided as a push-in or pull-out model. Push-in is important in preschool and lower elementary school, since being in the classroom is a good way of monitoring communication interaction, facilitating language when needed, and gleaning a general overview of the child's ability to advocate for his needs. In addition, being in the classroom gives the TOD hands-on information to share with other service providers and with parents.

As academics and language become more challenging, the pull-out model is preferable so that the TOD can preview and review academic material. TOD services are usually provided three to five times a week.

Speech-Language Pathology Services

The speech-language pathologist is a state-licensed individual who received generalized speech and language training in graduate school. Because delivering speech services to children who are deaf or hard of hearing requires specialized skills, the school pathologist or therapist usually needs support. There are speech-language pathologists and certified auditory-verbal therapists who specialize in teaching students who are deaf or hard of hearing. This learning helps children develop auditory skills to enable them to use hearing to learn language and who can provide training to the school's speech-language pathologist. An auditory-verbal therapist is knowledgeable in the application and management of technology, strategies, techniques, and procedures to enable youngsters who are deaf or hard of hearing to learn to listen and understand spoken language, and to use hearing to develop spoken language (Estabrooks, 2001).

Providing speech, language, and listening therapy in school will positively impact academic outcomes.

School speech services are usually offered three to five times a week. Most speech services are provided in a pull-out format, usually one on one, in a separate, quiet location. Some students receive group speech, where pragmatic skills are addressed during small group instruction. Understanding the importance of auditory therapy and helping the child maintain this skill is one of the keys to success in school.

Pitfall

- The TOD is responsible for the preview and review work. Therefore, the school speech therapists should not focus on preview and review during speech sessions. Even though school curriculum is the basis for language and vocabulary, listening therapy is still required, and the speech-language pathologist is typically the professional who offers auditory development.

The following additional related services are less common for the child who is deaf or hard of hearing.

Resource Room

Resource room services are provided by a certified, special education teacher, not a TOD. The resource room addresses fundamental academic skills in a small group setting. Some children receive this service when added support is needed in academic subjects because of additional disabilities that affect learning, or if there are too few TODs in a specific geographic region. Students are pulled out for this service, which will add time out of the classroom. Balancing pull-out time is important so that major classroom academics are not missed.

Teacher Assistant/Aide/Shadow/Intervention Assistant

This is an individual, who may or may not be a certified teacher, but is an adult who assists the child and the teacher in the classroom. He helps refocus the student who experiences behavioral issues and addresses academic concerns. Care and training are needed to insure that the assistant/aide/shadow does not interfere with teacher–student interaction. A child returning to the mainstream, who is dependent on the assistant/aide, will not have the appropriate student-teacher relationship. The classroom teacher, not the classroom assistant, needs to be the main focus for the child with hearing loss.

Interpreter

The student who participates in the general education setting usually has good communication skills and academic ability; however, group discussion or questions asked by students may require interpreting intervention. The interpreter may be used all day or for clarification purposes.

Sign Language

The sign language interpreter is knowledgeable in sign and preferably has RID (Registry of Interpreters for the Deaf) certification. Some children require the use of an interpreter consistently, since understanding the teacher is difficult for them. Other children who are developing auditory skills can use the sign language interpreter for clarification, as support. The sign language interpreter may also be used to reverse interpret for the teacher and other pupils in the class if the child who is deaf or hard of hearing has unintelligible speech.

Oral

The oral interpreter can be used with a child who has good lip reading skills. The interpreter sits close to the child and repeats the information spoken in the classroom so that the child can lip read. This type of interpreter may be helpful during group interactions, by repeating comments or questions of peers.

Cued Speech

Cued speech is a visual communication system of eight hand shapes or cues as an assist to lipreading. Although less common, a child trained to use Cued Speech would need a Cued Speech Interpreter in school full time (BEGINNINGS, 2005).

Controversial Point

- An educational interpreter needs to be sensitive to the needs of a child who is transitioning from a visual system to an auditory one. If the child uses an FM system and derives auditory benefit, the interpreter should be used for clarification purposes and to interpret questions or comments of classmates. Pointing to the individual who is speaking may be sufficient.

Counseling

Some children benefit from counseling services provided by a school psychologist or social worker. Transitioning to a mainstream environment may require support from a trained individual who is familiar with the social and emotional aspects of hearing loss. Being the only child in school with hearing loss may cause a sense of isolation. For secondary students, social issues are a major source of concern. Feeling different because of their hearing loss is prevalent within the adolescent population. In-school counseling and social skills groups or private therapy are helpful (see Chapter 29). Arranging for regular social activities with other children with hearing loss can also be helpful in dealing with social and emotional issues.

Educational Consultant

When a child transitions into elementary school, an educational consultant from a audiology center can provide training to district-based personnel (see Chapter 30). Consultation will cover assistive technology. In school, all children with hearing loss or auditory processing disorder require the use of an FM system that must be included on the IEP (see Chapter 20 for information about FM systems).

Special Consideration

- The FM system should be evaluated in every class, including specials. What works in one room or with one type of classroom setup, may not work in another.

Closed Captions

Whenever movies are shown in school, they need to be captioned. Children who are deaf or hard of hearing cannot understand all that is said in movies, and therefore should not be held responsible for the information unless the movie is captioned. Closed captions will benefit all children in class.

Classroom Modifications

All students who are deaf or hard of hearing need some modifications to participate in the general education curriculum. Some of these modifications are intended for school use, others are provided at home to enhance school performance. For a student who is deaf or hard of hearing, having modifications will create a means for equal access. The following are some examples of typical modifications listed on the IEP.

Preferential Seating

For many years, front and center seating was preferable. Listening up-close to the teacher and reading lips were necessary. Today, in most preschools and elementary schools, children are seated in clusters where collaboration and interaction are part of the learning experience. Preferential seating now becomes a place where the child who is deaf or hard of hearing has access to his peers, both auditorally and visually. The FM system will ensure hearing the teacher from any point in the classroom, so sitting directly in front of the teacher is no longer necessary. Movement from one area of the room to another as activities change is also part of preferential seating. The TOD or educational audiologist should analyze the classroom environment to help decide seat placement.

Acoustic Modifications

Due to poor acoustics, modifications are needed in all classrooms.

Wall-to-wall carpeting—Carpeting is a wonderful means of absorbing sound. However, many schools are concerned about allergens, dirt, and bugs and will not add carpeting as an acoustic modification. For any district that will provide wall-to-wall carpeting, it is a powerful means of reducing impulse sounds.

Area rugs—These can be placed in various parts of the classroom and can be easily cleaned. Impulse sound is reduced in a particular area, like the block corner, but an area rug does not offer the benefit of wall-to-wall carpeting.

Chair-foot covers—Tennis balls or products such as Hushhups, Quiet Feet, or Quiet Foot Chair Covers are placed on the legs of chairs, desks, and tables to reduce noise levels when there is a tile floor. They are not used to absorb sound, but to decrease the loud sounds associated with chair and desk movement.

Acoustic tiles and corkboards—These can be used on ceilings and walls to reduce reverberation (echo). They absorb sound and are relatively inexpensive.

Window covering—Drapes, curtains, blinds, or shades can help reduce reverberation.

Dropped ceilings—Many schools have high vaulted ceilings that are sources of reverberation. Dropping those ceilings and using acoustic ceiling tile produce a better sound environment and is the single most effective means of acoustic management in a classroom.

Static electricity reducers—Cochlear implants are electronic devices that can be affected by static electricity. When electrostatic discharge (ESD) occurs, cochlear implants are susceptible to damage to the speech processor program (Cochlear Americas, 2002). Static electricity reducers, including anti-static mats and screens for computers, wooden chairs substituted for plastic chairs, humidity control to decrease the possibility of static electricity buildup, and anti static-spray for carpets, mats, and other static causing materials, can be added to the child's IEP.

Modified Homework

Some students require too much time to complete homework assignments due to language, learning, or motor deficits. Modifying homework assignments is a means of eliminating repetitive, rote problems, such as computational examples in math. Extended time for long-term assignments may also be helpful.

> An extra set of books at home can be used to preview the next week's assignments in terms of vocabulary and concepts. These help the child with hearing loss and enhance reading skills for all children in class.
>
> Copy of class notes or study guides can be used before or during class, as well as for follow up during TOD sessions or at home. For older elementary students and secondary students, teachers' notes and study guides are extremely beneficial.

Test Accommodations

Students take tests throughout their school years. These exams may take the form of standardized state tests, schoolwide exams, or tests in school subjects. For youngsters who are deaf or hard of hearing, accommodations are necessary to give them an equal opportunity to demonstrate acquired knowledge and skills. The right of students with disabilities to appropriate test access and accommodations is also guaranteed under federal laws and regulations. Test accommodations must be listed on the IEP to be in effect. It is important that these test accommodations are carefully addressed at the IEP meeting for the following year, so that students are guaranteed their accommodation needs as soon as classes begin. Accommodations may include extended test-taking time (up to double time) to allow the student time to process information; administering state assessments over multiple days with state approval; taking tests in separate locations or in a small groups to permit children to get more assistance; special acoustics to be certain the child can hear all directions; directions, test passages, questions, items, and multiple-choices responses can be read aloud to the student who is deaf or hard of hearing when that student has difficulty reading for himself.

Note-Taking Systems

There are various note-taking systems for students with hearing loss. A scribe or adult may be needed for young students who have difficulty writing because of motor issues. A computer-assisted system can help students with hearing loss in the mainstream allowing the student to take detailed information home (Youdelman and Messerly, 1996).

CART (Computer-Assisted Real Time Translation) is the instant translation of the spoken word into English text using a stenotype machine, a notebook computer, and real-time software. A court reporter types what is said and the text appears on a computer monitor, TV, or projection screen (National Court Reporters Association, 2004). CART is

found in upper elementary, middle, and high schools, as well as in colleges and graduate programs.

Remote CART system is similar to CART, except the reporter is off site. The teacher wears a microphone that transmits information directly to the reporter. However, student comments and class discussion will be missed, unless the teacher repeats it all.

C-Print is another computer note-taking system. A trained operator produces text of spoken information in text-condensing strategies. The information may be a summarized translation of the content (NTID, 2003).

CAN (Computer Assisted Note Taking) uses two laptop computers. A professional note taker or good typist inputs all classroom interactions, which are transmitted to the student's laptop.

A student note taker who volunteers or is chosen by the teacher can provide notes for the student who is deaf or hard of hearing. Quality note taking is important.

Pearl

- Children with hearing loss have a much easier time in the classroom with appropriate access. Computer note-taking systems work effectively in schools and have given children a better sense of participation.

Anderson and Matkin (2007) have developed a table **(Table 26–1)** describing the possible impact of different degrees of hearing loss on understanding speech and language, social skills and needs, and required educational accommodations. It is a very useful document for all school personnel to use to assist in understanding the effect of

---

Table 26–1   Relationship of Hearing Loss to Listening and Learning Needs

16–25 dB Hearing Loss		
Possible Impact on the Understanding of Language and Speech	**Possible Social Impact**	**Potential Educational Accommodations and Services**
Impact of a hearing loss that is approximately 20 dB can be compared to ability to hear when index fingers are placed in your ears. Child may have difficulty hearing faint or distant speech. At 16 dB student can miss up to 10% of speech signal when teacher is at a distance greater than 3 feet. A 20 dB or greater hearing loss in the better ear can result in absent, inconsistent or distorted parts of speech, especially word endings (s, ed) and unemphasized sounds. Percent of speech signal missed will be greater whenever there is background noise in the classroom, especially in the elementary grades when instruction is primarily verbal and younger children have greater difficulty listening in noise. Young children have the tendency to watch and copy the movements of other students rather than attending to auditorily fragmented teacher directions.	May be unaware of subtle conversational cues that could cause him to be viewed as inappropriate or awkward. May miss portions of fast-paced peer interactions that could begin to have an impact on socialization and self-concept. Behavior may be confused for immaturity or inattention. May be more fatigued because of extra effort needed for understanding speech.	Noise in typical classroom environments impede child from having full access to teacher instruction. Will benefit from improved acoustic treatment of classroom and soundfield amplification. Favorable seating necessary. May often have difficulty with sound and letter associations and subtle auditory discrimination skills necessary for reading. May need attention to vocabulary or speech, especially when there has been a long history of middle ear fluid. Depending on loss configuration, may benefit from low power hearing aid with personal FM system. Appropriate medical management necessary for conductive losses. Inservice on impact of "minimal" 15–25 dB hearing loss on language development, listening in noise, and learning, required for teacher.

Table 26–1 *(Continued)*

26–40 dB Hearing Loss

Possible Impact on the Understanding of Language and Speech	Possible Social Impact	Potential Educational Accommodations and Services
Effect of a hearing loss of approximately 20 dB can be compared to ability to hear when index fingers are placed in ears therefore a 26–40 dB hearing loss causes greater listening difficulties than a "plugged ear" loss. Child can "hear" but misses fragments of speech leading to misunderstanding. Degree of difficulty experienced in school will depend upon noise level in the classroom, distance from the teacher, and configuration of the hearing loss, even with hearing aids. At 30 dB can miss 25–40% of the speech signal; at 40 dB may miss 50% of class discussions, especially when voices are faint or speaker is not in line of vision. Will miss unemphasized words and consonants, especially when he has high-frequency hearing loss. Often experiences difficulty learning early reading skills such as letter and sound associations. Child's ability to understand and succeed in the classroom will be substantially diminished by speaker distance and background noise, especially in the elementary grades.	Barriers begin to build with negative impact on self-esteem as child is accused of "hearing when he wants to," "daydreaming," or "not paying attention." May believe he is less capable because of difficulties understanding in class. Child begins to lose ability for selective listening, and has increasing difficulty suppressing background noise, causing the learning environment to be more stressful. Child is more fatigued from effort needed to listen.	Noise in typical class will impede child from full access to teacher instruction. Will benefit from hearing aids and use of a desktop or ear-level FM system in the classroom. Needs favorable acoustics, seating, and lighting. May need attention to auditory skills, speech, language development, speech reading, and support in reading and self-esteem. Amount of attention needed typically related to the degree of success of intervention before 6 months of age to prevent language and early learning delays. Teacher inservice training on impact of so called "mild" hearing loss on listening and learning to convey that it is often greater than expected.

41–55 dB Hearing Loss

Possible Impact on the Understanding of Language and Speech	Possible Social Impact	Potential Educational Accommodations and Services
Consistent use of amplification and language intervention before age 6 months increases the probability that the child's speech, language, and learning will develop at a normal rate. Without amplification, understands conversation at a distance of 3–5 feet, if sentence structure and vocabulary are known. The amount of speech signal missed can be 50% or more with 40 dB loss and 80% or more with 50 dB loss. Without early amplification the child is likely to have delayed or disordered syntax, limited vocabulary, imperfect speech production and flat voice quality. Addition of a visual communication system to supplement audition may be indicated, especially if language delays and/or additional disabilities are present. Even with hearing aids, child can "hear" but may miss much of what is said if classroom is noisy or reverberant. With personal hearing aids alone, ability to perceive speech and learn effectively in the classroom is at high risk. A personal FM system to overcome classroom noise and distance is typically necessary.	Barriers build with negative impact on self-esteem as child is accused of "hearing when he wants to," "daydreaming," or "not paying attention." Communication will be significantly compromised with this degree of hearing loss if hearing aids are not worn. Socialization with peers can be difficult, especially in noisy settings such as cooperative learning situations, lunch, or recess. May be more fatigued than classmates from effort needed to listen.	Consistent use of amplification (hearing aids + FM) is essential. Needs favorable classroom acoustics, seating, and lighting. Consultation/program supervision by a specialist in childhood hearing impairment to coordinate services is important. Depending on intervention success in preventing language delays, special academic support necessary if language and academic delays are present. Attention to growth of oral communication, reading, written language skills, auditory skill development, speech therapy, self esteem likely. Teacher inservice training required with attention to communication access and peer acceptance.

56–70 dB Hearing Loss

Possible Impact on the Understanding of Language and Speech	Possible Social Impact	Potential Educational Accommodations and Services
Even with hearing aids, child will typically be aware of people talking around him, but will miss parts of words said resulting in difficulty in situations requiring verbal communication (both one-to-one and in groups). Without amplification, conversation must be very loud to be understood; a 55-dB	If hearing loss was identified late and language delay was not prevented, communication interaction with peers will be significantly affected. Child will have greater difficulty socializing, especially in noisy	Full-time, consistent use of amplification (hearing aids + FM system) essential. May benefit from frequency transposition (frequency compression) hearing aids depending upon loss configuration. May require intense support in development of auditory, language, speech, reading, and

(Continued)

Table 26–1 (*Continued*)

loss can cause a child to miss up to 100% of speech information without functioning amplification. If hearing loss is not identified before one year of age and appropriately managed, delayed spoken language, syntax, reduced speech intelligibility, and flat voice quality is likely. Age when first amplified, consistency of hearing aid use, and success of early language intervention strongly tied to speech, language and learning development. Addition of visual communication system often indicated if language delays or additional disabilities are present. Use of a personal FM system will reduce the effects of noise and distance and allow increased auditory access to verbal instruction. With hearing aids alone, ability to understand in the classroom is greatly reduced by distance and noise.

settings such as lunch cooperative learning situations, or recess. Tendency for poorer self-concept and social immaturity may contribute to a sense of rejection; peer in service training helpful.

writing skills. Consultation and supervision by a specialist in childhood hearing impairment to coordinate services is important. Use of sign language or a visual communication system by child with substantial language delays or additional learning needs may be useful to access linguistically complex instruction. Note taking, captioned films, etc. accommodations often needed. Requires teacher inservice training.

71–90 dB & 91+ dB

Possible Impact on the Understanding of Language and Speech	Possible Social Impact	Potential Educational Accommodations and Services
The earlier the child wears amplification consistently with concentrated efforts by parents and caregivers to provide rich language opportunities throughout everyday activities or provision of intensive language intervention (sign or verbal), the greater the probability that speech, language, and learning will develop at a relatively normal rate. Without amplification, children with 71–90 dB hearing loss may only hear loud noises about one foot from ear. When amplified optimally, children with hearing ability of 90 dB or better should detect many sounds of speech if presented from close distance or via FM. Individual ability and intensive intervention prior to 6 months of age will determine the degree that sounds detected will be discriminated and understood by the brain into meaningful input. Even with hearing aids children with 71–90 dB loss are typically unable to perceive all high pitch speech sounds sufficiently to discriminate them or benefit from incidental listening, especially without the use of FM. The child with hearing loss > 70 dB may be a candidate for cochlear implants and the child with hearing loss > 90 dB will not be able to perceive most speech sounds with traditional hearing aids. For full access to language to be available visually through sign language or cued speech, family members must be involved in child's communication mode from a very young age.	Depending on success of intervention in infancy to address language development, the child's communication may be minimally or significantly affected. Socialization with hearing peers may be difficult. Children in general education classrooms may develop greater dependence on adults because of difficulty perceiving or comprehending oral communication. Children may be more comfortable interacting with peers who are deaf or hard of hearing due to ease of communication. Relationships with peers and adults who have hearing loss can make positive contributions toward the development of a healthy self-concept and a sense of cultural identity.	There is no one communication system that is right for all hard of hearing or deaf children and their families. Whether a visual communication approach or auditory/oral approach is used, extensive language intervention, full-time consistent amplification use, and constant integration of the communication practices into the family by 6 months of age will highly increase the probability that the child will become a successful learner. Children with late-identified hearing loss (after 6 months of age) will have delayed language. This language gap is difficult to overcome and the educational program of a child with hearing loss, especially those with language and learning delays secondary to hearing loss, requires the involvement of a consultant or teacher with expertise in teaching children with hearing loss. Depending on the configuration of the hearing loss and individual speech perception ability, frequency transposition (frequency compression) aids or cochlear implantation may be options for better access to speech. If an auditory/oral approach is used, early training is needed on auditory skills, spoken language, concept development and speech. If culturally deaf emphasis is selected, frequent exposure to deaf, American Sign Language users is important. Educational placement with other signing deaf or hard of hearing students (special school or classes) may be a more appropriate option to access a language-rich environment and free-flowing communication. Support services and continual appraisal of access to communication and verbal instruction is required. Note-taking, captioning, captioned films, and other visual enhancement strategies are necessary. Training in pragmatic language use and communication repair strategies helpful. Inservice training of general education teachers is essential.

Table 26–1   (*Continued*)

Unilateral Hearing Loss

Possible Impact on the Understanding of Language and Speech	Possible Social Impact	Potential Educational Accommodations and Services
Child can "hear" but can have difficulty understanding in certain situations, such as hearing faint or distant speech, especially if poor ear is aimed toward the person speaking. Will typically have difficulty localizing sounds and voices using hearing alone. The unilateral listener will have greater difficulty understanding speech when environment is noisy or reverberant, especially when normal ear toward the overhead projector or other competing sound source and poor hearing ear towards the teacher. Exhibits difficulty detecting or understanding soft speech from the side of the poor hearing ear, especially in a group discussion.	Child may be accused of selective hearing because of discrepancies in speech understanding in quiet versus noise. Social problems may arise as child experiences difficulty understanding in noisy cooperative learning, or recess situations. May misconstrue peer conversations and feel rejected or ridiculed. Child may be more fatigued in classroom from greater effort needed to listen, if class is noisy or has poor acoustics. May appear inattentive, distractible or frustrated, with behavior or social problems sometimes evident.	Allow child to change seat locations to direct the normal hearing ear toward the primary speaker. Student is at 10 times the risk for educational difficulties as children with two normal hearing ears and one third to one half of students with unilateral hearing loss experience significant learning problems. Children often have difficulty learning sound and letter associations in typically noisy kindergarten and 1st grade settings. Educational and audiologic monitoring is warranted. Teacher inservice training is beneficial. Typically will benefit from a personal FM system with low gain/power or a soundfield FM system in the classroom, especially in the lower grades. Depending on the hearing loss, may benefit from a hearing aid in the impaired ear.

Mid-Frequency Hearing Loss or Reverse Slope Hearing Loss
Mid-Frequency Hearing Loss or Reverse Slope

Possible Impact on the Understanding of Language and Speech	Possible Social Impact	Potential Educational Accommodations and Services
Child can "hear" whenever speech is present, but will have difficulty understanding in certain situations. May have difficulty understanding faint or distant speech, such as a student with a quiet voice speaking from across the classroom. The "cookie bite" or reverse slope listener will have greater difficulty understanding speech when environment is noisy or reverberant, such as a typical classroom setting. A 25–40 dB degree of loss in the low to mid-frequency range may cause the child to miss approximately 30% of speech information, if unamplified; some consonant and vowel sounds may be heard inconsistently, especially when background noise is present. Speech production of these sounds may be affected.	Child may be accused of selective hearing or "hearing when he wants to" because of discrepancies in speech understanding in quiet versus noise. Social problems may arise as child experiences difficulty understanding in noisy cooperative learning situations, lunch, or recess. May misconstrue peer conversations, believing that other children are talking about him. Child may be more fatigued in classroom setting due to greater effort needed to listen. May appear inattentive, distracted, or frustrated.	Personal hearing aids are important. but must be precisely fit to hearing loss. Child likely to benefit from a soundfield FM system, a personal FM system, or assistive listening device in the classroom. Student is at risk for educational difficulties. Can experience some difficulty learning sound and letter associations in kindergarten and 1st grade classes. Depending on degree and configuration of loss, child may experience delayed language development and articulation problems. Educational monitoring and teacher inservice training warranted. Annual hearing evaluation to monitor for hearing loss progression is important.

High-Frequency Hearing Loss

Possible Impact on the Understanding of Language and Speech	Possible Social Impact	Potential Educational Accommodations and Services
Child can "hear" but can miss important fragments of speech. Even a 25–40 dB loss in high-frequency hearing may cause the child to miss 20–30% of vital speech information if unamplified. Consonant sounds t, s, f, th, k, sh, ch likely heard inconsistently, especially in noise. May have difficulty understanding	May be accused of selective hearing because of discrepancies in speech understanding in quiet versus noise. Social problems may arise as child experiences	Student is at risk for educational difficulties. Depending upon onset, degree, and configuration of loss, child may experience delayed language and syntax development and articulation problems. Possible difficulty learning some sound and letter associations in kindergarten and 1st grade classes. Early evaluation of speech

(*Continued*)

Table 26–1   (*Continued*)

faint or distant speech, such as a student with a quiet voice speaking from across the classroom and will have much greater difficulty understanding speech when in low background noise and/or reverberation is present. Many of the critical sounds for understanding speech are high-pitched, quiet sounds, making them difficult to perceive; the words: cat, cap, calf, cast could be perceived as "ca," word endings, possessives, plurals and unstressed brief words are difficult to perceive and understand. Speech production may be affected. Use of amplification often indicated to learn language at a typical rate and ease learning.

difficulty understanding in noisy cooperative learning situations, lunch, or recess. May misinterpret peer conversations. Child may be fatigued in classroom from greater listening effort. May appear inattentive, distracted, or frustrated. Could affect self-concept.

and language skills is suggested. Educational monitoring and teacher inservice training is warranted. Will typically benefit from personal hearing aids and use of a soundfield or a personal FM system in the classroom. Use of ear protection in noisy situations is imperative to prevent damage to inner ear structures and resulting progression of hearing loss.

Fluctuating Hearing Loss

Possible Impact on the Understanding of Language and Speech	Possible Social Impact	Potential Educational Accommodations and Services
Of greatest concern are children who have experienced hearing fluctuations over many months in early childhood (multiple episodes with fluid lasting three months or longer). Listening with hearing loss that is approximately 20 dB can be compared to hearing when index fingers are placed in ears. This loss, or worse, is typical of listening with fluid or infection behind the eardrums. Child can "hear" but misses fragments of what is said. Degree of difficulty experienced in school will depend upon the classroom noise level, the distance from the teacher and the current degree of hearing loss. At 30 dB can miss 25–40% of the speech signal; child with a 40 dB loss associated with "glue ear" may miss 50% of class discussions, especially when voices are faint or speaker is not in line of vision. Will frequently miss unstressed words, consonants, and word endings.	Barriers begin to build with negative impact on self esteem as the child is accused of "hearing when he wants to," "daydreaming," or "not paying attention." Child may believe he is less capable because of understanding difficulties in class. Typically poor at identifying changes in own hearing ability. With inconsistent hearing, the child learns to "tune out" the speech signal. Children are judged to have greater attention problems, insecurity, distractibility, and lack self-esteem. Tend to be nonparticipative and distract themselves from classroom tasks; often socially immature.	Impact is primarily on acquisition of early reading skills and attention in class. Screening for language delays is suggested from a young age. Ongoing monitoring for hearing loss in school, communication between parent and teacher about listening difficulties, and aggressive medical management is needed. Will benefit from soundfield FM or an assistive listening device in class. May need attention to development of speech, reading, self-esteem, or listening skills. Teacher inservice training is beneficial.

Abbreviation: FM, frequency modulation.
(From Anderson and Matkin, 2007.)
© 1991, Relationship of Degree of Longterm Hearing Loss to Psychosocial Impact and Educational Needs, Karen Anderson & Noel Matkin, revised 2007 thanks to input from the Educational Audiology Association listserv.

hearing loss and to know what services might be needed. It is also very useful for audiologists, speech-language pathologists, and educators in clinical settings when making school recommendations, and for parents, to assist them in knowing what to request at IEP meetings. It offers an excellent summary of required services.

◆ Summary

The movement toward mainstreaming students who are deaf or hard of hearing is evolving. Because advances in technology and new legislation, mainstreaming is becoming the choice of many parents and their school districts.

Youngsters who have attended school in the mainstream have reported that advocating for their own needs, being responsible for their learning, and using communication aids in the classroom were of prime importance to a successful outcome. For children to succeed, schools need to have a team approach to learning, including having a TOD, who is the most important provider for students who are deaf or hard of hearing. For many school districts, finding quality service providers is the key to the child's positive educational outcome. TODs, speech-language pathologists, and mainstream staff must receive ongoing training through conferences, workshops, and networking to maximize the success of the child who is deaf or hard of hearing.

Having mainstream teachers who are sensitive to the academic, social, and emotional needs of the child with hearing loss will also make a difference. Willingness on the part of the school administration and staff, as well as creative thinking by everyone can help provide a positive outcome. Parents need to remain actively involved in their children's educational experience while continuing to advocate for them (Eriks-Brophy, 2006).

It is important to recognize the social and emotional consequences of oral success, and the ability to hear optimally with amplification and speak intelligibly. With changes in technology, hearing loss has become a more subtle disorder. A student who is deaf or hard of hearing may be the only one in school, and social isolation may be a concern (Luterman, 2006). Creating ways of helping schools to encourage greater inclusion within the mainstream will need to be addressed.

Although mainstreaming is the trend today, schools and programs for children who are deaf is still an option for families whose children require a more restrictive environment, for families who culturally make that choice, as well as for families who desire a greater peer affiliation for their children.

As educational options increase, parents have multiple choices for their children with hearing loss. With the right support within the chosen school placement, students have the opportunity for a happy, productive, and successful educational experience.

Discussion Questions

1. If a child receives a cochlear implant at one year of age, what types of educational options would be considered throughout his schooling and why?

2. What related services are needed for a student in the mainstream?

3. What are the three important acoustic modifications for classrooms and why?

4. What is the role for schools and programs for the deaf in the future?

5. Is there a place for sign language in the mainstream setting? Explain.

References

American Speech-Language-Hearing Association. (2005). Audiology Information Series. www.asha.org/members/deskref-journals/deskref/default.

American Speech-Language-Hearing Association. (2005). Acoustics in Educational Settings: Position Statement. www.asha.org/members/deskref-journals/deskref/default.

American Speech-Language-Hearing Association. (2006). Analysis of IDEA Part B Final Regulations. www.asha.org/about/legislation-advocacy/federal/idea.

Anderson, K. L., and Goldstein, H. (2004). Speech perception benefits of FM and infrared devices to children with hearing aids in typical classroom. ASHA, Language, Speech, and Hearing Services in Schools, 35, 169–184.

Berndsen, M. (2002). Preparing your implanted child for preschool. Loud & Clear, Advanced Bionics Corporation Publication, 1.

BEGINNINGS, For Parents of Children Who Are Deaf or Hard of Hearing, Inc. (2005). Raleigh, NC. Raleigh@beginningssvcs.com.

Brackett, D., and Maxon, A. (1986). Service delivery alternatives for the mainstreamed hearing-impaired child, ASHA, Language, Speech, and Hearing Services in Schools, 17, 115–125.

Chute, P. M., and Nevins, M. E. (2002). The parent's guide to cochlear implants. Washington, DC: Gallaudet University Press.

Cochlear Americas. (2002). Static electricity and cochlear implants, a teacher's guide to the Nucleus R Cochlear Implant system, pp. 70–75.

Dinnebeil, L. A., and McInerney, W. F. (2000). Supporting inclusion in community-based settings: the role of the "Tuesday morning teacher." Young Exceptional Children, 4 19–26.

Estabrooks, W (2001). 50 FAQ's about AVT. Toronto, Ontario, Canada. Learning to Listen Foundation.

Geers, A. (2002). Factors affecting the development of speech, language, and literacy in children with early cochlear implantation. ASHA Language, Speech, and Hearing Services in Schools, 33, 172–183.

Geers, A. (2003). Language skills of children with early cochlear implantation. Ear and Hearing, 24, 46S–58S.

Luterman, D. (2006). Children with hearing loss: reflections on the past 40 years. ASHA Leader, 6–7, 18–21.

Moore, J. A., and Teagle, H. F. B. (2002). An introduction to cochlear implant technology, activation, and programming. ASHA, Language, Speech, and Hearing Services in Schools, 33, 153–161.

National Court Reporters Association. (2004). Communication Access Information Center, National Court Reporters Foundation.

National Technical Institute for the Deaf, Rochester Institute of Technology. (2003). How Does C-Print Work? C-Print, Speech-to-Text System, Resource Guide.

Youdelman, K., and Messerly, C. (1996). Computer-assisted notetaking for mainstreamed hearing-impaired students, Volta Review, 98, 191–199.

Zwolan, T., and Sorkin, D. (2006). Cochlear implant collaborations aid school success. ASHA Leader, 11, 10–19.

Chapter 27

Working with Multicultural and Multilingual Families of Young Children with Hearing Loss

Ellen A. Rhoades

♦ Step 1—Engage in Introspection
♦ Step 2—Adopt a Family Systems Approach
♦ Step 3—Make a Commitment to Diversity
♦ Anchor Language Differences

   Interpreters

♦ Caregiver Intake Interview
♦ Learning a Second Language

   American Sign Language

Key Points

- Prejudices negatively affect the children we serve.

- A multicultural outlook should pervade the delivery of all clinical services.

- The audiologist must develop an effective alliance with parents.

- The child should learn the language spoken at home.

- Interpreters should be chosen with care.

- The audiologist should learn about each child's family culture.

- With parent commitment, children who are deaf can become bilingual.

Recent immigration trends have created dramatic changes in developed countries (Migration Policy Institute, 2006) that, of necessity, impact on services provided by audiologists and other auditory-based clinicians. An ideal family in Anglo-Western culture was that of a dual parent egalitarian structure stereotypically defined by the self-sufficient family's individualistic, competitive nature (Foster et al, 2003). But social changes have already resulted in minority groups collectively becoming the majority in a few parts of Anglo-Western countries (Maines, Abbady, and Benedick, 2006). Approximately half of America's children younger than 5 years are now considered racial or ethnic minorities (U.S. Census, 2006). Consequently, there is no dominant form

against which families can be measured or judged; family diversity is the norm (Baca Zinn and Eitzen, 2004).

Racism still prevails within majority Anglo-Western countries, and negatively affects children of color (Dunn, 2003; Lemos, 2005; Webster, 2004). Stereotypes drive prejudices; these emotions still cause discrimination that is unjustified or harmful behavior. Even when implicit, racism has a deleterious effect on the health, education, and psychosocial growth of children (Caughy et al, 2006; McKenzie, 2003; Tyler, Boykin, and Walton, 2006). On the whole, Anglo-Western culture has been disrespectful of diversity.

Multiculturalism, a social, intellectual, and moral movement, is an ethical force based on the goals of inclusion, social justice, and mutual respect (Fowers and Davidov, 2006). As such, multiculturalism is extraordinarily influential in psychology, education, and various allied health professions (Hwang, 2006; Tyler, Boykin, and Walton, 2006). Cultural, racial, and ethnic characteristics of each family have direct relevance to understanding specific domains of child development (Hughes et al, 2006). Such characteristics influence adult–child interactions, the way children are raised and educated, and long-term goals for them (Cabrera et al, 2006; Halgunseth, Ispa, and Rudy, 2006; Rodriguez and Olswang, 2003). Moreover, the ways that children play, socialize, learn, problem solve, and perceive the world are culturally grounded (Cole, Tamang, and Shrestha, 2006; Goneu, Mistry, and Mosier, 2000; Kobayashi, Glover, and Temple, 2006; Nisbett and Miyamoto, 2005; Suzuki and Aronson, 2003; Tudge et al, 2006). When clinicians better understand cultural differences, miscommunications and overrepresentation of minority students receiving special services may decrease (e.g., Crago et al, 1997).

Optimally effective, child-driven pediatric audiologists and early intervention clinicians are family centered and parent focused (Kargin, 2004), necessitating that service providers develop skills to meet the needs of diverse learners within diverse family contexts. To accomplish this level of intervention, it follows that audiologists must be knowledgeable and supportive of many family systems, cultures, and languages. Audiologists must first value diversity that is free from intolerance for people of various racial, ethnic, and religious backgrounds as well as varying sexual orientations and persons with disabilities. Only then can the strengths of each child's family be viewed as cultural capital (Woodrow, 2001); a deficit perspective is untenable.

Following is a discussion of three steps that clinicians can take toward developing a minimal level of competency in diversity: engage in introspection, adopt a family systems approach, and make a commitment to diversity.

◆ Step 1—Engage in Introspection

Clinicians serving children with hearing loss in North America are overwhelmingly from the traditional English-speaking Anglo-Western culture (Rhoades, Perigoe, and Price, 2004). The initial step, then, toward developing a minimal level of competency in diversity necessitates that audiologists first look within to better understand themselves, and to strive toward becoming nonjudgmental toward minority groups. Overcoming implicit racial biases and cultural attitudes requires that we first understand these attitudes for what they are (Dunham, Baron, and Benaji, 2006). Diversity-sensitive counseling challenges us to confront personal fears: myths, stereotypes, faulty assumptions, negative attitudes, and to redefine whiteness and the Eurocentric perspective (Watt et al, 2006). Awareness of our ignorance and subconscious beliefs can, in turn, cause us to be vigilant and to consciously not act on them; an ongoing concerted effort, facilitated by knowledge and understanding, must be made to develop tolerance.

Beyond self-analysis, interracial contact can be highly effective for reducing inherent biases (McGlothlin and Killen, 2006). Audiologists are encouraged to actively seek minority individuals to inquire about issues that directly bear on inherent biases. For example, to better understand others' experiences, ask people of different races and cultures what racism means to them. Shadow a minority child for at least a school day (Almarza, 2005). Read books by and about minority persons. Attend local cultural festivals and other celebratory events as well as those places of worship frequented by minority families.

Pitfall

- A professional's inherent racial biases and cultural misperceptions can negatively affect the delivery of services.

◆ Step 2—Adopt a Family Systems Approach

The second step toward developing a minimal level of competency in diversity is for audiologists to learn about basic family systems theory. Family systems theory has to do with the complex interrelationships and negotiations of each family member with others. An invisible web of complementary demands and expectations regulates family behavior. The family provides the primary context in which to view the young child who inhabits that context along with other social factors, all of whom are products and producers of culture (Tudge et al, 2000).

Essential terminology pertaining to the dynamics of family relationships should be understood (Christian, 2006; Kaczmarek, 2006). Reading a basic textbook on family systems theory can enable audiologists to at least recognize families that are clearly dysfunctional so that appropriate referrals to family therapists can be made (Graham, 2004; Minuchin and Fishman, 2004; Walker and Akister, 2004). Moreover, when audiologists are able to implement simple family supportive strategies, optimizing child potential and minimizing the secondary effects of hearing loss is more likely.

There are many simple strategies that audiologists can incorporate into their communications with the child's caregivers. One very effective strategy is that of mimicry, also known as mimesis, because it facilitates a family perceiving the clinician to be an ally. Mimicry occurs when an audiologist, while addressing a family, adopts that family's language level, mannerisms, communicative style, speech patterns, and familial colloquialisms. When conforming to the family's affective range, joining the family system and mutual rapport occurs (Bailenson and Yee, 2005; Graham, 2004; Robbins and Szapocznik, 2000; van Baaren et al, 2003).

Family relationships are dramatically altered in single-parent households and within impoverished families and in those whose children have disabilities (Naseef, 2001; Powers et al, 1995). Approximately 10% of parents and children have at least one disability. Children with disabilities are more likely to live with single women (Cohen and Petrescu-Prahova, 2006). Some parents are unemployed or in poor health; some children are abused or have many special needs. Nearly three quarters of America's children live in low-income or impoverished families, mostly with at least one employed parent. The majority of these children live in single-parent households, most of them children of color younger than 6 years (Chau, 2006). Impoverished at-risk families are likely to be driven by survival above and beyond any special needs, and they typically need a much stronger supportive network. Given that multicultural and multilingual families are part of this mix, a huge variety of childrearing practices presents to audiologists who must then seek an even wider base of professional and community collaboration.

♦ Step 3—Make a Commitment to Diversity

Beyond developing an awareness of and sensitivity to cultural differences, effective audiologists must operatively demonstrate cultural responsiveness (Association for Supervision and Curriculum Development, 2006). Just as there are differences in learning assumptions and principles between cultures (Woodrow, 2001), teaching strategies that are believed to promote learning in children from the Anglo-Western culture do not necessarily result in greater gains among children from minority cultures (Kolobe, 2004). Viewpoints as to whether teachers, clinicians, and audiologists are guardians of knowledge or facilitators of learning are culturally based.

As soon as all minority groups and languages represented in a possible caseload are identified, a pool of consultants and trained peer advocates from minority groups should be established (Turner and Lynas, 2000). Be nonjudgmental and show empathy when listening to parents; try to see the world as they see it. Communication obstacles are often culturally controlled and not in one's normal awareness. For example, before informing parents of a child's hearing loss, the culturally responsive audiologist can inquire about the family's belief system regarding disabilities (Salas-Provance, Erickson, and Reed, 2002). Learning about each child's family background can affect the clinician's choice of words in assessments; for example, immigrant children might not understand football, but the same child might understand soccer.

Furthermore, clinicians and audiologists who provide culturally relevant services can facilitate multicultural knowledge among all families, including those who are Anglo-Western. In addition to promoting interracial contact (Rutland et al, 2005), a simple technique for reducing prejudice and developing appreciation of diversity includes the consistent use of pictures and availability of children's books that positively feature children of color and multicultural folklore and holidays (Cameron et al, 2006). Children and their families are more likely to thrive when professionals demonstrate cross-cultural competence in how they think, feel, and behave.

♦ Anchor Language Differences

Language, a culturally based activity (Genesee, Paradis, and Crago, 2004), serves as an anchor for family cohesion, facilitates literacy, and promotes bilingualism (Macrory, 2006). Early exposure to the mother tongue is critical for the development of speech perception. The home language should be the child's language (Kohnert et al, 2005). When parents speak to their young children in a language in which they do not feel comfortable, the child receives a more restricted language exposure. Young children who have a strong grounding in their home language tend to perform better in

school (Petitto and Dunbar, 2006). Furthermore, abandoning a heritage language may have extensive personal, familial, religious, cultural, and academic implications that prove unfavorable for the child (Tabors, 1997; Eilers et al, 2006).

Assessing performance in the child's home language can be problematic if no normative-referenced standardized test is available in that language. A parent–report instrument that is available in several languages (e.g., Fenson et al, 1996), a culturally anchored parent–child interaction assessment (e.g., Bernstein et al, 2005), as well as developmental scales of functional communication can be used to monitor language progress and serve as yardsticks for normal development. Norm-referenced language assessment scores translated from English are invalid and should not be used as the basis for a child's Individual Education Plan, but they can be used as approximate guidelines to gather information along with the use of informal language samples and parent reports. When necessary, an interpreter can translate a test in advance and provide assistance in implementing alternative assessment procedures (Laing and Kamhi, 2003). Use of an interpreter and any other modifications are important when reporting test outcomes to the family.

Interpreters

Because most clinicians in North America speak only English (Rhoades, Price, and Perigoe, 2004), an interpreter is often needed for parents who speak another language. When enlisting the assistance of an interpreter, try to use the same one for the same family so that an ongoing relationship can be developed. Interpreters are selected for a variety of attributes, including honesty, reliability, neutrality, confidentiality, cultural proficiency, bilingual proficiency, and consistency in availability. Ideally, interpreters are of the same ethnicity as that of the family and are also familiar with the family's heritage culture (Turner and Lynas, 2000).

Before working with an interpreter, the audiologist should meet with the interpreter to gain rapport and set some ground rules such as the provision of exact translations for parents, and the avoidance of gestures and other cues that could unfairly assist the child during administration of audiologic tests. Audiologists should spend a few minutes orienting interpreters to the subject matter, procedures, and goals of audiologic services. These consultations involve discussion on the relevance of materials and language expressions to be used.

During these interpreted sessions, audiologists should face parents while talking to them, and interpreters should sit next to and slightly behind the audiologist, so that parents are more likely to face the audiologist (Lopez, 2002). Audiologists should avoid using slang, idioms, and metaphors while casually monitoring the process of interpreting, particularly watching that interpreters do not appear to be offering their own thoughts to parents. Subsequent to each treatment session, audiologists should review notes and progress and discuss any interpreting issues with the interpreter. Although family members are often used as interpreters when professional interpreters are unavailable, using them, especially children, in this capacity, is not a good idea, because real and potential family biases and relationships can negatively affect the audiologic session.

◆ Caregiver Intake Interview

From the outset, there needs to be a framework of information relevant to audiologic diagnosis and treatment that involves ascertaining the family's cultural and linguistic status as well as identifying the communicative style within the family system (Hughes et al, 2006). The best place to observe a child's proficiency in the home language is within the context of the home, where the child is most comfortable and can interact with family members. At the very least, the audiologist who does not speak the child's home language could observe the family's communicative style in the office or waiting room, noting fluency and variety of communication skills used by the child and the adults.

During the interview process, regardless of whether an interpreter is present, the audiologist should demonstrate warmth while initially avoiding prolonged eye or physical contact. In a trustworthy, compassionate, and personable manner, both closed-end and open-ended questions should be asked of caregivers, using pauses and silences to enable them time to think and respond.

Pearl

- Language is rooted in culture. Diversity is good.

◆ Learning a Second Language

Bilingualism is a treasured asset for child, family, and society. Globally, bilingualism is the rule rather than the exception. All languages are equal; that is, no one language is harder for children to learn than another (Pearson, 2007). The notion that confusion or delays occur when children learn two languages at the same time is a myth (Petitto, 2006). When children learn two languages during the first three years of life, the process is known as simultaneous bilingualism or bilingual first language acquisition (Genesee and Nicoladis, 2006). Although young bilingual children typically engage in some language mixing, it is quite normal and transitory and soon stabilizes into what is called code-switching. This mixing is rule-governed and responsive to nonlinguistic social requirements in bilingual conversations (Holowka, Brosseau-Lapre, and Petitto, 2002; Petitto et al, 2001; Yumoto, 1996).

A critical realization is that, within English-based cultures, the key to raising bilingual children is in establishing the minority language (Pearson, 2007; Eilers et al, 2006). Indeed, it is now becoming clear that children who are deaf or hard of hearing, but with access to soft conversational sound as a result of hearing technology, can become bilingual, that is, conversationally fluent in at least two spoken languages to a degree approximating that of normally hearing peers (Francis and Ho, 2003; Guiberson, 2005; Phillips, 1999; Waltzman et al, 2003). An English-based preschool environment can further strengthen the English being learned by the child in auditory-based therapy (Wilcox and Murphy, 2003).

The younger the child, the more likely that progress in learning English will be rapid (Petitto, 2006). However, it is imperative that the home language be continuously valued and strengthened; this is important for social and emotional growth and has benefits for intellectual growth as well (Pearson, 2007). With sufficient linguistic input in both languages from caregivers and clear linguistic boundaries between school and home, the young child can become fluent in two languages prior to kindergarten.

Special Consideration

- Parent commitment must be active and consistent to have their bilingual child retain over time a minority language.

Second language learning by children older than three years is known as the sequential or successive bilingual process. Undoubtedly, increasing age upon initiation of learning a second language necessitates greater commitment and effort from school and primary caregivers (Pearson, 2007). Moreover, the older the child when learning a second language, the less likely she will speak it like a native (Kuhl, Tsao, and Liu, 2003). However, that difficulty should not preclude having bilingualism as a goal for children taking advantage of optimal hearing technology.

Conversational fluency in any spoken language does not necessarily mean the child is ready for academic learning in that language. Typically, children need to master a language at least at the 4-year age equivalency level before they can begin grade school academic learning (Rhoades, 2003). Academic learning will best occur in the child's dominant language. If at all possible, it is important to assess the child in both English and the home language, even when one seems clearly more dominant than the other (Thordardottir, 2006). If the home language remains the child's dominant language, the child may be best served in a bilingual class or dual language school where code switching is encouraged (Macrory, 2006).

There are some circumstances, however, when initiating the process toward bilingualism may not be an appropriate goal for older children who are deaf. Neither the child's age nor cognitive status should be the decisive variable. Instead, much depends on these critical factors: (1) the child's accessibility to soft conversational sound; (2) the level of support of primary caregivers toward facilitating bilingualism; (3) significant neurophysiologic dysfunction; and (4) the intactness of the child's working memory (Ardila, 2003; Swanson, Saez, and Gerber, 2006).

Second language learners, particularly those engaged in the sequential bilingual process, may have greater difficulty listening in noisy environments (Mayo, Florentine, and Buus, 1997; Nelson et al, 2005; van Wijngaarden, Steeneken, and Houtgast, 2002; van Wijngaarden, 2001). Therefore, audiologists, teachers, and clinicians working with these children should take special care to minimize classroom noise and to ensure the availability of effective assistive hearing technologies that improve access to spoken language.

American Sign Language

Families with deaf parents may use American Sign Language (ASL) as their primary language. Children with normal hearing who grow up in homes where ASL is the primary language will hear the language of the larger community and will frequently become natural bilingual communicators (e.g., Petitto and Kovelman, 2003), often translating for their parents. However, children who are deaf and grow up in a home where ASL is the primary language may have a more difficult time learning a spoken language, because their primary language is not an auditory one (e.g., Bishop and Hicks, 2005; Seal and Hammett, 1995). If the goal is to teach these children to become fluent in English or in another spoken language, it will be important for the children to have sufficient exposure to a spoken language on a very consistent daily basis from infancy or, at the least, from preschool. This can be accomplished by having a family member, neighbor, or friend who speaks the language spend several hours each day providing good language modeling. Day care settings where a spoken language is used can also be of value. It is critical that all children who are deaf, including children in a home where ASL is the primary language, wear appropriately fit technology every day to be sure they are receiving good auditory exposure.

In the end, pediatric audiologists can evolve by paying attention to and embracing what is in front of them, that is, by being culturally and linguistically responsive. Audiologists can take responsibility for creating positive environments where initiatives for facilitating and supporting family diversity will flourish. A transformative cross-cultural multiprofessional and peer-mediated team approach in high-quality service delivery can then be implemented so that *all* children and their families will thrive, regardless of how they look, which cultural practices they maintain, or what languages they speak.

Discussion Questions

1. The young child with a hearing loss is often part of a minority group. How can implicit negative attitudes toward each minority group affect this child's performance when she is placed in the mainstream educational environment?

2. How can professional training institutions be reconceptualized to ensure that white Eurocentric audiologists understand the dynamic processes relevant to family life and, in turn, embrace diverse perceptions in content, methods, strategies, and assessment tools?

3. There are many advantages to being bilingual on many different levels. What are they, and how can parents be encouraged to ensure that their children do not lose the home language?

4. Parents and audiologists who do not speak the same language face many obstacles in the process of early intervention. What strategies can be implemented by members of the cross-cultural, multiprofessional, peer-mediated team that will facilitate effective professional–parent communication?

5. Cultural differences can be the most significant barriers to providing effective intervention services. How can the audiologist identify those barriers, and can those barriers be removed?

References

Almarza, D. J. (2005). Connecting multicultural education theories with practice: a case study of an intervention course using the realistic approach in teacher education. Bilingual Research Journal, 29, 527–539.

Ardila, A. (2003). Language representation and working memory with bilinguals. Journal of Communication Disorders, 36, 233–240.

Association for Supervision and Curriculum Development (2006). Conejos no ponen huevos (Rabbits don't lay eggs). Education Update, 48, 4–5.

Baca Zinn, M., and Eitzen, D. S. (2004). Diversity in families, 7th Ed. Boston: Allyn & Bacon.

Bailenson, J. N., and Yee, N. (2005). Digital chameleons: automatic assimilation of nonverbal gestures in immersive virtual environments. Psychological Science, 16, 814–819.

Bernstein, V. J., Harris, E. J., WeLaLa Long, C., Iida, E., and Hans, S. L. (2005). Issues in the multi-cultural assessment of parent–child interaction: an exploratory study from the early starting smart collaboration. Journal of Applied Developmental Psychology, 26, 241–275.

Bishop, M., and Hicks, S. (2005). Orange eyes: bimodal bilingualism in hearing adults from deaf families. Sign Language Studies, 5, 188–230.

Cabrera, N. J., Shannon, J. D., West, J., and Brooks-Gunn, J. (2006). Parental interactions with Latino infants: variation by country of origin and English proficiency. Child Development, 77, 1190–1207.

Cameron, L., Rutland, A., Brown, R., and Douch, R. (2006). Changing children's intergroup attitudes towards refugees: testing different models of extended contact. Child Development, 77, 1208–1219.

Caughy, M. O., Netties, S. M., O'Campo, P. J., and Lohrfink, K. F. (2006). Neighborhood matters: racial socialization of African American children. Child Development, 77, 1220–1236.

Chau, M. (2006). Low-income children in the United States: national and state trend data, 1995-2005. NY: National Center for Children in Poverty.

Christian, L. G. (2006). Understanding families: Applying Family Systems Theory to Early Childhood Practice. Young Children on the Web, January, 1-8. www.journal.naeyc.org/btj/200601/ChristianBTJ.pdf. Last accessed October 20, 2006.

Cohen, P. N., and Petrescu-Prahova, M. (2006). Gendered living arrangements among children with disabilities. Journal of Marriage and Family, 68, 630–638.

Cole, P. M., Tamang, B. L., and Shrestha, S. (2006). Cultural variations in the socialization of young children's anger and shame. Child Development, 77, 1237–1251.

Crago, M. B., Eriks-Brophy, A., Pesco, D., and McAlpine, L. (1997). Culturally-based miscommunication in classroom interaction. Language, Speech, and Hearing Services in Schools, 28, 245–254.

Dunham, Y., Baron, A.S., amd Benaji, M. R. (2006). From American city to Japanese village: a cross-cultural investigation of implicit race attitudes. Child Development, 77, 1268–1281.

Dunn, K. M. (2003). Racism in Australia: findings of a survey on racist attitudes and experiences of racism. Presented at The Challenges of Immigration and Integration in the European Union and Australia, 18-20 February conference, University of Sydney.

Eilers, R. E., Pearson, B. Z., and Cobo-Lewis, A. B. (2006). Social factors in bilingual development: the Miami experience. In E. Hoff and P. McCardle (Eds.), Childhood bilingualism (pp. 68–90). Clevedon, UK: Multilingual Matters.

Fenson, L., Dale, P. S., Reznick, et al. (1996). MacArthur communicative development inventories. San Diego: Singular Publishing Group.

Foster, S., Mudgett-Decaro, P., Bagga-Gupta, S., et al. (2003). Cross-cultural definitions of inclusion for deaf students: a comparative analysis. Deafness and Education International, 5, 1_19.

Fowers, B. J., and Davidov, B. J. (2006). The virtue of multiculturalism: personal transformation, character, and openness to other. American Psychologist, 61, 581–594.

Francis, A. L., and Ho, D. W. L. (2003). Case report: acquisition of three spoken languages by a child with a cochlear implant. Cochlear Implants International, 4, 31–44.

Genesee, F., and Nicoladis, E. (2006). Bilingual acquisition. In E. Hoff and M. Shatz (Eds.), Handbook of language development. Oxford UK: Blackwell.

Genesee, F., Paradis, J., and Crago, M. B. (2004). Dual language development and disorders. Baltimore: Paul H. Brookes.

Goneu, A., Mistry, J., and Mosier, C. (2000). Cultural variations in the play of toddlers. International Journal of Behavioral Development, 24, 321–329.

Graham, P. J. (2004). Cognitive behaviour therapy for children and families. Cambridge UK: Cambridge University Press.

Guiberson, M. M. (2005). Children with cochlear implants from bilingual families: considerations for intervention and a case study. Volta Review, 105, 29–40.

Halgunseth, L. C., Ispa, J. M., and Rudy, D. (2006). Parental control in Latino families: an integrated review of the literature. Child Development, 77, 1282–1297.

Holowka, S., Brosseau-Lapre, F., and Petitto, L. A. (2002). Semantic and conceptual knowledge underlying bilingual babies' first signs and words. Language Learning, 52, 205–254.

Hughes, D., Rodriguez, J., Smith, E. P., Johnson, D. J., Stevenson, H. C., and Spicer, P. (2006). Parents' ethnic-racial socialization practices: a review of research and directions for future study. Developmental Psychology, 42, 747–770.

Hwang, W. C. (2006). The psychotherapy adaptation and modification framework: application to Asian Americans. American Psychologist, 61, 702–715.

Kargina, T. (2004). Effectiveness of a family-focused early intervention program in the education of children with hearing impairments living in rural Areas. International Journal of Disability, Development, and Education, 51, 401–418.

Kaczmarek, L. A. (2006). A team approach: Supporting Families of Children with Disabilities in Inclusive Programs. Young Children on the Web, January, 1-10. www.journal.naeyc.org/btj/200601/KaczmarekBTJ.pdf. Last accessed October 18, 2006.

Kobayashi, C., Glover, G. H., and Temple, E. (2006). Cultural and linguistic influence on neural bases of "Theory of Mind": an fMRI study with Japanese bilinguals. Brain and Language, 98, 210–220.

Kohnert, K., Yim, D., Nett, K., Fong Kan, P., and Duran, L. (2005). Intervention with linguistically diverse preschool children. Language, Speech, and Hearing Services in Schools, 36, 251–263.

Kolobe, T. H. A. (2004). Childrearing practices and developmental expectations for Mexican-American mothers and the developmental status of their infants. Physical Therapy, 84, 439–452.

Kuhl, P. K., Tsao, F., and Liu, H. (2003). Foreign-language experience in infancy: effects of short-term exposure and social interaction on phonetic learning. Proceedings of the National Academy of Science, 100, 9096–9101.

Laing, S. P., and Kamhi, A. (2003). Alternative assessment of language and literacy in culturally and linguistically diverse populations. Language, Speech, and Hearing Services in Schools, 34, 44–45.

Lemos, G. (2005). The search for tolerance: challenging and changing racist attitudes and behaviour among young people. York, UK: Joseph Rountree Foundation.

Lopez, E. C. (2002). Recommended practices in working with school interpreters to deliver psychological services to children and families. In A. Thomas and J. Grimes (Eds.), Best practices in school psychology IV (pp. 1419–1432). Bethesda: National Association of School Psychologists.

McCrory, G. D. (2006). Bilingual language development: what do early years practitioners need to know? Early Years, 26, 159–169.

Maines, J., Abbady, T., and Benedick, R. (2006). Broward County is more diverse. Ft. Lauderdale Sun-Sentinel, August 15.

Mayo, L. F. H., Florentine, M., and Buus, S. (1997). Age of second-language acquisition and perception of speech in noise. Journal of Speech and Hearing Research, 40, 686–693.

McGlothlin, H., and Killen, M. (2006). Intergroup attitudes of European American children attending ethnically homogeneous schools. Child Development, 77, 1375–1386.

McKenzie, K. (2003). Racism and health. British Medical Journal, 326, 65–66.

Migration Policy Institute. (2006). Migration Information Source. Washington, DC. www.migrationinformation.org/GlobalData/. Last accessed January 4, 2008.

Minuchin, S., and Fishman, H. C. (2004). Family therapy techniques. Cambridge: Harvard University Press.

Naseef, R. A. (2001). Special children, challenged parents. Baltimore: Paul H. Brookes Publishing.

Nelson, P., Kohnert, K., Sabur, S., and Shawm, D. (2005). Classroom noise and children learning through a second language: double jeopardy? Language, Speech, and Hearing Services in Schools, 36, 219–229.

Nisbett, R. E., and Miyamoto, Y. (2005). The influence of culture: holistic versus analytic perception. Trends in Cognitive Sciences, 9, 467–473.

Pearson, B. Z. (2007). Social factors in childhood bilingualism in the U.S. Applied Psycholinguistics, 28, 399–410.

Petitto, L. A. (2006). How young monolingual and bilingual children acquire language. Presentation at Office of English Language Acquisition Summit, November 13, 2002, Washington, DC.

Petitto, L. A., and Dunbar, K. N. (2006). New findings from educational neuroscience on bilingual brains, scientific brains, and the educated mind. In K. Fischer and T. Katzir (Eds.), Building usable knowledge in mind, brain, & education. Cambridge, UK: Cambridge University Press.

Petitto, L. A., Katerelos, M., Levy, B., Tetrault, K., and Ferraro, V. (2001). Bilingual signed and spoken language acquisition from birth: implications for mechanisms underlying early bilingual language acquisition. Journal of Child Language, 28, 453–496.

Petitto, L. A., and Kovelman, I. (2003). The bilingual paradox: how signing-speaking bilingual children help us resolve bilingual issues and teach us about the brain's mechanisms underlying all language acquisition. Learning Languages, 8, 5–18.

Phillips, A. H. (1999). Retrospective study of 48 hearing impaired children who participated in MOSD parent infant and/or nursery programs (birth dates 1987–1993). In A. H. Phillips, I. M. Hoshko, T. Peled, J. Flanerty, M. Perusse, and S. Sully. Early intervention at the Montreal Oral School for the Deaf: Five companion studies. Research Reports presented to Interministerial Committee for the Health and Education Ministries, Government du Quebec.

Powers, A. R., Elliott, R. N., Patterson, D., Shaw, S., and Taylor, C. (1995). Family environment and deaf and hard-of-hearing students with mild additional disabilities. Journal of Childhood Communication Disorders, 17, 15–19.

Rhoades, E. A. (2003). Lexical-semantic and morpho-syntactic language assessment in auditory-verbal intervention: a position paper. Volta Review, 103, 169–184.

Rhoades, E. A., Price, F., and Perigoe, C. B. (2004). The changing American family and ethnically diverse children with multiple needs. Volta Review, 104, 285–305.

Robbins, M. S., and Szapocznik, J. (2000). Brief strategic family therapy. Juvenile Justice Bulletin, April, 1–11.

Rodriguez, B. L., and Olswang, L. B. (2003). Mexican-American and Anglo-American mothers' beliefs and values about child rearing, education, and language impairment. American Journal of Speech-Language Pathology, 12, 452–462.

Rutland, A., Cameron, L., Bennett, L., and Ferrell, J. (2005). Interracial contact and racial constancy: a multi-site study of racial intergroup bias in 3-5 year old Anglo-British children. Journal of Applied Developmental Psychology, 26, 699–713.

Salas-Provance, M. B., Erickson, J. G., and Reed, J. (2002). Disabilities as viewed by four generations of one Hispanic family. American Journal of Speech-Language Pathology, 11, 151–162.

Seal, B. C., and Hammett, L. A. (1995). Language intervention with a child with hearing whose parents are deaf. American Journal of Speech-Language Pathology, 4, 15–21.

Suzuki, L., and Aronson, J. (2003). The cultural malleability of intelligence and its impact on the racial/ethnic hierarchy. Psychology, Public Policy, and Law, 31, 320–327.

Swanson, H. L., Sáez, L., and Gerber, M. (2006). Growth in literacy and cognition in bilingual children at risk or not at risk for reading disabilities. Journal of Educational Psychology, 98, 247–264.

Tabors, P. O. (1997). One child, two languages: a guide for preschool educators of children learning English as a second language. Baltimore: Paul H. Brookes Publishing.

Thordardottir, E. (2006). Language intervention from a bilingual mindset. ASHA Leader, 11, 6–7, 20–21.

Tudge, J., Doucet, F., Hayes, S., et al. (2000). Parents' participation in cultural practices with their preschoolers. Psicologia: Teoria e Pesquisa, 16, 1–11.

Tudge, J. R. H., Doucet, F., Odero, D., Sperb, T. M., Piccinini, C. A., and Lopes, R. S. (2006). A window into different cultural worlds: young children's everyday activities in the United States, Brazil, and Kenya. Child Development, 77, 1446–1469.

Turner, S., and Lynas, W. (2000). Teachers' perspectives on support for under-fives in families of ethnic minority origin. Deafness and Education International, 2, 152–164.

Tyler, K. M., Boykin, A. W., and Walton, T. R. (2006). Cultural considerations in teachers' perceptions of student classroom behavior and achievement. Teaching and Teacher Education, 22, 998–1005.

U. S. Census Bureau (2006). www.census.gov/Press-Release/www/2006/nationalracetable3.xls. Last accessed October 20, 2006.

van Baaren, R. B., Holland, R. W., Steenaert, B., and van Knippenberg, A. (2003). Mimicry for money: behavioral consequences of imitation. Journal of Experimental Social Psychology, 39, 393–398.

van Wijngaarden, S. J. (2001). Intelligibility of native and non-native Dutch speech. Speech Communication, 35, 103–113.

van Wijngaarden, S. J., Steeneken, J. M., and Houtgast, T. (2002). Quantifying the intelligibility of speech in noise for non-native listeners. Journal of the Acoustical Society of America, 111, 1906–1916.

Walker, S., and Akister, J. (2004). Applying family therapy: a guide for caring professionals in the community. Lyme Regis, UK: Russell House Publishing.

Waltzman, S. B., Robbins, A. M., Green, J. E., and Cohen, N. L. (2003). Second oral language capabilities in children with cochlear implants. Journal of Otology and Neurotology, 24, 757–763.

Watt, S. E., Maio, G. R., Rees, K., and Hewstone, M. (2006). Functions of attitudes towards ethnic groups: effects of level of abstraction. Journal of Experimental Social Psychology, 43(3), 441–449.

Webster, E. (2004). Racism in South Africa: no easy walk to the rainbow nation. Codesria Bulletin, 1–2, 3–4.

Wilcox, M. J., and Murphy, K. M. (2003). Facilitating use of evidence-based language teaching practices in preschool classrooms. In L. Girolametto and E. Weitzman (Eds.), Enhancing caregiver language facilitation in childcare settings (pp. 8-1–8-10). Toronto: The Hanen Centre.

Woodrow, D. (2001). Cultural determination of curricula, theories and practices. Pedagogy, Culture and Society, 9, 5–27.

Yumoto, K. (1996). Bilingualism, code-switching, language mixing, transfer and borrowing: clarifying terminologies in the literature. Kanagawa Prefectural College of Foreign Studies, Working Papers, 17, 49–60.

Chapter 28

Counseling and Collaboration with Parents of Children with Hearing Loss

Jackson Roush and Garima Kamo

Key Points

- The stress and anxiety experienced by most parents at the time of diagnosis is a normal reaction to unfamiliar and unforeseen circumstances.

- Interactions between the audiologist and the family at the time of diagnosis can set the tone for future interactions.

- Identification of hearing loss in infancy puts parents in the position of receiving a diagnosis without the benefit of direct observation.

- Delivering difficult news requires careful consideration of how information is presented and the dialogue that follows.

- Parents' initial level of concern or emotional upheaval is usually unrelated to their child's type or degree of hearing loss.

- Audiologists need to be forthright in providing information to parents, but also willing to listen and reflect on their concerns and priorities.

- Inexperienced clinicians may provide more information than a family can comprehend, especially at the time of diagnosis.

- The support of other parents is vital to many families.

- Parents may experience ambivalent feelings throughout their child's early years, especially during periods of transition.

Historically, the diagnosis of hearing loss was a confirmation of what parents had suspected over a period of weeks or months. Now, with the widespread implementation of newborn screening, hearing loss is often identified in early infancy. Counseling at the time of diagnosis has always been important, but the role of the audiologist has been made more challenging by the need to address these issues soon after birth. Furthermore, identification of hearing loss in infancy puts parents in the difficult position of needing to accept the diagnosis without the benefit of direct observation. These realities, combined with the remarkable expansion of information available to many families through the Internet and other sources, require the audiologist to consider the emotional aspects of parent counseling while providing the information families need to be well-informed consumers and decision makers.

This chapter explores the audiologist's dual role of counselor and information provider within a family-centered framework. From the shared perspectives of a pediatric audiologist (JR) and the parent of a child with hearing loss (GK), we examine successful models for counseling and informing families as well as challenges and potential pitfalls.

◆ The Audiologist as Counselor and Informant

The early weeks and months following diagnosis are a time of conflict and emotional upheaval for most families. Not surprisingly, parents and family members differ in their reactions to these events. For some parents the diagnosis is a call to immediate action; for others, time and space are needed to reflect on the diagnosis and recommendations. Regardless of the families' initial reaction, it is important for the audiologist to recognize that most parents and family members are not emotionally disturbed but emotionally upset. Indeed, Luterman (1979) describes the distress and anxiety experienced by most parents as a normal response to unfamiliar and unforeseen circumstances. Consistent with that assumption, Clark and English (2004) characterize the audiologist's counseling role as one that is based on a well-patient model, with the goal of helping parents and family members acquire the support and information needed to attain a positive and constructive outlook.

What Does It Mean to Be Family Centered and Why Does It Matter?

Early intervention was, for many years, a child-focused endeavor designed to enhance developmental outcomes for young children with disabilities. The origin of the term family centered has been attributed to the field of health care in the 1960s as professionals attempted to provide a greater decision-making role for families (Trivette et al, 1995). Bronfenbrenner (1977) was among the first to apply the term to early intervention at a time when he and others sought to increase the level of parent participation in early education. Public Law 99–457, which was passed in the mid 1980s, established the Individualized Family Service Plan (IFSP) that, for the first time, required documentation of a family's strengths and needs, services to be provided, and specification of intended outcomes.

The years following implementation of PL 99–457, although better for families in many ways, have been characterized by inconsistency in how family-centered practices are defined and implemented. Since the 1990s, many professionals have advocated for a family-centered approach that focuses on the development of collaborative relationships between families and professionals (Trivette et al, 1995). Bailey et al (1998) emphasized the importance of examining family outcomes as well as those intended for the child, and Dunst (2000) proposed an expanded service-delivery model focusing on the social systems and environmental variables associated with

development-enhancing and family-strengthening consequences. This model includes children's learning opportunities, supports for parenting, and community supports provided within a family-centered framework. As suggested by Crais, Roy, and Free (2006), providing successful family-centered services does not require identification of the ideal or perfect set of practices. Rather, it requires recognition of the family's role in deciding and implementing those practices. With each reauthorization of what is now known as the Individuals with Disabilities Education Act (IDEA), a fundamental principle has been maintained: the importance of parental decision-making and individualized choices for families throughout the delivery of assessment and intervention services.

Support for this tenet can be found in the growing evidence of how family participation affects child outcomes. For families whose children are deaf or hard of hearing there is no better example than the work of Moeller (2000), who explored the relationship between age of enrollment in intervention and language outcomes at 5 years of age. She also studied the relationships between performance and various factors, including family involvement, degree of hearing loss, and nonverbal intelligence. Moeller's findings indicated that children enrolled earliest in intervention programs demonstrated significantly better vocabulary and verbal reasoning than later enrolled children. Interestingly, only two factors explained a significant amount of the variance: age of enrollment and the level of family involvement. In fact, family involvement explained the most variance after accounting for other variables.

Pearl

- Early enrollment in early intervention benefited all children who received services, but the most successful were those who also had high levels of family involvement (Moeller, 2000).

Applying Family-Centered Principles to Clinical Audiology

A family-centered approach requires careful examination of parent-professional communication and the dynamics of each context that brings parents and professionals together (Roush, 2001). Simeonsson et al (1996) describe the early services provided to families as an intervention cycle composed of discrete elements that include referral, assessment, intervention planning, service implementation, and follow-up. Each element involves a succession of encounters that children and families have with professionals, and each encounter is defined by mutual expectations, roles, and activities for families and service providers. Our encounters with children who are deaf or hard of hearing and their families include each component of this intervention cycle. Initially they revolve around the screening and diagnostic process and later with the selection and fitting of hearing instruments and the delivery of early intervention services. Along the way, professionals counsel families, provide information, and offer choices. For the audiologist, the parent-professional relationship often begins when an infant is referred from newborn screening. Other contexts include decisions regarding hearing aids or cochlear implants, and options for early intervention and school placement. The initial contacts during the early weeks and months following diagnosis may set the tone for future encounters and create a foundation for the interactions that follow (Roush, 2001).

Informing Families of Diagnostic Results

The audiologist's ever-increasing technological capability, combined with the remarkable expansion of universal infant hearing screening, has brought fundamental changes in how and when the diagnosis occurs. In contrast to earlier times when the audiologic assessment confirmed parental suspicions, the news now comes unexpectedly to many families. It is important to remember that physiologic evidence, such as auditory brainstem response test results, may be unequivocal to the audiologist. But in the absence of behavioral evidence, families may have difficulty comprehending or accepting the diagnosis. Clinicians must be prepared to respond to a broad range of questions and a variety of reactions to the news. There is no easy way to impart the diagnosis to families when testing reveals permanent hearing loss, but advice from other disciplines can be helpful. In his book, *How To Break Bad News*, Robert Buckman, an oncologist, characterizes the patient interaction as having two components: a divulging of information at the time of diagnosis and a therapeutic dialogue that follows (Buckman, 1992). Divulging information, according to Buckman, requires careful consideration and preparation of how the diagnosis will be presented. The therapeutic dialogue requires the clinician to listen carefully and respond appropriately to how information is received. Buckman offers a protocol that attempts to balance the inevitable limitations of time in most clinical settings with the need to consider, in a sensitive way, the impact of the news. The following strategies are adapted from Buckman (1992) and influenced by the writing of Luterman (1979; 1991). They are also shaped by the authors' own experiences as bearers and recipients of difficult news.

Preparation

The physical setting should be arranged to minimize physical discomfort and ensure privacy. This generally requires a quiet room where the door can be closed and where the counseling session can proceed without interruption. Once seated it is important to make introductions and establish who is present and their relationship to the family. Buckman recommends starting with a question (e.g., How are you doing?) to convey concern about the parents' feelings and to encourage a conversational tone.

Find Out What the Family Already Knows

Most families come with at least some knowledge or expectation regarding their children's hearing status. This may be

based on previous audiologic assessments or information they have acquired on their own.

Pearl

- Allowing the family to talk first not only sets a tone that encourages conversational interaction; it also gives the clinician an opportunity to assess the family's level of understanding and communicative style.

It is important for the clinician to listen carefully, making good eye contact and showing a genuine interest in what parents say, even if their knowledge is incomplete or incorrect. This is also an opportunity to evaluate their emotional state.

Determine What the Family Wants to Know

Luterman (1979) emphasizes the importance of meeting parents where they are at each point in time. In addition to delivering information clearly and accurately with sensitivity to the impact of this news, it is important to remember that the parents' level of emotional upheaval is unrelated to the child's degree of hearing loss. For some families the diagnosis of mild or even unilateral hearing loss may be emotionally traumatic. Parents typically have many questions regarding the cause of hearing loss, and how they should proceed with intervention (Roush, 2000).

Pitfall

- Inexperienced clinicians may be inclined to provide more information than the family can comprehend, especially at the time of diagnosis.

Share Information

Although many parents are emotionally upset at the time of diagnosis, most want a forthright explanation of the findings, a preliminary treatment plan, the prognosis, and services available to them (Buckman, 1992, Roush, 2000). Luterman (1979, 2001) and English (2002) emphasize the importance of differentiating content questions. Both are important, but the latter requires careful listening and reflection. At the time of diagnosis and during the early weeks and months, many of the questions asked by parents may appear on the surface to be seeking content information when, in fact, there is an underlying concern (Clark and English, 2004).

Listening for Affect

Carl Rogers was an influential 20th century psychologist and founder of the humanist approach to psychology. Over time he moved away from traditional psychotherapy aimed at changing or curing patients to an approach that sought ways to facilitate personal growth in his patients. He encouraged listening for affect in an effort to identify underlying intent and feelings. The following question is one that might be asked by the parent of an infant with hearing loss:

"Will it ever be possible for him to wear all-in-the-ear hearing aids?"

Content-level reply: "I'm afraid that wouldn't work very well for him because of problems with acoustic feedback and difficulty coupling with his FM system."

Affect-level reply: "It's not easy seeing all that hardware on your new baby, is it?"

The clinician is not forced to choose one response over another. Often the best approach is to provide an accurate and straightforward answer to the question, but also to recognize and acknowledge what may be an underlying question or concern.

Although it is important for the clinician to listen for affect, it is also important to recognize that parents want and need information, and the nature of the information they seek can change over time. At the time of diagnosis, Harrison and Roush (2002) found that many parents of newly identified child are especially interested in the etiology of the child's hearing loss and issues related to coping with the emotional aspects of the diagnosis. Many parents also want information about how and when their children will learn to listen and speak. However, the same respondents indicated somewhat different needs for information a few months following the diagnosis, with many turning greater attention to communication options, timelines for developing speech and language, responsibilities of early intervention providers, and legal rights of children with hearing loss (Harrison and Roush, 2002). Still, it is important to remember that each family is unique. Asking them what they want to know and what they hope to accomplish at each visit ensures that counseling and information are relevant to their current goals and priorities.

Pediatric audiologists face a variety of counseling situations, but in many ways the first visit, at the time of diagnosis, is the most challenging. Buchman (1992) suggests that the initial session include four specific objectives related to diagnosis, treatment, prognosis, and support. As a starting point the audiologist can use the information provided by the parents about what they already know to reinforce what was accurate in their interpretation. Recognizing that many

people retain few details once confronted with serious news, information must be delivered in small increments consisting of a frank but sincere statement of the facts followed by elaboration and explanation. Applied to the diagnostic audiology visit, the clinician might say: "Our testing indicates that Ben has a hearing loss in both ears. We were able to obtain reliable test results and I feel this diagnosis is accurate." This candid appraisal might be followed by a reassuring statement that indicates what can be done to help the child and family. Buchman emphasizes the importance of using plain English, avoiding technical language and frequently checking on reception and understanding: "Am I making sense?" "Does this seem reasonable to you?" Important points need to be restated to ensure comprehension, and the clinician must remember that the primary concerns of a parent at the time of diagnosis may be difficult to predict. It is not unusual for parents to ask questions that pertain to issues many years into the future. At our university hospital, the first question from one parent of an infant on the day of diagnosis was not about etiology or prognosis for developing speech, but about the implications of her daughter's deafness when she becomes an adolescent. The best response in a case like this might be to simply state that "it's impossible to know the outcome that far in the future," acknowledging that "it must be difficult not knowing what this will mean for her," but then assuring the family that much can and will be done to assist her and her child.

- Clinicians can blend the patient's agenda with their own, respecting the parents' issues and concerns but highlighting the most important recommendations and carefully checking for comprehension of the information provided.

Respond to the Patient's Feelings

There is considerable variability in how parents respond to news about their child's hearing loss. Reactions may be shaped by many factors, including the knowledge they bring with them, but their response to the diagnosis may also be affected by social or cultural factors. It is sometimes informative to ask the family if they have ever met a person who is deaf, or if they know someone with congenital hearing loss. There can be mistaken beliefs or unwarranted concerns based on limited contact with a person who is deaf or hard of hearing; conversely, there may be a more optimistic attitude if past experiences have been positive.

Most families do not have prior experience with congenital hearing loss, and for many the diagnosis is profoundly disturbing. Several authors have examined initial reactions and various stages that follow a serious diagnosis including disbelief, shock, anger, guilt, denial, and displacement or diversion of activities (Luterman, 1985, 2001; Moses, 1987; Buchman, 1992; Clark and English, 2004). Feelings of guilt may be especially acute and enduring, even if the etiology is beyond the parents' control. Most parents eventually come to a point of acceptance ,but for some, especially in the first few weeks following diagnosis, emotions may fluctuate between hope and despair. When parents appear distraught, and most are, Buckman (1992) advises adherence to three principles, adapted here for application to a parent/child with hearing loss:

1. **Don't promise anything you can't deliver**. Overassurance about the implications of deafness is misleading and condescending to families. It is important to be realistic, but also to assure families that much can and will be done.

2. **Allow the parent to express his concerns and feelings.** Encouraging an honest expression of emotions gives parents permission to be themselves. They will remember and appreciate this later.

3. **Let them know your relationship will continue—they're not in this alone.** More than anything at this early stage, families want to know they are in capable hands and that you will help guide them through the process.

The inexperienced clinician should not be surprised if some parents respond with tears to the diagnosis of hearing loss. A crying parent can be disturbing even to the experienced clinician, but it is important to recognize that for many people this is a natural reaction and often a beneficial one. Pausing in the dialogue and providing a tissue lets them know it is okay to express their feelings. Years later most parents will still remember that encounter. They will not recall the specific information conveyed, but most will remember how they were treated and whether the audiologist expressed genuine concern and compassion (Luterman, 2001).

Follow-Up and Follow-Through

The most successful counseling session is incomplete without a well-articulated plan based on mutual understanding of what needs to happen next. This includes the specific action items from the clinician's perspective but it must also acknowledge questions or concerns raised by the parents. Remembering again that most parents do not recall everything they are told, it is important for them to leave with information to take home, carefully selected handouts and literature, contact information for professional service providers and other families, and an appointment card for the next visit. At the conclusion it is always advisable to confirm that everyone is in agreement on the next steps. If it is a new diagnosis, some pediatric audiologists will invite parents to call if they have further questions before the next appointment. Many will.

◆ Decisions about Amplification and Cochlear Implantation

Providing information at the time of diagnosis is emotionally demanding for parents and clinicians. Adding to the pressure is a need to make important decisions soon after the diagnosis. The most recent position statements of the Joint Committee on Infant Hearing (JCIH 2000; 2007) recommend that infants without medical contraindications and whose families concur, begin use of amplification within one month after confirmation of the hearing loss. For nearly all parents this is a stressful and uncertain period with implications for the entire family. Most families are ready to proceed with amplification at the time of diagnosis, and many appear to gain a sense of relief knowing that an intervention plan is under way. But some families are not ready to proceed at that pace and may require additional time. Indeed, when parents were asked to indicate the optimal time interval from diagnosis to hearing aid fitting, Sjoblad et al (2001) found that nearly three fourths of the parents surveyed said 3 to 4 weeks, but approximately one fourth believed that 1 to 3 months was optimal. This finding illustrates the natural variability among families and the importance of not assuming that all will want to proceed at the same pace. However, it may also reflect the need for better counseling or peer support at the time of diagnosis. It may be that families who favored a longer delay lacked the information and support needed to proceed comfortably with hearing aid selection and fitting (Roush, 2001).

An issue rarely discussed but on the minds of most parents is the issue of appearance. Deafness is often described as an invisible handicap. This changes once the child is fitted with hearing aids. Sjoblad et al (2001) reported that more than half of the parent respondents in her survey expressed concern about the appearance of the devices. Nearly two thirds also expressed concerns about the perceived benefits of amplification. Fortunately, for more than half the respondents, perceptions about both appearance and benefit became more positive, and only a small number (fewer than 5%) felt less positive over time.

When acoustic amplification proves to be unsuccessful or of limited value, families are faced with decisions about cochlear implantation. In recent years the decision has expanded to include the issue of unilateral versus bilateral implantation. As criteria for cochlear implantation become more liberal, implanting ears with usable residual hearing will occur more frequently. Audiologists can support families by staying current with cochlear implant technology and candidacy to provide accurate information and to ensure timely referral when consideration of implantation is appropriate. For children who already have one implant, the issue of bilateral implantation can be difficult, especially if it means losing an ear with aidable residual hearing. Bilateral implantation is a relatively new option and there is evidence of beneficial outcomes, but there are also anecdotal reports of older children and adults who do well with bimodal hearing, the simultaneous use of a cochlear implant on one side and amplification on the other. Considering the complexity of preselection, assessment, surgical intervention, mapping, and unilateral versus bilateral implantation, families will be best served by a team of professionals who specialize in cochlear implants.

◆ Decisions about Early Intervention

Maximizing developmental language outcomes for young children with hearing loss requires that children be fit with appropriate technology and intervention soon after the hearing loss has been identified (Yoshinaga-Itano et al, 1998; Carney and Moeller, 1998; Moeller, 2000). But to make informed decisions about therapeutic intervention or special services, families need information that is objective, culturally sensitive, and considerate of their emotional state (Luterman, 1985; Luterman and Kurtzer-White, 1999; JCIH, 2000, 2007). Audiologists who work with infants and their families must be familiar with legislative mandates as well as state and local referral procedures. Moreover, they must provide unbiased information regarding options for intervention.

Pearl

- The most important issue is not necessarily the initial decisions made by families, but how freely they can modify their service and intervention plans as they acquire more information and greater confidence.

This entails a philosophical orientation that encourages families to make their own decisions and for professionals to support them in this process. Parents often seek advice from audiologists in making decisions regarding available intervention services. It is important for audiologists to recognize that legal and regulatory issues are unfamiliar to most parents. The audiologist must be well informed about eligibility criteria and know where to refer families for accurate unbiased information regarding options available to them. Reports intended for those agencies must be written in a manner that will facilitate eligibility for special services, environmental modifications, and provision of FM or other assistive technologies.

◆ Counseling the Parents of Older Children and Adolescents

Transitions in life can be stressful for any family, but they may be especially difficult when they involve a child with special needs. Important transitions for a child with hearing loss include home- to center-based services, early intervention to preschool, preschool to kindergarten, elementary to middle or high school, and transition at any age from a self-contained program to mainstream settings. The inevitable changes that occur with routines and personnel can bring anxiety to even the most secure and self-confident parent. Many parents report recycling previous emotions (grief, worry, frustration) as they face new challenges or confront new milestones. At age three, when transitioning from early intervention to school-based services, parents are often concerned about maintaining the quality and quantity of services they have had during the first three years. They are also anxious about life skills in a new setting. The transition to preschool or from preschool to kindergarten often entails noisy environments and teachers with little or no experience managing hearing aids and FM systems. Parents may worry about their children being left behind as classes move from room to room, or left out when children interact socially. As children progress through the elementary grades, the work is more challenging academically and many families feel the need for additional services. Children with hearing loss may get so focused on listening that comprehension lags. And the need to listen and learn is not limited to academic material. Flexer (1999) emphasizes the importance of overhearing pragmatic transactions as well as the incidental conversations that occur among children.

In middle school most children seek conformity. Although this can be a challenging time for the child and family, optimal communication is the key to maximizing academic and social success. Good acoustic environments rarely exist in the educational setting so it becomes imperative for the audiologist to collaborate effectively with parents and with school personnel to advocate for assistive technology and support systems. Once provided there needs to be ongoing management of the acoustic environment, appropriate microphone use, and modifications of communication style to optimize the child's receptive communication (Madell, 2001). The clinic-based audiologist can play a key role by ensuring that parents are aware of school-based services and to provide the documentation needed to make sure the child qualifies for assistive technology and special services. This is especially important as some states are revising IDEA eligibility criteria. The audiologist can assist parents in their advocacy efforts by making sure they understand the legal and regulatory issues that determine eligibility and maintenance of special services. This can be accomplished by the audiologist providing information directly or by referring the family to an appropriate agency, institution, or resource person. In that context the relationship between the parent and the audiologist is a collaborative one based on informational counseling essential to the acquisition of hearing instruments, assistive technologies, or support services.

◆ Other Sources of Information for Families

Audiologists and professional service providers were at one time the primary sources of information available to families. Today, many have access to information via the Internet, advocacy organizations, and other resources. Direct communication with other parents has expanded considerably in recent years and for many families represents a vital resource. There are also a growing number of states that provide family centered information and advocacy services.

Professional Support for New Families

For more than 20 years, a program based in North Carolina, Beginnings for Parents of Children who are Deaf or Hard of Hearing (www.beginningservices.com), has provided emotional support, unbiased information about communication and educational options, and technical assistance to parents whose children range in age from birth to 21 (Alberg, Wilson, and Roush, 2006). Beginnings also supports parents who are deaf or hard of hearing and whose children may or may not have hearing loss. The belief that parents should be the primary decision makers for their child is a guiding principle for Beginnings. When a child in North Carolina is diagnosed with a hearing loss, parents are informed about Beginnings and invited to talk with a parent educator. Audiologists are the primary source of referral, although anyone can make a referral. A parent educator is assigned to each family referred to Beginnings. Parents provide informed consent for parent educators to first contact the referral source to gain additional information regarding the family and their needs. The parent educator then meets with the family at a convenient time and place, usually in the family's home. Initially, home visits are intended to ensure that parents understand their child's hearing loss and to provide information regarding financial assistance, language development, communication options and early intervention services. Beginnings parent educators emphasize the importance of keeping appointments with the audiologist and they encourage parents to enroll their child as soon as possible in North Carolina's early intervention program, offering assistance if needed with the logistics of scheduling and transportation. The Beginnings model, which provides a bridge between the pediatric audiologist and early intervention providers, has been so successful it is now being replicated in several other states (Alberg, Wilson, and Roush, 2006).

Parent-to-Parent Support

Among the greatest gifts the pediatric audiologist can give to families is a direct link to other parents. Many experienced parents are willing to be available by phone or in person, and some are willing to initiate contact if desired by the family. Once parents are ready to connect with a larger circle of families, parent support groups can become an invaluable resource. In North Carolina a volunteer organization called HITCH-UP (Hearing Impaired Toddlers and Children Have Unlimited Potential), founded by parents and now active in several regions within the state, provides monthly support groups for families. Operated entirely by parents without public support, HITCH-UP plays an important role in providing peer support, exchange of information, and advice to professional organizations for improving and expanding services to families with children who are deaf or hard of hearing. The most effective support groups are often loosely structured, informal organizations that meet regularly, invite professionals to speak on topics of interest, and organize social functions throughout the year. It is comforting for families to know they are not alone and that they can interact with other families facing similar circumstances. One of the authors (GK) has drawn considerable strength from other families as well as satisfaction in seeing new families join and benefit from the collective experiences of many.

Internet Resources

Every year the Internet becomes a more important source of information for families. For many it is a primary resource for personal and health-related issues. An Internet search using the terms Hearing Loss in Children will produce hundreds of Web sites offering information on every aspect of hearing loss and its management. Needless to say, information from the Web varies in complexity and accuracy. A Web-based resource that has been especially helpful to families is www.babyhearing.org, developed at Boy's Town National Research Hospital with a grant from the National Institutes of Health. The site provides accurate, up-to-date information in English or Spanish, at a level most families can comprehend.

◆ Conclusion

Pediatric audiologists, especially those who work with newly identified infants and young children and their families, are called upon to serve as information providers and counselors. The role of informant often begins with an explanation of the diagnosis and options for audiologic intervention with amplification or cochlear implantation. In these technical matters families want and need an audiologist who is confident and self-assured, and willing and able to provide an accurate but understandable explanation of the findings and recommendations. But it is equally important for the audiologist to listen to families, their questions, their priorities, and their needs at each point in time. This requires the audiologist to serve as both counselor and confidant; roles that require, in addition to effective expressive communication, careful listening and reflection.

Families have access to a tremendous amount of information about their hearing loss. The pediatric audiologist can assist families by staying current with available resources, by identifying information that is accurate and up-to-date, and by making recommendations for how families can access and use available resources. Connecting parents with other parents is especially important. Where family resources are unsatisfactory or insufficient, audiologists can work with parents to establish better mechanisms for peer support and advocacy. They can empower families by promoting partnerships that encourage parents to assume responsibility for decisions that impact their children's educational and audiologic management. A few parents will be interested in working to make improvements at a systems level and some may even influence public policies and procedures. For all families, the audiologist can provide consultation and referral to appropriate institutions, informational resources, and advocacy groups. By recognizing the dual responsibility of information provider and counselor, and the importance of working collaboratively, the audiologist can facilitate the most important outcome: confident, well informed families capable of determining what is best for their child and comfortable knowing they will be supported and encouraged by their professional service providers.

Summary Pearls

- Families need hope based on the knowledge that much can and will be done to help them and their child.

- When delivering difficult news, give families an opportunity to respond and express their feelings; don't be afraid of a little silence.

- At the outset of each clinic appointment ask families what they are hoping to accomplish at that visit. Return to their priorities at the conclusion of the visit to determine if their goals were met and to confirm agreement on next steps.

- Observe parents interacting with their child and praise their efforts. Simple phrases: "Look how he responds to you!" are encouraging and empowering to parents.

Summary Pitfalls

- Providing too much information at one time can be overwhelming to parents.

- Delivering news in a manner that is overly positive fails to consider the seriousness of the situation.

- Delivering news in a manner that is negative or pessimistic can hinder the families' progress toward achieving a hopeful outlook for the future.

- Clinicians should not assume that they know how a family feels or what they want for their child. Trusting and collaborative relationships develop slowly over time.

Discussion Questions

- What does it mean to be family-centered? What if the parent's priorities or decisions differ from those of the audiologist?

- Some families are slow to accept the diagnosis and reluctant to move forward with the audiologist's recommendations. Although it is important to recognize that families need to move at their own pace, what factors might account for lack of acceptance and what might you do to help them?

References

Alberg, J., Wilson, K., and Roush, J. (2006). Statewide collaboration in the delivery of EHDI services. The Volta Review, 106, 259–274.

Bailey, D. B., McWilliam, R. A., Aytch Darkes, et al. (1998). Family outcomes in early intervention: a framework for program evaluation and efficacy research. Exceptional Children, 64, 313–328.

Bronfenbrenner, U. (1977). Toward an experimental ecology of human development. American Psychologist, 32, 513–521.

Buckman, R. (1992). How to break bad news: a guide for health care professionals. Baltimore: Johns Hopkins University Press.

Carney, A. E., and Moeller, M. P. (1998). Treatment efficacy: hearing loss in children. Journal of Speech Language and Hearing Research, 41, S61–84.

Clark, J., and English, K. (2004). Counseling in audiologic practice. Boston: Allyn and Bacon.

Crais, E. R., Poston Roy, V., and Free, K. (2006). Parents' and professionals' perceptions of the implementation of family-centered practices in child assessments. American Journal of Speech-Language Pathology, 15, 365–377.

Dunst, C. J. (2000). Revisiting "Rethinking early intervention." Topics in Early Childhood Special Education, 20, 95–104.

English, K. (2002). Counseling children with hearing impairment and their families. Boston: Allyn and Bacon.

Flexer, C. (1999). Facilitating hearing and listening in young children. San Diego: Singular Publishing Group.

Harrison, M., and Roush, J. (2002) Information for families with young deaf and hard-of-hearing children: reports from parents and pediatric audiologists. In R. Seewald and J. Gravel (Eds.), A sound foundation through early amplification, Proceedings of the Second International Conference (pp. 233–251). United Kingdom: St. Edmundsbury Press.

Joint Committee on Infant Hearing Year 2000 Position Statement. (2000; 2007).

Luterman, D. (1979). Counseling parents of hearing impaired children. Boston: Little, Brown.

Luterman, D. (1985). The denial mechanism. Ear and Hearing, 6, 57–58.

Luterman, D. (1991). Counseling the communicatively disordered and their families. Austin: Pro-Ed.

Luterman, D. (2001). Counseling persons with communication disorders and their families (4th ed.). Austin: Pro-ed.

Luterman, D., and Kurtzer-White, E. (1999). Identifying hearing loss: parents' needs. American Journal of Audiology, 8, 13–18.

Luterman, D. M. (1995). Counseling for parents of children with auditory disorders. In R. Roeser and M. Downs (Eds.), Auditory disorders in school children (3rd ed., pp. 352–362). New York: Thieme.

Madell, J. (2001). Assistive listening technology for infants and young children with hearing loss. In E. Kurtzer-White and D. Luterman (Eds.), Early childhood deafness (pp. 73–94).

Moses, K. (1987). The impact of childhood disability: the parent's struggle. Ways Magazine, Spring issue.

Moeller, M. P. (2000). Early intervention and language development in children who are deaf and hard of hearing. Pediatrics, 106, E43, 1–9.

Roush, J. (2000). Implementing parent–infant services: advice from families. In R. Seewald (Ed.), A sound foundation through early amplification (pp. 159–165). Phonak, AG.

Roush, J. (2000) What happens after screening? Hearing Journal, Special Issue: Universal Newborn Hearing Screening, Philadelphia: Lippincott Williams and Wilkins, 53, 56–60.

Roush, J. (2001). Staying family centered. In E. Kurtzer-White and D. Luterman (Eds.), Early childhood deafness Timonium, MD: York Press, 49–62.

Roush, J. (2000). Implementing parent-infant services: advice from families. In R. Seewald (Ed.), A sound foundation through early amplification Stafa, Switzerland: Phonak, AG, 159–165.

Simeonsson, R. J., Huntington, G. S., Sturtz-McMillen, J., Haugh-Dodds, A., Halperin, D., and Zipper, I. (1996). Services for young children and families: evaluating intervention cycles. Infants and Young Children, 9, 31–42.

Sjoblad, S. Harrison, M., Roush, J., and McWilliams, R. (2001). Parents' reactions and recommendations after diagnosis and hearing aid fitting. American Journal of Audiology, 10, 24–31.

Trivette, C. M, Dunst, C.J, Boyd, K., and Hamby, D. W. (1995). Family-oriented program models, helpgiving practices, and parental control appraisals. Exceptional Children, 62, 237–248.

Yoshinaga-Itano, C., Sedey, A., Coulter, D.K., and Mehl, A. L. (1998). Language of early and later identified children with hearing loss. Pediatrics, 102, 1161–1171.

Chapter 29

Educating and Counseling Children and Teens with Hearing Loss

Kris English

♦ **Teaching and Counseling in the 21st Century**

Audiologists as Teachers

Audiologists as Counselors

♦ **Teaching and Counseling Younger Children**

Additional Resources

♦ **Teaching and Counseling Middle- and High-School Teens**

Teaching and Counseling in a Group Format

Case Study

Analysis

♦ **Do We See a Red Flag?**

♦ **Conclusion**

Key Points

1. Educating children about hearing loss requires an updated understanding of how people learn.

2. Counseling children and teens about living with hearing loss requires audiologists to know the answer to the question, "Who owns this hearing loss?"

3. Most materials designed to teach children about hearing loss can also be used as a springboard to counseling conversations about their reactions and concerns about living with hearing loss.

4. If the audiologist suspects that a child has a more complicated learning or emotional problem than a hearing loss can account for, the audiologist must convey those concerns to parents and to an appropriate specialist.

Audiologists are uniquely qualified to teach children and teens about their hearing loss, and to provide counseling support for psychological or emotional reactions associated with hearing loss. This chapter will describe how audiologists can educate and counsel children with hearing loss from elementary school age to the teen years.

♦ Teaching and Counseling in the 21st Century

Audiologists as Teachers

Before we begin, it is important to update our thinking about "teaching." Traditionally, this process implies that the adult talks while the child listens. This approach assumes that when words are spoken by the adult, the child will understand and remember those words, and translate them into meaningful concepts (i.e., will learn).

However, research indicates that this assumption is flawed. When measured by outcomes, the "teaching-by-telling/learning-by-listening" approach tends to result in unimpressive results. Children who merely listen to lectures or directions will soon forget most of what was said, and will usually not generalize what they do remember to other situations (National Research Council, 2000).

On the other hand, when learners are actively engaged in their own learning, they demonstrate more desirable outcomes. When learners participate in problem-solving, discussion, role-playing, research, "thinking out loud" activities, building, creating, or writing, they are more likely to understand new content because they discover connections to previously learned content. Those connections help them remember the new content longer, and apply that content to novel situations. Although not a new idea (see Dewey, 1938), recent neurological evidence now supports the use of active learning: compared with listening only, "learning by doing" results in more neural activity and the creation of more synaptic connections, which allow the brain to function more efficiently (Zull, 2002).

With this evidence in mind, this chapter provides an in-depth suggestion designed to engage the school-aged child and the teen as active learners, and a short list of additional resources for each group. Audiologists will note that this approach will also require them to reconsider their role as teacher, here held to be less a "sage on the stage" and more a "guide on the side."

Audiologists as Counselors

We also need to update the concept of counseling as it applies to audiology. Until recently, counseling and explaining were considered synonymous. However, counseling actually has two domains: informational counseling (explaining content, or teaching as we discussed earlier), and personal adjustment counseling (Kennedy and Charles, 2001). Neither domain was effectively addressed in audiology training in the past, but, as audiology evolves into a doctoral-level profession, most graduate programs now include counseling in their curriculums (English and Weist, 2005).

Personal support counseling in pediatric settings attempts to help children understand their reactions to living with hearing loss, and to accept themselves as persons with impaired hearing. The principles of audiologic counseling have much in common with active learning: rather than telling children how they should feel or act or think or believe, audiologists should develop strategies to help children explain to themselves how they perceive the world and their lives. By describing out loud (by voice or sign) how she thinks and feels, a child is now better able to understand those thoughts and feelings, and thus takes the first step in learning how to handle them.

During this process, audiologists-as-counselors must resist playing the role of rescuer. It is very tempting to take over with advice and action plans, or try to help children feel better. In all aspects of counseling, practitioners are reminded to ask themselves, "Who owns this problem?" Individuals must assume responsibility of owning a problem before assuming the responsibility of addressing the problem. In audiology, we must routinely ask ourselves, "Who owns this hearing loss?" (Clark and English, 2004). For the population under consideration, the answer for younger children is, "The child and parents." As children become teens, the ownership of their hearing loss must gradually transition from parents to the teens.

This chapter will therefore also include a discussion on how to help children and teens own their hearing loss as they acquire new information about hearing. Blending informational and personal adjustment counseling into the same activities is not only efficient; it is also a natural process. All learners have emotional and psychological reactions to the material they are learning, particularly when the instructional material is about themselves. It is both expeditious and logical to discuss what one is learning, and

how one thinks, feels, and believes about that learning, at the same time.

> **Pitfall**
>
> - It may seem more efficient to an audiologist to assume a directive (telling) role rather than a facilitative one when teaching or counseling children. Consider the time spent as an investment in the future: the long-term goal is to help the child develop independence, confidence, and strategies to succeed, and these goals are acquired only with practice and support. They cannot be taught by telling.

◆ Teaching and Counseling Younger Children

One of the most useful materials available to the audiologist is a curriculum called "Knowledge Is Power–KIP" (Martilla and Mills, 2002). This program provides lessons designed to help children understand their hearing loss, hearing aids, assistive devices, and more. Lessons are written in both an introductory and an advanced level, so that the audiologist can present the same material in more depth as the child becomes older.

Each lesson has specific learning objectives to reflect increasing interest in obtaining measurable outcomes. The curriculum contains crisp graphics to explain the function of hearing aids and cochlear implants, Web pages for assistive devices and legislation information, information about telephone relay services, and auditory testing, including otoacoustic emissions and auditory brainstem response.

Each lesson also includes pretests and posttests to measure learning, and take-home letters asking parents or caregivers to review content with their child. This review surely helps the parent as well as the child, and hopefully helps both parent and child feel comfortable talking about hearing problems. In addition, a page on hearing aid care is provided to serve as a stand-alone handout for a child who would like to develop a presentation for her class.

Earlier it was mentioned that we might strive to combine instruction and counseling into the same activities. The KIP curriculum provides resources to do just that. A section called "Our Stories" has contributions from children and young adults with hearing loss, and their own words are used. No editing was done to clean up syntax and grammar. Children can be encouraged to read "Our Stories," and either write their own stories, or discuss the stories in KIP: Are there similarities to their own experiences? Are there lessons to learn? What would they want to ask the author? What would they want to add to the stories?

The section titled "Coping, Part 1" asks children to consider big questions such as "How do you feel about your hearing loss?" "Does your family accept your hearing loss?"

"Who do you talk to when you have a problem?" Topics about responsibility for communication problems and friendships are open for consideration, and KIP gives a framework for the audiologist to bring them to the fore.

The section called "Coping, Part 2" provides a helpful introduction about how audiologists might help children recognize that negative beliefs ("I should not have to wear this hearing aid") can create barriers for themselves, affecting how they feel and ultimately how they act. A set of activities is provided to help children identify how they do think about circumstances, and then how they can change those thoughts.

Special Consideration

- Although counseling is now part of most audiology training programs, it is not uncommon for an audiologist to feel unprepared for these kinds of conversations. In that situation, it is recommended that an appropriate professional be contacted for help. A school counselor, social worker, or psychologist could provide invaluable support, but may also need specialized information from the audiologist to meet children's needs.

Additional Resources

Following is a short list of other materials audiologists can use for teaching and counseling. Each resource provides opportunities to share new information as well as to listen for a child's thoughts and feelings.

- The Hearing Performance Inventory for Children (Giolas, Maxon, and Kessler, 1997) addresses school listening challenges. Pictures of different scenarios help children identify the problems faced in the classroom and describe their strategies in solving the problems and their confidence levels in doing so.

- Listening Inventories for Education (LIFE) (Anderson and Smaldino, 1998) addresses school listening challenges and collects perceptions from teachers. Children can learn more about their hearing loss as they consider their challenges and learn how those challenges are perceived by others.

- I Start/You Finish (English, 2002) is an open-ended activity that will address what the child chooses to talk about. Children complete "stem phrases" such as "I am happy when..." "I am sad when..." "The thing I like most in the world is..." "The thing I would most like to change is..." "Because I have hearing loss..."

- Time Out! I Didn't Hear You (Palmer et al, 1996) addresses participation in sports. As with the other suggestions named above, this manual presents a range of listening challenges, with solutions that can focus on teaching and personal adjustment.

♦ Teaching and Counseling Middle- and High-School Teens

It may surprise the reader to learn that few materials are available for the audiologist who wants to continue teaching and counseling children as they reach their teen years. However, one tool has been expressly designed for this purpose. It is called the Self-Assessment of Communication—Adolescents (SAC-A) (Elkayam and English, 2003), and it was modified from an instrument originally designed for adults. The original SAC (Schow and Nerbonne, 1982) is a popular self-assessment tool because it is short, addresses multiple domains, and has a version that a significant other (SO) can complete. A comparison of the two reports leads to insights regarding the stressors, thoughts, and feelings of both patient and significant other. The ensuing conversation is often the first time both parties communicate with each other about specific challenges associated with hearing loss.

The SO version of the SAC-A is to be completed by a good friend (the Significant Other Assessment of Communication—Adolescent [SOAC-A]). Both instruments have 12 questions about how the teen with hearing loss functions, how the teen feels about her hearing loss, and what others might have mentioned about her hearing loss. For example, are there problems communicating with one person? A small group? Listening to entertainment? Does the teen feel left out or upset when it's hard to hear, or does it seem people often get the wrong impression because of the hearing loss?

To use the SAC-A and the SOAC-A as a teaching and counseling tool, the audiologist would first ask if the teen is interested in completing the SAC-A, and have a friend complete the SOAC-A. As with most self-assessment administrations, the two parties are not likely to be in full agreement with their answers. Depending on the teen's preference, the audiologist can ask the teen to expand on answers in the friend's presence, or in private. The audiologist can learn if the teen is experiencing problems, understands the problems, or needs help solving them. Is the problem something technology can improve? Is the teen aware of the technology (or relevant communication repair strategy)? Is the teen aware of a solution but unwilling to make a change at this time?

Pearl

- The audiologist can be mindful of a counseling maxim: "Help is defined by the recipient." Although it is tempting to provide every solution possible to the teen, the teen must declare what help is desired. The audiologist's first role is to serve as a sounding board, then to convey trust in the teen's own ability to find solutions to many of these problems, before "leapfrogging" into problem-solving mode (Stone, Patton, and Heen, 1999).

Anecdotal evidence indicates that many teens do not have a friend they can approach to help with this activity. If this is the case, the audiologist should take extra care to be readily available to the teen, and to watch for the possible need to refer to a professional counselor (Stepp, 2000).

Teaching and Counseling in a Group Format

The counseling activity described above is likely to be a one-on-one conversation between teen and audiologist. However, the benefits of group and peer interaction are well known, especially for teens, and the audiologist may decide to capitalize on the dynamics of a group format to help teens tackle the challenges of living with hearing loss.

In keeping with the philosophy expressed throughout this chapter that help is defined by the recipient, it is recommended that the audiologist conduct a teen education/counseling group in a format similar to that described by Hickson (2007). Rather than predeveloping a lecture or presenting packaged material, the audiologist allows the members of the group to set the agenda. The audiologist might feel uncomfortable about releasing this kind of control, so she should be clear that the goals are to help teens (1) express their thoughts and reactions to living with hearing loss; (2) develop some insights about their thoughts and reactions; (3) learn a helpful strategy or two; and (4) obtain a sense of support from others who have the same experiences. These are teen-centered goals, and therefore not goals that an audiologist can teach. Teens need to actively engage in the process to achieve those goals.

How would such a program be managed? A basic overview would include these steps: Once teens are seated and introductions are made, the audiologist models a teen-centered approach from the beginning by informing the group members that they will determine the topics for discussion. To keep the focus on hearing, they can be asked to complete a statement such as, "Because I have hearing loss..." The audiologist writes each response on a chalkboard or big piece of paper. If teens do not know and trust each other yet, they may prefer to write their thoughts on a piece of paper; these are then read aloud but anonymously. When responses are similar or overlapping, they can be clustered together thematically. The audiologist then directs the group to consider all the responses and ask, "As a group, what are our top three concerns today?" The group must prioritize from the choices and acknowledge that not all topics will be addressed.

When the top three topics are identified, the audiologist facilitates the discussion with the following three prompts:

♦ As a group, what do we know about each topic (i.e., develop common ground)?

♦ What might explain the situation (develop group insights)?

♦ What would help the situation (problem-solving)? Note that problem-solving is not attempted until teens feel understood, and until they are given the opportunity to understand the underlying concerns.

Case Study

A group of teens indicates that Topic #1 was "Because I have hearing loss... I feel left out most the time." The audiologist first asks, "As a group, what do we know about feeling left out? What does it look like, what does it feel like?" Possible answers might be: never being asked for a date; not receiving any text messages or phone calls; rarely being included in trips to the movies; having only one friend when most people seem to have several, etc. As the teens describe their observations and experiences, the audiologist will give teens the floor as much as possible. To ensure that outcome, when each teen is finished speaking, it is particularly helpful to ask the teen to call on the next speaker, rather than the audiologist doing so. This strategy helps the teens talk to each other instead of only to the expert adult.

When it is clear that the group has fully addressed the first question, the audiologist asks the second question: "What might explain why teens with hearing loss feel left out?" Possible answers might include: persons with normal hearing do not understand hearing loss; people with hearing loss have less energy for socializing; teens with hearing loss may be self-conscious about making social mistakes and that could make others uncomfortable, etc.

When all possible insights are expressed, the final question is, "There is much agreement in this group about the experiences of feeling left out and why that might happen. What would help the situation?" Some teens are natural problem solvers; other teens benefit from observing that skill. Each group member should describe one strategy they will try to improve their situation.

Now the group moves on. Topic #2 is "Because I have a hearing loss... I have to work 10 times harder at schoolwork than other kids." The audiologist again facilitates the discussion with the same questions: What do we know about learning with hearing loss? What might explain the situation? What would help the situation? And so on.

Analysis

Were the goals of this teen group met? Let's review: The goals were to help teens (1) express their thoughts and reactions to living with hearing loss; (2) develop some insights about their thoughts and reactions; (3) learn a helpful strategy or two; and (4) obtain a sense of support from others who have the same experiences. In this case study, the audiologist organized the teen meeting in such a way that all teens had the chance to talk, share, vent, commiserate, learn, and engage in problem solving. If the teens were polled after the session, it is likely they would affirm that these goals were indeed met.

♦ Do We See a Red Flag?

Clearly, the interactions described above take the audiologist and child beyond the superficial "Are your hearing aids working OK?" relationship. Now that we are genuinely talking and listening, we may notice that a child's learning style is affected not only by the hearing loss, but by other traits as well (attention span, logic, knowledge base, memory skills, for instance). The audiologist should discuss these observations with the classroom teacher, since that professional may have attributed all learning challenges to the hearing loss alone.

Additionally, during these interactions, conversations are inherently more personal and may lead to new self-disclosures. That change also brings a new responsibility: we may now perceive that a child is experiencing more than the expected problems of living with hearing loss. Even when the audiologist is not sure about the concerns, she must work with the site's referral process to ensure that a professional counselor becomes involved.

♦ Conclusion

When adults plan their teaching, they often ask themselves, "What am I going to cover (talk about)?" Although typical, this approach gives no attention to the learner's role in the process. Instead of that question, audiologists involved with instruction and counseling should ask themselves, "What is the child going to do?" If the answer is, "Listen and take notes," the instruction must be redesigned! A learner-centered approach will result in more learning, so the answer needs to be, "The child will do" something, such as

♦ write a story

♦ describe anatomy to a parent

♦ find information on new devices and share it with friends

♦ conduct a survey

♦ interview a peer about friendships

The time available to teach and counsel children is usually limited, so the audiologist will want to use that time as effectively as possible. Audiologists who engage in this level of support will find it to be a highlight of their career.

Discussion Questions

1. Describe a time when you participated in an exceptionally positive learning experience. Why was experience memorable? What did the designer of that instruction do to ensure that you understood and remembered the content? Describe your emotional or psychological response to that learning experience. Was that response important?

2. Children must feel a sense of safety before they open up to (learn) new information. Are children with hearing loss comfortable talking to their audiologists? What barriers might exist, and what can audiologists do to remove those barriers?

3. Stepp (2000) wrote that teens need support from three groups: peers, parents, and other adults, such as youth group leaders, coaches, and teachers. The role of other adults is to endow teens with confidence so that they can gradually disconnect from parents and develop autonomy with increasing self-direction. Do audiologists typically relate to teens with hearing loss as influential other adults? Why or why not?

References

Anderson, K., and Smaldino, J. (1998). Listening Inventories for Education (LIFE). Educational Audiology Association. 800-460-7322. www.edaud.org.

Clark, J. G., and English, K. (2004). Audiologic counseling: helping patients and families adjust to hearing loss. Boston: Allyn & Bacon.

Dewey, J. (1938). Experience and education. New York: Macmillan & Co.

Elkayam, J., and English, K. (2003). Counseling adolescents with hearing loss with the use of self-assessment/significant other questionnaires. Journal of the American Academy of Audiology, 14, 485–499.

English, K. (2002). Counseling children with hearing impairment and their families. Boston: Allyn & Bacon.

English, K., and Weist, D. (2005).Proliferation of AuD degrees found to increase training in counseling. Hearing Journal, 58, 54–58.

Giolas, T., Maxon, A., and Kessler, A. (1997). Hearing Performance Inventory for Children (HPIC). Educational Audiology Association. 800-460-7433.www.edaud.org. Last accessed

Hickson, L. (2007). Pull out an "ACE" to help your patients become better communicators. Hearing Journal, 60, 10–16.

Kennedy, E., and Charles, S. (2001). On becoming a counselor: a basic guide for nonprofessional counselors. New York: Consortium.

Martilla, J., and Mills, M. (2002). Knowledge is power. Educational Audiology Association. 800-460-7322. www.edaud.org.

National Research Council. (2000). How people learn: brain, mind, experience and school. Washington, DC: National Academy Press.

Palmer, C., Butts, C., Lindley, G., and Snyder, S. (1996). Time out! I didn't hear you. Educational Audiology Association. 800-460-7433. www.edaud.org. Last accessed

Schow, R., and Nerbonne, M. (1982). Communication screening profile: use with elderly patients. Ear and Hearing, 3, 135–147.

Stepp, L. (2000). Our last best shot: guiding our children through early adolescence. New York: Riverhead Books.

Stone, D., Patton, B., and Heen, S. (1999). Difficult conversations: how to discuss what matters most. New York: Viking Press.

Zull, J. (2002).The art of changing the brain: enriching the practice of teaching by exploring the biology of learning. Sterling, VA: Stylus Publishing.

Chapter 30

Facilitating Clinic–School Coordination

Meredith Berger and Susan Cheffo

Key Points

- The following characteristics and methods contribute to a positive clinic–school partnership; support, communication, and information sharing.

- Effective communication between agencies can occur in a variety of ways.

- The sharing of information benefits both the clinic and the school as they work together to meet a child's needs.

When a child is diagnosed with a hearing loss, two separate entities converge in his life—one is medical and the other one is educational. Too often, these entities remain independent of one another, to the detriment of the child. However, a strong partnership between the clinic which provides audiologic, otologic, and other medical services, and the school that provides educational support can bridge the gap between medical and educational management of hearing loss.

♦ The Educational Consultant in the Clinic

Ideally, each clinic and hospital working with children with hearing loss should employ an educational consultant or coordinator who acts as the liaison between the clinic and the school. This person is usually a certified teacher of the deaf/hard of hearing (TOD) who is knowledgeable about hearing loss, current technology, and communication options. This qualified individual also should be well informed about the educational needs of children who are deaf or hard of hearing and about the education system itself. In clinics without an educational consultant, a speech language pathologist, social worker, or audiologist may need to step into this role. That is, someone who is employed by the community-based clinic needs to be responsible for developing a partnership with schools to share information and advance the child's interests.

In addition to the knowledge an educational consultant possesses, several strategies facilitate a successful school–clinic partnership:

♦ Understand the roles of the various school professionals.

♦ Cultivate a relationship with school professionals, including administrators, classroom teachers, and related service providers.

♦ Support and respect the various professionals and their unique roles in the child's education.

♦ Listen effectively to the concerns of the school professionals.

♦ Understand that the child with the hearing loss is one of many children for whom the educators are responsible.

♦ Provide flexible options and choices to address problems.

♦ Discuss information with school professionals before putting observations and suggestions in writing.

Pearl

- Strong interpersonal skills are key to creating a positive working relationship with schools. Providing a pat on the back and offering encouragement will keep the doors open at schools, allowing the educational consultant continued entry. A harmonious relationship between the clinic and school will result in a successful educational outcome for the student.

◆ Establishing Communication

When the child first comes under the care of the clinic, the parents should be asked for information about his educational history, current school placement, provision of related services such as speech-language pathology and TOD, and the frequency of delivered services. It is important that the clinic know the primary educational contact at the school, that person's title or role, and contact information (Cheffo, 2003). At times, the person whom the parents identify as the primary contact may not be the person in a position to make major changes, but may be the person who the parents feel knows the child best.

When first making contact with the school, the clinician should be cognizant of the roles and politics within the school hierarchy and attempt to follow the chain of command. This protocol may vary from school to school. For example, if the parents indicate that the classroom teacher is the best person to speak with regarding the child, a call of introduction to the principal before asking to speak with the teacher is appropriate. In other schools, there may be a case manager or guidance counselor who should be spoken to first. Although this line of command may seem time consuming, following the proper procedures will ultimately create a more positive, open, and effective relationship.

◆ Exchange of Information

Although the clinic staff possesses a great deal of information about hearing loss and about the child, the exchange of information between clinic and school is not one-sided. Professionals in the school are knowledgeable about expectations for typically developing hearing peers and have a great deal of information about the child who is deaf or hard of hearing since they are with him almost daily. Specifically, school personnel are in a unique position to provide feedback to the clinic about

- the consistency of hearing aid/cochlear implant use
- family involvement
- current educational environment and demands
- areas or situations in which the child is demonstrating difficulty
- changes in behavior or responses after amplification or mapping adjustments
- unexpected changes in performance or in academic-social functioning (Zwolan, 2006)

The school providers and decision makers are not experts in hearing loss. Some school districts have an educational audiologist who can offer information to school staff. Usually this individual is contracted out by that district. Other districts use the TOD to provide the necessary information to staff. Information needed by the school district to appropriately meet the child's needs includes

- general information about hearing loss
- the child's type and degree of hearing loss
- how the hearing loss effects the child at various levels of education
- the type of technology (hearing aids and/or cochlear implants) used
- frequency modulation (FM) systems including when and how to use them
- how to use and troubleshoot all technologies used by the child
- the management plan that the clinic has or is developing for hearing aid trials, FM use, and frequency of follow-up visits to the clinic
- therapy strategies and approaches, such as acoustic highlighting, closed set versus open set listening, and preview and review of academic curricula
- ways of developing and monitoring appropriately high expectations for academic success

Communication between the clinic and school team members needs to occur in order for coordination to be effective; however, contact between the school and clinic cannot take place without parental permission. The Health Insurance Portability and Accountability Act regulations followed by hospital-based personnel, and confidentiality regulations followed by the schools require a signed release from the child's legal guardian before any communication is shared. Once the release is signed, phone, face-to-face, and written communications are all generally acceptable ways of giving out information. E-mail should be used within the boundaries of current communication regulations. Many facilities do not permit e-mail communication of patient information because of security concerns. All communication exchanges should be documented through chart notes and logs.

Often, classroom teachers and school-based therapists have limited access to the telephone during the school day, which can make communication challenging. Because school and clinic personnel juggle busy schedules, creative communication is often needed to stay in touch. After the initial contact has been made with or by the school, there are numerous ways information can be obtained and shared: via fax, through phone conversations or teleconferences, through secure e-mail, notebooks, logs, and in-person during site visits.

◆ Types of Reports

In educational and clinical environments, regular reports are generated. Reports commonly generated by the schools include

- Individual Education Plan (IEP) or Individual Family Service Plan (IFSP)
- IEP progress reports
- related service reports
- academic report cards
- academic progress reports

The clinic also produces reports describing the child including

- hearing evaluation reports, including the audiogram and a description of the child's performance with technology
- speech, language, and functional listening evaluations
- cochlear implant programming reports

Before an appointment at the clinic, information about the child's functional performance and emerging educational issues can be effectively communicated through a brief note from the school staff to the clinic staff. The child's speech perception/misperception competencies provided by the speech-language pathologist (SLP) or TOD will help the clinical audiologist adjust the cochlear implant or hearing aid settings. After an adjustment to the settings of a hearing aid or a cochlear implant program, the clinical audiologist should report these changes to the school personnel. Information about audiologic test results should then be transmitted back to the school. In addition to information about how the child is performing with the technology, it will be useful for the clinic to tell the school how to use the different programming positions on the technology. For example, if one of the program positions on the hearing aid or cochlear implant is set for FM use, the school must be informed. In the case of cochlear implants, if the programs are set to increasing loudness, the school should be given some direction about when to move the device to the next louder setting.

For a child who has recently been implanted, the cochlear implant audiologist will plan how and when a child will progress through the mapping programs. The educational team then will play a prominent role in implementing the cochlear implant plan, and providing feedback to the clinic regarding the child's progress. The implant programs are frequently set so that each successive program is increasingly loud, and the cochlear implant audiologist will provide information in the programming report to tell the school staff when to change the programs. Sometimes the decision about when to change the cochlear implant program will be based on length of use; at other times, implant program changes will be based on the child's performance. For an educational team with little or no experience, the educational consultant from the clinic can train school personnel in how to participate in this part of the implanted child's development.

Pitfall

- When a child goes to the cochlear implant center, the TOD and SLP at the school need to receive a copy of the programming report. A summary page of the child's various implant programs, volume, and sensitivity should be included, as well as information about when the child should be switched from one program to the next. Parents need to give this report to the school, but they do not always do so. Finding ways for the school to gain implant information in a timely manner can be challenging. If the school does not know information about implant speech processor settings and adjustments, there is the potential that the child will not be listening appropriately.

In addition, the school-based educational audiologist will be interested in information from the clinic about hearing aid or implant programs that are designated for FM use, the mixing ratio of environmental microphone and FM microphone, and feedback on the type of FM system to use. (See Chapter 20 on FM Systems and Chapter 19 for the section on FM with Cochlear Implants.)

◆ Team Meetings

Children receiving special education support under the Early Intervention Program (birth to three years of age) have services specified as a result of meetings that occur several times a year (refer to Chapter 24 on early intervention). The meeting generates a document known as the IFSP. Children aged 3 to 21 have program accommodations specified annually at an IEP meeting (refer to Chapter 23 about education laws). At the IFSP or IEP meeting, the education team meets to determine services, school placement options, goals, accommodations, and assistive technology. Members of the team usually include the early intervention coordinator or committee chairperson, the parents or guardians, a psychologist, related service providers such as the SLP, educational audiologist, and, for a school-age child, a regular education teacher. Either the school district or the parents can request that a representative of the clinic participate as part of the team. Although the clinic has information that will assist the educational team as they consider a child's needs, clinic personnel are often unavailable to appear at meetings. Teleconferences can be the next best thing. Even when the educational team has documents and reports from the clinic before the meeting, they often lack the experience or knowledge to interpret the information and recognize the implications for the child's learning.

Other, less formal meetings may be conducted to discuss the child's overall progress and functioning or to discuss a concern. Having these informal meetings provides a forum for addressing concerns and insures that each member of the team has access to the same information. Although having all parties in the same room for meetings is most effective, it is possible to conduct this type of exchange through a teleconference.

◆ School–Clinic Visits

When possible, visits to the clinic by school personnel provide a view of the child, which they might not otherwise have. Even for those educators who have experience working with children with hearing loss, it is often an enlightening experience to observe the techniques used by pediatric audiologists. Seeing a youngster perform during highly structured, controlled, auditory situations reveals an aspect of the child that they cannot see in the school environment. This audiologic information can lead to a change in the type or structure of therapy targeted at skills being assessed during clinic appointments. The school staff often leaves the clinic with a deeper understanding of the technical aspects of how children are evaluated, how hearing aids are selected, how an implant works, and what to expect from the child in the classroom. In addition, a clinic visit gives school personnel an appreciation for the parental commitment and work involved with raising a child with a hearing loss.

When an educational consultant is part of the clinic staff, she may make periodic visits to the school. The parents, the school, or the clinic can initiate these visits. Clinic to school visits can occur for a variety of purposes:

◆ To observe the child

◆ To provide an in-service

◆ To participate in IEP/IFSP meetings

◆ To assess the current or future educational placements

The most common school visits are scheduled to observe the child in class and in therapy to understand how a child performs at school. During these observations, the educational consultant will look at the physical and acoustic characteristics of the school environment, and the strategies employed by the teacher and child during formal and informal activities. Visits may also include in-service workshops for staff regarding hearing loss, technology, and strategies to assist the child who is deaf or hard of hearing in learning.

Allowing sufficient time for discussion and questions following an observation or in-service training, and providing contact information to enable school personnel to address future questions is essential for developing a true coordination between the school and the clinic. A follow-up written summary of the visit including suggestions and recommendations that were discussed and any additional concerns or remaining questions is also helpful.

Special Consideration

- Since there is no health insurance coverage for educators from a hospital clinic, cost of the school visit must be covered in other ways. If the in-service or observation is written on the child's IEP, the district can be asked to pay for this consultant service. Consultant responsibilities and fees will need to be determined at the IEP meeting.

◆ Postsecondary Education

Individuals with disabilities can remain in secondary education programs through age 21. Some students may do so because they have additional or significant disabilities. Other students may need more time to complete educational requirements, but will ultimately enter the work force or attend college or vocational school. Although there are resources within the schools (e.g., guidance counselors and state agencies such as statewide vocational and educational service programs) to assist with transition planning, valuable information about available services for those with hearing loss can be provided by the clinic to individual, vocational counselors, and college personnel.

The clinic staff may be asked to talk to prospective colleges or admissions counselors on behalf of college-bound students. If the student is 18 years or older, the student, not the parents, is responsible for giving consent for the release of information. Generally, colleges have an office for disabled student services and consider the needs of the person with a disability independently of admission to the college. The college-bound student should be made aware of this office and of how to contact the office. As with all other communications, the student must sign a release to give permission for the clinic and the college to share information. The student will also need to give the disabled student services office permission to share information about his disability with the professors and other college staff members.

The clinic's role usually involves providing verification that the student does indeed have hearing loss that affects education, describing the hearing loss, and providing information about the accommodations that are needed to enable the student to access and participate in education. Any letter drafted for the purpose of recommending needed accommodations should include

- a brief summary of the individual's degree of hearing loss and type of technology used

- classroom accommodations needed: teacher's notes, preferential seating, CART (computer access real time translation) performed by a trained court reporter.

- assistive technology needed: FM system, decoder, visual alarms in the dorm

- testing accommodations needed: extended test time, repetition for orally presented directions and listening comprehension sections, quiet environment (see Chapter 26 for further details).

Pearl

- The IEP from the student's last year of high school contains information about his hearing loss, modifications, and testing accommodations that will be needed for college. It is important to be aware that the IEP may not reflect the most appropriate technology for a college student. The clinic audiologist can be a good resource for the university.

◆ Summary

Lack of coordination between the community-based clinic and the school district is a common problem that, if not solved, can sabotage the child's progress. The purpose of this chapter has been to present issues and strategies for formulating a positive community–school working relationship for the benefit of the child.

Children who are diagnosed with a hearing loss will experience better audiologic and educational management that leads to improved outcomes if the clinic and the school make a commitment to share information with each other. A strong relationship between the school and the clinic is characterized by frequent communication and respect for the role each plays in the child's development.

Discussion Questions

1. Why are communication and collaboration between the clinic and the school important?

2. Describe the steps to initiate communication with the school for a child newly identified with hearing loss.

3. What information does the clinic have that the school needs? What information does the school have that the clinic needs?

4. What are the most effective ways that the educational consultant or clinician can communicate with the school? Describe a situation in which you could use one of these communication methods.

References

Cheffo, S. (2003) Working together: the educational consultant and the school. Audiology Today-Focus Topic, 5–6.

Cheffo, S., and Dawson, D. (2004). Working together: the clinical educational consultant and the school. Volta Voices, 11, 36–37.

Giangreco, M. (2000). Related services research for students with low-incidence disabilities: implications for speech-language pathologists in inclusive classrooms. Language Speech & Hearing Services in School, 31, 230–239.

Marge, D., and Marge, M. (2006). Critical next steps for infants and toddlers with hearing loss. Volta Voices 13, 46–47.

Marge, D., and Marge, M. (2005). Beyond newborn hearing screening: meeting the educational and health care needs of infants and young children with hearing loss in America. Report of the National Consensus Conference on Effective Educational and Health Care Interventions for Infants and Young Children with Hearing Loss, September 10–12, 2004. Syracuse, New York: Department of Physical Medicine and Rehabilitation, SUNY Upstate Medical University.

Part V

Disorders Requiring Special Consideration

Chapter 31

Managing Children with Mild and Unilateral Hearing Loss

Sarah McKay

- ♦ **Background**
- ♦ **Educational, Speech-Language and Social-Emotional Impact of Minimal Hearing Loss**
  - Unilateral Hearing Loss
  - Mild Conductive Hearing Loss
- ♦ **Psychoacoustic Effects**
- ♦ **Audiologic Considerations**

- ♦ **Amplification Options**
  - Fitting a Binaural Hearing Loss
  - Fitting a Unilateral Hearing Loss
  - Use of Frequency Modulation Devices
- ♦ **Additional Information**
  - Counseling Parents
- ♦ **Conclusion**

Key Points

- Children with mild hearing loss and unilateral hearing loss (UHL) are at risk for academic, speech and language, and social-emotional difficulties.

- Current universal newborn hearing screening technologies do not identify a significant proportion of infants with milder degrees of hearing loss (both unilateral and bilateral). Efforts to detect children with these forms of hearing loss must continue throughout early childhood.

- Audiologists need to feel that electrophysiologic and behavioral test results are valid estimates of hearing sensitivity before initiating amplification options for children with mild and unilateral hearing loss.

- An increased number of children with mild hearing loss and UHL are being identified in their first weeks of life. Audiologists will need to choose management options for their patients, sometimes based solely on evidence gathered from older children. Ongoing research initiatives will continue to shape future best practice guidelines.

The topics of mild hearing loss and UHL are not new to the profession of audiology, but they have been receiving renewed attention. Before universal newborn hearing screening (UNHS) was implemented, the average age of identification of hearing loss was 30 months, and many children with mild hearing loss and UHL were often not identified until they were school aged (Joint Committee on

Infant Hearing (JCIH), 2000; Brookhuser, Worthington, and Kelly, 1991). Speech and language delays, which were more apparent in children with greater degrees of hearing loss, were often more subtle in children with mild hearing loss or UHL. However, for a significant number of children, these degrees of hearing loss have been found to have adverse affects on academic achievement, speech and language development, and social-emotional wellness.

It is now estimated that 95% of children are being screened in their first weeks of life (JCIH, 2007). Research supports best outcomes for children with hearing loss when intervention is in place in the first year of life (Moeller, 2000; Yoshinaga-Itano et al, 1998). Audiologists who work with children with mild hearing loss and UHL face three major challenges: (1) Evidence suggests that UNHS technologies are sensitive to identifying moderate or greater degrees of hearing loss, but some children with milder degrees of hearing loss are not being identified by these methods; (2) Although electrophysiologic and behavioral tests allow audiologists to fit children with moderate or greater degrees of hearing loss with amplification, audiologists may not feel confident about fitting an infant with mild hearing loss or UHL with hearing aids based on electrophysiologic measures alone (see Chapter 6 for information about behavioral evaluation of infants); (3) Because children with these forms of hearing loss have not typically been identified until they are school aged and subsequent research was concentrated on this age group, best practice guidelines for management of infants and young children with mild hearing loss and UHL are currently not available.

♦ Background

The results of various studies on the incidence and prevalence of mild hearing loss and UHL, as well as the types of difficulties that children with these forms of hearing loss encounter, are relevant to management and will be discussed. To proceed with a discussion about mild hearing loss and UHL, the terms must first be defined. Both mild hearing loss and UHL sometimes fall under the umbrella term of minimal hearing loss. Although there may be similarities in the impact of the two forms of hearing loss, the audiologist should not assume that the impact and subsequent management strategies will be the same for both.

For the purposes of this chapter, mild bilateral hearing loss is defined as permanent, established behavioral pure tone air conduction thresholds between 20–40 dB hearing level (HL) at 500, 1000 and 2000 HZ. UHL is defined as a permanent behavioral, pure tone average (PTA) (air conduction thresholds – 500, 1000, 2000Hz) at any level 20 dB HL or greater in the affected ear. Average pure tone thresholds in the good ear are better than or equal to 15 dB HL (Bess, Dodd-Murphy, and Parker, 1998). There is great variability in the accepted definitions and descriptions of mild hearing loss and UHL. These differences affect subsequent reports on incidence and outcomes.

The incidence of UHL is about 1/1000 (Prieve et al, 2000). If the incidence is divided into categories of babies who were in the neonatal intensive care unit (NICU) and well-baby nursery (WBN), the incidence is 3.2/1000 and 0.41/1000, respectively. These numbers might not accurately reflect the number of children with mild hearing loss or UHL. The incidence of bilateral mild hearing loss in the newborn population is difficult to obtain because traditional screening protocols may be less sensitive. Gravel, White, Johnson et al (2005) have estimated the incidence of mild permanent bilateral and mild UHL in the newborn population to be 0.55/1000.

The prevalence of minimal SNHL (including mild bilateral hearing loss and UHL) in the school-aged population has been reported to be about 54/1000—much greater than in the newborn population. The prevalence of mild hearing loss and UHL was 1 and 3%, respectively (Bess, Dodd-Murphy, and Parker, 1998). These numbers demonstrate the need for ongoing screening procedures throughout early childhood.

As mentioned earlier, differences in the definition of mild hearing loss and UHL may affect reported incidence and prevalence rates. Also, differences or discrepancies in incidence and prevalence rates may be due to hearing loss missed by current screening protocols, lack of follow-up of high-risk infants, and progressive or late-onset hearing loss resulting from infections, illnesses, trauma or noise (CDC National Workshop on Mild and UHL Proceedings, 2005).

♦ Educational, Speech-Language and Social-Emotional Impact of Minimal Hearing Loss

Minimal hearing loss (a term that includes mild hearing loss and UHL) has been described as an invisible acoustic filter

(Flexer, 1995). If a teacher or caregiver is not informed that a child has mild or UHL, they may never know. Although audiologists may be familiar with the difficulties that children with minimal hearing loss could experience, these difficulties are not always conveyed to parents as conditions to warrant great concern.

Pitfall

- The very term *mild* denotes a lack of alarm, a feeling of a condition that will have little impact. The use of the *mild* or *minimal* term can have a ripple effect beyond the parents. Physicians, teachers, and other caregivers may have the impression that the hearing loss is not significant, and thus will require minimal attention or intervention.

Traditional classification of hearing loss has described the degree of hearing loss and the loss's handicapping effect. When handicapping effect is taken into account, mild hearing loss might negatively affect a child's language development by affecting subtle speech cues such as prosody, stress patterns, and grammatical rules (Northern and Downs, 2002).

Anderson and Matkin (1998) found that in a classroom, a child with a 30 dB hearing loss can miss 25–40% of the speech signal, and a child with a hearing loss of 35–40 dB can miss as much as 50% of classroom discussions. This hearing problem is compounded when the speaker's voice is at greater distance, when there is excessive competing noise, or when the speaker is not in the child's line of vision.

Bess, Dodd-Murphy, and Parker (1998) conducted a study on 1228 children in grades three, six, and nine who had minimal hearing loss (including mild hearing loss and UHL). They reported that children in the third grade scored significantly lower than normal hearing peers on the Comprehensive Test of Basic Skills (4th Edition). An alarming 37% of children with minimal sensorineural hearing loss (SNHL) had failed at least one grade in school. Finally, children in all three grades showed greater difficulty in the areas of behavior, energy, stress, social support, and self-esteem. These areas were measured by the COOP Adolescent Chart Method (Dartmouth Primary Care Cooperative Information Project COOP; Nelson et al, 1987). This tool evaluates a child's functional status in a variety of domains. If children are missing a large percentage of the speech signal in addition to subtle speech cues, it is easy to understand how self-esteem and other behavioral areas would be affected. Children with minimal hearing loss can become fatigued by the constant effort needed to listen, and their behaviors can be misinterpreted as being inattentive or aloof.

Unilateral Hearing Loss

Oyler, Oyler and Matkin (1987) made the following statement about the audiology profession's response to UHL:

"Historically, the involvement of hearing health professionals in the management of children with unilateral hearing loss has been limited. The conventional approach was to identify the cause of the hearing loss and then to assure the parents that there would be no handicap" (p. 18). The results of germinal studies in the area of children with UHL as well as attention by agencies such as the Centers for Disease Control and Prevention (2005) have illuminated the need to help children with UHL.

Children with UHL are at risk for academic delays. In studies of grade failure, children with UHL were 10 times more likely to fail a grade than their normal hearing peers, and a significant number of children required resource assistance or special services (Bess and Tharpe, 1986; Oyler, Oyler, and Matkin, 1988). In a more recent study, English and Church (1999) found that grade failure and retention is no longer a recommended educational practice. They found that 54% of children with UHL received individualized special education services.

Some studies have indicated that children with UHL are at risk for speech and language delays. Kiese-Himmell (2002) found that the average age for first words for babies with UHL was within normal limits (12.7 months); however, the average age for first two-word utterances was significantly delayed (23.5 months). Children with severe to profound UHL have been found to have a lower full-scale intelligence quotient score on the Wechsler Intelligence Scale for Children-Revised (WISC-R) than children with lesser degrees of UHL (Culbertson and Gilbert, 1986; Klee and Davis-Dansky, 1986). For an in-depth review of the educational and speech language consequences of UHL, Please refer to Lieu (2004).

Mild Conductive Hearing Loss

The impact of childhood conductive hearing loss is often minimized. Although conductive hearing loss can be caused by a variety of conditions such as cerumen, perforated tympanic membrane, cholesteatoma, and atresia/microtia, the most common cause of conductive hearing loss in children is otitis media (OME) (Northern and Downs, 2002) The American Academy of Family Physicians, Clinical Practice Guideline: Otitis Media With Effusion, 2004 states that in the first year of life, more than 50% of children will experience OME, increasing to more than 60% by two years of age. Although many episodes resolve spontaneously within three months, about 30 to 40% of children have recurrent OME, and 5 to 10% of those episodes last one year or longer. Pediatricians may be more reluctant to initially prescribe antibiotics because of increased rates of antibacterial resistance. Northern and Downs (2002) reported that the average air conduction threshold of children with a documented middle ear infection was 27 dB HL and degree of hearing loss was about 10 dB worse when both ears had abnormal middle ear conditions. When you add the percentage of children who have fluctuating or temporary conductive hearing loss as the result of OME to the aforementioned 5.4% school-aged children with permanent minimal hearing loss, the total number of children with some degree of hearing loss is staggering.

Pearl

- Parents of a child with SNHL (including mild and unilateral) should be advised to be particularly vigilant about OME. They should be made aware of the symptoms and encouraged to have their child checked by their pediatrician if they suspect a problem. Middle ear fluid will likely have a cumulative effect on a child with SNHL. The added hearing loss caused by the fluid could mean the difference between hearing speech and not hearing speech. It also will be beneficial to inform the child's pediatrician of this negative impact.

◆ Psychoacoustic Effects

Binaural advantages (of normal hearing in both ears) include localization, binaural summation, and binaural release from masking. Localization is affected most significantly in individuals with UHL because they do not have the benefit of interaural time and intensity cues (Bess et al, 1986). Binaural release from masking allows an individual with normal hearing in both ears to "filter out noise" and thus to better hear the speech signal. For children who do not have normal hearing in both ears, the difficulty in noise is compounded because they do not yet have a language base to fill in the gaps in running speech. Binaural summation is the increased perception of loudness when sound is heard by two normal hearing ears rather than just one. Psychophysics is covered in Chapter 16 and binaural advantages are covered in Chapters 17 and 18.

◆ Audiologic Considerations

As mentioned, UNHS test protocols are not designed to identify more mild forms of hearing loss less than 35 to 40 dB (ASHA, 2006). Automated auditory brainstem response testing (aABR) usually has a 35 dB pass/refer criteria. When distortion product or transient otoacoustic emissions (OAEs) are employed, the result of present OAEs indicates normal cochlear outer hair cell function and hearing sensitivity better than about 35 to 40 dB (ASHA, 2006). Johnson et al (2005) found that when a two-step, two-technology hearing screening protocol (OAEs and aABR testing) was used, 80% of infants with later confirmed diagnosis of bilateral mild hearing loss or ULH were not identified (using a pass/refer criteria). Employing more sensitive electrophysiologic testing technologies would probably yield more false-positive results with subsequent effects on patients, parents, audiologists, and hospitals. This increased false-positive rate would likely affect the cost effectiveness of screening as well. Gravel et al (2005) advocate ongoing research in this area before global changes are made in public policy. They suggest searching for other opportunities for ongoing screening of young children, such as having screening routinely performed by the child's primary care physician. This leaves audiologists with the responsibility of educating physicians about which children are at risk for progressive hearing loss as well as stressing the importance of listening to parents' concerns about speech and language development or hearing problems.

In the event that electrophysiologic test results indicate mild hearing loss, the audiologist may not feel as though they have obtained enough information to confidently fit that child with amplification. The American Academy of Audiology (AAA) Pediatric Amplification Protocol advocates obtaining frequency-specific air and bone conduction ABR thresholds before fitting amplification on infants. In addition, this document states that acoustic immittance measures, including tympanometry and middle ear reflexes and OAEs, are necessary to determine the type and configuration of hearing loss. Even if an audiologist has obtained all of these results, it may be difficult to move forward without also having behavioral audiologic test results. (See Chapter 6 for a discussion on behavioral testing for infants.)

Pearl

- There may be times when an audiologist has identified a mild hearing loss or UHL in an infant, but does not feel comfortable moving forward with amplification until obtaining more precise frequency/ear specific behavioral audiometric results. In this scenario parents can be counseled about how to create the best listening environments for their child. Proximity of an infant to her parent is a benefit. Often a parent is holding an infant, and with slight modifications in the position of the baby, an improved speech-to-noise ratio can be achieved. Parents should also be counseled about raising their voice slightly and reducing unneeded background noise (such as a dishwasher or TV).

As an example, let us take a 3-month-old infant with an average ABR threshold of 30 dB nHL. This child would likely have passed the newborn screen, and may have present OAEs which, in this case, provide no useful information about precise degree of hearing loss. Often audiologists must employ correction factors to estimate hearing loss from ABR results This correction is of minimal consequence to the decisions made for a child with ABR thresholds at 60 dB nHL, but has an impact on decisions audiologists make about children with minimal hearing loss.

Another consideration in moving forward with amplification is bone conduction results. Does the audiologist feel confident that a conductive component does not exist? Behavioral test results should include ear- and frequency-specific testing. Immittance measurements should be completed at every visit. Fortunately, the proximity of infant to parent in the first 6 months of life is optimal. Difficulties that children with hearing loss experience when attempting to listen from a distance and in the presence of noise will be less likely with infants.

Another tool that may be particularly helpful in directing management choices for children with mild hearing loss or UHL is the use of functional auditory measures/outcome measures. These paper and pencil survey tools allow a child, child's parent or teacher to make observations about the child's auditory behaviors in different listening environments. (Refer to **Table 5–4** in Chapter 5 for a listing and summary of functional auditory tests.) If an audiologist or parent is on the fence about whether to fit with hearing aids, results of functional auditory measures may provide the information needed to move forward. In addition to assisting in decisions about management, discussing the results of these functional measures can serve as a valuable springboard for counseling and interaction.

◆ Amplification Options

Hearing aids, which alert teachers to children with greater degrees of hearing loss, are not always recommended or chosen for children with mild hearing loss or UHL. Even if the audiologist recommends amplification, parents may hold off to see if the child experiences difficulties.

Controversial Issue

- We know that about 35% of children with mild hearing loss or UHL will encounter academic difficulties. This means that about 65% of children will not. We do not yet have a tool to predict which children will encounter these difficulties and which will not. Parents, however, may need to make decisions about intervention such as hearing aids and special services. They may be forced to decide whether to wait and see if problems develop (which in turn could cause intervention to be failure-based) or to be proactive.

The AAA Pediatric Amplification Protocol (2003), addressed the fitting of amplification on children with UHL and minimal to mild hearing loss in its Special Consideration section. The following statement is relevant to the discussion: "The decision to fit a child with unilateral hearing loss should be made on an individual basis, taking into consideration the child's or family's preference as well as audiologic, developmental, communication, and educational factors (p. 3). . . .Children with minimal to mild hearing loss should be considered candidates for amplification and/or personal frequency modulation (FM) system or soundfield systems for use in school" (p.4).

Fitting a Binaural Hearing Loss

For children with mild bilateral SNHL, binaural amplification is recommended. This fitting will provide the binaural advantages mentioned earlier (i.e., head shadow effect, binaural squelch and binaural summation). As previously discussed, the audiologist should feel confident about the frequency-specific thresholds obtained (both air and bone conduction) before fitting a child with mild hearing loss. The Pediatric Amplification Protocol advocates the use of prescriptive methods such as desired sensation level (DSL) to establish targets for gain and output, and verification methods using real-ear measures, such as real-ear to coupler difference (RECD) to ensure that targets are being met and that a child is not being over- or underamplified.

Fitting a Unilateral Hearing Loss

The fitting of a hearing aid for children with UHL is not as straightforward as with children with bilateral hearing loss. To the author's knowledge, there is no evidence about whether babies with UHL benefit from being fit with a hearing aid early. The use of a hearing aid on school-aged children with moderately severe or better hearing in the impaired ear has met with considerable success as indicated by subjective rating scales (Kiese-Himmel, 2002; McKay, 2002). Degree and configuration of hearing loss are important factors when deciding whether to fit a child with UHL. With a lesser degree of hearing loss, it may be possible to achieve a more balanced sense of hearing between the ears. Balance of sound is simply not possible with severe or profound UHL.

Amplification systems that may not be appropriate for young children with UHL are the CROS (contralateral routing of signal) hearing aid and the bone-anchored hearing apparatus (BAHA). The CROS system picks up sound from the impaired side via a microphone and delivers it via a hard wire or FM signal to the normal hearing ear. Although the CROS was found to be useful in quiet situations, especially in cases where the signal originates on the side of the impaired ear, it can actually be detrimental if noise is introduced to the normal hearing ear via the microphone on the impaired side (Kenworthy, Klee, and Tharpe, 1990). A CROS system should not be considered until a child is old enough to choose the listening environments in which she might benefit. The CROS system should therefore not be considered for very young children.

The BAHA was originally intended for individuals with conductive or mixed hearing loss, but has also recently been marketed for those with UHL. Because of issues related to anatomical maturation of the temporal bone, the BAHA is FDA-approved only for use in children older than five years. For individuals with conductive hearing loss, the BAHA provides the signal to both cochleas via bone conduction. For a child with atresia or permanent conductive hearing loss, the BAHA may be an excellent option. The premise of fitting a BAHA on a person with severe or profound UHL is to allow transcranial delivery of the signal from a microphone on the impaired side via bone conduction the normal hearing ear. A device which also employs transcranial delivery of signal is the transcranial CROS aid. In this scenario, an individual is fit with a high-powered, deep fitting in-the-ear (ITE) or behind-the-ear (BTE) aid on the impaired ear which generates enough output to stimulate the contralateral cochlea.

To the author's knowledge, there are no reports to date on the use or efficacy of transcranial fitting on children with severe or profound UHL. One could speculate that the introduction of noise from the impaired side to the normal hearing ear would have a similar impact on a child to that of the CROS aid. More evidence is needed on the efficacy of the BAHA and the transcranial CROS for children with UHL.

Use of Frequency Modulation Devices

The benefit of FM technology in this population has been well documented (Flexer, 1995; Kenworthy, Klee, and Tharpe, 1990; Tharpe, Ricketts and Sladen, 2004; Updike, 1994). Improving the signal-to-noise ratio for a child who is developing language is clearly an advantage. As with the aforementioned studies, most evidence is with the school-aged population. In the infant/toddler population, one must creatively consider which listening situations could benefit from the use of FM, such as while a child is in a stroller or car seat or during instructional time in a daycare or preschool environment. Loaner FM banks in conjunction with parent education have met with success (Gabbard, 2004). Another factor to consider is the best choice of routing of the FM signal. If a child already has a hearing aid, one may choose to couple an FM receiver to the hearing aid. Another option is to couple the FM to the normal hearing ear via an ear-level FM system. Personal and soundfield FM systems may also be an option. Ricketts and Tharpe (2004) found that for school-aged children with mild hearing loss, the most significant improvements were seen with binaural ear-level FM placement. Decisions about the most appropriate FM option must be made on an individual basis. As a child approaches school age or if she is already receiving early intervention services, it is recommended that such decisions be coordinated with her educational audiologist or hearing support teacher.

♦ Additional Information

Parents and teachers of children with mild hearing loss and UHL should be provided with written information. This information should include an explanation of tests, additional recommended evaluations (i.e., medical, speech-language, early intervention), information about how to best help a child with mild hearing loss or UHL at home, in daycare settings, or at school, and additional resources (see Appendix 31–1). Medical management of children with hearing loss is discussed in Chapter 3. One additional factor to keep in mind for children diagnosed with UHL is the possible progression of unilateral to bilateral hearing loss. Inner ear anomalies have been found to be most likely in children with UHL (Coticchia et al, 2006; Bamiou et al, 1999). Although the hearing loss is unilateral, the inner ear anomalies may be bilateral.

Counseling Parents

Information should also be provided to parents about how to best help their child at home or in the classroom. The

Appendix 31–1   Ways for Parents to Help a Child with Mild or Unilateral Hearing Loss at Home

- Try to make eye contact when speaking to your child.
- Get your child's attention before talking to her.
- Help your child localize sound if she looks like she is having difficulty.
- Look for cues that your child understands what you are saying.
- Raise your voice slightly and face he when you are at a greater distance (another room).
- Make the home listening friendly. Try to reduce things that cause unneeded noise. Use carpeting and cloth curtains. Use corkboards instead of magnetic boards. Replace buzzing fluorescent lights. Operate noisy appliances (dishwasher, washing machine) when your child is not home or is sleeping.
- If your child has hearing loss in one ear, always be aware of where her normal hearing ear is facing. It should always be facing you or those talking to her. Think about this when your child is at dinner, in the car, etc.
- Do not have the TV or radio on while eating dinner or at other times when you are talking with your child.
- Create a quiet listening environment while your child is watching TV.
- Do not give your child instructions from another room. She will likely hear your voice, but not understand what you are saying.
- If your child wears a hearing aid, make sure it is functioning properly at all times. Hearing aids that do not work are much worse than no hearing aids at all.
- Teach your child's siblings things that you have learned about helping her.

Ways to Help a Child with Mild or Unilateral Hearing Loss at School

- Teach your class speaking and listening etiquette (one person talks at a time, everyone listens).
- Always make sure that the student is seated in close proximity to you (within six feet) and if she has hearing loss in one ear, that the normal hearing ear is facing you, and is in close proximity to you.
- Always make sure that your student is not near a noise source such as the hallway, HVAC vents, and computers. If she has hearing loss in one ear, make sure that her normal hearing ear does not face the noise source.
- Be aware of your student's placement relative to the other students. Other students' responses and contributions add to the educational experience.
- Try to get your student's attention by calling her name before giving oral instructions.
- Try to give written instructions in conjunction with oral instructions.
- Ensure optimal lighting.
- Try not to speak with your back to the student.
- Have a pre-understood nonverbal cue to use with your student (i.e., a tap on the shoulder to regain attention).
- Give your student a note buddy.
- Provide visual aids; however, do not place your student next to a slide or LCD projector.
- Allow your older student to record lectures.
- Teach your student to advocate for herself by saying for example, "Can you repeat that?"
- Make sure one person talks at a time during a class discussion. Draw attention to the speaker.
- During group time, separate groups and place noisy groups off on their own.
- Train volunteers to be good communication models. This is particularly important with student teachers and parent volunteers. Parents should not be talking to children or other parents while the teacher is giving instructions.
- Take interest in your student's hearing aid or FM system. Understand the use and care of the device.

recommendation of preferential seating simply does not suffice. Caregivers of these children need to have an understanding of the types of difficulties they can encounter and an explanation of why they encounter them. Once families have an understanding, they can begin to implement their own strategies to help the child.

Parents should be encouraged to be good language models for their child. The audiologist can share strategies for parents to minimize background noise in the home and be acoustically aware of the child's listening environments. They should also be informed about the importance of appropriate placement of the child in communication situations (such as placing a child with hearing loss in the left ear behind the driver's seat in the car so that their normal hearing ear will be facing the passengers). Similar information should be given to teachers on how to create an acoustically friendly classroom for the child and employ strategies to promote ease of listening. Degree-specific brochures with useful strategies are available from the

Pearl

- In some cases, particularly of very young children with mild hearing loss or UHL, the audiologist may be on the fence about amplification. As parents look to professionals for answers, it is difficult to admit that we may not know what will be best. It often comes back to the choice of "Let's wait and see" versus "Let's be proactive." Providing parents with information (written, online resources, other parents) helps them to feel empowered and to make informed decisions about their child. In some cases the wait and see choice may be the best choice for that child. An audiologist can feel confident that she has provided parents with information about the difficulties experienced with the hearing loss, guidelines for normal speech and language development, and strategies for use at home and at school to help their child.

Educational Audiology Association (www.edaud.org and in Chapter 26.). Examples of information/strategies to provide to parents and teachers of children with mild or UHL can be found in **Appendix 31–1**.

♦ Conclusion

Children with mild hearing loss and UHL are at risk for academic, speech-language, and social-emotional difficulties. Since the implementation of UNHS, more children with these forms of hearing loss will be identified in their first weeks of life; however, until new UNHS protocols are employed with proven sensitivity and specificity, many infants with mild hearing loss will continue to be missed by UNHS. We know that children with hearing loss who receive intervention by the age of 6 months have the best outcomes. Although we do not yet know which children are at greatest risk for difficulties, early identification provides a previously nonexistent window of opportunity for audiologists and other caregivers to serve children with mild hearing loss and UHL. Subsequently, care can be proactive instead of failure

based. Until more evidence is gathered to support best practice guidelines, audiologists can continue to make choices that may have positive impacts on speech-language and auditory development. They can continue to provide parents and other caregivers with strategies of how to give a child with mild or UHL the best chance for success.

Discussion Questions

1. Should UNHS technologies be more sensitive to milder degrees of hearing loss? List the possible impacts.

2. What types of audiologic recommendations should be made after a baby is identified with mild hearing loss or UHL, and what factors go into decisions about recommendations?

3. What nonaudiologic recommendations can be made after a baby is identified with mild hearing loss or UHL?

4. What are the future research needs in the area of children with mild hearing loss and UHL? How may future research guide the choices audiologists make for their patients with mild and UHL?

References

The American Academy of Audiology. (2003). Pediatric Amplification Protocol. www.audiology.org/professionals/position. Last accessed February 1, 2005.

American Academy of Family Physicians, American Academy of Otolaryngology-Head and Neck Surgery, and American Academy of Pediatrics Subcommittee on Otitis Media With Effusion. (2004). Clinical Practice Guideline: Otitis Media with Effusion. May 03, 2004

Bamiou, D. E., Savy, L., O'Mahoney, C., Phelps, P., and Sirimanna, T. (1999). Unilateral sensorineural hearing loss and its aetiology in childhood: the contribution of computerized tomography in aetiological diagnosis and management. International Journal of Pediatric Otolaryngology, 51, 91–99.

Bess, F. H., Dodd-Murphy, J. D., and Parker, R. A. (1998). Children with minimal sensorineural hearing loss: prevalence, educational performance, and functional health status. Ear and Hearing, 17, 1–11.

Bess, F. H., and Tharpe, A. M. (1986). Case history data on unilaterally hearing impaired children. Ear and Hearing, 7, 14–17.

Brookhauser, P. E., Worthington, D. W., and Kelly, W. J. (1991). Unilateral hearing loss in children. Laryngoscope, 101, 1264–1272.

The Centers for Disease Control and Prevention (2005). Proceedings of the National Workshop on Mild and Unilateral Hearing Loss. www.cdc.gov. Last accessed

Coticchia, J., Gokhale, A., Waltonen, J., and Sumer, B. (2006). Characteristics of sensorineural hearing loss in children with inner ear anomalies. American Journal of Otolaryngology–Head and Neck Medicine and Surgery, 27, 33–38.

Culbertson, J. L., and Gilbert, L. E. (1986). Children with unilateral sensorineural hearing loss: cognitive, academic and social development. Ear and Hearing, 7, 38–42.

Directors of Speech and Hearing Programs in State Health and Welfare Agencies (2003). www.cdc.gov/ehdi. Last accessed August 18, 2006.

English, K., and Church, G. (1999). Unilateral hearing loss in children: an update for the 1990s. Language, Speech and Hearing Services in Schools, 30, 26–31.

Flexer, C. (1995). Classroom management of children with minimal hearing loss. Hearing Journal, September, 10–13.

Gabbard, S. (2004) The use of FM technology for infants and young children. ACCESS: Achieving Clear Communication Employing Sound Solutions, 93–97.

Gravel, J., White, K., Johnson, J., Widen, J., Vohr, B., and James, M. (2005). A multisite study to examine the efficacy of the otoacoustic emission/automated auditory brainstem response newborn hearing screening protocol: recommendations for policy, practice, and research. American Journal of Audiology, 14, 217–228.

Joint Committee on Infant Hearing: year 2007 position statement: principles and guidelines for early hearing detection and intervention programs. Pediatrics, 120(4): 898–921.

Kenworthy, O. T., Klee, T., and Tharpe, A. M. (1990). Speech recognition ability of children with unilateral sensorineural hearing loss as a function of amplification, speech stimuli and listening condition. Ear and Hearing, 11, 264–270.

Kiese-Himmel, C., (2002). Unilateral senorineural hearing impairment in childhood: Analysis of 31 consecutive cases. International Journal of Audiology, 41, 57–63.

Klee T., and Davis-Dansky, E. (1986). A comparison of unilaterally hearing-impaired children and normal-hearing children on a battery of standardized language tests. Ear and Hearing, 7, 27–37.

Lieu, J. E. (2004) Speech-language and educational consequences of unilateral hearing loss in children. Archives of Otolaryngology Head and Neck Surgery, 130, 524–530.

McKay, S. (2002). To aid or not to aid: children with unilateral hearing loss. Poster presentation at the Annual AAA Convention. Philadelphia, PA.

Moeller, M. P. (2000). Early intervention and language development in children who are deaf and hard of hearing. Pediatrics, 106.

Nelson, E. C., Wasson, J., Kirk, J., et al. (1987). Assessment of function in routine clinical practice: description of the COOP chart method and preliminary findings. Journal of Chronic Diseases, 40, 55S–63S.

Northern, J., and Downs, M. (2002). Hearing in children (5th ed.). Baltimore: Williams & Wilkins.

Oyler, R. F., Oyler, A. L., and Matkin, N. D. (1987). Warning: a unilateral hearing loss may be detrimental to a child's academic career. Hearing Journal, September, 18–22.

Oyler, R. F., Oyler, A. L., and Matkin N.D. (1988). Unilateral hearing loss: demographics and educational impact. Language, Speech Hearing Services in Schools, 19, 201–209.

Prieve, B., Dalzell, L., Berg, A., et al. (2000). The New York state universal newborn hearing screening demonstration project: outpatient outcome measures. Ear and Hearing, 21, 104–117.

Ricketts, T. A., Tharpe, A. M. (2005). Directional microphone technology for children. *A sound Foundation Through Early Amplificaton 2004*: *Proceedings of the Third International Conference*. Sewald, R. C. and Bamford, J. (eds.). Great Britain: Cambrian Printers, 143–153.

Tharpe, A. M., Ricketts, T., and Sladen, D. (2003). FM Systems for children with minimal to mild hearing loss. ACCESS: Achieving Clear Communication Employing Sound Solutions, Fabry, D. and Johnson C. D. (eds.). 191–197.

Updike, C. D. (1994). Comparison of FM auditory trainers, CROS aids and personal amplification in unilaterally hearing impaired children. Journal of the American Academy of Audiology, 5, 204–209.

Yoshinage-Itano, C., Sedey, A., Coutter, D., and Mehl, A. (1998). Language of early—and later—identified children with hearing loss. Pediatrics, 102(5): 161–771.

Chapter 32

Managing Infants and Young Children with Auditory Neuropathy

Laura Austin Duffy and Kevin H. Franck

♦ **Diagnosis**

♦ **Recommendations and Management Team**

Audiology—Follow-Up
Auditory Brainstem Response
Immittance
Otoacoustic Emissions
Pure Tone Audiometry
Hearing Aids and Cochlear Implants
Otolaryngology

Ophthalmology
Genetics
Neurology
Neonatal Follow-Up
Early Intervention/Educational Consultation
Speech-Language Pathology
Family Wellness

♦ **Summary**

Key Points

1. The management of young patients with auditory neuropathy includes close audiologic monitoring, repeated use of outcomes measures, and a multidisciplinary team approach.

2. The multidisciplinary team approach includes the parent, audiologist, otolaryngologist, geneticist, ophthalmologist, neurologist, neonatal follow-up team, counselor, speech-language pathologist, and early intervention provider or teacher of the hearing impaired.

Young children diagnosed with auditory neuropathy call for a specific agenda of management. This chapter focuses on a plan tailored specifically to infants and young children with confirmed or suspected auditory neuropathy. These recommendations include close audiologic monitoring with a heavy reliance on outcome measures, a team approach of professionals familiar with hearing loss, the inclusion of a neurologist or neonatal follow-up team, and a family wellness program.

♦ Diagnosis

Germinal articles about the diagnosis of auditory neuropathy were primarily about children and adults in whom full audiograms, including word recognition, could be measured (Starr et al, 1996, 1998; Starr, Sininger, and Pratt, 2000). Many of the patients showed a variety of audiometric configurations. Audiologists dealing with infants who are younger than 6 months or developmentally delayed may have objective test results as the only audiologic information available at diagnosis. This varied clinical presentation will not be apparent because behavioral pure tone threshold and speech discrimination data may not be available. (Chapter 6 of this text includes a discussion of behavioral testing of infants younger than 6 months.)

Auditory neuropathy is suspected in an infant or young child as a result of specific electrophysiologic test findings. Typical test results include absent or grossly abnormal auditory brainstem responses (ABRs) with cochlear microphonic and evoked otoacoustic emissions (EOAE). Despite normal tympanometry, immittance shows absent or elevated middle ear muscle reflex (MEMR) thresholds (Berlin et al, 2005). Behavioral audiometry results can vary from being within normal limits to suggesting a profound hearing loss.

Efficacy of amplification is variable, given behavioral audiometric results (Rance et al, 1999).

Although the audiologic description of auditory neuropathy may be straightforward, there likely are a variety of underlying pathologies that are not limited to those of the auditory nerve as the name would imply. Many organic disorders of the central nervous system may produce an abnormal ABR in the presence of normal peripheral hearing sensitivity (Rapin and Gravel, 2006). EOAE responses confirm the function of outer hair cells, but not inner hair cells.

Children with auditory neuropathy fall in one of two categories:

+ Children with the above-described objective results who exhibit behavioral audiometric responses that are consistent with a profound hearing loss. These are the patients who would be categorized as deaf before otoacoustic emission testing. Audiologic intervention has included powerful amplification, which typically resulted in limited auditory skills. Cochlear implantation has become an option for these patients. This group likely does not have any form of neuropathy, but rather has a dysfunction of inner hair cells (Amatuzzi et al, 2001; Rodriguez-Ballesteros et al, 2003).

+ Children have similar objective test results but variable audiograms and worse-than-expected success with amplification. This group might have a pathology of the inner hair cells, auditory nerve or central auditory system. Some researchers have posited that this group experiences a lack of neural synchrony, and they use a diagnosis of auditory dys-synchrony (Berlin et al, 2002).

+ Starr et al (1996, 1998, 2000) described a final category of individuals who developed pathologies of the auditory nerve as well as other neurons).

+ Recommendations and Management Team

Several initial evaluations and recommendations should be obtained to supplement audiologic findings. These include medical consultations by otolaryngology, ophthalmology, genetics, neurology, and neonatal follow-up. In addition to a schedule of audiologic follow-up, involvement of speech-language pathology, early intervention (specialized with deaf and hearing impaired education), and family mental health support are indicated. The following sections describe typical recommendations from each of these disciplines of the care team.

Audiology—Follow-Up

The conflicting audiologic test results established at diagnosis call for close audiologic monitoring involving a battery of tests and various habilitation techniques.

Auditory Brainstem Response

The cochlear microphonic is important to identify as a means of ruling out sensory hearing loss when click ABR responses are absent or poorly defined at high intensity levels. If the initial auditory neuropathy diagnosis is determined before six months of age, repeating the ABR between three and six months of age is recommended. Gestational age and middle ear status should be considered when repeating the ABR. Sedation risk and avoidance of sedation for ABR procedures may also determine when a repeat ABR will be completed. Since many patients identified with suspected auditory neuropathy may have been premature or suffered perinatal insult, abnormal ABR findings may be indicative of a global issue of the nervous system. Infants who were born preterm or who were identified before three months of age and who show these conflicting test results may need repeated ABR measures to cross check behavioral responses after six months of age. If the ABR waveform is absent and continues to show the same result after a repeated measure at a later gestational age, testing most likely will not need to be repeated unless behavioral responses improve or patients are unable to perform behavioral test tasks because of developmental delays. Patients who continue to show improvements in the ABR waveform may need several ABRs every 6 to 12 months to cross check these ABR changes closely.

> **Pitfall**
>
> + Otitis media can negatively affect OAE, immittance, and ABR results. If middle ear status is not taken into consideration, misdiagnosis of the hearing loss is highly possible.

Immittance

Immittance testing includes tympanometry and evaluation of middle ear muscle reflexes (MEMRs). Tympanometry should be performed using a 1000 Hz probe tone for patients younger than six months. Acoustic reflex testing should be completed using a 660-Hz probe tone for infants younger than four months. Immittance testing should be attempted at every audiology visit. Reflex data should be measured at least once for diagnostic purposes in the presence of normal middle ear status. Tympanometry should be performed with the appropriate probe tone at each visit to monitor middle ear status. (See Chapter 13 for a complete discussion of middle ear measurement.)

Otoacoustic Emissions

EOAE data, including distortion product and transient evoked responses, are typically present or normal in patients with auditory neuropathy. Responses that are initially present at diagnosis can disappear over time, or may be absent because of middle ear effusion, negative pressure, cerumen or debris in the ear canal, or inappropriate probe fit or calibration. The EOAE data yield information about the cochlea. It is important to document this information when no response is obtained at the limits of the equipment with the ABR to rule out any preneural activity. The cochlear microphonic can also serve this function. Otoacoustic emissions should be completed in conjunction with ABR testing and should be repeated at future visits in conjunction with behavioral and immittance testing.

Pure Tone Audiometry

Visual reinforcement audiometry (VRA) testing can be attempted at about 5 months to obtain threshold information in the soundfield and with insert earphones (See Chapter 7 for more information on VRA and Chapter 6 for information on behavioral observation audiometry.) Once the patient is developmentally ready for VRA testing, frequent sessions may be necessary to obtain ear specific and frequency specific data. Monitoring every 2 to 4 months at this point forward may be indicated based on the child's test reliability, middle ear status, and developmental status.

Hearing Aids and Cochlear Implants

Young patients who show consistent threshold responses with testing using VRA techniques can be considered candidates for amplification and frequency modulation (FM) systems and can be evaluated for cochlear implantation candidacy. We strongly recommend that hearing aids be fit using threshold information obtained from VRA testing. Hearing aids can be obtained from a loaner bank if possible to complete a trial before purchasing. Outcome measures should be completed before and after the hearing aid trial. Close communication is also encouraged among the parents, audiologist, early intervention providers, and the speech-language pathologist to monitor progress with technology and to document observations of the child's auditory behaviors. The trial should be long enough so that the child is able to tolerate the hearing aids for most of his waking hours. FM systems should also be considered alone or in conjunction with hearing aids.

Cochlear implantation may be considered when a child is not making adequate gains in auditory skill development despite proper amplification. Families are encouraged to attend a cochlear implant information meeting at any time following diagnosis. The information meeting is an opportunity for a family to ask questions and obtain general information about cochlear implantation so that they can determine if a cochlear implant would be an option for their child.

A patient who has shown behavioral responses consistent with severe to profound hearing loss, who is not benefiting from hearing aids, and whose parents are interested in having him develop spoken language, is eligible for cochlear implant surgery at 12 months of age. A patient who shows consistent behavioral test results in the moderate range may or may not become a candidate; however, he may require a longer trial period with traditional amplification before being considered as a candidate for cochlear implantation. If

after age two years, the child is still not developing auditory and speech skills, and lack of improvement in hearing test results has been documented, he is then a candidate for cochlear implantation.

Outcomes measures should be an integral part of audiologic follow-ups, and should be obtained at all visits. Close monitoring of auditory development is crucial in supporting decisions regarding amplification. Outcome measures are especially important in managing patients with developmental delay and when behavioral data are sparse.

Otolaryngology

A pediatric otolaryngology consultation is recommended when any permanent hearing loss is identified. Auditory neuropathy is considered to be a significant hearing loss (JCIH, 2007). Therefore, the otolaryngologist organizes the search for the cause of the hearing loss, evaluates middle ear status, looks for syndromic features, and oversees a medical workup.

The medical workup may consist of laboratory testing and imaging. Imaging may include magnetic response imaging (MRI) and computerized tomography scanning. The MRI would be most sensitive to ruling out a space occupying lesion, and absence or underdevelopment of the eighth cranial nerve. A medical workup is especially critical for ruling out other causes for the audiologic test results that lead to a suspicion of auditory neuropathy. Follow-up visits will be designated by the physician based on findings and middle ear status. (See Chapter 3, Medical Evaluation and Management of Hearing Loss in Children.)

Pearl

- Families have the potential to become overwhelmed with the number of appointments they need to attend when a child is diagnosed. An involved and informed primary care physician is the key to providing support to families by reiterating results, making referrals, and offering encouragement that supports family choices. The audiologist can take the first step by contacting the child's pediatrician or medical home and providing information needed to offer support.

Ophthalmology

Any vision impairment needs to be ruled out when hearing loss is identified because of its importance for communication and its effect on the infant's or child's overall development. In suspected cases of auditory neuropathy, a visual communication approach is an option. Visual communication approaches can be used alone or in conjunction with spoken language, and good visual abilities need to be confirmed for these approaches. Cases where a severe visual impairment is identified or the potential for visual impairment is evident, communication modes relying heavily on visual input may not be options. It is crucial to identify any visual condition early so that a choice for a communication approach can be made as soon as possible, and early intervention and education services can be tailored appropriately. Follow-up visual monitoring will be determined by the physician, and more information can be obtained in the medical work-up section of this text. (See Chapter 3, Medical Evaluation and Management of Hearing Loss in Children.)

Genetics

When auditory neuropathy is suspected, a genetics evaluation is warranted because neuropathy is viewed as a significant hearing loss that may be related to other health problems. For example, DFNB9 is a nonsyndromic recessive deafness caused by a gene mutation in OTOF. OTOF provides the genetic code for otoferlin, a protein found in normal auditory systems. Patients with this genetic form of hearing loss may have electrophysiologic test results similar to those with suspected auditory neuropathy (Loundon et al, 2005). (See Chapter 2 for a complete discussion of the genetics of hearing loss.)

Special Consideration

- Negative family attitudes about genetic testing may delay ruling out this diagnosis, or ruling out other diagnoses for any child with permanent hearing loss. In addition, at the time of publication of this book there may still be limited availability of clinics currently testing for OTOF.

Neurology

The literature suggests that classic cases of auditory neuropathy may actually be Friedrich's ataxia, Charcot-Marie-Tooth disease, or a hereditary sensory motor neuropathy that can occur in adults and older children (Starr et al, 1996). Young patients with suspected auditory neuropathy warrant the expertise of a pediatric neurologist to rule out these other conditions. The professional will determine the frequency of follow-up. Often these neurological conditions are not evident in the infant population and the diagnosis of auditory neuropathy may be presumptive. Younger patients with suspected auditory neuropathy may have endured several coexisting medical conditions such as prematurity, jaundice, or cerebral palsy (Madden et al, 2002).

Neonatal Follow-Up

The concept of a neonatal follow-up program is to facilitate care for premature and high-risk infants following neonatal intensive care discharge. Many of these infants have multiple medical problems, and coordination of medical visits, therapies, and treatments is a useful service for parents and guardians. The other purposes of the neonatal follow-up program are to track the development of high-risk infants, to publish research, and to serve as a resource for the medical

community about needs, intervention, and outcomes of high-risk infants.

Infants and children with suspected auditory neuropathy are considered eligible for this follow-up service because of their health problems and because of the auditory neuropathy. Infants are evaluated at the ages of 3, 6, 12, 18, and 24 months, and annually until five years of age. Each of these sessions includes medical and behavioral history, physical evaluation, neuromuscular evaluation, nutritional assessment, psychological assessment, social needs assessment, and physical therapy evaluation as needed (Franck et al, 2002).

Pearl

- Many families, do not have access to all of these services. If the audiologist takes the time to find a child neurologist, neonatologist, and developmental pediatrician who are accessible and willing to become knowledgeable of the diagnosis of neuropathy, all parties, especially the patient and family, will benefit.

Early Intervention/Educational Consultation

A child younger than three years should be served by a professional who has knowledge of children and infants who present with hearing loss. These professionals provide counseling, therapy, and monitoring of the infant or young child's progress, and can supply information about the effects of hearing loss on child development. The investigation of communication options should be explored with the help of the audiologist and early intervention provider. A manual mode that follows the English language syntax would be an appropriate visual-based mode. All communication options should be presented to the family (Berlin et al, 2005; Stredler-Brown, 2002). The family should make the decision for their child based on their needs and on the child's response to auditory stimulation.

Speech-Language Pathology

A speech-language pathologist who has experience working with children who are deaf or hard of hearing is a valuable resource. A speech-language pathologist will be able to set appropriate speech, language, and auditory goals and facilitate the development of these goals. Information from the speech-language pathologist can be used to monitor progress with amplification, and to determine the need for a cochlear implant.

Special Consideration

- A family will encounter many professionals who do not know about the diagnosis of auditory neuropathy. The audiologist has the responsibility of providing information about the diagnosis and appropriate follow-up of the condition.

Family Wellness

The prognosis is unknown for infants diagnosed with suspected auditory neuropathy. Unlike typical sensorineural hearing losses, the severity measured by the ABR and audiogram provides a poor estimation of the child's functional auditory ability and success with amplification. Several children in the population diagnosed with auditory neuropathy have also survived a perinatal insult, and as a result, have ongoing medical issues that also need to be addressed. A family wellness program addresses the stressors caused by ongoing illnesses combined with hearing loss.

The family wellness program provides support and addresses the unique needs of this population through individual counseling sessions and parent seminars in a safe and confidential environment. A mental health counselor is available as needed to provide encouragement, information, or to assist in finding additional counseling services.

A referral to a family wellness program by the managing audiologist is suggested if there is a concern about significant parental stress, disruption in family function, or if the child's daily function is disrupted as a result of her hearing condition. The overall goal of a family wellness program is to strengthen the parents' confidence in their ability to make important decisions, and to assist the family in finding and learning new information independently.

♦ Summary

The management of infants and young children with auditory neuropathy does not rely on the audiologist alone, but rather requires a team approach. The management team includes the audiologist, parents, otolaryngologist, ophthalmologist, neurologist, neonatal follow-up, family wellness, speech-language pathology, and educator of the hearing impaired.

Discussion Questions

1. What treatment choices would be appropriate audiologic intervention for a child with auditory neuropathy who is younger than 6 months?

2. What would a neonatal follow-up program for infants with auditory neuropathy look like?

3. What is the role of a mental health counselor for families affected by auditory neuropathy?

References

Amatuzzi, M. G., Northrop, C., Liberman, M. C., et al. (2001). Selective inner hair cell loss in premature infants and cochlea pathological patterns from neonatal intensive care unit autopsies. Archives of Otolaryngology–Head Neck Surgery, 127, 629–636.

Berlin, C. I., Hood, L. J., Morlet, T., Rose, K., and Brashears, S. (2002). Auditory neuropathy / dys-synchrony: its many forms and outcomes. Seminars in Hearing, 23, 209–214.

Berlin, C. I., Hood, L. J., Morlet, T., et al. (2005). Absent or elevated middle ear muscle reflexes in the presence of normal otoacoustic emissions: a universal finding in 136 cases of auditory neuropathy/dys-synchrony. Journal of the American Academy of Audiology, 16, 546–553.

Franck, K., Rainey, D., Montoya, L., and Gerdes, M. (2002). Developing a multidisciplinary clinical protocol to manage pediatric patients with auditory neuropathy. Seminars in Hearing, 23, 225–237.

Joint Commission on Infant Hearing, year 2007 position statement: Principles and guidelines for early hearing detection and interention programs. Pediatrics, 120(4): 898–921.

Loundon, N., Marcolla, A., Roux, I., et al. (2005). Auditory neuropathy or endocochlear hearing loss? Otology & Neurotology, 26, 748–754.

Madden, C., Rutter, M., Hilbert, L., Greinwald, J. H., and Choo, D. I. (2002). Clinical and audiological features in auditory neuropathy. Archives Otolaryngology–Head and Neck Surgery, 128, 1026–1030.

Rance, G., Beer, D. E., Cone-Wesson, B., et al. (1999). Clinical findings for a group of infants and young children with auditory neuropathy. Ear and Hearing, 20, 238–252.

Rapin, I., and Gravel, J. S. (2006). Auditory neuropathy: a biologically inappropriate label unless acoustic nerve involvement is documented. Journal of the American Academy of Audiology, 17, 147–150.

Rodriguez-Ballesteros, M., del Castillo, F. J., Martin, Y., et al. (2003). Auditory neuropathy in patients carrying mutations in the otoferlin gene (OTOF). Human Mutation, 22, 451–456.

Starr, A., Picton, T. W., Sininger, Y., Hood, L. J., and Berlin, C. I. (1996). Auditory neuropathy. Brain, 119, 741–753.

Starr, A., Sininger, Y., Winter, M., Derebery, M. J., Oba, S., and Michalewski, H. J. (1998). Transient deafness due to temperature-sensitive auditory neuropathy. Ear and Hearing, 19, 169–179.

Starr, A., Sininger, Y. S., and Pratt, H. (2000). The varieties of auditory neuropathy. Journal of Basic and Clinical Physiology and Pharmacology, 11, 215–230.

Stredler-Brown, A. (2002). Developing a treatment program for children with auditory neuropathy. Seminars in Hearing, 23, 239–249.

Appendix

Position Papers and Policy Statements

- American Academy of Family Physicians, American Academy of Otololaryngology–Head and Neck Surgery, and American Academy of Pediatrics Subcommittee on Otitis Media With Effusion. (2004). *Clinical Practice Guideline: Otitis Media with Effusion. May 03, 2004*

- American Academy of Pediatrics. (2002). The Medical Home Policy Statement. *Pediatrics 110(1).* Retrieved Dec. 18, 2002 from http://www.aap.org/policy/s060016.html.

- American National Standards Institute. (S12.60–2002). *Acoustical Performance Criteria, Design Requirements, and Guidelines for Schools.* New York: American National Standards Institute (ANSI S12.60).

- American National Standards Institute (ANSI). (1997). *American national standards methods for calculation of the speech intelligibility index.* New York: American National Standards Institute.

- American Speech-Language-Hearing Association (1997). *Guidelines for audiologic screening.* Rockville, MD: ASHA.

- American Speech-Language-Hearing Association. (2002). *Guidelines for fitting and monitoring FM systems.* Available at http://www.asha.org/members/deskref-journals/deskref/default.

- American Speech-Language-Hearing Association. (2004a). *Guidelines for the audiologic assessment of children from birth to 5 years of age.* Available at http:// www. asha. org/ members/deskref-journals/deskref/default.

- American Speech-Language-Hearing Association. (2004b). *Cochlear implants.* Available at http://www.asha.org/members/deskref-journals/deskref/default.

- American Speech-Language-Hearing Association. (2005). *Guidelines for addressing acoustics in educational settings.* Available at http://www.asha.org/members/deskref-journals/deskref/default.

- American Speech-Language-Hearing Association (2005). *(Central) Auditory Processing Disorders.* Available at http://www.asha.org/members/deskref-journals/deskref/default

- American Speech-Language-Hearing Association (2005). *(Central) Auditory Processing Disorders—The Role of the Audiologist [Position statement].* Available at http://www.asha.org/members/deskref-journals/deskref/default.

- American Speech-Language-Hearing Association. (2006*). Roles, knowledge, and skills: Audiologists providing clinical services to infants and young children birth to 5 years of age.* Available at http://www.asha.org/members/deskref-journals/deskref/default.

- Centers for Disease Control and Prevention (CDC). (2004). *National EHDI Goals.* Retrieved June 14, 2004 from http://www.cdc.gov/ncbddd/ehdi/nationalgoals.htm

- Colorado Infant Hearing Advisory Board and Membership of the Screening, Assessment, and Early Intervention Task Forces (2003). *Guidelines for Infant Hearing Screening, Audiologic Assessment, and Early Intervention* (Colorado Infant Hearing Advisory Committee). Denver, CO: Colorado Department of Public Health and Environment.

- Joint Committee on Infant Hearing (2007). Year 2007 position statement: Principles and guidelines for early hearing detection and intervention programs. Pediatrics; 102(4): 893–921.

- Marge, D.K. & Marge, M. (2005). *Beyond newborn hearing screening: Meeting the educational and health care needs of infants and young children with hearing loss in America.* Report of the National Consensus Conference on Effective Educational and Health Care Interventions for Infants and Young Children with Hearing Loss, September 10–12, 2004. Syracuse, New York: Department of Physical Medicine and Rehabilitation, SUNY Upstate Medical University.

- National Center for Hearing Assessment and Management (NCHAM). (2006). *Criteria for infants and toddlers with hearing loss to be eligible for early intervention services under IDEA.* Retrieved December 15, 2006, from http://www.infanthearing.org.

- National Center for Hearing Assessment and Management (NCHAM). (2007b.) *Policy Statements Regarding Newborn Hearing Screening.* Retrieved April 27, 2007 from http://www.infanthearing.org/policystatements/index. html.

- NPL. (2005). Newborn hearing screening program (NHSP) ABR Reference levels for stimulus calibration. from http://www.npl.co.uk/acoustics/research/theme1/reportret. pdf

- Offeciers, E., Morera, C., Müller, J., Huarte, A., Shallop, J., & Cavallé, L. (2005). International consensus on bilateral cochlear implants and bimodal stimulation. *Acta Oto-Laryngologica* 125: 918–919.

- Pediatric Amplification Guideline: Position Statement of the American Academy of Audiology. (2004*). Audiology Today, 16(2)*, 46–53.

- Red Book. (2006). *2006 Report of the committee on infectious diseases.* Elk Grove Village, IL: American Academy of Pediatrics.

- The Centers for Disease Control and Prevention (2005). *Proceedings of the National Workshop on Mild and Unilateral Hearing Loss.* Available on www.cdc.gov.

◆ (Educational) Audiology Websites

- www.audiology.org
- www.edaud.org
- www.asha.org

◆ Children with Hearing Loss: General Information

- www.hearingjourney.com
- www.voicefordeafkids.com
- www.agbellacademy.org
- www.agbell.org
- www.oraldeafed.org
- www.nciohio.com
- www.listen-up.org
- http://www.johntracyclinic.org
- www.ncbegin.org
- http://www.handsandvoices.org
- http://www.babyhearing.org
- www.childrenshearing.org

◆ Literacy Information

- www.nationalreadingpanel.org/publications/researchread. htm
- http://www.trelease-on-reading.com

◆ Infant-Toddler Information Websites

- http://dltk-teach.com
- http://www.naturallearning.com/fingerplays.shtml
- http://www.preschoolexpress.com/toddler_station.shtml

- http://www.drjean.org
- http://www.listen-up.org (auditory enrichment and developmental normative milestones)

◆ Literature Websites

- http://www.magickeys.com: on-line books for both young and advanced readers
- http://www.readinga-z.com: printable books; first 30 are free; $29.95/yr.-subscrip.
- Log onto famous author Web sites: http://www.kevin-henkes.com; http://www.eric-carle.com
- http://www.readwme.com: Shari Robertson and Helen Davig's Web site for Read With Me! Stress-Free Strategies for Building Language and Literacy (2002). Available from Thinking Publications.com. Phone: 1–800–225-GROW

◆ Education Laws

- Individuals with Disabilities Education Improvement Act of 2004, 20 U.S.C. § 1400 *et seq.* (2004).
- No Child Left Behind Act of 2001. Education. Intergovernmental Relations. 20 USC 6301 et. seq. note.
- President's Commission on Excellence in Special Education. (2002). *A new era: Revitalizing special education for children and their families.* Washington, DC: U.S. Department of Education.
- Rehabilitation Act Amendments of 1992, P.L. 102–569. (1992, October 29). *United States Statutes at Large*, 106, 4344–4488.
- Rehabilitation Act of 1973, P.L. 93–112. (1973, September 26). *United States Statutes at Large*, 87, 355–394.
- Technology-Related Assistance to Individuals with Disabilities Act of 1988, P.L. 100–407, 29 U.S.C.; 2201 *et seq.* (1997).
- U.S. Department of Education (1995). *Seventeenth annual report to Congress on the implementation of the individuals with disabilities education act.* Washington, DC: U.S. Government Printing Office.
- U.S. Department of Health, Education, and Welfare. (August 23, 1977). Rules and regulations for the administration of the education of all handicapped children act, *Federal Register* (Part IV), 42, 163.
- United States Department of Education. (1991). *Public Law 102–119, The Disability Education Act, P* (IDEA, Part H).

Index

Note: Page numbers followed by *f* and *t* indicate figures and tables, respectively.